Advances in Intelligent Systems and Computing

Volume 915

The series "Advances in Intelligent Systems and Computing" contains publications on theory, applications, and design methods of Intelligent Systems and Intelligent Computing. Virtually all disciplines such as engineering, natural sciences, computer and information science, ICT, economics, business, e-commerce, environment, healthcare, life science are covered. The list of topics spans all the areas of modern intelligent systems and computing such as: computational intelligence, soft computing including neural networks, fuzzy systems, evolutionary computing and the fusion of these paradigms, social intelligence, ambient intelligence, computational neuroscience, artificial life, virtual worlds and society, cognitive science and systems, Perception and Vision, DNA and immune based systems, self-organizing and adaptive systems, e-Learning and teaching, human-centered and human-centric computing, recommender systems, intelligent control, robotics and mechatronics including human-machine teaming, knowledge-based paradigms, learning paradigms, machine ethics, intelligent data analysis, knowledge management, intelligent agents, intelligent decision making and support, intelligent network security, trust management, interactive entertainment, Web intelligence and multimedia.

The publications within "Advances in Intelligent Systems and Computing" are primarily proceedings of important conferences, symposia and congresses. They cover significant recent developments in the field, both of a foundational and applicable character. An important characteristic feature of the series is the short publication time and world-wide distribution. This permits a rapid and broad dissemination of research results.

** Indexing: The books of this series are submitted to ISI Proceedings, EI-Compendex, DBLP, SCOPUS, Google Scholar and Springerlink **

More information about this series at http://www.springer.com/series/11156

Mostafa Ezziyyani
Editor

Advanced Intelligent Systems for Sustainable Development (AI2SD'2018)

Volume 5: Advanced Intelligent Systems for Computing Sciences

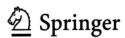 Springer

Editor
Mostafa Ezziyyani
Faculty of Sciences and Techniques
Abdelmalek Essaâdi University
Tangier, Morocco

ISSN 2194-5357 ISSN 2194-5365 (electronic)
Advances in Intelligent Systems and Computing
ISBN 978-3-030-11927-0 ISBN 978-3-030-11928-7 (eBook)
https://doi.org/10.1007/978-3-030-11928-7

Library of Congress Control Number: 2018968381

This Springer imprint is published by the registered company Springer Nature Switzerland AG
The registered company address is: Gewerbestrasse 11, 6330 Cham, Switzerland

Preface

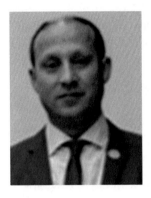

Overview

The purpose of this volume is to honour myself and all colleagues around the world that we have been able to collaborate closely for extensive research contributions which have enriched the field of Applied Computer Science. Applied Computer Science presents a appropriate research approach for developing a high-level skill that will encourage various researchers with relevant topics from a variety of disciplines, encourage their natural creativity, and prepare them for independent research projects. We think this volume is a testament to the benefits and future possibilities of this kind of collaboration, the framework for which has been put in place.

About the Editor

Prof. Dr. **Mostafa Ezziyyani,** IEEE and ASTF Member, received the "Licence en Informatique" degree, the "Diplôme de Cycle Supérieur en Informatique" degree and the PhD "Doctorat (1)" degree in Information System Engineering, respectively, in 1994, 1996 and 1999, from Mohammed V University in Rabat, Morocco. Also, he received the second PhD degree "Doctorat (2)" in 2006, from Abdelmalek Essaadi University in Distributed Systems and Web Technologies. In 2008, he received a Researcher Professor **Ability Grade. In 2015, he receives a PES grade —the highest degree at Morocco University.** Now he is a Professor of Computer Engineering and Information System in Faculty of Science and Technologies of Abdelmalek Essaadi University since 1996.

His research activities focus on the modelling databases and integration of heterogeneous and distributed systems (with the various developments to the big data, data sciences, data analytics, system decision support, knowledge management, object DB, active DB, multi-system agents, distributed systems and mediation). This research is at the crossroads of databases, artificial intelligence, software engineering and programming.

Professor at Computer Science Department, Member MA laboratory and responsible of the research direction Information Systems and Technologies, he formed a research team that works around this theme and more particularly in the area of integration of heterogeneous systems and decision support systems using WSN as technology for communication.

He received the first WSIS prize 2018 for the Category C7: ICT applications: E-environment, First prize: MtG—ICC in the regional contest IEEE - London UK Project: "World Talk", The qualification to the final (Teachers-Researchers Category): Business Plan Challenger 2015, EVARECH UAE Morocco. Project: «Lavabo Intégré avec Robinet à Circuit Intelligent pour la préservation de l'eau», First prize: Intel Business, Challenge Middle East and North Africa—IBC-MENA. Project: «Système Intelligent Préventif Pour le Contrôle et le Suivie en temps réel des Plantes Médicinale En cours de Croissance (PCS: Plants Control System)», Best Paper: International Conference on Software Engineering and New Technologies ICSENT'2012, Hammamat-Tunis. Paper: «Disaster Emergency System Application Case Study: Flood Disaster».

He has authored three patents: (1) device and learning process of orchestra conducting (e-Orchestra), (2) built-in washbasin with intelligent circuit tap for water preservation. (LIRCI) (3) Device and method for assisting the driving of vehicles for individuals with hearing loss.

He is the editor and coordinator of several projects with Ministry of Higher Education and Scientific Research and others as international project; he has been involved in several collaborative research projects in the context of ERANETMED3/PRIMA/H2020/FP7 framework programmes including project management activities in the topic modelling of distributed information systems reseed to environment, Health, energy and agriculture. The first project aims to propose an adaptive system for flood evacuation. This system gives the best decisions to be taken in this emergency situation to minimize damages. The second project aims to develop a research dynamic process of the itinerary in an events graph for blind and partially signet users. Moreover, he has been the principal investigator and the project manager for several research projects dealing with several topics concerned with his research interests mentioned above.

He was an invited professor for several countries in the world (France, Spain Belgium, Holland, USA and Tunisia). He is member of USA-J1 programme for TCI Morocco Delegation in 2007. He creates strong collaborations with research centres in databases and telecommunications for students' exchange: LIP6, Valencia, Poitier, Boston, Houston, China.

He is the author of more than 100 papers which appeared in refereed specialized journals and symposia. He was also the editor of the book "New Trends in Biomedical Engineering", AEU Publications, 2004. He was a member of the Organizing and the Scientific Committees of several symposia and conferences dealing with topics related to computer sciences, distributed databases and web technology. He has been actively involved in the research community by serving as reviewer for technical, and as an organizer/co-organizer of numerous international and national conferences and workshops. In addition, he served as a programme committee member for international conferences and workshops.

He was responsible for the formation cycle "Maîtrise de Génie Informatique" in the Faculty of Sciences and Technologies in Tangier since 2006. He is responsible too and coordinator of Tow Master "DCESS - Systèmes Informatique pour Management des Entreprise" and "DCESS - Systèmes Informatique pour Management des Enterprise". He is the coordinator of the computer science modules and responsible for the graduation projects and external relations of the Engineers Cycle "Statistique et Informatique Décisionnelle" in Mathematics Department of the Faculty of Sciences and Technologies in Tangier since 2007. He participates also in the Telecommunications Systems DESA/Masters, "Bio-Informatique" Masters and "Qualité des logiciels" Masters in the Faculty of Science in Tetuan since 2002.

He is also the founder and the current chair of the blinds and partially signet people association. His activity interests focus mainly on the software to help the blinds and partially signet people to use the ICT, specifically in Arabic countries. He is the founder of the private centre of training and education in advanced technologies AC-ETAT, in Tangier since 2000.

Mostafa Ezziyyani

Contents

Intelligent Reservation Systems Based on MAS & Data Mining Method

Oum Elhana Maamra$^{(\boxtimes)}$ and Mohamed-Khireddine Kholladi$^{(\boxtimes)}$

Mathematical Department and Computer Science,
University El-Oeud, El Oued, Algeria
hanaoumelhana@gmail.com, kholladi@yahoo.fr

Abstract. The basic concepts of reservation system and management system are discussed in this paper. The proposed "intelligent reservation system that is based on a combination of multi-agents system and data mining techniques makes intelligent reservation decisions whether to accept or reject a new client's request for reservation needed services. In the first step of the proposed model. These reservation strategies are developed using integer aggregate results database (ARD) with multi-agent system, it consists of the following agents: Client Agent, Stock Agent, Agent Station, Aggregation Agent and Agent Response. We preprogrammed our system to apply data mining methods in a distributed way to retrieve information requested by client, the result obtained is a local model of each station the latter sends to the aggregator to obtain the final model that represents the customer response. The purpose of our proposal is to reduce response time and resource consumption by storing responses in ARD.

Keywords: Multi-agent · Data mining · Intelligent reservation system

1 Introduction

Data mining is a generic term for a family of analysis tools particularly suited to the exploitation of large masses of data. Data mining makes it possible, in particular, to search for structures that are difficult to identify and correlations which are not very noticeable with more conventional statistical analysis techniques.

The important question in the field of Data Mining is to be able to answer the question: which tool should we use for which problem?

Depending on the type of problem, there are many competing Data Mining methods. A general consensus seems to emerge to recognize that no method outperforms the others because they have all their specific strengths and weaknesses. It seems more advantageous to cooperate methods. Data mining is the heart of the EDC process. This phase uses multiple methods from statistics, machine learning, pattern recognition or visualization. These methods can be divided into three categories:

- Visualization and description methods;
- Classification and structuring methods;
- And methods of explanation and prediction.

© Springer Nature Switzerland AG 2019
M. Ezziyyani (Ed.): AI2SD 2018, AISC 915, pp. 1–12, 2019.
https://doi.org/10.1007/978-3-030-11928-7_1

For that we choose the global Distribution System, (GDS) are electronic reservations management platforms that allow customers to know in real time the stock status of the various suppliers of tourism products (airlines, rail and sea, hotel chain, car rental companies, tour operators, etc.) and reserve remotely.

Computer reservation systems (CRS) allow you to reserve a resource or a service in time for a person or a group. These systems are integrated in real estate (room, conference room, tennis court, conference room), transport (car, train, boat, plane), tools (saw, crane) under form of provision (rental, loan) from a specified time slot with, as the case may be, the option of one or more persons.

Our approach based on the multi agent system and data mining to reserve all the elements born for tourism in complex, useful and dynamic data structures. The client can access the system through a platform.

In our system customers are divided into two types People and, Travel Agencies: have privileges for example it can book for several people in various conditions. In both cases, after the registration, the customer receives the registration confirmation letter, which includes the cost of the trip from the transfer and residence according to his request, confirming his registration to pay the fees within twenty-four hours if he does not pay the fees his application will be canceled.

In this paper, we analyzed related work of reservation system and we proposed intelligent system for reservation based on multi-agent system, we analyzed different reservation model, and we discuss the performance of each one. The contribution of the paper is as:

1. We analyzed reservation system existent in Literature and we proposed model of reservation system based on MAS.
2. Proposed architecture of reservation system.
3. The rest of the paper is organized as follows, Sect. 2 describes related work about reservation system, In Sect. 3, all detailed of our contribution. Decision and conclusion are in Sects. 4 and 5, respectively.

2 Related Work

The internet has become an integral part of a modern society helping revolutionize how businesses are conducted and our personal lives, the used of Internet has led to the emergence of a variety of electronic services, e-services. Electronic ticket, or e-ticket, is an example of such a class of e-services. E-tickets give evidence to their holders to have permission to enter a place of entertainment, use a means of transportation, or have access to some Internet services. Users can get the e-tickets by purchasing them from a web server, or simply receiving from a vendor, or from another user who previously acquired them. E-tickets can be stored in desktop computers or personal digital assistants for future use [1].

For that we study the related works, among them we can quote the works of:

2.1 System of Reservation

In 2014 Oloyede propose a bus reservation system in Nigeria was developed using Extensible Hypertext Markup Language (XHTML), PHP Hypertext Preprocessor (PHP), Ajax, Cascading Style Sheet (CSS), and JavaScript. The system has a relational database modeled by Structure Query Language (SQL) [2].

In 2014 Ogirima propose an Online computerized Hotel Management System (HMS), the system has a relational database modeled by Structure Query Language (SQL). The author describe his system and presented comparison of Online HMS and Manual Hotel Management System. The result indicates that users prefer online Hotel management to conventional Hotel management Services in terms of ease of use, accessibility and security in the study area [3].

In other work 2010, the author proposed an intelligent agent-based hotel search and booking system that will undertake the bulk of the search and booking of hotels for various users. The system provided users with the ability to enter some criteria for the search and then perform the search base on those criteria and book the most appropriate hotel base on the user's confirmation. These are carried out using JADE-LEAP on user's mobile device [4].

In 2014, Bemile proposed online Hotel Reservation System that allows customers to make inquiries online and book for services providing the required details. Of the system feature make sure that potential guests get the correct information, such as room rates and hotel location. It adopts the virtual tour feature in the Shangri-La Hotel in Singapore. The tools developed this system are Apache, MySQL and PHP was used for the server programming which is basically queries used to link the website to the database [5].

Other work, Bhagat proposed perceptive car parking booking system with IOT technology. The system of Bhagat consists of different modules like server, database, user application and parking slot arrangement. The mechanism of parking slot it is an Arduino UNO and Ultrasonic sensor. Arduino is used for managing ultrasonic sensor and entry gate. The ultrasonic sensor is useful for detecting the car position. When user will scan QR code at the parking slot that time user will be charged or pay for a time duration which is user already mention at the slot booking time through android application. A user must first download the android application in his android mobile phone. After user must goes only one time for registration with specific id (using AADHAR CARD no. or License no.) using the application. Then registered user information is sent to the server system and data stored in the database. The parking slot information is also stored in the database which is always updated, and servers manages and updates this information and keep sending notification to the user after parking slot booking. For manage parking locations and user database system, the authors provide a website for the Admin user [6].

In Table 1, we compare the president's works of the online reservation system such that the comparison lines are Search and booking method, multidimensional model and Domain application

As a general summary, the majority works that deal with the reservation system used for search and booking the classic method (Query SQL) and used the simple database. A domain of application of this works is a part of our system.

Table 1. Comparison between different systems

Works	Online reservation system such		
	Search and booking method	Multidimensional model	Domain application
Oloyede [2]	Request SQL	Non	Bus reservation
Ogirima [3]	Request SQL	Non	Online computerized hotel management
Sankaranarayanan [4]	Intelligent agent	Non	Hotel search and booking
Bemile [13]	Request SQL	Non	Hotel reservation
Bhagat [6]	Arduino UNO and Ultrasonic sensor	Non	Perceptive car parking booking

2.2   Data Base

In 2003 Vrdoljak propose a method for building an XML data warehouse from the Web. They are based on XML schemas that write and validate the source data. The method involves extracting XML schemas from data sources, building and transforming these schemas into data graphs, identifying the facts, and finally building a logical XML schema that validates the data in the warehouse. The authors implement a prototype that takes an XML schema as input and outputs a logical schema of the warehouse [7].

The method of Rusu in 2005 is based on the XQuery2 language to build an XML data warehouse. The proposed method covers the processes of extracting, transforming, aggregating, and integrating XML data into the warehouse. All of these steps are based on the XQuery language and aim to minimize duplication and errors in the warehouse data [8].

In 2006 Boussaid define themselves as a warehouse by an XML schema. The authors implement a prototype, named X-Warehousing, for storing complex data. The user analysis requirements as well as the source XML documents are represented by XML schemas. These patterns are transformed into attribute trees. The method then applies pruning and/or grafting functions on these trees to construct a final attribute tree that represents the warehouse schema. In this type of a warehouse, each fact, as well as the corresponding dimensions, is stored in an XML document. The resulting XML document set constitutes an XML data cube. The authors define this set as a context of analysis [9].

Park in 2005, offer a platform for online analysis of XML documents named XML-OLAP. The authors rely on an XML data warehouse where the facts are represented by a collection of XML documents and each dimension by another collection of XML documents. Authors represent each fact by an XML document. This representation is inspired by that adopted by Nassis. In 2005, an XML document of a dimension collection stores an instance of the hierarchy of a dimension. The authors claim that this eliminates the join operations between the hierarchical levels of a dimension. To query the XML data warehouse the authors propose a multidimensional expression language: XML-MDX [10].

In 2009 Zanoun proposed a neural approach that reduces the data cube fragmentation by building a new representation space. It consists of eliminating irrelevant exogenous variables by minimizing connections and selecting non-applicable individuals to mitigate the negative effect of sparse by organizing the cells of a data cube [11].

Bentayeb in 2007 proposes a UML meta model describing complex data in the form of complex object classes according to the object paradigm. A complex object is composed of different basic elements according to the type of data to which they belong (text, image, sound, video, materialized relational view). After instantiation of the meta model, the obtained UML model can be translated directly into XML logical schema, whether it is expressed using a DTD or using the XML-Schema language. Finally, the XML logic model is translated into a physical model as XML documents. From the logical model and complex data, valid XML documents are generated. These can be finally stored either in a native XML database or in a relational database via a mapping process. The relational model obtained at the end of this process defines low-level links, to define the semantic links between the different documents the authors use the techniques of the data mining that aid to the multi-dimensional modeling of the complex data [12].

In the following table we compare the president's works of the databases such that the comparison lines are Multidimensional model, Data type and Representation of facts and dimensions.

As a general summary the work that deals with the storage of XML data varies by their approach to building the warehouse and cover more or less the various stages of the storage process: ETL (Extraction, Transformation and Loading), modeling and analysis. Some propose to process the data directly from their sources, others favor the loading into a data warehouse modeled by a star schema. Some also offer analysis operators specific to XML data. This work is summarized in Table 2. The symbol "+" indicates that an approach deals with a step in the storage process.

Table 2. Comparison between different approaches

Works	Databases		
	Multidimensional model	Data type	Representation of facts and dimensions
Vrdoljak [7]	–	Web	–
Rusu [8]	+	Heterogeneous	+
Park [10]	+	Heterogeneous	+
Boussaid [5]	+	Heterogeneous	–
Bentayeb [12]	+	Heterogeneous	+
Zanoun [11]	+	Cube	+

3   Methodologies

The tourist agencies are the only link between the countries which guarantees the traveler's comfort and safety in his journey and travel, the manual use of ticket reservation is presently very strenuous and also consumes a lot of time.

For example the services in case of a hotel, we generally want to choose the best hotel in prime sites, with modern facilities, clean environment, and affordable rates. This can be time-consuming and sometimes costly when doing this on our own physical or using human agents. The advent of the World Wide Web or internet (as we know) changed the landscape of communication and the way we conduct business dramatically, allowing us to reach beyond boundaries once separated by miles of oceans. Information that one took days and in some cases weeks, can now be received in a matter of seconds, This technology has grown significantly over the years and has been interfaced with other technologies such as smart phones, PDAs and other forms of wired and wireless networking devices, propagating the ability to receive information and conduct business on the go at the finger tip. With this background in mind we have proposed a digital tourism agency, the customer is allowed to book travel from any place and at any time according to him conditions required and in a short time [3, 13].

Our system includes an aggregate results database as requested by the customers that is when the user enters the booking request status the answer is immediate. The presence of these collected results helps speed up the customer service. this database managed by a task manager that connects with workstations which manage distributed and different databases for hotels, airports, land transport stations as well as tour guides and on the other hand with clients. Figure 1 shows the architecture of our system.

3.1   Task Manager

The task manager of our study is a multi-agent system intelligent (instead of the human agent) to perform similar search and booking activities that can improve the speed of the search and reduce cost significantly, but the question here is why the multi-agent system, and what is the agent?

Definition of agent. An agent is called a physical or virtual entity has these features [14]:

1. who is able to act in an environment,
2. who can communicate directly with other agents,
3. that is driven by a set of trends (in the form of individual goals or a function of satisfaction, or even survival, which it seeks to optimize),
4. who has own resources,
5. who is able to perceive (but in a limited way) his environment,
6. which only has a partial representation of this environment (and possibly none),
7. who has skills and offers services,
8. who can possibly reproduce,
9. whose behavior tends to meet its objectives, taking into account the resources and expertise at its disposal, and in terms of its perception, representations and the communications it receives.

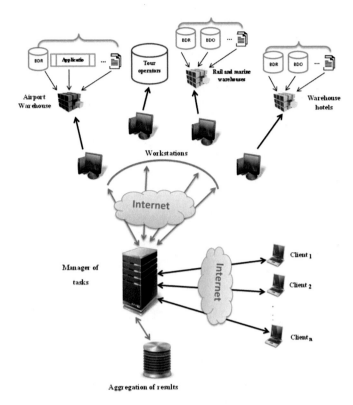

Fig. 1. Architecture of our system

Agents enjoy autonomy. This means that they are not driven by commands from the user (or another agent), but by a set of trends that can take the form of individual goals to fulfill.

He has the opportunity to answer yes or no to requests from other agents. It therefore has a certain freedom of maneuver, which differentiates it from all similar concepts, which they call "objects", "software modules" or "processes". But autonomy is not only behavioral, it is also about resources. To act, the agent needs a number of resources: energy, CPU, amount of memory, access to certain sources of information, etc. These resources are both what makes the agent not only dependent on his environment, but also, by being able to handle these [14].

Definition of multi-agent system. A multi-agent system (SMA) is a system composed of the following elements [14]:

- An environment E, that is to say a space generally having a metric.
- A set of objects O. These objects are located, that is to say that, for any object, it is possible, at a given moment, to associate a position in E. These objects are passive, c that is, they can be perceived, created, destroyed and modified by agents.

- A set of agents, which are particular objects (A ⊆ O), which represent the active entities of the system.
- A set of relations R which unite objects (and thus agents) between them.
- A set of Op operations that allow A's agents to perceive, produce, consume, transform, and manipulate O objects.
- Operators to represent the application of these operations and the reaction of the world to this attempt to change, which will be called the laws of the universe.

Our task manager is multi-agent system composed of the following agents: Client Agent, Stock Agent, Agent Station, Aggregation Agent and Agent Response.

Communication Between Agents

Communications between our manager's agents through the exchange of Different messages, Fig. 2 represents this communication.

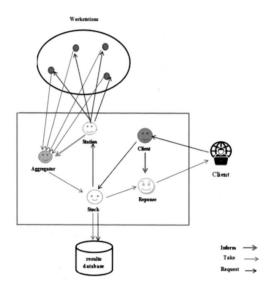

Fig. 2. Communication between agents in our task manager

Communication Scenario Between Agents

- *Client Agent.* Receives the message from clients, and sends this message to the store and informs the response agent.
- *Agent stock.* receives the client agent message, then searches the BR, if the result exists sending the response to the response agent, else sending the message to the agent station.
- *Station Agent.* Merges the message to the workstation, and informs the Aggregation Agent.
- *Aggregator agent.* Receives and aggregates responses, and sends responses to the stock agent.

- *Stock Agent.* Sends a copy of the results to the client agent, and stores another copy in the results database.
- *Response Agent.* Receives the stock agent message, and sends the response to the client.

3.2   B. Work Stations

The work stations of our study are warehouses of different and distributed data, we apply the methods of data mining for extraction of data requested by the customer. The question asked here for what to use the methods of excavations?

Now a day's large quantities of data are being accumulated up to millions or trillions of bytes of data. Data mining, the extraction of hidden predictive information from large databases, is a powerful new technology with great potential to help companies focus on the most important information in their data warehouses. The automated, prospective analyses offered by data mining move beyond the analyses of past events provided by retrospective tools typical of decision support systems. Data mining tools can answer business questions that traditionally were too time-consuming to resolve [15].

For our system we have a four work stations:

- Hotel Work Stations: allows extracting hotel knowledge requested by the customer.
- Airport Work Stations: allows you to extract the knowledge of the aircraft schedule requested by the customer.
- Tour operator workstations: allows extracting the tour operator knowledge requested by the customer.
- Railway and marine railway stations: allows you to extract the knowledge of the railway and maritime requested by the customer.

Figure 3 represents apply of Work stations.

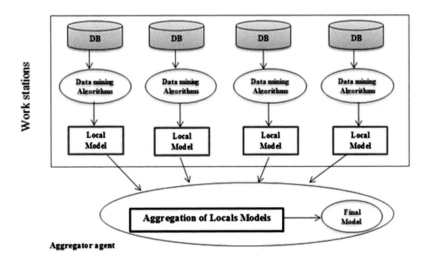

Fig. 3. Apply of work stations

To extract the knowledge that requested by the customer,

1. Each station applies data mining algorithms in complex data warehouses;
2. The result obtained is a local model of each station;
3. Each station sends this model to the aggregator to obtain the final model.

3.3   Data Warehouses

The data warehouses of our system are complex because they contain heterogeneous data from various sources to facilitate the use of these warehouses; we seek to propose a restructuring of these data.

3.4   Customers

In our system customers are divided into two types People and, Travel Agencies: have privileges for example it can book for several people in various conditions. In both cases, after the registration, the customer receives the registration confirmation letter, which includes the cost of the trip from the transfer and residence according to his request, confirming his registration to pay the fees within twenty-four hours if he does not pay the fees his application will be canceled.

4   Expected Result

Data mining, or data mining, is the set of methods and techniques intended for the exploration and analysis of computer databases (often large), automatically or semi-automatically, in order to detect in these data rules, associations, unknown or hidden trends, particular structures rendering most of the useful information while reducing the amount of data [16]. The purpose of this knowledge represent in:

- describe the current behavior of the data and/or,
- Predict the future behavior of the data.

These points make it possible to predict the customer's requests, which help us to create the database collected from the various data warehouses.

On the other hand, A multi-agent system consists of a set of computer processes taking place at the same time, thus of several agents living at the same time, sharing common resources and communicating with each other. The key point of multi-agent systems lies in the formalization of the coordination between the agents [17].

Thus, an SMA is a system composed of an environment; a set of objects in the environment that can be perceived, created, destroyed and modified by agents; a set of agents able to perceive, produce, consume, transform and manipulate the objects of the environment; a set of communications uniting agents and finally an administrator responsible for controlling the activation of agents [9].

This information confirms to us the importance of a multi-agent system in our project because it achieves the constant mobility of information under the agents' systems.

5 Conclusion

In this paper, we have proposed a new architecture of reservation system. The proposed architecture is based on MSA & data mining method for finding the optimized the time to retrieve information from a large, heterogeneous and distributed database to minimize the waste of network resources and maximize interaction with a user. The perspective of this work we make a restructuring on data warehouses then we choose the method of data mining that we will apply on the databases to extract the information.

References

1. Saleem, H., Ali Khan, M.Z., Afzal, S.: Mobile agents: an intelligent multi-agent system for mobile phones. J. Comput. Eng. IOSRJCE. ISSN: 2278-0661, Sept–Oct 2012
2. Oloyede, M.O., Alaya, S.M., Adewole, K.S.: Development of an online bus ticket reservation system for a transportation service in Nigeria. J. Comput. Eng. Intell. Syst. **5**(12), ISSN 2222-1719 (2014)
3. Ogirima, S.A.O., Awode, T.R., Adeosun, O.O.: Online computerized hotel management system. J. Comput. Biosci. Eng., ISSN: 2348-7321, 2 Apr 2014
4. Sankaranarayanan, S.: Intelligent agent based hotel search & booking system. In: 9th WSEAS International Conference on Telecommunications and Informatics, ISSN: 1790-5117 (2010)
5. Boussaid, O., Messaoud, R.B., Choquet, R., Anthoard, S.: X-warehousing: an XML-based approach for warehousing complex data. In: 10th East-European Conference on Advances in Databases and Information Systems, ADBIS 2006. Lecture Notes in Computer Science, vol. 4152, pp. 39–54. Springer, Thessaloniki, Greece (2006)
6. Bhagat, S.S., Bagul, A.D., Patil, P.N., Dahale, S.A.: Perceptive car parking booking system with IOT technology. Int. Res. J. Eng. Technol. IRJET, ISSN: 2395-0072, Feb 2018
7. Vrdoljak, B., Banek, M., Rizzi, S.: Designing web warehouses from XML schemas. In: 5th International Conference on Data Warehousing and Knowledge Discovery, DaWaK 2003. Lecture Notes in Computer Science, vol. 2737, pp. 89–98. Springer, Prague, Czech Republic (2003)
8. Rusu, L.I., Rahayu, J.W., Taniar, D.: A methodology for building XML data warehouse. Int. J. Data Warehous. Min. **1**(2), 67–92 (2005)
9. Boussaid, O., Bentayeb, F., Darmont, J., Rabaseda, S: Towards complex data warehousing structuring, integration and analysis. In: RSTI-ISI. Semistructured databases, vol. 8(0), pp. 79–107 (2003)
10. Park, B.K., Han, H., Song, I.Y.: XML-OLAP: a multidimensional analysis framework for XML warehouses. In: 7th International Conference on Data Warehousing and Knowledge Discovery, DaWaK 2005. Lecture Notes in Computer Science, vol. 3589, pp. 32–42. Springer (2005)
11. Zanoun, N., Atmani, B., Adellouhab, F.Z.: Towards a reorganization of cubes of data by a neuronal approach dedicated to visualization. In: 4th Edition of the Conference on Advances of Decisional Systems, pp. 1–16 (2009)
12. Bentayeb, F., Darmont, J., Udrea, C.: Efficient integration of data mining techniques in database management systems. In: 8th International Database Engineering and Applications Symposium, IDEAS 2004. IEEE Computer Society, Coimbra, Portugal, pp. 59–67, July 2004

13. Bemile1, R., Achampong, A., Danquah, E.: Online hotel reservation system. Int. J. Innov. Sci. Eng. Technol., ISSN 2348-7968, Nov 2014

14. Ferber, J.: Les Systèmes Multi Agents: Vers Une Intelligence Collective, pp. 26–29. Enter Edition, 513p (1995)

15. Sangeetha, K.V., Rajeshwari, P.: Data mining and warehousing. J. Comput. Appl. **5** (EICA2012-1), ISSN: 0974-1925 (2012)

16. Kantardzic, M.: Data Mining-Concepts, Models, Methods, and Algorithms. IEEE Press, Piscataway, NJ, USA (2003)

17. Klusch, M.: Information agent technology for the internet: a survey. In: Fensel, D. (ed.) J. Data Knowl. Eng. Spec. Issue Intell. Inf. Int. **36**(3) (2001)

A Lightweight Ciphertext-Policy Attribute-Based Encryption for Fine-Grained Access Control

Hassan El Gafif[✉], Naima Meddah, and Ahmed Toumanari

National School of Applied Sciences, Ibn Zohr University, Agadir, Morocco
hassan.elgafif@edu.uiz.ac.ma

Abstract. With the expansion of data, companies start to look for new efficient and cheap alternatives to store, share and manage their data. In this regard, cloud storage services appeared to fill this gap by providing a huge amount of computing resources ensuring data availability and efficient data management with low cost due to the pay-as-you-go payment-model adopted by cloud providers. However, by outsourcing their sensitive data (financial data, health records ...), companies will no longer be in control of them, so this arises big challenges related to the confidentiality and data security against attackers (in case of compromised cloud servers) and even against curious cloud providers. Therefore, encrypting data before outsourcing them is the only way that gives to the data owners the control over their data. However, using traditional public key cryptography in a data-sharing context produces an unnecessary communication and computation overhead since for each targeted user, the data owner needs to encrypt a copy of data with the corresponding user's public key. To fix this problem, many attribute-based encryption (ABE) schemes were proposed. In the ABE model, the encryption process is done based on the attributes instead of a unique public key, and users with matching attributes can decrypt the ciphertext, so data owners in this model don't need to generate many copies of the same data as in the traditional cryptosystems. However, these schemes still require a huge computational power and communication cost since they are based on expensive bilinear pairing and modular exponentiation operations. We propose a lightweight version of the Ciphertext-Policy Attribute-Based Encryption (CP-ABE) using elliptic curve cryptography and scalar point multiplications, instead of bilinear pairings and modular exponentiations, to ensure a fine-grained access control with less computation cost and shorter keys and ciphertexts. The results show that our scheme improves the execution efficiency and requires a low-cost communication and storage.

Keywords: Cloud computing · Fine-grained access control · Elliptic curve cryptography · Attribute-Based encryption

1 Introduction

Cloud Computing, according to NIST, "is a model for enabling convenient, on-demand network access to a shared pool of configurable computing resources (e.g., networks, servers, storage, applications, and services) that can be rapidly provisioned and released

© Springer Nature Switzerland AG 2019
M. Ezziyyani (Ed.): AI2SD 2018, AISC 915, pp. 13–23, 2019.
https://doi.org/10.1007/978-3-030-11928-7_2

with minimal management effort or service provider interaction" [1]. These computing resources are provided in three main service models:

- Software as a Service (SaaS): Amazon S3, Salesforce ...
- Platform as a Service (PaaS): Microsoft Azure, Google AppEngine ...
- Infrastructure as a Service (IaaS): Amazon EC2 ....

Recently, many enterprises started to migrate toward outsourcing their business to the cloud to benefit from its attractive features, such as:

- On-demand self-service: computing resources are provisioned to the user as needed automatically without requiring human interaction.
- Broad network access: resources are accessible anywhere at any time using any type of connected devices (e.g., mobile phones, tablets, laptops, and workstations).
- Data availability: data will be replicated in geographically distributed datacenters so that users can access their data anytime and anywhere, and data will not be lost in case of disasters.
- Resources availability: Virtualization, load balancing and scheduling techniques adopted by cloud architectures make resources appear to the user to be unlimited and available in any quantity at any time.
- Transparency: resources usage can be monitored, controlled, and reported, providing transparency for both the provider and consumer of the utilized service.
- Low cost: resources will be provisioned as needed, so this model resolves the problem of overprovisioning and underprovisioning encountered in the traditional hosting solutions. In addition, the consumer will pay only the amount of resources he used (pay-as-you-go). Cloud computing solutions uncover the factors of 5 to 7 decrease in cost of resources compared to traditional data centers [2].
- No up-front commitment: users can start small and as long as their business grows up, they can use more resources easily without any intervention [3, 4].

However, although these interesting features of cloud computing solutions, users still hesitant of outsourcing their data. This is due to the fact that data owners will no longer be in control of their data when they are outsourced and this arises confidentiality and data security challenges against attackers compromising cloud servers and curious cloud providers who can easily access to data which are in a plain form. To prevent this problem, data owners must encrypt their data before outsourcing them. However, when a data owner wants to share its data with a group of users, traditional encryption schemes will no longer be useful, because the data owner will need to get all public keys of those users and encrypt many copies of the same data, each copy will be encrypted with the corresponding user's public key, so this generates a huge overhead in term of storage of ciphertexts and communication of public keys. Sahai and Waters proposed a new cryptosystem concept to overcome the traditional cryptography's limitation, it's called Attribute-Based Encryption (ABE) [5]. In this new cryptosystem, secret keys and ciphertexts are generated based on a set of attributes. Therefore, data will be encrypted one time with a set of attributes and only users with matching attributes will be able to decrypt the ciphertext. Two main variants of ABE scheme were proposed: Key Policy Attribute-Based Encryption (KP-ABE) [6] and Ciphertext-Policy Attribute-Based Encryption (CP-ABE) [7]. In the KP-ABE, the data owner encrypts data using his own attributes and the trusted authority generates secret keys for users based on their access policies. However, in the CP-ABE the data owner encrypts data using an access policy and the trusted authority generates secret keys for users based on their own attributes.

Organization. The rest of our paper will be organized as follows. In Sect. 2, we will discuss related works. Section 3 will be dedicated to present the preliminaries related to the proposed ABE scheme. We present the highlights of our system model in Sect. 4. We then show and analyze the performance results of our scheme and other existing solutions in Sect. 5. Finally, we conclude in Sect. 6.

2 Related Work

Sahai and Waters [5] were the first to propose a one-to-many encryption scheme based on attributes as a generalization of the existing Identity-Based Encryption (IBE) model that uses the identity (a string of characters) of the user to encrypt data instead of the public key. In the ABE scheme, data are encrypted using a set of attributes (which replaces the identity in the IDE schemes) and then the private key is generated based on the user's set of attributes, so only users with attributes matching the ciphertext's embedded attributes can decrypt the ciphertext and get data.

Two main schemes were proposed based on the abovementioned work; Goyal, Pandey, Sahai, and Waters introduced the first one under the name of Key-Policy Attribute-Based Encryption (KP-ABE) which is suitable for the query applications, such as pay TV system, audit log, targeted broadcast, and database access. In this scheme, a monotonic access structure is used to generate the secret key. The second is called Ciphertext-Policy Attribute-Based Encryption (CP-ABE), it was proposed by Bethencourt, Sahai, and Waters. Contrarily to the KP-ABE, in CP-ABE, the monotonic access structure is used to encrypt data so it is adapted for access control applications, such as social networking site access and electronic medical systems.

Subsequently, many contributions have been done based on these two main schemes. Cheung and Newport [8] proposed a provably secure CP-ABE which supports a non-monotonic access policy using negative attributes but in the other side, in this scheme the lengths of ciphertext and secret key increase linearly with the number of attributes in the universe of attributes which makes the basic CP-ABE proposed by Bethencourt, Sahai and Waters more efficient. Ibraimi et al. [9] provided a new CP-ABE solution to ensure a fine-grained access control with less computation overhead using an n-ary tree instead of threshold secret sharing. Ostrovsky et al. [10] proposed a scheme with a non-monotonic access structure where the secret keys are labeled with a set of attributes including positive and negative attributes. Comparatively, the ABE scheme with non-monotonic access structure can express a more complicated access policy. Unfortunately, this mechanism doubles the size of the ciphertext and secret key and adds encryption/decryption overheads at the same time. Subsequently, Attrapadung and Imai [11] proposed a Dual-Policy ABE scheme which allows key-policy and ciphertext-policy to act on encrypted data simultaneously. Many other works [12–15] were done to improve the security of the existing CP-ABE schemes, but almost all the existing schemes, to the best of our knowledge, are based on bilinear pairing and modular exponentiation operations which are proved to be computationally expensive.

Our contribution. We provide a lightweight version of CP-ABE using elliptic curves instead of bilinear pairing operations. Elliptic curves provide the same security-level as the RSA and other exponential-based encryption schemes using shorter keys [16]. Therefore, the generation and management of keys in our scheme will be more efficient than the aforementioned schemes and their variants that use bilinear pairing operations.

3 Preliminaries

In this section, we will define some preliminaries related to the elliptic curve cryptography and ABE cryptosystem related techniques.

3.1 Elliptic Curve Cryptography (ECC)

Elliptic curve cryptography is a public-key cryptography which is based on the elliptic curves defined over a finite field Fq (Galois field) such that Fq is whether a prime field (where q is a prime number) or a binary field (q = 2 m). Victor Miller and Neal Koblitz are the first to introduce it in 1985. There are many elliptic curves over finite field Fq. For instance, an elliptic curve can be defined as follows:

$$E(F_q) = E(Z_p) = \left\{(x, y) \in Z_p^2 \middle| y^2 = x^3 + ax + b\right\}, \tag{1}$$

where a, b are any elements in Fq that satisfy $4a^3 + 27b^2 \neq 0$.

The group operation in E(Fq) is the addition of points, and it is defined geometrically as follows: As illustrated in Fig. 1, we take two points P and Q in E(Fq), then we draw the line L joining P and Q (we take the tangent to E at P, if P = Q). L intersects the elliptic curve at a third point R. The addition of P and Q is the point –R (the symmetric point of R about the x-axis) and we note: P + Q = −R.

If P = −Q, the result of the addition P + Q is O and it's called the point at infinity. O is the zero element of E(Fq), which means: for every point P in E(Fq), P + O = P. The multiplication of a scalar and a point P is nothing more than repeatedly adding the same point P. So, we note: k.P = P + P + ⋯ + P (if k = 0, k.P = O). We call the number of points in E(Fq) the order of the curve and we represent it as #E. However, the order of a point P is the smallest positive integer n that produces: n.P = O.

As we know, cryptographic algorithms are implemented in a cyclic group. However, elliptic curves are not cyclic in general. In this regard, we select a point G ∈ E(Fq) whose order is a large prime number n and we generate a subgroup

$$\langle G \rangle = \{k.G | k \in Z_n\} = \{G, 2G, \ldots, nG = 0G = O\} \subset E(F_q) \tag{2}$$

Like in the RSA, the security in ECC is based on the Elliptic Curve Discrete Logarithm Problem (ECDLP) which is the equivalent of the Discrete Logarithm Problem in the

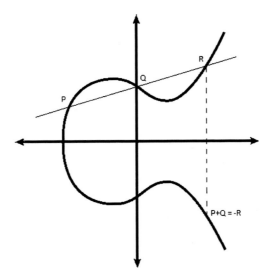

Fig. 1. Addition of points in the elliptic curve

RSA, and it means that it's hard to get the number k for given Q and P such that: Q = k.P. The fact that there is no efficient algorithm to resolve the ECDLP is called Elliptic Curve Discrete Logarithm Assumption.

3.2 Secret Sharing Schemes

Secret Sharing Schemes (SSS) aim to share a secret S among n parties by giving every party a share Si such that:

- using k or more shares S_i, we can easily reconstruct the secret S
- using $k - 1$ or less shares S_i, it's impossible to know anything about the secret S.

Shamir proposed the first construction for secret sharing schemes where the access structure is a threshold gate [17]. To share a secret S $\in$ Zp (where p is a prime) among n parties such that t + 1 colluding parties are required to reconstruct the secret, we define a t-degree polynomial $P(x) = \sum_{0 \leq j \leq t} a_i x^i$ where a_0 = S and for i $\neq$ 0, a_i is a random positive integer in Zp. Then, we give every party the share S_i = P(i). Any group J of t + 1 parties can compute the secret S using the Lagrange interpolation:

$$S = P(0) = \sum_{j \in J} \triangle_j(0).P(i) \tag{3}$$

where $\triangle_j(x) = \prod_{j \in J, j \neq i} \frac{x-j}{i-j}$ is called the Lagrange coefficient.

Subsequently, many other threshold secret sharing schemes were introduced [18, 19]. However, Benaloh and Leichter [20] proved that even if threshold schemes have found many applications in recent years, there are many other secret sharing applications which do not fit into the model of threshold schemes. For example, if we want to divide a secret S among four participants A, B, C, and D so that either A together with B can reconstruct the secret or C together with D can reconstruct the secret, then threshold schemes are provably insufficient. Therefore, they proposed a new generalized secret sharing scheme, which uses a tree-access structure instead of a threshold.

In the ABE schemes, a secret S is shared using a tree-access structure where the leaves (the parties) are associated with the attributes. Therefore, users need to have a minimum number of attributes satisfying the access structure to get the secret S.

3.3 Access Structure

Definition 1 (*Access Structure* [21]). Let $\{P1, P2, ..., Pn\}$ be a set of parties. A collection $\mathbb{A} \in 2^{\{P1,P2,...,Pn\}}$ is monotone if $\forall B, C$: if $B \in \mathbb{A}$ and $B \subseteq C$ then $C \in \mathbb{A}$. An access structure (respectively, monotone access structure) is a collection (respectively, monotone collection) $\mathbb{A}$ of non-empty subsets of $\{P1, P2, ..., Pn\}$, i.e., $\mathbb{A} \in 2^{\{P1,P2,...,Pn\}} \backslash \{\phi\}$. The sets in $\mathbb{A}$ are called the authorized sets, and the sets not in $\mathbb{A}$ are called the unauthorized sets.

In the ABE schemes, the access structure represents the access policy, where the parties are the attributes. Thus, the access structure $\mathbb{A}$ contains the authorized sets of attributes. Our construction uses a monotone access structure like the basic CP-ABE scheme.

4 Proposed Scheme

Our lightweight scheme is based on the basic CP-ABE model. Therefore, it consists of four main algorithms, which are executed by the system components as shown in Fig. 2:

- Setup: This algorithm is executed by the Trusted Authority (TA) to initialize the parameters (the elliptic curve, the generator...) that will be used in the system. It outputs a public key (PK) and a master secret key (MK).
- KeyGen (Au, MK): when the TA receives a request from the user, it executes this algorithm which takes user's set of attributes (Au) and the MK as inputs and generates user's secret key (SK).
- Encrypt (M, Ac, PK): the data owner executes the Encrypt algorithm to get the ciphertext (C) which is the encryption of the data M with an access policy Ac using the PK generated in the setup phase by the TA.
- Decrypt (C, SK, PK): This algorithm is executed by the data user. It takes as input the ciphertext (C) and the user's secret key (SK) along with the public key (PK) and it gives as output the data M if and only if the user's attributes (Au) satisfies the access policy (Ac) defined by the data owner.

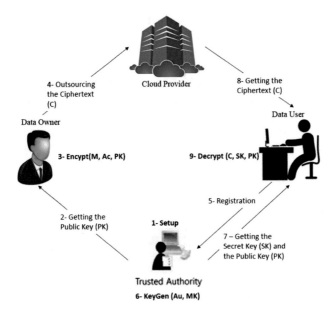

Fig. 2. System model of the LCP-ABE

5 Performance Analysis

In this section, we will compare our scheme with the existing CP-ABE based schemes in term of communication and computational overheads. To do that, we will apply the comparison approach used in [22]. Therefore, the first thing we have to do is to define and unify the comparison metrics.

5.1 Comparison Metrics

Communication Overhead Metrics. The communication overhead depends on the length of the transmitted messages. In the ABE schemes, the transmitted messages are ciphertext, public key, and private key. So the metrics we will use to compare the communication overhead of our schemes are the lengths of those three elements. Since the existing ABE schemes are based on modular exponentiation, they are called RSA-based ABE schemes and our scheme is called an ECC-based scheme. According to [16], elliptic curve cryptography has longer bit security than RSA, which means that ECC guarantees the same security-level with shorter keys compared to RSA. There-fore, to compare our ECC-based scheme with RSA-based schemes, we will fix a security level and use it as the unit to measure the length of our metrics. We will assume that the length of the value generated by the hash function is equal to the length of data which is equivalent to the security-level l = 160-bits. Therefore, the size of the private key is l and the size of the public key is 2 l since the public key is a point of the elliptic curve, which has two coordinates with a length of l for each of them. On the other hand, the size of keys of the 1024-bit RSA based ABE schemes is 6.4 l and the size of an element of G2 is 12.8 l. The ciphertexts and private keys in ABE schemes include the attributes set. However, for the sake of comparison, all ABE schemes to be compared with are assumed to be with the same attributes set, so the length of attributes can be ruled out from the length of ciphertext and secret key.

Computational Overhead Metrics. The computational overhead is caused by the operations: Encryption, decryption, hash, bilinear mapping, arithmetic and logic operations. The most expensive operation is bilinear mapping followed by the encryption and decryption operations. The rest of operations will not be considered in our comparison since they are negligible compared with the abovementioned operations. In the RSA-based public key encryption schemes, the most expensive operation is modular exponentiation and all other operations can be ignored. In the other side, the most expensive operation In an ECC-based public key scheme is point-scalar multiplication and all other operations can be ignored. Therefore, the computational overhead caused by public key based encryption and decryption can be measured by modular exponentiation or point-scalar multiplication. In addition, according to [22], one bilinear mapping is about 20 point scalar multiplication and one modular exponentiation is equivalent to 2 point scalar multiplication, so obviously we will use the point-scalar multiplication as the unit to measure the computational overhead.

Data used in Tables 1 and 2 were taken from [23] and converted using the abovementioned conversions for the purpose to have unified metrics. (Security-level l for the communication comparison, and point scalar multiplication M for the computation comparison.)

Table 1. Communication overhead comparison

Scheme	Ciphertext size	Public key size	Private key size
Bethencourt et al. [7]	$(2|A_c|+3)6.4$ l	32 l	$(2|A_U|+1)6.4$ l
Waters [24]	$(2|A_c|+3)6.4$ l	$(n+4)6.4$ l	$(|A_U|+2)6.4$ l
Cheung and Newport [8]	$(n+3)6.4$ l	$(3n+3)6.4$ l	$(2n+1)6.4$ l
Lewko et al. [15]	$(2|A_c|+3)6.4$ l	$(n+4)6.4$ l	$(|A_U|+2)6.4$ l
Ibraimi et al. [9]	$(|A_c|+3)6.4$ l	$(n+3)6.4$ l	$(|A_U|+1)6.4$ l
Our scheme	$(4|A_c|+6)$ l	6 l	$(2|A_U|+1)$ l

Legend |*| Number of elements in *, A_c Access Policy, A_U User's set of attributes, n Number of attributes in the universe of attributes, l Security level

Table 2. Computational overhead comparison

Scheme	Encryption	Decryption
Bethencourt et al. [7]	$(4|A_c|+5)M$	$(40|A_U|+4|S|+4)M$
Waters [24]	$(8|A_c|+5)M$	$46|A_U|M$
Cheung and Newport [8]	$(2n+5)M$	$22(n+1)M$
Lewko et al. [15]	$(8|A_c|+5)M$	$46|A_U|M$
Ibraimi et al. [9]	$(2|A_c|+5)M$	$22(|A_U|+1)M$
Our scheme	$(2|A_c|+3)M$	$(2|A_U|+|S|+1)M$

Legend |*| Number of elements in *, A_c Access Policy, A_U User's set of attributes, n Number of attributes in the universe of attributes, M Point scalar multiplication, S Satisfied nodes

5.2 Comparison Analysis

In order to study the efficiency of our scheme, we will compare it with other existing CP-ABE based schemes. We did not use KP-ABE based schemes in our comparison because KP-ABE and CP-ABE are dedicated to different types of applications as we mentioned in the introduction. Hence, we limit our comparison to CP-ABE based schemes. The communication overhead comparison results are shown in Table 1. Table 2 presents the computational overhead comparison results.

From Table 1, it's obvious that the ciphertexts generated by [7, 15, 24] are longer than the ciphertext generated by [9]. We admit that the number of attributes (n) in the universe of attributes is always bigger than the number of attributes in the access policy $(|Ac|)$. Therefore, [8] generates longer ciphertexts than [9] which, in turn, generates longer ciphertexts than our scheme since $(|Ac| + 3)6.41 > (|Ac| + 1.5)41$. In the public key length's view, it's clear that our scheme is the most efficient scheme. The private key size in [8] is bigger than the private key size in [7] since the number of attributes in the universe of attributes is bigger than the user's set of attributes' size. In addition, generates private keys that are 6.4 times longer than the private key generated in our scheme. The schemes [9, 15, 24] have approximately the same private key size which equals $(2|A_U| + 2)3.21$ which is approximately 3.2 times longer than the private keys in our scheme. Therefore, our scheme is the most efficient scheme in term of communication overhead.

From Table 2, we notice that the encryption algorithms in [15, 24] are the most expensive followed by [7]. The encryption algorithm in [9] is considered to be more efficient than [8] since the number n is bigger than $|A_c|$ as we mentioned in the previous paragraph. Therefore the encryption algorithm used in our scheme is the most efficient followed by [9] with a little difference. In the other side, we obviously notice that the decryption algorithm in our scheme requires less computation power than [7]. Cheung and Newport's scheme [8] (respectively, Ibraimi et al's scheme [9]) will be more efficient than our scheme if and only if the number of satisfied nodes (S) in the access policy is much bigger than 20 times the size of the universe of attributes (respectively, the number of user's attributes) which is not satisfied in the wide real cases. In the same way, Waters' and Lewko et al's schemes can be more efficient than our scheme only if the number of satisfied nodes (S) in the access policy is bigger than 44 times the number of user's descriptive attributes. It is clear that these conditions are not frequently satisfied in the real cases. Therefore, the decryption operation in our scheme is also considered more efficient than the other schemes.

6 Conclusion

We created a new lightweight CP-ABE scheme that provides a fine-grained access control with more efficiency compared to the existing pairing-based CP-ABE schemes. Our system allows policies to be expressed as any monotonic tree access structure and is resistant to collusion attacks. However, our scheme is not suitable for dynamic systems where users and attributes can be revoked, and the fact that the keys are generated by only one trusted authority makes our scheme vulnerable if an attacker gets into the trusted authority server and gets the master key. Therefore, in the future, it will be interesting to extend our scheme to a user/attribute-revocable scheme with multi-authority.

Acknowledgements. This work is supported by the National Center for Scientific and Technical Research's (CNRST) scholarship M.06/4.

References

1. Mell, P., Grance, T.: The NIST definition of cloud computing recommendations of the National Institute of Standards and Technology. Natl. Inst. Stand. Technol. Inf. Technol. Lab. **145**, 7 (2011)
2. Armbrust, M., et al.: A view of cloud computing: clearing the clouds away from the true potential and obstacles posed by this computing capability. Commun. ACM **53**(4), 50–58 (2010)
3. Zhang, Q., Cheng, L., Boutaba, R.: Cloud computing: state-of-the-art and research challenges. J. Internet. Serv. Appl. **1**(1), 7–18 (2010)
4. Armbrust, M., Fox, A., Griffith, R., Joseph, A., Katz, R.H.: Above the clouds: a Berkeley view of cloud computing. University of California, Berkeley, Technical Report UCB, pp. 07–013 (2009)
5. Sahai, A., Waters, B.: Fuzzy identity-based encryption. In: Eurocrypt, pp. 457–473 (2005)
6. Goyal, V., Pandey, O., Sahai, A., Waters, B.: Attribute-based encryption for fine-grained access control of encrypted data. In: Proceedings of the 13th ACM Conference on Computer and Communications Security—CCS'06, p. 89 (2006)
7. Bethencourt, J., Sahai, A., Waters, B.: Ciphertext-policy attribute-based encryption. In: Proceedings of the IEEE Symposium on Security and Privacy, pp. 321–334 (2007)
8. Cheung, L., Newport, C.: Provably secure ciphertext policy ABE. In: Proceedings of the 14th ACM Conference on Computer and Communications Security, CCS 2007, pp. 456–465 (2007)
9. Ibraimi, L., Tang, Q., Hartel, P., Jonker, W.: Efficient and provable secure ciphertext-policy attribute-based encryption schemes. In: Lecture Notes in Computer Science (Including Subseries Lecture Notes in Artificial Intelligence and Lecture Notes in Bioinformatics). LNCS, vol. 5451, pp. 1–12 (2009)
10. Ostrovsky, R., Sahai, A., Waters, B.: Attribute-based encryption with non-monotonic access structures. In: Proceedings of the 14th ACM Conference on Computer and Communications Security—CCS'07, p. 195 (2007)
11. Attrapadung, N., Imai, H.: Dual-policy attribute based encryption. In: Lecture Notes in Computer Science (Including Subseries Lecture Notes in Artificial Intelligence and Lecture Notes in Bioinformatics). LNCS, vol. 5536, pp. 168–185 (2009)
12. Nishide, T., Yoneyama, K., Ohta, K.: Attribute-based encryption with partially hidden encryptor-specified access structures. In: Lecture Notes in Computer Science (Including Subseries Lecture Notes in Artificial Intelligence and Lecture Notes in Bioinformatics). LNCS, vol. 5037, pp. 111–129 (2008)
13. Emura, K., Miyaji, A., Nomura, A., Omote, K., Soshi, M.: A ciphertext-policy attribute-based encryption scheme with constant ciphertext length. In: Lecture Notes in Computer Science (Including Subseries Lecture Notes in Artificial Intelligence and Lecture Notes in Bioinformatics). LNCS, vol. 5451, pp. 13–23 (2009)

14. Herranz, J., Laguillaumie, F., Ràfols, C.: Constant size ciphertexts in threshold attribute-based encryption. In: Lecture Notes in Computer Science (Including Subseries Lecture Notes in Artificial Intelligence and Lecture Notes in Bioinformatics). LNCS, vol. 6056, pp. 19–34 (2010)

15. Lewko, A.B., Okamoto, T., Sahai, A., Takashima, K., Waters, B.: Fully secure functional encryption: attribute-based encryption and (hierarchical) inner product encryption. In: Eurocrypt, vol. 02, no. subaward 641, pp. 62–91 (2010)

16. Martínez, V.G., Encinas, L.H., Sanchez-Avila, C.: A survey of the elliptic curve integrated encryption scheme. Secur. Manag. **2**(2), 495–504 (2010)

17. Shamir, A., Shamir, A.: How to share a secret. Commun. ACM **22**(1), 612–613 (1979)

18. Kothari, S.C.: Generalized Linear Threshold Scheme. In: Lecture Notes in Computer Science (Including Subseries Lecture Notes in Artificial Intelligence and Lecture Notes in Bioinformatics). LNCS, vol. 196, pp. 231–241 (1985)

19. Asmuth, C., Bloom, J.: A modular approach to key safeguarding. IEEE Trans. Inf. Theory **29**(2), 208–210 (1983)

20. Benaloh, J., Leichter, J.: Generalized secret sharing and monotone functions. Advances in Cryptology—CRYPTO'88, vol. 403, pp. 27–35 (1988)

21. Beimel, A.: Secure schemes for secret sharing and key distribution. Tech. Inst. Technol. Fac. Comput. Sci. (1996)

22. Yao, X., Chen, Z., Tian, Y.: A lightweight attribute-based encryption scheme for the internet of things. Future Gener. Comput. Syst. **49**, 104–112 (2015)

23. Pang, L., Yang, J., Jiang, Z.: A survey of research progress and development tendency of attribute-based encryption. Sci. World J. **2014**, 13 (2014)

24. Waters, B.: Ciphertext-Policy Attribute-Based Encryption: An Expressive, Efficient, and Provably Secure Realization, vol. 6571 (2006), pp. 1–25 (2011)

Generate a Meta-Model Content for Communication Space of Learning Management System Compatible with IMS-LD

Mohammed Ouadoud[1]([⊠]) and Mohamed Yassin Chkouri[2]

[1] LIROSA Lab, Faculty of Sciences, UAE, Tetouan, Morocco
mohammed.ouadoud@gmail.com
[2] SIGL Lab, National School of Applied Sciences, UAE, Tetouan, Morocco

Abstract. The context of this work is that of designing an IMS-LD meta-model for communication space of a Learning Management System (LMS). Our approach is to first think about the conditions for creating a real IMS-LD meta-model for communication space between learners, and designing the IT environment that supports this space. In this paper, we try to adapt the IMS-LD model with a communication meta-model for Learning Management System based on the social constructivism. This adaptation will go through three stages. Firstly, the development of a communication meta-model of LMS. Secondly, the study of correspondence between the developed meta-model and IMS-LD model. Finally, their transformation to IMS-LD meta-model.

Keywords: LMS · Communication space · IMS-LD · eLearning platform · Designing an IMS-LD meta-model

1 Introduction

ELearning is promoted through educational platforms: integrated systems offer a wide range of activities in the learning process. Teachers use the platforms to monitor or evaluate the work of students. They use LMS to create courses, tests, etc. However, the LMS eLearning platforms do not offer personalized services and therefore do not take into account the aspects of personalization such as the level of knowledge, interest, motivation and goals of learners. They access the same resource set in the same way.

In fact, we present an easy communication meta-model of LMS to create and administer the educational content online. This tool allows the generation and editing structures of websites through database rather than pedagogical models, with a variety of choices that ensures better adaptation to the teaching of the course and learning style. Therefore, it is necessary to find a method to model all LMS types. In order to modeling the communication space of LMS we have based ourselves upon the IMS-LD specification focusing on learning theory that was judged the most important and relevant to our modeling, namely the social constructivism. Then, this learning theory which have inspired for a long time the design of computer applications are combined and put into perspective with several emergent pedagogical functionalities to build an original modeling for our communication space of LMS. Reveals that this proposed

© Springer Nature Switzerland AG 2019
M. Ezziyani (Ed.): AI2SD 2018, AISC 915, pp. 24–39, 2019.
https://doi.org/10.1007/978-3-030-11928-7_3

modeling that is presented to readers here looks for ways to leverage technology for learning by considering users as being human actors and not human factors [1].

The IMS-LD specification or instructional design engineering uses pedagogical concepts, allowing to model learning units. IMS-LD takes into account a wide variety of teaching models it is there its flexibility. A course plan extract of a general or specific database can be modeled with IMS-LD, through the description of the different roles, activities, environments, methods,[1] properties, conditions and notifications. It is used to transform the course plans into formal learning units (UOL) that can be performed with an IMS-LD editor based on an engine such as Coppercore [2]. These executable units can be designed from the beginning using an editor such as Reload [3].

During the last decade, the LMS eLearning platforms have evolved considerably. However, several modeling of LMS platforms has been developed previously [4–8], but they have been abandoned because platforms' life cycle is changing apace. Therefore, we have conducted a comparative and analytical study on free e-learning platforms based on an approach of evaluating the e-learning platforms quality [9–12]. Based on these various research works, which seemed to us incomplete, we proposed a modeling portrait of a designing an IMS-LD communication model for LMS platform. This latter is anthropocentric and relies on a learning conception that is located at the intersection of the most used learning theory. Indeed, the idea is to orient the design work research towards a great and optimal compatibility between the services offered by eLearning platforms and the needs of all users, particularly learners, for better optimization of online learning.

To concretize our modeling work, we present in the section "Theoretical approach, concepts and related work" the different theories of learning used for the modeling of this space, namely the social constructivism. We also present the e-learning specification Learning Management Systems—Learning Design (IMS-LD) and related work. Next, in "transformation rules" section, we present the ATL transformation language to perform the transformation between the developed meta-model and IMS-LD model. We also determine in this section, the reasons why, we did not use the ATL language for transformation of models. Finally, we present in the section "Model-driven engineering", the modeling Driven Architecture (MDA). Thus, we try to adapt the proposed meta-model of the communication space to the equivalent IMS-LD model.

2 LMS and Activity Spaces

2.1 Activity Spaces

The learning management system consists of different activity spaces for activities of teaching and learning [13–15]. Each model represents a space, in these spaces, both teachers and learners can have:

- Disciplinary information space. In disciplinary information space, teachers or tutors can export content from the LMS as IMS/SCORM conformant Content Packages

---

[1] The word "method" used by IMS-LD means the unfolding of the scenario.

that can be viewed offline, or imported into the LMS. Entire courses or individual course units can be packaged for viewing or redistribution.

- Communication space. Communication is the act of conveying intended meanings from one entity or group to another using mutually understood signs and semiotic rules. Learners can communicate with others through their Inbox using LMS's private mail, through the discussion forums or the chat rooms.
- Collaboration space. Collaboration is the process of two or more people or organizations working together to realize or achieve something successfully [16]. Collaboration requires leadership, although the form of leadership can be social within a decentralized and egalitarian group [17]. Teams that work collaboratively can obtain greater resources, recognition and reward when facing competition for finite resources.
- Sharing space. Sharing space or exchange space, it allows discussing, to define and to follow the implementation of collaborative projects of one or several courses.
- Evaluation space. Evaluation is a process where learners are assessed to determine their suitability to take a course. The learners' aptitudes are determined by a variety of techniques including interviews, group exercises, presentations, examinations and psychometric testing.
- Production space. In production space, the teacher or tutor can create notifications, and assess the productions undertaken by learners.
- Self-management space. Self-management is the management of an LMS by the administrators themselves. The customizations are decentralized as much as possible and the sharing of tasks between all the users (administrators, coordinators, teachers, tutors, and learners) is done equitably.
- Assistance space. Assistance designates the action of bringing help or relief. It is about providing aid, support or relief in all matters.

2.2 Benefits of LMS

The LMS on which we increasingly rely as a means of learning have a considerable potential in the construction of knowledge and competence development. Thanks to the different services offered by these e-learning platforms, individuals can access and use interactively the multiple sources of information available to them everywhere, at all times. They can also compose customized training programs and thus develop their abilities to the highest level of their potential, according to their needs [18].

Based on the work of De Vries [19], the main pedagogical functions that may be assigned to the LMS as computer applications for learning are:

- Presenting information,
- Providing exercises,
- Really teaching,
- Providing a space of exploration,
- Providing a space of exchange between educational actors (learners, teachers, tutors…).

These different pedagogical functions, that correspond to one or many learning theories, allow the learner to acquire individual and collective knowledge according to the type of interaction that takes place between him/her and the sources of information made at his/her disposal. In practice, each individual has a set of tasks to deal with such as:

- Consulting and reading the pedagogical resources,
- Realizing the interactive exercises,
- Exploring the learning environment,
- Solving the problem situations,
- Discussing via synchronous and asynchronous tools of communication.

3 Theoretical Approach, Concepts and Related Work

3.1 LMS and the Social Constructivism

The social constructivism is the fruit of the development of learning theories under the influence of some researchers, particularly Lev Vygotski in 1934 [20, 21], who wanted to depart from the behaviorism by integrating other factors that are able to positively influencing the knowledge acquisition. Thus, new ideas emerged in connection with the possible interaction of individuals with the environment.

The social constructivism outlines learning by construction in a community of learners. In this light, learners are expected to interact with the available human resources (teachers, tutors, other learners…) in the proposed learning environment. In this way, the learners' psychological functions increase through social cognitive conflicts that occur between them. These conflicts lead to the development of the zone of proximal development[2] [23] and thus facilitate the acquisition of knowledge.

Learning is seen as the process of acquisition of knowledge through the exchange between teachers and learners or between learners. These latter learn not only through the transmission of knowledge by their teacher but also through interactions [24]. According to this model, learning is a matter of the development of the zone of proximal development: this zone includes the tasks that learners can achieve under the guidance of an adult; they are not very tough or so easy. The development of this zone is a sign that the learners' level of potential development increases efficiently [22].

The teacher's role is to define precisely this zone in order to design suitable exercises for learners. Furthermore, designing collaborative tasks, which involve discussions and exchange (socio-cognitive conflicts) between learners is so important in this model. Errors are considered as a point of support for the construction of new knowledge.

Based on the social constructivism approach (Fig. 1), the design of the LMS was oriented towards integrating online communication and collaboration tools. In practice, a wide range of platforms, particularly the social constructivist ones, proposes a set of

---

[2] "The distance between actual development level as determined by independent problem solving and the level of potential development as determined through problem solving under adult guidance or in collaboration with more capable peers [22, p. 86]".

tools, which allow sharing, exchanging and interacting in synchronous and asynchronous mode such as blogs, wikis, forums....

In summary, the ideas of social constructivist authors have highlighted the social nature of learning. Other authors have taken one-step further by emphasizing the distribution of intelligence between individuals and the environment. Furthermore,

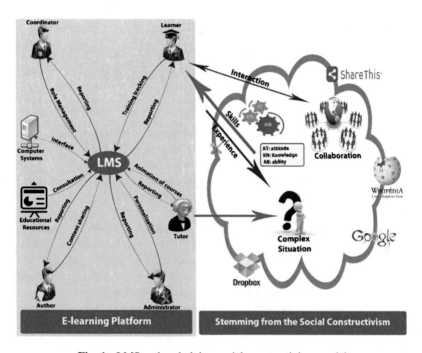

Fig. 1. LMS and underlying social constructivism model

considering that learning occur in a social context is no longer enough to ensure deep learning. Indeed, working in groups can affect negatively the quality of learning if these following conditions are not taken into consideration: Learning styles, the way groups are formed, interaction modality, and the characteristics of tasks.

3.2 Instructional Management Systems—Learning Design

There are several eLearning specifications, for example: SCORM,[3] DCMI,[4] IMS-SS[5] or IMS-CP.[6] Among these, IMS-LD, one of the last publications, seeks to incorporate pedagogical flexibility and complements certain aspects treated by others.

IMS-LD was published in 2003 by the IMS/GLC. (Instructional Management Systems Global Learning Consortium: Consortium for global learning management systems with training, the original name when IMS was started in 1997 Instructional Management Systems project) [25, 26]. Reminds us of its origins: the source (EML[7]) of the proposed language was assessed by the European Committee for Standardization (CEN) in a comparative study of different SRMS [26, 27], as best suited to satisfy the criteria definition of an EML. EML is defined by CEN/ISS as *"an information aggregation and semantic model describing the content and processes involved in a unit of learning from an educational perspective and in order to ensure the reusability and interoperability."* [26, 28] In this context, the North American IMS consortium undertook a study and provided a specification of such a language, giving birth in February 2003, the Learning Design specification V1.0 (IMS-LD). She adds that proposal, largely inspired EML developed by [26, 29] (OUNL) provides a conceptual framework for modeling a Learning Unit and claims to offer a good compromise between on the one hand to the generic implement a variety of instructional approaches and secondly, the power of expression that allows an accurate description of each learning unit.

This specification allows us to represent and encode learning structures for learners both alone and in groups, compiled by roles, such as "learners" and "Team" (cf. Fig. 2) [26] We can model a lesson plan in IMS-LD, defining roles, learning activities, services and many other elements and building learning units. The syllabus is modeled and built with resources assembled in a compressed Zip file, then started by an executable ("player"). It coordinates the teachers, students and activities as long as the respective learning process progresses. A user takes a "role" to play and execute the activities related to in order to achieve a satisfactory learning unit. In all, the unit structure, roles and activities to build the learning scenario to be executed in a system compatible with IMS-LD.

IMS-LD does not impose a particular pedagogical model, but can be used with a large number of scenarios and pedagogic models, demonstrating its flexibility. Therefore, IMS-LD is often called a meta-pedagogic model. Previous eLearning ini-

---

[3] **SCORM**: Sharable Content Object Reference Model. Available at https://www.adlnet.gov/adl-research/scorm/.

[4] **DCMI**: Dublin Core Metadata Initiative. Available at http://dublincore.org/.

[5] **IMS-SS**: Instructional Management Systems—Simple Sequencing. Available at https://www.imsglobal.org/simplesequencing.

[6] **IMS-CP**: Instructional Management Systems-Content Packaging. Available at https://www.imsglobal.org/content/packaging.

[7] **EML**: Educational Modelling Language.

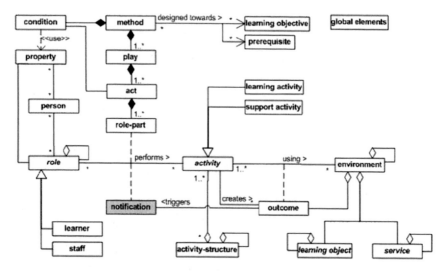

Fig. 2. The conceptual model of instructional management systems—learning design [26]

tiatives claim to be pedagogically neutral, IMS-LS is not intended to pedagogical neutrality, but seeks to raise awareness of eLearning on the need for a flexible approach.

IMS-LD has been developed for eLearning and virtual classes, but a course face to face can be done and integrated into a structure created by this specification, as an activity of learning or support activity. If the ultimate goal to create rich learning units, with support to achieve the learning objectives by providing the best possible experience, face-to-face meetings, and any other learning resource are permitted such as video conferencing, collaborative table or any field action research.

IMS-LD uses the theatrical metaphor, which implies the existence of roles, resources and learning scenario itself: one room is divided into one or more acts and conducted by several actors who can take on different roles at different times. Each role is to carry out a number of activities to complete the learning process. In addition, all roles must be synchronized at the end of each act before processing the next act.

3.3   Related Works

A great deal of research is focused in one way or another on the platforms' engineering for distance education, including LMS. For example Chekour [20], presented a synthesis of the main learning theories in the digital era, namely: the behaviorism, the cognitivism, the constructivism and the social constructivism. El-Mhouti [21] highlighted the ICT use in the service of active pedagogies, based on the social constructivist approach, the principles that structure the instructional design approaches, and the assessment of the social constructivist activities.

These works, among many others, emphasized the contribution of learning theories in the design and development of learning systems. The direct application of each of these theories allows particularly providing supporting methods for the design and development of LMS. The hybridization of the learning theories that we presented in this paper as an original conceptual model has allowed us to design a new LMS whose benefit resides essentially in the richness of the proposed functionalities in a way that fits the needs of all its final users: teachers and learners.

Furthermore, several research [30–32] had for goal to implement and present the functionalities of LMS platforms (such as Moodle) and their possibilities to effectively manage users assessment approach (teachers and/or learners) within training institutions. Moreover, in the framework of the European project Mediasite [33], a reference model for the process for distance learning has been developed. This theoretical framework has led to the integration of several applications (video-conferencing, document manager, portal...) in order to define an electronic training platform for online communication and/or collaboration.

In addition, much work has been done in the field of collaborative learning and IMS-LD specification. For example, Dyke [34] explains how models' socio-cognitive interaction are related to the properties of collaborative tools. Ferraris [35] expresses collaborative learning scenarios by teachers animating virtual classrooms to promote the re-use and share teaching practices. He proposes an approach led by the models in accordance with the recommendations of the Model Driven Architecture OMG. He presents a meta-model based on IMS-LD enhanced by the concepts of participation model to capture the richness of the interactions inherent in collaborative activities. Moreover, El-Moudden [28, 36] proposes a designing an IMS-LD model for collaborative learning. His approach is to first think about the conditions for creating a real collective activity between learners, and designing the IT environment that supports these activities.

On the other hand, other research aimed at proposing the modeling of new units, approach, architecture, or adaptive, flexible and interactive e-learning devices. For example, Sadiq proposed the modeling of learning units on eLearning platforms, which relies on the application of the standard IMS-LD in the production of adaptive learning units [4].

Based on these various research works, which seemed to us incomplete, we proposed a modeling portrait of a designing an IMS-LD communication meta-model for LMS platform. For us, this is not the same case and the same vision as our modelization is more general, it aims on one hand to create an LMS from which teachers can animate virtual groups for the re-use and sharing of teaching practices and on the other hand, the re-use of the content created in other frameworks. Indeed, the idea is to orient the design work research towards a great and optimal compatibility between the services offered by eLearning platforms (LMS) and the needs of all users, particularly learners, for better optimization of online learning.

4 Transformation Rules

4.1 Atlas Language Transformation (ATL)

In their operational ATL, Canals et al. use [36, 37]. State that to deal with the transformation of models; it is difficult and cumbersome to use object languages since we spend so much effort to the development of transformation definitions of the framework for the set work. The use of XSLT as a language if it is more direct and adapted by rest against difficult to maintain [36, 37]. We follow their choice by focusing on the implementation of approaches centered on the MDA (Model Driven Architecture), MDE (Model Driven Engineering) and QVT (Queries View Transformation) tools. Query/View/Transformation (QVT) [36, 38] is a standard defined by the OMG. This is a standardized language to express model transformations. QVT is not advanced sufficiently now in its definition for Queries and View aspects. Against transformation by the appearance expressed by MDA approach has resulted in various experiments (e.g. Triskell, ATL...) in both academic and commercial levels. To determine the transformation, it is necessary to have tools of transformations. These are based on language transformations must respect the QVT standard [36, 38] proposed by the OMG [36, 39]. There is an offer of free tools (ATL, MTF, MTL, QVTP, etc.) and commercial (e.g. MIA). We chose ATL[8] from the provision of free tools, to the extent that only ATL has a spirit consistent with OMG/MDA/MOF/QVT [36, 37].

4.2   ATL Description

Atlas Transformation Language (ATL) has been designed to perform transformations within the MDA Framework proposed by the OMG [36, 40, 41]. The ATL language is mainly based on the fact that the models are first-class entities. Indeed, the transformations are considered models of transformation. Since the transformations are considered themselves as models, we can apply their transformations. This possibility of ATL is considered an important point. Indeed, it provides the means to achieve higher order transformations (HOT Higher-Order Processing) [36, 41]. A higher-order transformation is a transformation, including source and target models that are themselves transformations. As ATL is among the languages model transformation respecting the QVT [38] standard proposed by OMG [39], we describe its structure in relation to this standard (QVT).

The study of the abstract syntax of the ATL language is to study two features provided by this language more than rules changes. The first feature, navigation, allows studying the possibility of navigation between meta-models sources and targets. The second feature, Operations, used to describe the ability to define operations on model elements. Finally, the study of the transformation rules is used to describe these types of rules, how they are called and the type of results they return.

- Navigation [36, 39, 40] this feature is offered by ATL language (Object Constraint Language). Navigation is allowed only if the model elements are fully initialized. The elements of the target model cannot be definitively initialized at the end of the execution of the transformation. Therefore, the navigation in the ATL can only be made between elements of the model (or meta-model) source and model (or meta-model) target.
- Operations: [36, 40] this feature ATL is also provided by the OCL (Object Constraint Language). In OCL, operations can be defined on the elements of the model.

---

[8] **ATL**: Atlas Transformation Language.

ATL takes this opportunity to OCL to allow defining operations on elements of the source model and the transformation model [36, 39].

The transformation rules: there are several types of transformation rules based on how they are called and what kind of results they return (cf. Fig. 3).

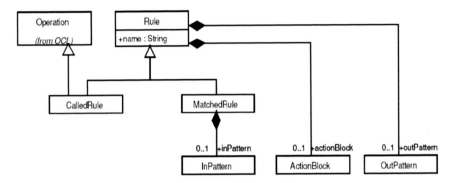

Fig. 3. ATL transformation rules [36]

CalledRule [40] rule explicitly called by its name and by setting its parameters.

MatchedRule [40] rule executed when a guy (InPattern) scheme is recognized in the source model.

The result of a rule may be a set of predefined models (OutPattern) or a block of mandatory (ActionBlock). If the rule is MatchedRule type and if its result is a set of elements of the target model (OutPattern), it was named declarative. If it is CalledRule type whose result is a block of statements, it is then called procedure. Combinations of rules (declarative and imperative) are called hybrid rules [39].

4.3   Synthesis

In this research, we try to adapt the model IMS-LD with a communication meta-model supporting LMS. This adaptation will go through three stages, first the development of a communication meta-model; secondly, the study of correspondence between the developed meta-model and IMS-LD model and their transformation to IMS-LD meta-model that reduced the MDA approach in a transformation that is based on the rules implemented in the ATL language. However, we will talk about the IT design of our LMS communication meta-model without using the transformation that is based on the rules implemented in the ATL language, because we have detected the same problems as in El-Moudden's works [28, 36]. In IMS-LD, we do not have the opportunity to build a Course, which consists of several Chapters. For this, there is at this level a semantic loss. Frankly, we find that there are the real problems of semantic loss during the transformation of our communication meta-model to an IMS-LD meta-model with the ATL language.

5 Model-Driven Engineering

5.1 Modeling Driven Architecture (MDA)

In November 2000, the OMG in the field of software engineering consortium of over 1000 companies, has initiated the process MDA [OMG MDA], the concepts-oriented models rather than object-oriented. The Model Driven Architecture MDA [OMG MDA] offers the power of abstraction, refinement and different views of the models. This standard has to add a new way to design applications by separating business logic from business, any technical platform to increase the reuse of previously developed code, reducing development time and facilitating the integration of new technology [42]. It gives the opportunity to develop independent model platforms and implementation [43] environment. MDA is used to separate two extreme views of the same system [44]:

- Its functional specifications on the one hand.
- Its physical implementation on the other hand.

Including several aspects of the life of the software, namely its tests, its quality requirements, the definition of successive iterations, etc. The MDA architecture consists of four layers. In the center, there is a UML (Unified Modeling Language) standard MOF (Meta-Object Facility) and CWM (Common Warehouse Meta-model). The second layer contains the XMI (XML Metadata Interchange) standard for dialogue between the middleware (Java, CORBA, .NET, and Web services). The next layer refers to the services to manage events, transaction security, and directories. The last layer offers specific frameworks in scope (Telecommunications, medicine, electronic commerce, finance, etc.) A designer to create his own application can use UML as it can use other languages. So, according to this architecture independent technical context, MDA proposes to structure the front needs to engage in a transformation of this functional modeling technical modeling while testing each product model [44]. This application model is to be created independently of the target implementation (hardware or software). This allows greater reuse of patterns. MDA is considered an approach with the ambition to offer the widest possible view of the life cycle of the software, not content with only its production. Moreover, this is intended overview described in a unified syntax. One of the assumptions underlying the MDA is that the operationalization of an abstract model is not a trivial problem. One of the benefits of MDA is to solve this problem [45]. MDA proposes to design an application through software chain is divided into four phases with the aim of flexible implementation, integration, maintenance and test:

- The development of a computer model without concern (CIM: Computer Independent Model).
- The manual transformation into a model in a particular technological context (PIM: Platform Independent Model).
- The automatic transformation into a pattern associated with the target implementation of the platform (PSM: Platform Specific Model) model to be refined.
- Its implementation in the target platform.

5.2   Correspondence Between the Terminology of IMS-LD and that of the Communication Meta-Model

The majority of classes designed in our communication meta-model for LMS correspond perfectly with the IMS-LD model, which makes possible their transformations to it. The transformation of models is a technique aims to put links between models in order to avoid unnecessary reproductions.

In Table 1, we have tried to collect all the communication meta-model classes for LMS and their equivalent at the IMS-LD.

Table 1. Correspondence between the terminology of IMS-LD and that of the communication meta-model

Communication meta-model	IMS-LD
Activity	Activity
Learning activity	Learning activity
Social networking, survey, videoconferencing, chat and messaging	Support activity
Role, and features	Role
Members	Person
Coordinator, teacher, and tutor	Staff
Learner	Learner
Objective	Learning objective
Activity space	Environment
Course and chapter	Learning object
Communication space	Services

6   Designing a Communication Meta-Model for LMS Based on IMS-LD

In our research, we propose a meta-model for a communication space designed to achieve the needs of LMS platform, and the needs of teachers and learners. Therefore, we establish the following diagram as a first proposal of a communication meta-model for LMS platform.

Indeed, we will talk about the IT design of our communication meta-model for LMS. This led us to develop our meta-model in which we will eventually identify the features of the constituent entities of our meta-model in which we specify the different classes of our modeling.

Teachers, tutors, and learners can promote sharing experiences through the meta-model tools presented in Fig. 4 and these following technological advances:

- Social Networking. All LMS users can develop a network of contacts, create and join interest groups, set up a network profile, and link any of the thousands of remote gadget applications into their networking environment. Photos can be shared across courses, or through the social networking area.

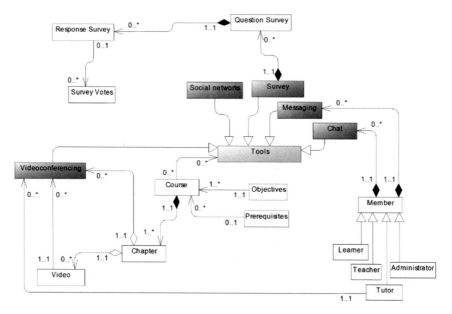

Fig. 4. Proposition of an conceptual meta-model of the communication space

- Messaging. Teachers, tutors, and learners can send bulk message to course members, assistants, or both. Insert tokens to customize messages for each individual user.
- Survey. This module provides an Amazon-style 5-star rating system for courses. Each user can give a rating and the total is displayed in the block. Administrators can connect to survey module instances on the same course from the block, to add a "Review" survey.
- Videoconferencing is a web conferencing system for distance education. The goal of the module is to enable universities, and colleges deliver a high-quality learning experience to remote learners. The latter supports real-time sharing of slides, audio, video, chat, and desktops.
- Chat. This module uses a block to list all online users that are part of all courses. A user who is subscribed to, can open a chat window on the bottom of the page.

7   Conclusion and Perspectives

In our work, we are on the way to the design and modeling a meta-model content for communication space of Learning Management System compatible with IMS-LD. This design is based on active teaching learner-centered, and as an example of the pedagogy, we opted for theory as a basis for teaching this communication space of LMS, namely the social constructivism. The latter, that allows us to reach a teaching object through the implementation of the courses that are divided into tasks performed by students collaboratively or individually. To achieve a goal, we need to reach the model validation step, which is one of the tasks to be performed in our future work; also, we seek a framework that will guide us better to start the development part.

References

1. Henri, F., Rabardel, P., Pastré, P. (eds.): Modèles du sujet pour la conception. Toulouse. Int. J. ELearn. Dist. Educ. **22**(1), 101–106 (2005). Octares Éditions, 260p., Aug 2007
2. Alfanet Project: CopperCore V 3.3. CopperCore is one of the OUNL's contributions to the Alfanet project, Nov 2008
3. Bolton: RELOAD Project: Editor. The University of Bolton, The University of Strathclyde and JISC, United Kingdom (2005)
4. Sadiq, M., Talbi, M.: Modélisation des unités d'apprentissage sur des plates-formes de formation à distance. Association EPI, Mar 2010
5. Tonye, E.: Modeling a framework for open and distance learning in sub-Saharan African countries. frantice.net, numéro 2, Dec 2010
6. Chouchane, K.: Modélisation et réalisation d'une approche pour le m-learning. In: Magister en Informatique Option Système d'Informatique et de Communication (SIC), Université Hadj Lakhdar, Batna, Algérienne (2012)
7. Brunel, S., Girard, P., Lamago, M.: Des plateformes pour enseigner à distance: vers une modélisation générale de leurs fonctions. In: AIP Primeca 2015, La Plagne, France (2015)
8. née Dahmani Farida, B.: Modélisation basée ontologies pour l'apprentissage interactif—application à l'évaluation des connaissances de l'apprenant. Ph.D. dissertation in computer science, Computer Science Department, Mouloud Mammeri University of Tizi-Ouzou, Algeria, 28 Nov 2010
9. Ouadoud, M., Chkouri, M.Y., Nejjari, A., El Kadiri K.E.: Studying and analyzing the evaluation dimensions of eLearning platforms relying on a software engineering approach. Int. J. Emerg. Technol. Learn. (iJET) **11**(1), 11–20 (2016). 10p. http://dx.doi.org/10.3991/ijet.v11i01.4924
10. Ouadoud, M., Chkouri, M.Y., Nejjari, A., Kadiri, K.E.E.: Studying and comparing the free eLearning platforms. In: 2016 4th IEEE International Colloquium on Information Science and Technology (CiSt), pp. 581–586 (2016). http://dx.doi.org/10.1109/CIST.2016.7804953
11. Ouadoud, M., Chkouri, M.Y., Nejjari, A., El Kadiri, K.E.: Exploring a recommendation system of free eLearning platforms: functional architecture of the system. Int. J. Emerg. Technol. Learn. (iJET) **12**(02), 219–226 (2017). https://doi.org/10.3991/ijet.v12i02.6381
12. Ouadoud, M., Chkouri, M.Y., Nejjari, A.: LeaderTICE: a platforms recommendation system based on a comparative and evaluative study of free E-learning platforms. Int. J. Online Eng. (iJOE) **14**(01), 132–161 (2018). https://doi.org/10.3991/ijoe.v14i01.7865
13. Ouadoud, M., Nejjari, A., Chkouri, M.Y., El-Kadiri, K.E.: Learning management system and the underlying learning theories. In: Innovations in Smart Cities and Applications, pp. 732–744 (2017). https://doi.org/10.1007/978-3-319-74500-8_67
14. Ouadoud, M., Nejjari, A., Chkouri, M.Y., Kadiri, K.E.E.: Educational modeling of a learning management system. In: 2017 International Conference on Electrical and Information Technologies (ICEIT), pp. 1–6 (2017). http://dx.doi.org/10.1109/EITech.2017.8255247
15. Ouadoud, M., Chkouri, M.Y., Nejjari, A.: Learning management system and the underlying learning theories: towards a new modeling of an LMS. Int. J. Inf. Sci. Technol. (iJIST) **2**(1), 25–33 (2018)

16. Martinez-Moyano, I.J.: Exploring the dynamics of collaboration in interorganizational settings. In: Creating a Culture of Collaboration: The International Association of Facilitators Handbook (2006)
17. Spence, M.U.: Graphic design: collaborative processes. a course on collaboration, theory and practice. In: Art 325: Collaborative Processes. Fairbanks Hall, Oregon State University, Corvallis, Oregon (2005)
18. Paquette, G.L.: Ingénierie Pédagogique: Pour Construire l'Apprentissage en Réseau. PUQ (2002)
19. Marquet, P.: Lorsque le développement des TIC et l'évolution des théories de l'apprentissage se croisent. Savoirs 9, 105–121 (2005). https://doi.org/10.3917/savo.009.0105
20. Chekour, M., Laafou, M., Janati-Idrissi, R.: L'évolution des théories de l'apprentissage à l'ère du numérique. Association EPI, Feb 2015
21. El Mhouti, A., Nasseh, A., Erradi, M.: Les TIC au service d'un enseignement-apprentissage socioconstructiviste. Association EPI, Jan 2013
22. Vygotsky, L.S.: Mind in Society: The Development of Higher Psychological Processes, revised edn. Harvard University Press, Cambridge (1978)
23. Wake, J.D.: Evaluating the organising of a collaborative telelearning scenario from an instructor perspective œ an activity theoretical approach. Ph.D. dissertation in computer science, Department of Information Science, University of Bergen, Dec 2001. Thèse de doctorat
24. Doise, W., Mugny, G.: Le développement social de l'intelligence, vol. 1. Interéditions, Paris (1981)
25. Lejeune, A.: IMS Learning Design: Étude d'un langage de modélisation pédagogique, Revue Distances et Savoirs, vol. 2
26. Burgos, D., Arnaud, M., Neuhauser, P., Koper, R.: IMS Learning Design. Association EPI, Dec 2005
27. CEN/ISS WS/LT, Learning Technologies Workshop: Survey of Educational Modelling Languages (EMLs). Version 1, Sept 2002
28. El-Moudden, F., Khaldi, M., Aammou, S.: Designing an IMS-LD model for collaborative learning. IJACSA 1(6), 42–48
29. Koper, R.: Modeling Units of Study from a Pedagogical Perspective, the Pedagogical Meta-Model Behind EML (2001)
30. Benslimane, M., Zine, O., Derouich, A., Talbi, A.: Proposition et implémentation sur Moodle d'une approche de conception d'un cours en ligne: cas d'un cours d'algorithmique. In: Workshop International sur les Approches Pédagogiques & ELearning (2016)
31. Zoubaidi, X., Ait Daoud, M., Namir, A., Talbi, M., Nachit, B.: La formation de formateurs d'éducateurs du préscolaire: mise en place d'un dispositif de formation à distance. Association EPI, Jan 2014
32. Chemsi, G., Radid, M., Sadiq, M., Talbi, M.: Une plate-forme d'évaluation des enseignements et des formations à distance: EVAL-EFD. Association EPI, Sept 2011
33. Bechina, A., Keith, B., Brinkschulte, U.: Mediasite: une nouvelle plate-forme dédiée à l'enseignement à distance. In: IRES 2001, 07 July 2005
34. Dyke, G., Lund, K.: Implications d'un modèle de coopération pour la conception d'outils collaboratifs, Dec 2006
35. Ferraris, C., Lejeune, A., Vignollet, L., David, J.-P.: Modélisation de scénarios pédagogiques collaboratifs (2005)
36. El-Moudden, F., Aammou, S., Khaldi, M.: A tool to generate a collaborative content compatible with IMS-LD. Int. J. Softw. Web Sci. 11(1), 01–08, Dec 2014–Feb 2015

37. Canals, A., Le Camus, C., Feau, M., Jolly, G., Bonnafous, V., Bazavan, P.: Une utilisation opérationnelle d'ATL: L'intégration de la transformation de modèles dans le projet TOPCASED. In: Génie logiciel, pp. 21–26 (2005)
38. OMG/RFP/QVT MOF 2.0 Query/Views/Transformations RFP. OMG, Object Management Group, 28 Oct 2002
39. Bézivin, J., Dupé, G., Jouault, F., Pitette, G., Rougui, J.E.: First experiments with the ATL model transformation language: Transforming xslt into xquery. In: OOPSLA 2003 Workshop, Anaheim, California (2003)
40. ATLAS Group LINA and INRIA Nantes: Atlas transformation language. ATL user manual —version 0.7. Technical report. INRIA University of Nantes, Feb 2006
41. Combemale, B., Rougemaille, S.: ATL—Atlas Transformation Language. Master 2 Recherche SLCP, Module RTM edn (2005)
42. Boulet, P., Dekeyser, J.L., Dumoulin, C., Marquet, P.: Mda for soc embeddeb systems design, intensive signal processing experiment. In: SIVOESMDA Workshop at UML 2003, San Francisco, Oct 2003
43. Thi-Lan-anh, D., Olivier, G., Houari, S.: Gestion de modèles: définitions, besoins et revue de littérature. In: Premières Journées sur l'Ingénierie Dirigée par les Modèles, pp. 1–15. Paris, France, 30 June–1 July 2005
44. Clave, A.: D'UML à MDA en passant par les métas modèles. Technical report, La Lettre d'ADELI no. 56 (2004)
45. Caron, P.A., Hoogstoel, F., Le Pallec, X., Warin, B.: Construire des dispositifs sur la plateforme moodle—application de l'ingénierie bricoles. In: MoodleMoot-2007, Castres, France, 14–15 Jun 2007

Designing an IMS-LD Model for Communication Space of Learning Management System

Mohammed Ouadoud[1][(⊠)] and Mohamed Yassin Chkouri[2]

[1] LIROSA Lab, UAE, Faculty of Sciences, Tetouan, Morocco
mohammed.ouadoud@gmail.com
[2] SIGL Lab, UAE, National School of Applied Sciences, Tetouan, Morocco

Abstract. The context of this work is that of designing an IMS-LD model for communication space of a Learning Management System (LMS). Our work is specifically in the field or seeking to promote, by means of information technology from a distance. Our approach is to first think about the conditions for creating a real communication space for LMS between learners, and designing the IT environment that supports this space. In this paper, we try to adapt the IMS-LD model with a communication model for LMS based on the social constructivism. This adaptation will go through three stages. Firstly, the development of an LMS model. Secondly, the study of correspondence between the developed model and IMS-LD model. Finally, their transformation to IMS-LD model.

Keywords: LMS · Communication space · IMS-LD · eLearning platform · Designing an IMS-LD model

1 Introduction

In the 20th century, there was an international movement in favor of eLearning integration in higher education. This movement has been operationalized due to the variety of the educational offer by universities, which most have opted to diversify knowledge dissemination platforms to meet the needs of their target public.

ELearning is promoted through educational platforms: integrated systems offer a wide range of activities in the learning process. Teachers use the platforms to monitor or evaluate the work of students. They use learning management systems (LMS) to create courses, tests, etc. However, the LMS eLearning platforms do not offer personalized services and therefore do not take into account the aspects of personalization such as the level of knowledge, interest, motivation and goals of learners. They access the same resource sets in the same way.

In fact, we present an easy communication model of LMS to create and administer the educational content online. This tool allows the generation and editing structures of websites through database rather than pedagogical models, with a variety of choices that ensures better adaptation to the teaching of the course and learning style. Therefore, it is necessary to find a method to model all LMS types. In order to modeling the

© Springer Nature Switzerland AG 2019
M. Ezziyyani (Ed.): AI2SD 2018, AISC 915, pp. 40–54, 2019.
https://doi.org/10.1007/978-3-030-11928-7_4

communication space of LMS we have based ourselves upon the IMS-LD[1] specification focusing on learning theory that was judged the most important and relevant to our modeling, namely the social constructivism. Then, this learning theory which have inspired for a long time the design of computer applications are combined and put into perspective with several emergent pedagogical functionalities to build an original modeling for our communication space of LMS. This reveals that this proposed modeling that is presented to readers here looks for ways to leverage technology for learning by considering users as being human actors and not human factors [1].

The IMS-LD specification or instructional design engineering uses pedagogical concepts, allowing to model learning units. IMS-LD takes into account a wide variety of teaching models it is there its flexibility. A course plan extract of a general or specific database can be modeled with IMS-LD, through the description of the different roles, activities, environments, methods,[2] properties, conditions and notifications. It is used to transform the course plans into formal learning units (UOL) that can be performed with an IMS-LD editor based on an engine such as Coppercore [2]. These executable units can be designed from the beginning using an editor such as Reload [3].

During the last decade, the LMS eLearning platforms have evolved considerably. However, several modeling of LMS platforms have been developed previously [4–8], but they have been abandoned because platforms' life cycle is changing apace. Therefore, we have conducted a comparative and analytic study on free e-learning platforms based on an approach of evaluating the e-learning platforms quality [9–12]. Based on these various research works, which seemed to us incomplete, we proposed a modeling portrait of a designing an IMS-LD communication model for LMS platform. This latter is anthropocentric and relies on a learning conception that is located at the intersection of the most used learning theory. Indeed, the idea is to orient the design work research towards a great and optimal compatibility between the services offered by eLearning platforms and the needs of all users, particularly learners, for better optimization of online learning.

To concretize our modeling work, we present in the section "Theoretical approach, concepts and related work" the different theories of learning used for the modeling of this space, namely the social constructivism. We also present the ATL transformation language to perform the transformation between the developed model and IMS-LD model. We also determine in this section, the reasons why, we did not use the ATL language for transformation of models. Next, we present in "Instructional Management Systems—Learning Design" section, the IMS-LD online learning specification. Then, we present in the section "Designing an IMS-LD model of communication space", the use case diagram of the communication space. Thus, we try to adapt the class diagram model of the communication space to the equivalent IMS-LD model.

---

[1] **IMS-LD:** Instructional Management Systems-Learning Design. Available at https://www.imsglobal. org/learningdesign.

[2] The word "method" used by IMS-LD means the unfolding of the scenario.

2 LMS and Activity Spaces

The learning management system consists of different activity spaces for activities of teaching and learning [13–15]. Each model represents a space, in these spaces, both teachers and learners can have a:

- Disciplinary information space. In disciplinary information space, teachers or tutors can export content from the LMS as IMS/SCORM conformant Content Packages that can be viewed offline, or imported into the LMS. Entire courses or individual course units can be packaged for viewing or redistribution.
- Communication space. Communication is the act of conveying intended meanings from one entity or group to another using mutually understood signs and semiotic rules. Learners can communicate with others through their Inbox using LMS's private mail, through the discussion forums or the chat rooms.
- Collaboration space. Collaboration is the process of two or more people or organizations working together to realize or achieve something successfully [16]. Collaboration requires leadership, although the form of leadership can be social within a decentralized and egalitarian group [17]. Teams that work collaboratively can obtain greater resources, recognition and reward when facing competition for finite resources.
- Sharing space. Sharing space or exchange space, it allows discussing, to define and to follow the implementation of collaborative projects of one or several courses.
- Evaluation space. Evaluation is a process where learners are assessed to determine their suitability to take a course. The learners' aptitudes are determined by a variety of techniques including interviews, group exercises, presentations, examinations and psychometric testing.
- Production space. In production space, the teacher or tutor can create notifications, and assess the productions undertaken by learners.
- Self-management space. Self-management is the management of an LMS by the administrators themselves. The customizations are decentralized as much as possible and the sharing of tasks between all the users (administrators, coordinators, teachers, tutors, and learners) is done equitably.
- Assistance space. Assistance designates the action of bringing help or relief. It is about providing aid, support or relief in all matters.

3 Theoretical Approach, Concepts and Related Work

3.1 LMS and the Social Constructivism

The social constructivism is the fruit of the development of learning theories under the influence of some researchers, particularly Lev Vygotski in 1934 [18, 19], who wanted to depart from the behaviorism by integrating other factors that are able to positively influencing the knowledge acquisition. Thus, new ideas emerged in connection with the possible interaction of individuals with the environment.

The social constructivism outlines learning by construction in a community of learners. In this light, learners are expected to interact with the available human resources (teachers, tutors, other learners ...) in the proposed learning environment. In this way, the learners' psychological functions increase through social cognitive conflicts that occur between them. These conflicts lead to the development of the zone of proximal development[3] [21] and thus facilitate the acquisition of knowledge.

Learning is seen as the process of acquisition of knowledge through the exchange between teachers and learners or between learners. These latter learn not only through the transmission of knowledge by their teacher but also through interactions [22]. According to this model, learning is a matter of the development of the zone of proximal development: this zone includes the tasks that learners can achieve under the guidance of an adult; they are not very tough or so easy. The development of this zone is a sign that the learners' level of potential development increases efficiently [13].

The teacher's role is to define precisely this zone in order to design suitable exercises for learners. Furthermore, designing collaborative tasks, which involve discussions and exchange (socio-cognitive conflicts) between learners is so important in this model. Errors are considered as a point of support for the construction of new knowledge.

Based on the social constructivism approach (Fig. 1), the design of the LMS was oriented towards integrating online communication and collaboration tools. In practice, a wide range of platforms, particularly the social constructivist ones, proposes a set of tools, which allow sharing, exchanging and interacting in synchronous and asynchronous mode such as blogs, wikis, forums ....

In summary, the ideas of social constructivist authors have highlighted the social nature of learning. Other authors have taken one-step further by emphasizing the distribution of intelligence between individuals and the environment. Furthermore, considering that learning occur in a social context is no longer enough to ensure deep learning. Indeed, working in groups can affect negatively the quality of learning if these following conditions are not taken into consideration: Learning styles, the way groups are formed, interaction modality, and the characteristics of tasks.

3.2 Atlas Language Transformation (ATL)

In their operational ATL, Canals et al. use [23, 24]. State that to deal with the transformation of models; it is difficult and cumbersome to use object languages since we spend so much effort to the development of transformation definitions of Framework for the set work. The use of XSLT as a language if it is more direct and adapted by rest against difficult to maintain [23, 24]. We follow their choice by focusing on the implementation of approaches centered on the MDA (Model Driven Architecture), MDE (Model Driven Engineering) and QVT (Queries View Transformation) tools. Query/View/Transformation (QVT) [24, 25] is a standard defined by the OMG. This is

---

[3] "The distance between actual development level as determined by independent problem solving and the level of potential development as determined through problem solving under adult guidance or in collaboration with more capable peers [20, p. 86]".

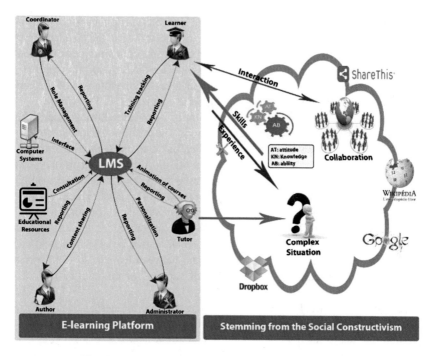

Fig. 1. LMS and underlying social constructivism model

a standardized language to express model transformations. QVT is not advanced sufficiently now in its definition for Queries and View aspects. Against transformation by the appearance expressed by MDA approach has resulted in various experiments (e.g. Triskell, ATL …) in both academic and commercial level. To determine the transformation, it is necessary to have tools of transformations. These are based on languages transformations must respect the QVT standard [24, 25] proposed by the OMG [24, 26]. There is an offer of free tools (ATL, MTF, MTL, QVTP, etc.) and commercial (e.g. MIA). We chose ATL (Atlas Transformation Language) from the provision of free tools, to the extent that only ATL has a spirit consistent with OMG/MDA/MOF/QVT [23, 24].

3.3   Related Works

A great deal of research is focusing in one way or another on the platforms engineering for distance education, including LMS. For example Chekour [18], presented a synthesis of the main learning theories in the digital era, namely: the behaviorism, the cognitivism, the constructivism and the social constructivism. El-Mhouti [19] highlighted the ICT use in the service of active pedagogies, based on the social constructivist approach, the principles that structure the instructional design approaches, and the assessment of the social constructivist activities.

These works, among many others, emphasized the contribution of learning theories in the design and development of learning systems. The direct application of each of these theories allows particularly providing supporting methods to the design and development of LMS. The hybridization of the learning theories that we presented in this paper as an original conceptual model has allowed us to design a new LMS whose benefit resides essentially in the richness of the proposed functionalities in a way that fits the needs of all its final users: teachers and learners.

Furthermore, several research [27–29] had for goal to implement and present the functionalities of LMS platforms (such as Moodle) and their possibilities to effectively manage users assessment approach (teachers and/or learners) within training institutions. Moreover, in the framework of the European project Mediasite [30], a reference model for the process for distance learning has been developed. This theoretical framework has led to the integration of several applications (video-conferencing, document manager, portal...) in order to define an electronic training platform for online communication and/or collaboration.

In addition, much work has been done in the field of collaborative learning and IMS-LD specification. For example, Dyke [31] explains how models socio-cognitive interaction are related to the properties of collaborative tools. Ferraris [32] expresses collaborative learning scenarios by teachers animating virtual classrooms to promote the re-use and share teaching practices. He proposes an approach led by the models in accordance with the recommendations of the Model Driven Architecture OMG. He presents a meta-model based on IMS-LD enhanced by the concepts of participation model to capture the richness of the interactions inherent in collaborative activities. Moreover, El-Moudden [24, 33] proposes a designing an IMS-LD model for collaborative learning. His approach is to first think about the conditions for creating a real collective activity between learners, and designing the IT environment that supports these activities.

On the other hand, other research aimed at proposing the modeling of new units, approach, architecture, or adaptive, flexible and interactive eLearning devices. For example, Sadiq proposed the modeling of learning units on eLearning platforms, which relies on the application of the standard IMS-LD in the production of adaptive learning units [4].

Based on these various research works, which seemed to us incomplete, we proposed a modeling portrait of a designing an IMS-LD Model for LMS platform. For us, this is not the same case and the same vision as our modelization is more general, it aims on one hand to create a LMS from which teachers can animate virtual groups for the re-use and sharing of teaching practices and on the other hand, the re-use of the content created in other frameworks. Indeed, the idea is to orient the design work research towards a great and optimal compatibility between the services offered by eLearning platforms (LMS) and the needs of all users, particularly learners, for better optimization of online learning.

4   Instructional Management Systems—Learning Design

There are several eLearning specifications, for example: SCORM,[4] DCMI,[5] IMS-SS[6] or IMS-CP.[7] Among these, IMS-LD, one of the last publications, seeks to incorporate pedagogical flexibility and complements certain aspects treated by others.

IMS-LD was published in 2003 by the IMS/GLC. (Instructional Management Systems Global Learning Consortium: Consortium for global learning management systems with training, the original name when IMS was started in 1997 Instructional Management Systems project) [34, 35]. Reminds us of its origins: the source (EML[8]) of the proposed language was assessed by the European Committee for Standardization (CEN) in a comparative study of different SRMS [35, 36], as best suited to satisfy the criteria definition of an EML. EML is defined by CEN/ISS as *"an information aggregation and semantic model describing the content and processes involved in a unit of learning from an educational perspective and in order to ensure the reusability and interoperability."* [33] In this context, the North American IMS consortium undertook a study and provided a specification of such a language, giving birth in February 2003, the Learning Design specification V1.0 (IMS-LD). She adds that proposal, largely inspired EML developed by [35, 37] (OUNL) provides a conceptual framework for modeling a Learning Unit and claims to offer a good compromise between on the one hand to the generic implement a variety of instructional approaches and secondly, the power of expression that allows an accurate description of each learning unit.

This specification allows us to represent and encode learning structures for learners both alone and in groups, compiled by roles, such as "learners" and "Team" (cf. Fig. 2) [35] We can model a lesson plan in IMS-LD, defining roles, learning activities, services and many other elements and building learning units. The syllabus is modeled and built with resources assembled in a compressed Zip file then started by an executable ("player"). It coordinates the teachers, students and activities as long as the respective learning process progresses. A user takes a "role" to play and execute the activities related to in order to achieve a satisfactory learning unit. In all, the unit structure, roles and activities build the learning scenario to be executed in a system compatible with IMS-LD.

---

[4] **SCORM**: Sharable Content Object Reference Model. Available at https://www.adlnet.gov/adl-research/scorm/.

[5] **DCMI**: Dublin Core Metadata Initiative. Available at http://dublincore.org/.

[6] **IMS-SS**: Instructional Management Systems-Simple Sequencing. Available at https://www.imsglobal.org/simplesequencing.

[7] **IMS-CP**: Instructional Management Systems-Content Packaging. Available at https://www.imsglobal.org/content/packaging.

[8] **EML**: Educational Modelling Language.

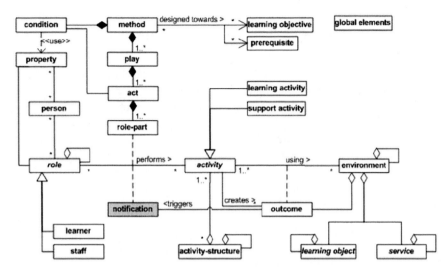

Fig. 2. The conceptual model of instructional management systems—learning design [35]

IMS-LD does not impose a particular pedagogical model but can be used with a large number of scenarios and pedagogic models, demonstrating its flexibility. Therefore, IMS-LD is often called a meta-pedagogic model. Previous eLearning initiatives claim to be pedagogically neutral, IMS-LS is not intended to pedagogical neutrality but seeks to raise awareness of eLearning on the need for a flexible approach.

IMS-LD has been developed for eLearning and virtual classes, but a course face to face can be done and integrated into a structure created with this specification, as an activity of learning or support activity. If the ultimate goal to create rich learning units, with support to achieve the learning objectives by providing the best possible experience, face-to-face meetings, and any other learning resource are permitted such as video conferencing, collaborative table or any field action research.

IMS-LD uses the theatrical metaphor, which implies the existence of roles, resources and learning scenario itself: one room is divided into one or more acts and conducted by several actors who can take on different roles at different times. Each role is to carry out a number of activities to complete the learning process. In addition, all roles must be synchronized at the end of each act before processing the next act.

5   Designing an IMS-LD Communication Model for LMS

In our work, we tried to design an LMS model of learning online, beginning with the study of the IDM approach, (Model based Engineering) based on four stages of implementation:

- The development of a model without IT preoccupation (CIM: Computer Independent Model);
- Its manual transformation into a model in a particular technological environment (PIM: Platform Independent Model);

- The automatic transformation into a model associated with the target implementation platform (PSM: Platform Specific Model) model must be refined;
- Its implementation in the target platform.

In this section, we will talk about the IT design of our LMS model without using the same approach that we have adopted in previous works, because we have detected the real problems of semantic loss during the transformation of the model.

This led us to develop our model through the outline of the diagram in which we will eventually identify the features of the constituent entities of our model and the class diagrams in which we will specify the different classes' constituents our LMS model.

5.1 Use Case Diagram

The use case diagrams identify the functionality provided by the model (use case); users interact with the system (actors), and the interactions between them. The main objectives of the use case diagrams are:

- Provide high-level view of the model.
- Identify users ("actors") of the model.
- Define the roles of the actors in the model.

Table 2 describes the service function for each actor.

Here are the use case diagram (cf. Fig. 3) of the model representing the external actors who will interact with the system and how they will use it.

5.2 Correspondence Between the Terminology of IMS-LD and that of the Communication Model

In this research, we try to adapt the model IMS-LD with a communication model supporting LMS. This adaptation will go through three stages, first the development of a LMS communication model, secondly, the study of correspondence between the developed model and IMS-LD model and their transformation to IMS-LD model that reduced the MDA approach in a transformation that is based on the rules implemented in the ATL language. However, we will talk about the IT design of our LMS communication model without using the transformation that is based on the rules implemented in the ATL language, because we have detected the same problems as in El-Moudden's works [24, 33]. In IMS-LD, we do not have the opportunity to build a Project, which consists of several Projects. For this, there is at this level a semantic loss. Frankly, we find that there are the real problems of semantic loss during the transformation of our communication model to an IMS-LD model with the ATL language.

Consequently, the majority of classes designed in our LMS communication model correspond perfectly with the IMS-LD model, which makes possible their transformation to it. The transformation of model is a technique aims to put links between models in order to avoid unnecessary reproductions. In Table 1, we have tried to collect all the classes of LMS communication model and their equivalent at the IMS-LD.

Table 1. Correspondence between the terminology of IMS-LD and that of the communication model

Communication model	IMS-LD
Activity	Activity
Learning activity	Learning activity
Social networking, survey, videoconferencing, chat and messaging	Support activity
Role, and features	Role
Members	Person
Coordinator, teacher, and tutor	Staff
Learner	Learner
Objective	Learning objective
Activity space	Environment
Course and chapter	Learning object
Communication space	Services

5.3 Class Diagram IMS-LD

In our work, we will try to create a communication model based on the theoretical study of our current work and allows simultaneously to ensure its projection to the model, on top of that we will try to recognize our communication model with the IMS-LD model, this compatibility will not be a direct way c to d, one will use the same terminology IMS-LD for all classes of our proposed LMS communication model, there is an equivalent class in the IMS-LD, which will greatly help us in the implementation level. We present in Table 1 the different classes of our communication model and the IMS-LD model.

In the following, we propose communication model to achieve the needs of LMS platform, and the needs of teachers and learners. Therefore, we establish the following class diagram (cf. Fig. 4) as a proposal of communication model for LMS platform. Teachers, tutors, and learners can promote collaboration experiences through these following technological advances:

- Social Networking. All LMS users can develop a network of contacts, create and join interest groups, set up a network profile, and link any of the thousands of remote gadget applications into their networking environment. Photos can be shared across courses, or through the social networking area.
- Messaging. Teachers, tutors, and learners can send bulk message to course members, assistants, or both. Insert tokens to customize messages for each individual user.

Table 2. Table function description

Actor	Function	Description
Learner	Consult the course	The learner can view the course, prerequisites, and its objectives at any time
	View documents	Learners read the downloaded documents
	Initiate discussions	The learner can start discussions
	Upload documents	The learner can upload documents
	Download documents	The learner can download the documents
Tutor	Manage groups	The tutor adds, modifies or deletes groups
	Assign students to groups	The tutor can assign learners to groups
	Initiate discussions	The tutor can start discussions
	Set tasks	The tutor can set tasks
	Assign tasks	The tutors can assign tasks to learners
	Support the learners	Tutor can keep tracking of learners
Teacher	Create courses	The teacher can create courses
	Set prerequisites	The teacher can set prerequisites for course
	Set objectives	The teacher can set objectives for course
	Upload documents	The teacher can upload documents
	Download documents	Teachers can download the documents
	Planning of teaching resources	The teacher must planning of teaching resources
Administrator	Set in place groups	The administrator can set in place the classes' groups
	Management of the courses	The administrator can management of the courses
	Manage access rights	The administrator can manage the access rights of teachers and learners
Coordinator	Manage teachers	The coordinator adds, modifies, or deletes a teacher
	Monitoring of teachers' activities	The coordinator can monitoring of teachers' activities
	Assignment of courses to tutors	The coordinator can assignment of courses to tutors according to the specialty of each one

- Survey. This module provides an Amazon-style 5-star rating system for courses. Each user can give a rating and the total is displayed in the block. Administrators can connect to survey module instances on the same course from the block, to add a "Review" survey.

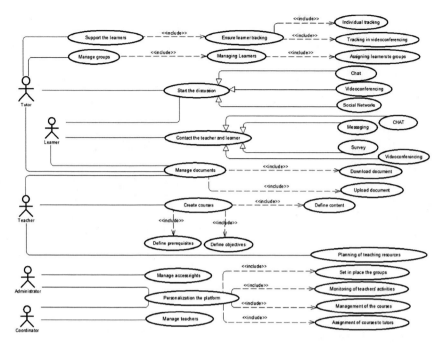

Fig. 3. Use case diagram of communication space

- Videoconferencing is a web conferencing system for distance education. The goal of the module is to enable universities, and colleges to deliver a high-quality learning experience to remote learners. The latter supports real-time sharing of slides, audio, video, chat, and desktops.
- Chat. This module uses a block to list all online users that are part of all courses. A user who is subscribed to, can open a chat window on the bottom of the page.

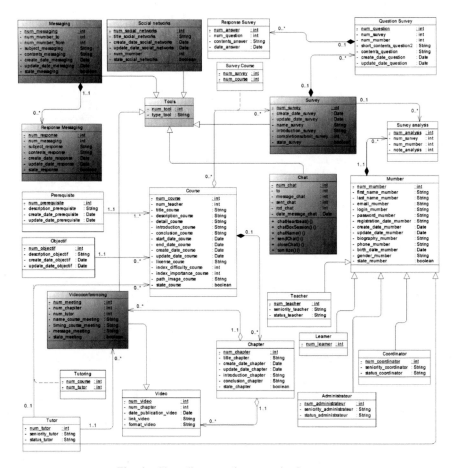

Fig. 4. Class diagram of communication space

6   Conclusion and Perspectives

In our work, we are on the way to the design and modeling a meta-model content for communication space of Learning Management System compatible with IMS-LD. This design is based on active teaching learner-centered, and as an example of the pedagogy, we opted for theory as a basis for teaching this communication space of LMS, namely the social constructivism. The latter, that allows us to reach a teaching object through the implementation of the courses that are divided into tasks performed by students collaboratively or individually. To achieve a goal, we need to reach the model validation step, which is one of the tasks to be performed in our future work; also, we seek a framework that will guide us better to start the development part.

References

1. Henri, F., Rabardel, P., Pastré, P. (eds.): Modèles du sujet pour la conception. Toulouse. Int. J. eLearn. Dist. Educ. **22**(1), 101–106 (2005). Octares Éditions, 260p., Aug 2007
2. Alfanet Project: CopperCore V 3.3. CopperCore is one of the OUNL's contributions to the Alfanet project, Nov 2008
3. Bolton: Reload Project: Editor. The University of Bolton, The University of Strathclyde and JISC, United Kingdom (2005)
4. Sadiq, M., Talbi, M.: Modélisation des unités d'apprentissage sur des plates-formes de formation à distance. In: Association EPI, Mar 2010
5. Tonye, E.: Modeling a framework for open and distance learning in sub-Saharan African countries. Frantice.net, Numéro 2, Dec 2010
6. Chouchane, K.: Modélisation et réalisation d'une approche pour le m-learning. In: Magister en Informatique Option Système d'Informatique et de Communication (SIC), Université Hadj Lakhdar, Batna, Algérienne (2012)
7. Brunel, S., Girard, P., Lamago, M.: Des plateformes pour enseigner à distance: vers une modélisation générale de leurs fonctions. In: AIP Primeca 2015, La Plagne, France (2015)
8. née Dahmani Farida, B.: Modélisation basée ontologies pour l'apprentissage interactif— application à l'évaluation des connaissances de l'apprenant. Ph.D. dissertation in computer science, Computer Science Department, Mouloud Mammeri University of Tizi-Ouzou, Algeria, 28 Nov 2010
9. Ouadoud, M., Chkouri, M.Y., Nejjari, A., El Kadiri, K.E.: Studying and analyzing the evaluation dimensions of eLearning platforms relying on a software engineering approach. Int. J. Emerg. Technol. Learning (iJET) **11**(1), 11–20 (2016). 10p. http://dx.doi.org/10.3991/ijet.v11i01.4924
10. Ouadoud, M., Chkouri, M.Y., Nejjari, A., Kadiri, K.E.E.: Studying and comparing the free eLearning platforms. In: 2016 4th IEEE International Colloquium on Information Science and Technology (CiSt), pp. 581–586 (2016). http://dx.doi.org/10.1109/CIST.2016.7804953
11. Ouadoud, M., Chkouri, M.Y., Nejjari, A., El Kadiri, K.E.: Exploring a recommendation system of free eLearning platforms: functional architecture of the system. Int. J. Emerg. Technol. Learn. (iJET) **12**(02), 219–226 (2017). https://doi.org/10.3991/ijet.v12i02.6381
12. Ouadoud, M., Chkouri, M.Y., Nejjari, A.: LeaderTICE: a platforms recommendation system based on a comparative and evaluative study of free e-learning platforms. Int. J. Online Eng. (iJOE) **14**(01), 132–161 (2018). https://doi.org/10.3991/ijoe.v14i01.7865
13. Ouadoud, M., Chkouri, M.Y., Nejjari, A.: Learning management system and the underlying learning theories: towards a new modeling of an LMS. Int. J. Inf. Sci. Technol. (iJIST) **2**(1), 25–33 (2018)
14. Ouadoud, M., Nejjari, A., Chkouri, M.Y., El-Kadiri, K.E.: Learning management system and the underlying learning theories. In: Innovations in Smart Cities and Applications, pp. 732–744 (2017). https://doi.org/10.1007/978-3-319-74500-8_67
15. Ouadoud, M., Nejjari, A., Chkouri, M.Y., Kadiri, K.E.E.: Educational modeling of a learning management system. In: 2017 International Conference on Electrical and Information Technologies (ICEIT), pp. 1–6 (2017). http://dx.doi.org/10.1109/EITech.2017.8255247
16. Martinez-Moyano, I.J.: Exploring the dynamics of collaboration in interorganizational settings. In: Creating a Culture of Collaboration: The International Association of Facilitators Handbook (2006)

17. Spence, M.U.: Graphic design: collaborative processes. A course on collaboration, theory and practice. Art 325: collaborative processes. Fairbanks Hall, Oregon State University, Corvallis, Oregon (2005)
18. Chekour, M., Laafou, M., Janati-Idrissi, R.: L'évolution des théories de l'apprentissage à l'ère du numérique. Association EPI, Feb 2015
19. El Mhouti, A., Nasseh, A., Erradi, M.: Les TIC au service d'un enseignement-apprentissage socioconstructiviste. Association EPI, Jan 2013
20. Vygotsky, L.S.: Mind in Society: The Development of Higher Psychological Processes, revised edn. Cambridge: Harvard University Press (1978)
21. Wake, J.D.: Evaluating the organising of a collaborative telelearning scenario from an instructor perspective œ an activity theoretical approach. Ph.D. dissertation in computer science, Department of Information Science, University of Bergen. Thèse de doctorat, Dec 2001
22. Doise, W., Mugny, G.: Le développement social de l'intelligence, vol. 1. Interéditions, Paris (1981)
23. Canals, A., Le Camus, C., Feau, M., Jolly, G., Bonnafous, V., Bazavan, P.: Une utilisation opérationnelle d'ATL : l'intégration de la transformation de modèles dans le projet TOPCASED. In: Génie logiciel, pp. 21–26 (2005)
24. El-Moudden, F., Aammou, S., Khaldi, M.: A tool to generate a collaborative content compatible with IMS-LD. Int. J. Softw. Web Sci. 11(1), 01–08, Dec 2014–Feb 2015
25. OMG/RFP/QVT MOF 2.0 Query/Views/Transformations RFP. OMG, Object Management Group, 28 Oct 2002
26. Bézivin, J., Dupé, G., Jouault, F., Pitette, G., Rougui, J.E.: First experiments with the atl model transformation language: transforming xslt into xquery. In: OOPSLA 2003 Workshop, Anaheim, California (2003)
27. Benslimane, M., Zine, O., Derouich, A., Talbi, A.: Proposition et implémentation sur Moodle d'une approche de conception d'un cours en ligne: cas d'un cours d'algorithmique. In: Workshop International sur les Approches Pédagogiques & eLearning (2016)
28. Zoubaidi, X., Ait Daoud, M., Namir, A., Talbi, M., Nachit, B.: La formation de formateurs d'éducateurs du préscolaire: mise en place d'un dispositif de formation à distance. Association EPI, Jan 2014
29. Chemsi, G., Radid, M., Sadiq, M., Talbi, M.: Une plate-forme d'évaluation des enseignements et des formations à distance: EVAL-EFD. Association EPI, Sept 2011
30. Bechina, A., Keith, B., Brinkschulte, U.: Mediasite: une nouvelle plate-forme dédiée à l'enseignement à distance. IRES 2001, 07 Jul 2005
31. Dyke, G., Lund, K.: Implications d'un modèle de coopération pour la conception d'outils collaboratifs, Dec 2006
32. Ferraris, C., Lejeune, A., Vignollet, L., David, J.-P.: Modélisation de scénarios pédagogiques collaboratifs (2005)
33. El-Moudden, F., Khaldi, M., Aammou, S.: Designing an IMS-LD model for collaborative learning. IJACSA 1(6), 42–48
34. Lejeune, A.: IMS learning design: étude d'un langage de modélisation pédagogique. Rev. Dist. Savoirs 2, 409–450 (2004)
35. Burgos, D., Arnaud, M., Neuhauser, P., Koper, R.: IMS learning design. In: Association EPI, Dec 2005
36. CEN/ISS WS/LT, Learning Technologies Workshop: Survey of Educational Modelling Languages (EMLs). Version 1, Sept 2002
37. Koper, R.: Modeling Units of Study from a Pedagogical Perspective, the Pedagogical Meta-Model Behind EML (2001)

A Smart Cascaded H-Bridge Multilevel Inverter with an Optimized Modulation Techniques Increasing the Quality and Reducing Harmonics

Babkrani Youssef$^{(\boxtimes)}$, Naddami Ahmed, and Hilal Mohamed

Department of Electrical Engineering, Faculty of Science and Technical,
University of Hassan 1st, Settat, Morocco
y.babkrani@gmail.com

Abstract. The world community relied heavily on fossils energies but just after the big oil crisis the use of renewable energy has greatly increased and has become the main interest of many countries for its many advantages such as: minimal impact on the environment, renewable generators requiring less maintenance than traditional ones and it has also a great impact on economy. It is easy to get charmed by the advantages of using the renewable resources but we must also be aware of their disadvantages. One of the major disadvantages is that the renewable energy resources are intermittent and thus they have led scientists to develop new semiconductor power converters among which are the multilevel inverter. In this paper a new smart multi-level inverter is proposed so as to increase its levels according to the user's needs and also to avoid the impact of shades and the intermittence on photovoltaic panels. We also propose a modification on the multicarrier aiming to reduce the harmonics. This modification introduces a sinusoidal wave compared with trapezoidal multi-carrier to generate the pulses. In order to obtain the line voltages and the total harmonic distortions (THD) MATLAB/SIMULINK is used.

Keywords: Phase disposition (PD) · Phase opposition disposition (POD) · Alternative phase opposition disposition (APOD) · Total harmonics distortion (THD) · Cascaded H bridge · Smart Multi-level inverter

1 Introduction

The world around us has changed considerably over the past 20 years. As fossil fuels have become more expensive and tougher to find and also because energy fuels related activities have led to significant environmental damages [1]. Thus it is wiser decision for governments all around the word to reduce their dependency on such traditional types of energy and replace it by other sources of energy that can be safer cheaper cleaner and renewable, solar energy is undeniably one of these sources, using solar radiation to produce the heat and electricity [2].

Solar energy demand has grown by 25% annually during the past 20 years [3]. However, it utilization has met different difficulties witch has led researchers to find

© Springer Nature Switzerland AG 2019
M. Ezziyyani (Ed.): AI2SD 2018, AISC 915, pp. 55–68, 2019.
https://doi.org/10.1007/978-3-030-11928-7_5

new, more efficient technologies one of them is the multilevel inverter used in medium and high voltage [1].

Multilevel inverters are gaining celebrity for Photovoltaic (PV) systems due to the reduced total harmonics distortions of the output signal and the low voltage stress of power switches. It produces almost a sinusoidal voltage at the output [4].

In addition, two-level inverters are exposed to thermal stresses created by converting the full voltage imposed by the continuous source, so the performance and lifetime of its components are actually affected.

Among the diverse multilevel structures, cascaded H-bridge multilevel is found to be attractive for our smart inverter because it uses the same technology in series "full H-Bridges" to produce inverted AC from separate DC sources [5].

This paper presents a proposition of a smart cascaded h-bridge multi-levels inverter with the possibility of increasing the levels according to the need of the user.

Multiple multi-carrier SPWM methods for cascaded h-bridge are analyzed and compared with the conventional SPWM technique. Those carriers are being implemented with different sinusoidal dispositions PD, POD and APOD and with different frequencies.

2   Multi-level Inverter

2.1   Induction Motors

Big electric energies uses include advanced power electronics inverter to encounter the high demands. As a result, multilevel voltage inverter has been presented as an alternative in high power and medium voltage circumstances [6]. A multilevel converter not only attains high power assessments, but also it increases the performance of the whole structure in terms of harmonics [7]. Many present schemes incorporate the use of induction motors as main source for traction in electric vehicles, those driver require advanced power electronic inverters, to attain their high power demands.

The multilevel voltage inverters structure allows them to grasp this high voltage requirement without the usage of transformers [8], especially high voltage vehicle drives where electromagnetic interference (EMI) and low total harmonic distortion (THD) of the output voltage are vital.

The general utility of the multilevel inverter is to create a desired voltage from multiple levels of dc voltages, for this reason, multilevel inverters can easily deliver the high power necessary to large electrical Vehicles, hybrid Vehicles or any motor inverter technology used mainly in areas of high energy consumption such as air conditioning.

Cascade inverters are perfect for an induction motor this configuration gives many advantages such as [9]:

(1) It makes induction motor safer/handy for induction motor power system.
(2) No electromagnetic interference.
(3) Higher efficiency is attained compared to low voltage motors.
(4) Low voltage switching devices are used.
(5) No unbalance charge problem in drive mode or charge mode.

2.2 Basic Structure

A cascaded multilevel inverter is a power electronic device made to create a desired AC voltage from several of DC voltages the structure is composed of several H-bridges converters in series connection as given in Fig. 1 it got many advantages it can reach high voltage and high power without transformers and with a remarkable improvement of the spectral quality [10].

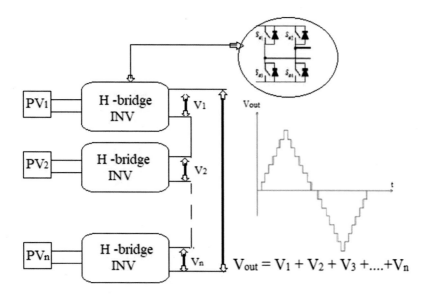

Fig. 1. Structure of a cascaded H bridge

The voltage levels L of the cascaded H inverter is defined by L = 2 N + 1, where N is the number of DC sources

The more H inverters are used the more levels of the output waveform are created and the shape becomes approximate to sinusoidal waveform.

The output voltage can be expressed as:

Vout = V1 + V2 + V3 + ··· + Vn. Each full bridge inverter can generate three levels −Vdc, 0 and +Vdc.

2.3 Carrier-Based Modulation Schemes

Most carrier-based PWM schemes for cascaded H-bridge multi-level inverters descend from the carrier disposition scheme [11] For an L level cascaded inverter, L-1 triangular carriers is used with the same frequency and amplitude so that they fully occupy the range. A single reference sinusoidal signal with low frequency is been continuously compared with each carrier to determine the switched device.

Three carrier disposition PWM strategies are well known and referenced [2]:

- Phase disposition (PD), carriers are in the same phase Fig. 2a, b.
- Phase opposition disposition (POD), carriers above zero are 180° phase shifted with those below.
- Alternative phase opposition disposition (APOD), where the carriers are alternately 180° phase shifted.

In this paper, different multi-carrier shapes (**Triangular, Trapezoidal**) are used and the performances are analyzed to prove the best techniques.

The results are obtained when using those techniques with different sinusoidal dispositions PD PWM, POD PWM and APOD PWM.

Equation (1) for trapezoidal carrier can be inserted in DSP defined as:

Where A is the amplitude and T is the period of the carrier signal.

(a)

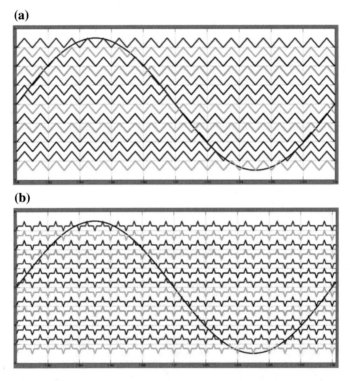

(b)

Fig. 2. a Triangular multi-carriers with phase disposition (PD) arrangement. **b** Trapezoidal multi-carriers with phase disposition (PD) arrangement

$$U(t) = \begin{cases} \frac{t}{t1}\left(\frac{A}{2}\right) & 0 \le t < t1 \\ A/2 & t1 \le t < t2 \\ \left[\frac{t-t2}{t3-t2}\right]\left(\frac{A}{2}\right) + A/2 & t2 \le t < t3 \\ \left[\frac{t4-t}{t4-t3}\right]\left(\frac{A}{2}\right) + A/2 & t3 \le t < t4 \\ A/2 & t4 \le t < t5 \\ \left[\frac{t-t6}{t5-t6}\right]\left(\frac{A}{2}\right) & t5 \le t < t6 \end{cases} \tag{1}$$

3 The Total Harmonic Analyze

The total harmonic distortions (THD) are evaluated through all the modulation techniques and for various frequencies.

To acquire the spectrum of the output voltage (THD) Fast Fourier Transform (FFT) is applied [12]. The THD is calculated using the following Eq. (2):

$$THD = \frac{\sqrt{\sum_{n=2}^{\infty} v_n^2}}{v_1} \tag{2}$$

where:

n   is the harmonic order.

v_n is the root mean square (RMS) value of the nth harmonic component.

v_1 is the (RMS) value of the fundamental component.

The output voltage wave-forms Fig. 3 and the total harmonic distortions Fig. 4a, b are acquired for both types of multi-carriers.

Table 1, resumes all harmonics distortion results for both multi-carrier techniques with different frequencies.

It confirms that the best performance for triangular carriers is when phase disposition with 2 kHz frequency is used and after using the trapezoidal carriers better results are obtained with a gain of 1.28%.

So it is clear that this new modification is best suited for Cascaded Multi-Level with the improvement of the output signal quality which makes it more suitable for both standalone and grid connected systems.

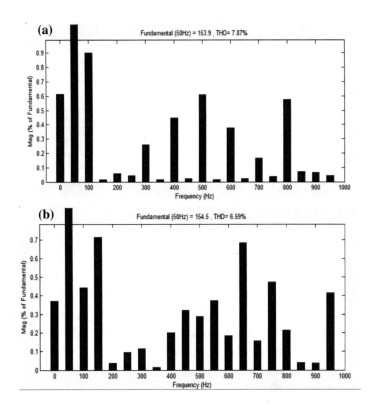

Fig. 3. **a** FFT analysis of the output using triangular carriers. **b** FFT analysis of the output using modified trapezoidal carriers

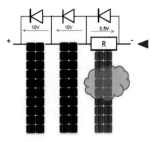

Fig. 4. Effect of shades on photovoltaic panels

4 Smart Multi-level Inverter

4.1 Shades

In most solar photovoltaic (PV) systems it contains about 6–30 panel, to encounter the voltage necessities of the system's inverter, solar arrays are usually alienated into

Table 1. The harmonic distortion analyses

Techniques	Frequencies (kHz)	Dispositions		
		Phase Dispositions (%)	Phase opposite disposition (%)	Alternative phase opposite disposition (%)
Triangular	1	8.27	8.28	9.45
	2	7.87	8.68	8.14
Trapezoid	1	6.71	7.39	7.20
	2	6.59	7.06	6.74

strings of solar panels but those strings are usually consisted form more than one single panel [4].

If shade is on even one of the panels in the string, the output of the entire string will be reduced to nearly zero [13] for as long as the shadow stands there. In some cases, a shadow does not essentially need to descent on a whole panel, even just one cell could crush the output of the panel and turn off the entire string and becomes a receiver that will heat up and lead to a loss of production or even worse Fig. 5.

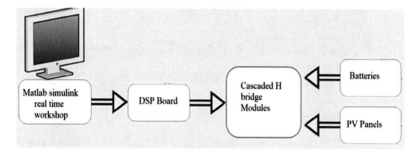

Fig. 5. Smart cascaded system

The smart multilevel inverter Fig. 6 proposed in this paper will have the possibility of increasing levels of the output according to the need of the user mainly according to the number of continuous DC sources available and also according to the power desired. In this way it will allow every solar panel in the system to operate independently and the total energy system will not be excessively affected by any shaded panels and at the same time it can be replaced by a storage battery.

The user will have multiple of h-bridge cards Fig. 7, those cards can be inserted in another card with slots to increase the levels; the number of inserted card must be the same as the continuous sources disposed.

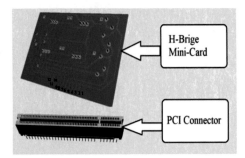

Fig. 6. H-bridge cards

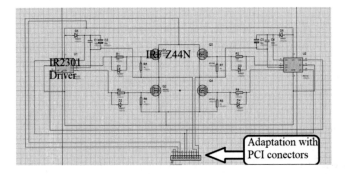

Fig. 7. H bridge with MOSFET drivers

4.2 H-Bridge with Driver

An output pulse (+5 V) of a microcontroller is generally sufficient to drive a MOSFET dedicated to small signal. However, two problems arise when working with more powerful MOSFETs:

- The control signal of the 3.3 V or 5 V microcontrollers is not often enough. It is necessary to apply at least 8–12 V to completely ignite the MOSFET which can cause their destruction [13].
- Without drivers MOSFET switching can cause a feedback to the control circuit, while the drivers are designed to handle this problem.

Since we will convert voltages higher than +30 V we will need drivers (IR2304) in our circuits, it will maximize the switching speed by injecting current so that the MOSFET spends the least possible time in transition time, and so we will have a minimum waste of energy and heat on components.

For simulation purposes, Proteus ISIS was used Fig. 7 to simulate the H-bridge system alongside the MOSFET drivers, with microcontroller programming and all switching devices (Fig. 8).

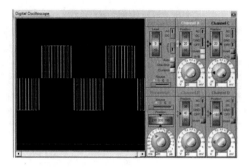

Fig. 8. The output voltage of the H-bridge inverter

5 Experimental Results

As for Experimental results, the output voltage designed for the system is 230 AC supply Fig. 9c. In order to reach it the input supply used is 34 V for each different inverter stages, for all switching devices MOSFETs IRF 44ZN are utilized in order to obtain high efficiency over an extensive load range. The DSP controller or arduino-mega is used to generate the switching pulses for switches based on POD, APOD and PD arrangements for PWM. The carrier signals above and below zero are levels shifted to realize PD, POD and APOD signals. And to generate the pulses required for the MOSFET switches these signals are been compared continuously with the reference sinusoidal signal.

When the inverter starts working, the microcontroller generates a 5 V signal to detect the number of cards inserted. Then, a code of 7 digits received will be equivalent to the number and the location of each card. For example, the reception of 0000001 code means that only one card is inserted and the location of the card is in the first slot.

After the testing, the program to produce the switching pulses will be generated corresponding to the code listed and will keep functioning until the inverter's shutdown.

As for relays Fig. 9b it will let the current flow if there is no h-bridge card inserted.

For every h-bridge card the following equipment's is needed (Table 2).

The experimental prototype is illustrated on Fig. 9a along with the PCB layout for every h-bridge card.

According to this system, Phase disposition multi-carrier modulation techniques are used and the output and the performances are analyzed. Figure 9b shows the suggested smart multi-level inverter system made up to analyze the performances of a cascaded fifteen levels inverter.

This system is devised into four major parts:

Part 1: Pulses Inputs, where Multi-carrier PWM techniques are inserted (The Command part).
Part 2: DC inputs where, Photo-voltaic DC sources or batteries are used (DC inputs).

(a)

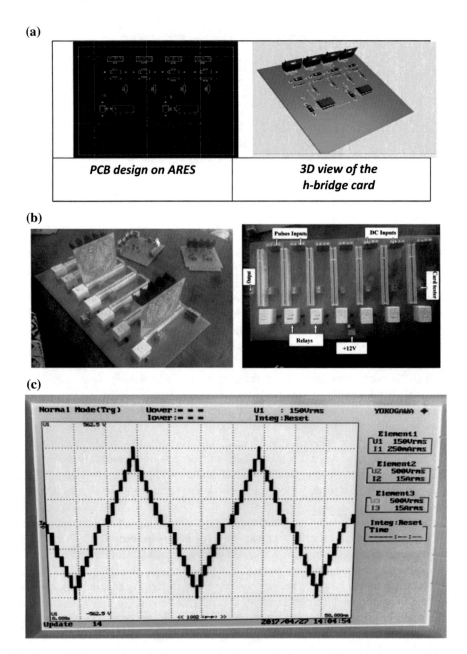

(b)

(c)

Fig. 9. **a** PCB layout for h-bridge cards. **b** Suggested smart multi-level inverter. **c** Voltage output of fifteen multi-level inverter

Table 2. H-bridge materiels

Quantities	Materials
4	10R resistors
4	10R resistors
2	33 uF/16 V capacities
2	IR2304 drivers or IR2301
4	IRF Z44N transistors
6	1N4007 diodes

Part 3: Relays will let the current flow if there is no h-bridge card inserted.
Part 4: The output voltage after DC conversion (AC output).

For experimental application. The PWM scheme was executed in MOSFETs IRFZ44N using an Arduino Mega 2560 and for better comparison, the same configurations are used in the simulation and experimentation. The output voltage waveform is shown in Fig. 9c. It can be seen that the experimental result match with simulation. A comparison between the cascaded topology of a seven and a fifteen multi-level inverter is done and the results are shown in Table 3, Fig. 10 which clearly shows the percentage reduction in the total harmonic distortion by increasing the number of levels "N".

6 Results Interpretation

Table 3, Fig. 11 resumes all harmonics distortion results for the seven and fifteen level inverters.

Table 3. THD values

PWM techniques	Seven level (%THD) (%)	Fifteen level (%THD) (%)
PD	18.00	7.87
POD	18.35	8.62
APOD	18.15	8.14

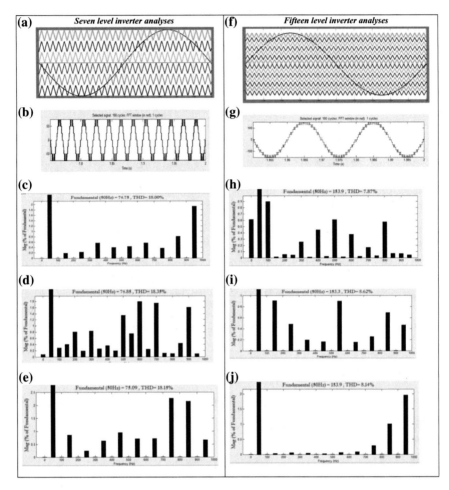

Fig. 10. **a** Multi-carriers PD arrangement for a seven level inverter. **b** Seven multi-level inverter output signal. **c** Seven multi-level inverter THD analysis of PD. **d** Seven multi-level inverter THD analysis of POD. **e** Seven multi-level inverter THD analysis of APOD. **f** Multi-carriers POD arrangement for a fifteen level inverter. **g** Fifteen multi-level inverter output signal. **h** Fifteen multi-level inverter THD analysis of PD. **i** Fifteen multi-level inverter THD analysis of POD. **j** Fifteen multi-level inverter THD analysis of APOD

The comparative THD analysis of seven and fifteen multilevel inverters is achieved using several multicarrier PWM techniques, Phase Disposition (PD), Phase Opposition Disposition (POD) and Alternative Phase Opposition Disposition (APOD) techniques are applied. From the above analysis, it is noticed that increasing the number of level "N" increase greatly the quality of the output signal by reducing the total harmonic distortion, so it clear that increasing levels makes it more suitable for applications where electromagnetic interference (EMI) and low total harmonic distortion (THD) of the output voltage are vital.

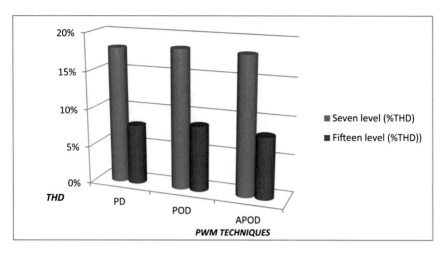

Fig. 11. THD analysis for the line voltages

7 Conclusion

The SPWM control scheme for the fifteen level cascaded H bridge inverter has been presented in this paper The PD PWM method has given the better results for all types of carriers, The results illustrate that after modifying the carriers better results can be obtained.

The smart multilevel inverter suggested will allow every solar panel in the system to operate independently and the total energy system will not be extremely affected by shades or some intermittence".

A comparative study of a seven and fifteen multi-level inverter is done to illustrate the great improvement of the quality signal due to the N level of the multi-inverter.

It is clear that this new scheme is best suited for Cascaded Multi-Level with the improvement of the output signal quality which makes it more suitable for both standalone and grid connected systems.

References

1. Xiao, B., Hang, L., Mei, J., Riley, C.: Modular cascaded H-bridge multilevel PV inverter with distributed MPPT for grid-connected applications. IEEE Trans. Ind. Appl. **51**(2), 1722–1731 (2015)
2. Wang, L., Zhang, D., Wang, Y., Wu, B.: Power and voltage balance control of a novel three-phase solid-state transformer using multilevel cascaded H-bridge inverters for microgrid applications. IEEE Trans. Power Electron. **31**(4), 3289–3301 (2016)
3. Letha, S.S., Thakur, T., Kumar, J.: Harmonic elimination of a photo-voltaic based cascaded H-bridge multilevel inverter using PSO (particle swarm optimization) for induction motor drive. Energy **107**, 335–346 (2016)

4. Dabbaghjamanesh, M., Moeini, A.: High performance control of grid connected cascaded H-bridge active rectifier based on type II-fuzzy logic controller with low frequency modulation technique. Int. J. Electr. Comput. Eng. (Yogyakarta) **6**(2), 484–494 (2016)
5. Sastry, J., Bakas, P., Kim, H., Wang, L.: A marinopoulos—evaluation of cascaded H-bridge inverter for utility-scale photovoltaic systems. Renew. Energy **69**, 208–218 (2014)
6. Selvamuthukumaran, R., Garg, A.: Hybrid multicarrier modulation to reduce leakage current in a transformerless cascaded multilevel inverter for photovoltaic systems. IEEE Trans. Power Electron. **30**(4), 1779–1783 (2015)
7. Gupta, V.K., Mahanty, R.: Optimized switching scheme of cascaded H-bridge multilevel inverter using PSO. Int. J. Electr. Power Energy Syst. **64**, 699–707 (2015)
8. Karasani, R.R., Borghate, V.B.: A three-phase hybrid cascaded modular multilevel inverter for renewable energy environment. IEEE Trans. Power Electron. **32**(2), 1070–1087 (2017)
9. Prabaharan, N., Palanisamy, K.: Analysis and integration of multilevel inverter configuration with boost converters in a photovoltaic system. Energy Convers. Manag. **128**, 327–342 (2016)
10. Yu, Y., Konstantinou, G., Hredzak, B.: Operation of cascaded H-bridge multilevel converters for large-scale photovoltaic power plants under bridge failures. IEEE Trans. Ind. Electron. **62**(11), 228–7236 (2015)
11. Kakosimos, P., Pavlou, K., Kladas, A., Manias, S.: A single-phase nine-level inverter for renewable energy systems employing model predictive control. Energ. Convers. Manag. **89**(1), 427–437 (2015)
12. Coppola, M., Di Napoli, F., Guerriero, P.: An FPGA-based advanced control strategy of a grid-tied PV CHB inverter. IEEE Trans. Power Electron. **31**(1), 806–816 (2016)
13. Krishnan, G.V., Rajkumar, M.V., Hemalatha, C.: Modeling and simulation of 13-level cascaded hybrid multilevel inverter with less number of switches. Int. J. Innov. Stud. Sci. Eng. Technol. (IJISSET) **2**(11), ISSN 2455-4863 (2016)

Approaches and Algorithms for Resource Management in OFDMA Access Mode: Application to Mobile Networks of New Generation

Sara Riahi[✉] and Ali Elhore

Department of Computer Science, Faculty of Sciences, Chouaib Doukkali University, PO Box 20, 24000 El Jadida, Morocco
riahisaraphd@gmail.com

Abstract. The increased need for speed and mobility is the cause of the rapid evolution of mobile radio systems during the last decade. In mobile radio communication systems for broadband (e.g. UMTS, HSDPA, WiMax, LTE, ... etc.), an intense research activity on optimization and radio resource management techniques (RRM Radio Resource Management) is conducted. Management and resource optimization are two themes dealt with separately. This study achieves two goals: achieving an overview of different methods and approaches for allocation of radio resources and focus on the optimization algorithms dedicated to the allocation of resources in the single cell case by deploying one of the most promising access technologies in terms of speed called OFDMA.

Keywords: OFDMA · Radio resources · Adaptive and random allocation · Optimization algorithms · Bandwidth allocation · Assigning subcarriers

1 Introduction

In this paper, we present a detailed study of the different methods and techniques of resource allocation on the downlink OFDMA. This is mainly to spread the subcarriers and the available power between different users in a cell. OFDMA is a promising candidate for broad band access networks post 3G (e.g. IEEE 802.16, WiMax, LTE ...). This technique is characterized by its ability to support large numbers of users with variable characteristics (QoS flow rate). In mobile radio communication systems for broadband, An intense research activity on optimization and radio resource management techniques (RRM Radio Resource Management) is conducted. These scalable communication systems can incorporate multimedia services in addition to traditional voice services and data. Research on these communication technologies aimed at improving the quality of service (QoS: Quality of Service) and therefore minimize the losses in terms of resources [1]. Traditionally, management and resource optimization are two themes treated separately. In fact, different methods radio resource management based optimization algorithm under QoS constraints has been proposed. This makes management and resource allocation issues far from fully resolved and remains a focus of research. The goal of the optimization problem can be to minimize the transmitted

© Springer Nature Switzerland AG 2019
M. Ezziyani (Ed.): AI2SD 2018, AISC 915, pp. 69–84, 2019.
https://doi.org/10.1007/978-3-030-11928-7_6

power, to maximize the total throughput of users, maximize fairness or to minimize the number of users, which do not reach their minimum throughput $\left(r_u^0, r_{u,b}^0 \right)$. In the following sections, we recall the relationship between the power and optimize the radio channel quality [2]. The present paper is organized as follows: In the first section, we present the principle of random allocation methods. In the second section of this paper, we will present a state of the art on the various problems related to optimizing the adaptive allocation of subcarriers and powers available between users in the single cell case. The third section will be reserved for highlighting a key from the adaptive allocation approach that defined the determination of the number of subcarriers required for each user and the assignment of subcarriers to users according to their needs.

2 Methods of Resource Allocation

Two types of allocation are often considered in the literature [3]. The first is the random allocation methods and the second focuses on adaptive allocation methods.

2.1 Random Allocation Methods

In a randomized OFDMA system, each user allocated in a random manner a set of n sub-carriers, which may be different from one user to another. The challenge of this method is that multiple users can choose the same sub-carriers, resulting in transmission of disturbances. Therefore, having a variable number of users generates a number of subcarrier collisions in proportional to the number of user and consequently an unsatisfactory transmission rate [4]. However, this type of system admits its own advantages, such as the non-necessity of a subcarrier allocation protocol for users, since every user knows his subcarriers and the base station (BS) knows the subcarriers of each user [5] (Fig. 1).

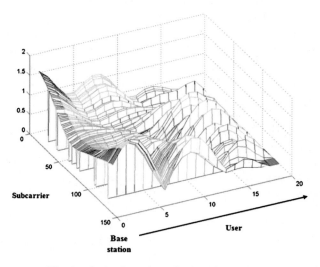

Fig. 1. Optimal number of subcarriers per user

2.2   Adaptive Allocation Methods

In this section we look at the principle problem of adaptive allocation of radio resources. Several studies were performed in a single cell OFDMA context. The word allowance means the arrangement of subcarriers and powers available between users [6]. Often in an optimization problem, constraints are related and can be expressed in terms of minimum flow, each user must ensure, in order to be satisfied. Each user is therefore subject to QoS constraints, in relation to its mobility. We denote QoS, the ability to provide a service according to the requirements of response time and bandwidth [7] (Fig. 2).

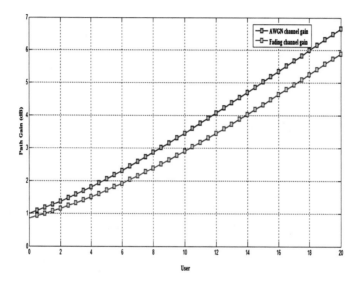

Fig. 2. The gain of gaussian and fading channel for 20 users

The main objectives of the optimization problem can be either [8]:

- Minimizing the transmitted power (Optimization MA).
- Maximization of total users rate (Optimization RA).
- An optimization of the fairness (max-min).
- Minimizing the number of unsatisfied users (Minimization of failure: Outage).

2.3   Optimization Problem with Constraints

The optimization problem with radio resources constraints OFDMA is a problem that seeks to minimize the transmitted power and in this case is treated the optimization case so-called "MA" (Margin Adaptive Optimization) or to maximize the overall throughput of users in a cell and in which case the problem is said to be "RA" (Rate Adaptive Optimization). This type of optimization problem (RA) is the main object of our study. A constraint on the individual rate, ensuring each user is placed in these two types of problem. Another type of problem is also presented in the literature [9]. This is a problem that treats the optimization of fairness among different users. In this case, the problem is called "max-min". Finally, the last type of optimization problem, whose main objective is to minimize the number of unmet user, not having reached its minimum rate. This type of problem is known by the minimization of the failure (Outage).

2.3.1   Optimization in MA (Margin Adaptive)

Objective

In this case of optimization, we try to minimize the total power transmitted P_{tr}, under a minimum flow constraint $r_{u,b}^0$ to be guaranteed for all users [10]. With:

$$P_{tr} = \sum_{b=1}^{B} \sum_{u=1}^{U} P_{u,b}(r_{u,b}), \quad and\ (1 \leq u \leq U),\ (1 \leq b \leq B) \tag{1}$$

Formulation of the problem

The problem is expressed as:

$$\begin{cases} \min_{\underline{r}} P_{tr}(\underline{r}) \\ \underline{r} \geq \underline{r}^0 \\ \underline{r} = (r_{1,1}, \ldots, r_{u,b}, \ldots, r_{U,B}) \\ \underline{r}^0 = (r_{1,1}^0, \ldots, r_{u,b}^0, \ldots, r_U^0) \end{cases} \tag{2}$$

2.3.2   RA Optimization (Rate Adaptive)

Objective

The objective of the RA optimization problem is to maximize the total throughput $r_{u,b}^0$ users with conditions on the transmitted maximum power (fixed power budget) and possibly the minimum rates for each individual user [11].

Formulation of the problem

The problem is therefore expressed as follows:

$$\begin{cases} \max \sum_{b=1}^{B} \sum_{u=1}^{U} r_{u,b} \\ P_{tr}^{(b)} \prec P_{tr}, \max, (1 \leq u \leq U), (1 \leq b \leq B) \\ (\underline{r}) \geq \underline{r}^0 \end{cases} \tag{3}$$

2.3.3   Optimization of Fairness (Max-Min)

Band equity refers to the allocation of an equal amount of frequency resources to different users. This type of optimization does not guarantee users any quality in terms of throughput [12]. The goal of the fairness optimization problem can be, to maximize the minimum bit rate among users or to minimize the number of users who do not reach their minimum throughput $\left(r_u^0 r_{ub}^0\right)$.

Objective

To be able to benefit from a total fairness of rate, we can maximize the lowest rate among the users.

Formulation of the fairness issue

The problem can be formulated as follows:

$$\begin{aligned} \max_A \left(\min_u \left(r_{u,A}\right)\right) \\ P_{tr} \prec P_{tr,Max} \end{aligned} \tag{4}$$

2.3.4   Outage Minimization

Objective

In this optimization problem, we try to minimize the number of users who have not reached their instream rate $r_{u,b}^0$ is designated by the unsatisfied users. In general, these users will not be blocked, but they are given what is called probability of failure (Outage Probability:P_{outage}). This probability is expressed as the ratio between the number of dissatisfied users and the total number of users [13].

Formulation of the outage problem

$$\begin{cases} \min\left(P_{outage}\right), r \prec r_u^0 \\ P_{outage} = \frac{\text{Number of unsatisfied users}}{\text{Total number of users}} \end{cases} \tag{5}$$

3   Approaches Related to Optimization Algorithms

There are two main approaches. Called "Approach A" and "Approach B ", each admits his own principle, despite the existence of similarities between the two [14]. Recall that in our study, the main objective is the allocations of resources in OFDMA, that is, make a distribution of subcarriers and power available between users in a cell. The basic principle of the approach A, lies the fact of considering that the assignment of subcarriers (step 1) and the power allocation (step 2) are two steps which are performed separately [15]. As for the approach B, the basic principle is that the allocation of subcarriers and power allocation are present together (or joint). Most of the algorithms used for solving a RA optimization problem, are type A (approach A). All the algorithms of type B (approach B), solve a problem of type MA (Fig. 3).

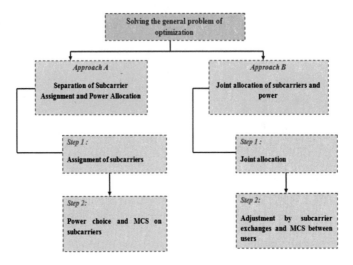

Fig. 3. Structures of resource allocation algorithms

In both approaches (A and B), stage 1 (the band allocation), represents a common point, it is to determine the number of subcarriers required for each user. In addition to its main objective, this first step can also be two options. In the first (option 1), the number of subcarriers per user is unknown, whereas in the second (option 2), the number of subcarriers per user, turns out to be an important parameter and must necessarily be known [16].

3.1 Approach A

3.1.1 Allocation of Subcarriers
It is recalled that this phase involves two stages; namely the allocation of the frequency band and allocating subcarriers to users according to their demand. These two steps can be done in a nested (option 2) or separate way (option 1). Remember also, that the approach in A, the allocation of subcarriers and power allocation are two separate steps [17].

Option 1: Distinct

In option 1, band allocation and subcarrier assignment represent two separate (or separate) steps. That is, knowledge of the number of subcarriers to be assigned to a user is necessary. The determination of the number of subcarriers to be assigned to a user represents the first sub-step of the assignment. The second sub-step will then be the assignment of the sub-carriers.. This approach is often used in cases where a minimum rate $r_{u,b}^0$ to be achieved for each user is needed. The sub-steps 1 and 2 may be described as follows:

The band allocation: Two alternatives are taken into account in the allocation of the band. The first consists in considering an MCS (Modulation and Coding Scheme) and only in this case the relationship between the minimum rate and the number of subcarriers is direct. As for the second alternative, called adaptive modulation, where there are several MCSs [18].

Assignment of subcarriers: The optimal solution is obtained with the Hungarian algorithm, used in many fields because it solves allocation problems with minimizing a cost. The latter deemed slow in its execution time in real time, is based on the principle of a rigid estimation to assess the number of subcarriers per user.

Option 2: Embedded

In the step of allocating subcarriers, Option 2 is to join the band allocation and assignment of subcarriers. This approach is often used in the case where the stress on the individual flow rates can be ignored.

Opportunistic problem: its basic principle is to maximize the total throughput of users without imposing constraints on the individual rates. The user with the best channel gain (CgNR), will be assigned a subcarrier. Given that solves a RA optimization problem; the type A (approach A), the number of subcarriers is unknown a priori [19].

Problem of fairness in rate: the research carried out in this context, are intended to maximize the lowest rate among the users. What defines a problem "max-min".

RA problem with constraint: the basic principle of this is to maximize the total throughput of users with constraints on the maximum power and minimum rates $r^0_{u,b}$ individual for each user.

3.1.2 Power Allocation

This step represents the second task of the approach A. The power allocation is a step for determining the power level of each subcarrier. A uniform distribution of power level is proving to be more popular than the water-filling [20]. Two different problems are to be solved in this approach, either a problem in RA or a problem in MA.

3.2 Approach B

The basic principle of B approach is to allocate the subcarriers and power allocation simultaneously (joint). The two main steps in this approach are:

- Step 1: make a subcarrier allocation and power allocation of the subcarriers (choice of MCS).
- Step 2: often there, it is to reduce the transmitted power.

Approach B may also include two options (Option 1 and 2).

3.2.1   Joint Allocation of Subcarriers and Power

Option 1

The number of subcarriers (N_u) is not known a priori. In Option 1, two approaches were identified, namely:

- Conflict resolution approach.
- Progressive spectrum allocation.

The first approach is based on an algorithm called "bit loading". The base station (BS) built a list of best subcarriers for each user, allowing it to achieve an easy way its minimum rate r_0^u. As the number of bits provided on each of subcarriers, it will be calculated by the same sub-described algorithm. The notion of subcarriers "conflict" means the subcarriers that are not yet affected by the list than the BS built and will be processed by a report CgNR descending medium [21].

Option 2

The number of subcarriers (N_u) is known. This option is used to classify the subcarriers for each user by decreasing CgNR or by increasing power in the case of a fixed MCS.

3.2.2   Improved Transmitted Power

This step consists in calculating the power reduction factor that is noted $p(u_1; u_2)$ for each user pair $(u_1; u_2)$. Indeed inadequacy of the approach B, the resolution of the problem is not obvious if an RA problem without constraints.

3.3   Optimality and Opportunity Approaches

In approach A, the subcarrier assignment phase (step 1) is broken down into two stages: the allocation of the band and allocating subcarriers. These two steps can be performed either in a nested manner (Option 1), or separate (option 2). The notion of "flexible" or "rigid" estimation in Step 1 of Approach A is required accordingly. In the case where the band allocation is separate from the assignment of subcarriers, there is N_u the number of subcarriers necessary for the user u and N the total number of available subcarriers: In the case of solving a problem without RA type constraints on individual rates, global optimality is produced by separating the assignment of subcarriers and power allocation (approach A) [22].

4   Adaptive Allocation Algorithm

The technique of adaptive allocation based on relatively new and intuitive ideas, but has experienced a real growth as an advanced resource management technique. The proposed strategies are sufficiently complete structure to solve an optimization problem with or without constraints [23].

4.1 Resource Allocation Algorithms

It is assumed in a wireless environment, there are users with a SNR (Signal to Noise Ratio) smaller than others. As a result, these users tend to consume more power. Once each user had the necessary subcarriers to meet the required minimum rate, given the remaining subcarriers to users who have the smallest SNR to minimize the transmission power required. In what follows, we describe some algorithms using the SNR of each user to determine the number of sub-carriers allocated to each user.

4.1.1 Algorithm BABS

Known as BABS (Bandwidth Assignment Based on SNR), this algorithm starts to allocate to each user the minimum number of subcarriers he needs. If the total number of requested subcarriers exceeds the total number of subcarriers available N, it eliminates users who have the minimum of the allocated subcarriers.

$$\begin{cases} \sum_{u=1}^{N} N_u \prec N : \textit{Flexible estimation} \\ \sum_{u=1}^{N} N_u = N : \textit{Rigid estimation} \end{cases} \qquad (6)$$

When we arrive at a number of subcarriers lower than N, or if we have not exceeded N, we begin to allocate additional subcarriers to users who, in fact the addition of an additional sub-carrier will have a decrease of the transmitted maximum power

4.1.2 MBABS Algorithm

MBABS is a modified version of the algorithm BABS (modified BABS). The idea of this algorithm is to eliminate the user whose required number of subcarrier is the closest (greater than or equal to) the difference between the number of subcarrier requested by the system and the available number [24]. To assess the optimality of BABS and MBABS A comparative study was conducted. The latter has noted that the rate per subcarrier adjusted by the BABS is less important than the modified adjusted BABS. This is because to eliminate broadband users who consume more subcarriers and probably represent a minority compared to those with a lower rate. These broadband users accordingly release more resources to other users [25].

4.1.3 HBABS Algorithm (Hybrid BABS)

The HBABS algorithm is a contribution that is to provide a new technique for determining the number of subcarriers in the case of an optimization problem in RA. Consequently, a new hybrid strategy is proposed based on the allocation algorithms of the BABS band and MBABS, adapted to the constraints of the problem RA. This algorithm determines the number of subcarriers per user. The constraint on the individual rates is always taken into account [26].

4.1.4 BARE Algorithm (Based on Bandwidth Allocation Rate Estimated)

BARE represents an alternative to the algorithms to determine the number of subcarriers by user in RA. This algorithm makes it possible to increase the number of subcarriers of a user under bit rate constraint. BARE seeks to minimize the difference between the estimated flow rate and the minimum flow rate of each user. For this, the algorithm modifies the bandwidth of $i(u)$, which is assigned to a user u. Where $\underline{i} = (i(u))_u$ is the difference between the estimated rate and the required minimum rate is called gap. The vector represents the number of subcarriers of the users in the BARE algorithm. For u user, the difference between the estimated rate and the desired minimum rate depends on the bandwidth $i(u)$ received [27]:

$$gap(u, i(u)) = r_{est}(u, i(u)) - r_u^0 \tag{7}$$

Indeed, when adjusting the minimum rate, the algorithm finds a feasible BARE minimum rate lower than the BABS and throughput obtained by BARE algorithm is higher than that of the BABS.

4.2 Algorithms for Allocating Subcarriers

Once the number of subcarriers per user is determined, the allocated subcarriers should be specified, taking into account the channel status. Various algorithms have been proposed; namely Rate Craving Greedy (RCG) and Amplitude Craving Greedy (ACG), RPO (Rate Profit Optimization) [28] (Fig. 4).

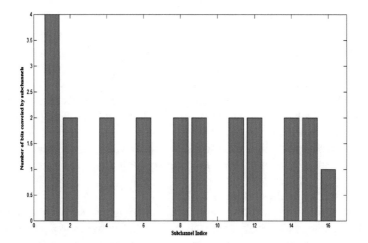

Fig. 4. Number of bits transmitted by the subchannels

4.2.1 Rate Craving Greedy (RCG)

The proposed algorithm aims to maximize throughput in the case of an optimization problem of the RA types. The steps of the algorithm are as follows [26]:

- Initializing a distribution A_k of sub-carriers for the different users. We give e.g. subcarriers to users who have the greatest gain.
- For all users k such that the number of subcarriers in the distribution exceeds the number of subcarriers allocated ($\#A_k \succ m_k$), removing a subcarrier and it is given to the user who has the highest rate among the all the users who have not yet allocated all their subcarriers (Fig. 5).

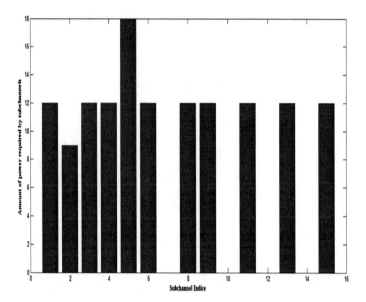

Fig. 5. Amount of power required by the sub-channels in dB

4.2.2 Amplitude Craving Greedy (ACG)

The ACG algorithm. It is an opportunistic algorithm whose number of subcarriers of each user is limited to N_u. At each stage a subcarrier is fixed, the algorithm allocates subcarrier n to the user who has the best channel gain ($CgNR$) and has not yet reached its number of subcarriers N_u. The algorithm stops when no more of subcarriers to be allocated. The main limitation of this algorithm is the processing order of subcarriers [29] (Fig. 6).

4.2.3 Rate Profit Optimization (RPO)

The best subcarrier of users is determined. In the absence of conflict, the subcarriers are allocated. Otherwise, the sub-carrier is assigned to the one with the best profit there. A user who has received N_u subcarriers is no longer competing for a subcarrier. The algorithm ends when all subcarriers are assigned. The RPO goal is to avoid blindly allocating a subcarrier at its best user [27]. When multiple users have a better common subcarrier, the second best of each subcarrier is estimated [29] (Fig. 7).

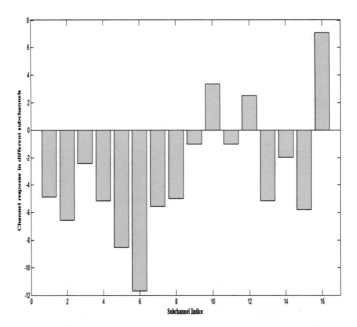

Fig. 6. Channel response in different subchannels

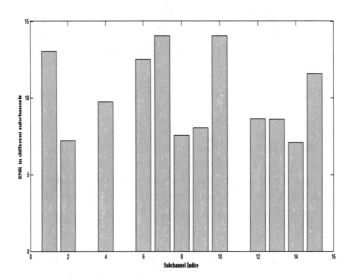

Fig. 7. SNR of different subchannels

5   Simulation and Analysis of Results

There is provided an adaptive resource allocation algorithm that minimizes the total power while maintaining a minimum flow rate per user. This minimization is performed with the proviso that the power transmitted for each user does not exceed a certain predetermined maximum value. As the conditions on the rate and power are per user, then this algorithm can be used for the uplink and downlink: For the UpLink, there is a constraint on the power transmitted for each user. In this work, we present an algorithm that takes into account the requirements of throughput and individual power users.

The base station controller allocates each user to a set of subcarriers corresponding to the flow rate and the power requested. Information for this controller will be the SNR which will be valid after the channel estimation in the base station. It is assumed that the duration of the impulse response does not exceed the length of the guard interval; the channel is of course broken down into several sub-channels which are independent and mutually orthogonal. On the channel, there was an addition of Gaussian noise. Once each user had the necessary subcarriers to meet the required minimum rate, given the remaining subcarriers to users who have the smallest SNR to minimize the transmission power required. Our method uses the SNR of each user to determine the number of subcarriers allocated to each user. This method starts by allocating to each user the minimum number of subcarriers he needs. If the total number of requested subcarriers exceeds the total number of available sub-carriers, we will remove users who have the minimum of allocated subcarriers, SNR smaller than the other (Fig. 8).

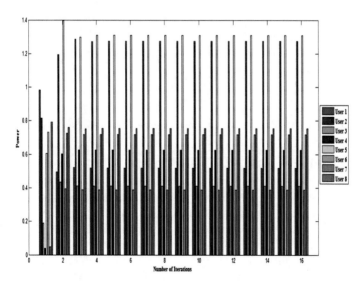

Fig. 8. Evolution of the power versus Number of iterations, fairness optimization

When we arrive at a number of subcarriers less than the number of available subcarriers, or if it is not already exceeded, the additional subcarriers are started to be allocated to the users who, in the case of adding an additional subcarrier, have a maximum transmitted power decrease. After determining the number of subcarriers that each user is allocated, it should be clear the allocated subcarriers, taking into account the channel state. We begin to allocate subcarriers to users who have the greatest gain of the channel for these subcarriers (Fig. 9). Each user allocates these subcarriers and once they are allocated, it will not be able to allocate more. It initializes a distribution of subcarriers to different users, it gives the subcarriers to users who have the greatest gain. For users such as the number of subcarriers in the distribution exceeds the number of allocated subcarriers. Removing a subcarrier and it is given to the user who has the highest rate among all users who have not allocated all their subcarriers.

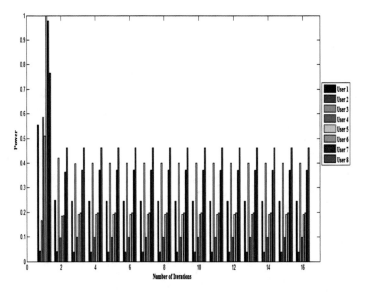

Fig. 9. Evolution of the power versus number of iterations, SINR optimization

6   Conclusion

This paper is a study of the different methods and techniques of management and allocation of resources in the single cell case in OFDMA mode. Two famous optimization problems often treated in the literature were presented; namely the problem in MA and RA. The first is to minimize the total transmitted power, while the second tends to maximize the total throughput of users in the cell with constraint on the power budget. We focused our study to the optimization problem. It was possible to highlight a key from the adaptive allocation approach that defined the determination of the number of subcarriers required for each user and the assignment of subcarriers according to users their need. The following criteria which have been made are allocating power, flow rates and the fact that a subcarrier can be allocated only by a single user. It has been possible to have allocation algorithms which give as output the subcarriers allocated by each user, so as to satisfy the conditions on the flow rates and the power.

Acknowledgements. We would like to thank the CNRST of Morocco (I012/004) for support.

References

1. Zappone, A., Sanguinetti,L., Bacci, G., Jorswieck, E., Debbah, M.: A framework for energy-efficient design of 5G technologies (2015)
2. Chang, T.-S., Feng, K.-T., Lin, J.-S., Wang, L.-C.: Green resource allocation schemes for relay-enhanced MIMO-OFDM networks. IEEE Trans. Vehicular Technol. **62** (2013)
3. Naghibi, F.: Uplink Resource Scheduling in Dynamic OFDMA Systems. Communication Systems, Sweden (2008)
4. Chen, M., Huang, J.: Optimal resource allocation for OFDM uplink communication: a primal-dual approach. In: Conference on Information Sciences and Systems (CISS) (2008)
5. Yin, H., Liu, H.: An efficient multiuser loading algorithm for OFDM-based broadband wireless systems. In: Proceedings of IEEE Globecom, Nov 2000
6. Yaqot, A., Hoeher, P.A.: efficient resource allocation in cognitive networks. In: Vehicular Technology. IEEE (2017)
7. Ahmadi, H., Chew, Y.H., Chai, C.C.: Multicell multiuser OFDMA dynamic resource allocation using ant colony optimization. Institute for Infocomm Research, Agency for Science (2011)
8. Nogueira, M.C., et al.: QoS aware schedulers for multi-users on OFDMA downlink: optimal and heuristic. In: 8th IEEE Latin-American Conference on Communications (LATINCOM), Medellin (2016)
9. Narmanlioglu, O., Zeydan, E.: Performance evaluation of schedulers in MIMO-OFDMA based cellular networks. In: 2017 25th Signal Processing and Communications Applications Conference (SIU), Antalya (2017)
10. Tseng, S.-C., Huang, C.-W., Lu, T.-L., Chiang, C.-T., Wei, W.-H.: A field-tested QoS scheduler for diverse traffic flows over mobile networks. In: Wireless and Optical Communication Conference (2015)
11. Sonia, Khanna, R., Kumar, N.: Load balancing efficiency improvement using hybrid scheduling algorithm in LTE systems. Wireless Personal Commun. (2017)
12. Da, B., Ko, C.C.: A new scheme with controllable capacity and fairness for OFDMA downlink resource allocation. In: IEEE (2007)
13. Yang, L., Yang, H.C.: GSECps: a diversity technique with improved performance-complexity tradeoff. In: IEEE Global Telecommunications Conference, vol. 6 (2005)
14. Zelikman, D., Segal, M.: Reducing interference in vanets. IEEE Trans. Intell. Transport. Syst. **16**(3) (2015)
15. Bianzino, A., Chaudet, C., Rossi, D., Rougier, J.: A survey of green networking research. IEEE Commun. Surveys Tuts. **14**(1) (2012)
16. Li, L., Goldsmith, A.: Capacity and optimal resource allocation for fading broadcast channels—part I: ergodic capacity. IEEE Trans. Inform. Theory **47**, 1083–1102 (2001)
17. Gueguen, C., Baey, S.: Opportunistic access schemes for multiuser OFDM wireless networks. Radio Commun. (2010)
18. Park, D.C., Yun, S.S., Kim, S.C., Shin, W., Kim, H., Lim, K.: Distributed data scheduling for OFDMA based wireless mesh networks (2011)

19. IEEE 802.16m 2011 Part 16.: Air interface for broadband wireless access systems, advanced air interface. IEEE 802.16m, May 2011
20. Eslami, M., Krzymien, W.: Efficient transmission schemes for multiuser MIMO downlink with linear receivers and partial channel state information. EURASIP J. Wirel. Commun. Netw. **2010**, 572675 (2010)
21. Nagaraj, S., Khan, S., Schlegel, C.: On preamble detection in packet-based wireless networks. In: IEEE Ninth International Symposium on Spread Spectrum Techniques and Applications (2006)
22. Caire, G., Jindal, N., Kobayashi, M., Ravindran, N.: Multiuser MIMO achievable rates with downlink training and channel state feedback. IEEE Trans. Inform. Theory **56**(6), 2845–2866 (2010)
23. Ayoub, H., Assaad, M.: Scheduling in OFDMA systems with outdated channel knowledge. In: 2010 IEEE International Conference on Communications, Cape Town, South Africa (2010)
24. Zhang, X., Wang, W.: Multiuser frequency-time domain radio resource allocation in downlink OFDM systems: capacity analysis and scheduling methods. Comput. Elect. Eng. **32**, 118–134 (2006)
25. Kaewmongkol, K., Jansang, A., Phonphoem, A.: Delay-aware with resource block management scheduling algorithm in LTE. In: Computer Science and Engineering Conference (2015)
26. Pietrzyk, S., Janssen, G.J.M.: Multiuser subcarrier allocation for QoS provision in the OFDMA systems. In: Proceedings of VTC 2002, vol. 2 (2002)
27. Bhooma, G., Kokila, S., Jayanthi, K., Jagadeesh Kumar, V.: A digital instrument for venous muscle pump test. In: Proceedings of IEEE International Instrumentation and Measurement Technology Conference, China, May 2011
28. Zhou, S., Zhang, K., Niu, Z., Yang, Y.: Queuing analysis on MiMO systems with adaptive modulation and coding. In: IEEE International Conference on Communications (2008)
29. Kim, K., Han, Y., Kim, S.-L.: Joint subcarrier and power allocation in uplink OFDMA systems. IEEE Commun. **9**(6) (2005)

A New Efficient Technique to Enhance Quality of Service in OLSR Protocol

Moulay Hicham Hanin[1]([✉]), Youssef Fakhri[1], and Mohamed Amnai[2,3]

[1] Department of Computer Sciences, Faculty of Science,
Laboratory in Computer Science and Telecommunications
(LARIT), Kenitra, Morocco
haninone@gmail.com,
fakhri-youssef@univ-ibntofail.ac.ma
[2] Engineering Laboratory and Process Optimization of Industrial Systems
(LIPOSI), National School of Applied Sciences, Khouribga, Morocco
mohamed.amnai@uhp.ac.ma
[3] Team Networks and Telecommunications Faculty of Science,
Research Laboratory in Computer Science and Telecommunications
(LARIT), Kenitra, Morocco

Abstract. A routing protocol, in Mobile ad hoc networks (MANETs) use global information about the network topology and communication links to handle the data exchange between communication nodes. Several architectures and protocols have been defined to optimize transmission data between nodes. OLSR (Optimized Link State Routing) was proposed owing to Multipoint Relays (MPRs) that reduce the number of redundant retransmissions while diffusing a broadcast message in the network. In this paper we propose a new efficient mechanism, named F-QMPR-OLSR to select MPRs in OLSR protocol, which use two methods. The first use fuzzy systems based three quality of service (QoS) metrics as inputs: Buffer Availability, Stability and SINR (Signal to Interference plus Noise Ratio) and return as output the high efficient selection of MPRs. The second is to adjust the value of a node's willingness parameter to best perform and improve network lifetime, and therefore it can improve the network transmission capacity. Implementation and simulation experiments with Network Simulator NS2 are presented in order to validate our contribution. The results show that F-QMPR-OLSR achieves a significant improvement of data packets exchange quality in term of QoS.

Keywords: MANET · OLSR · QOLSR · QMPR · Fuzzy logic · SINR stability · Buffer

1 Introduction

A mobile ad hoc network (MANET) [1] is formed of wireless equipment and mobile who self-organize without the help of any infrastructure. So, this type of network is particularly useful in military, search, rescue and other tactical situations. Each node in MANET must forward traffic and hence act as a route [2]. So, keep up routing information and forwarding packets by nodes are a challenging task [3].

© Springer Nature Switzerland AG 2019
M. Ezziyyani (Ed.): AI2SD 2018, AISC 915, pp. 85–97, 2019.
https://doi.org/10.1007/978-3-030-11928-7_7

Topology-based routing techniques use global information about the network topology and communication links to handle the data exchange between communicating nodes. In fact, link states and routing tables are exchanged between neighbors to discover and maintain routes between a source and destination. There are vast of methods suggested so outlying for routing in MANET [1, 4–8]. In many of the proposals, and other related to MANET routing protocols are classified as reactive, proactive and hybrid [9]. In the reactive protocol the path is locate and used accordingly as and when there is a need for packet transmission. Hence, the name on-demand routing protocol is also give to this class. Proactive protocol on the other hand maintains a routing table and hence called table-driven protocol because of existence of routing table. The hybrid protocol is combination of proactive and reactive protocol.

Flooding is a key networking operation in ad hoc multiservice, used for the dissemination of data packets and able to operate in a dynamic network, even in the absence of (or not relying on) precise information about the network topology. In OLSR [10] proactive protocols, flooding is for acquiring or disseminating topological information. In its most basic form, flooding consists of requiring every router in the network to retransmit each received packet exactly once over all of its interfaces. OLSR [4] is based on the periodic flooding of control information using special nodes acting as Multipoint Relays (MPRs) to maintain fresh routes to destinations.

The data packets transmission in demands low data loss, low delay and high network lifetime. Consequently, for good transmission quality, it is essential to taking into a account multiple quality of service (Qos).

To this end, we propose, in this article an extension of MPR selection algorithm, named F-QMPR-OLSR (fuzzy based quality of service OLSR). Like original MPR selection algorithm of OLSR, F-QMPR-OLSR use fuzzy based quality of service. Rather than using enough propitious quality metrics in MPR selection algorithm, F-QMPR-OLSR uses a new routing metric based on multiple quality metrics to find the high quality of MPR selection in terms of QoS (QMPR) [5]. Finally, F-QMPR-OLSR propose a modification of willingness parameter to improve network lifetime.

The remaining of this paper is structured as follows: Sect. 2 presents a Survey related work. In Sect. 3 we discuss the improvements made to MPR selection. Describes approach with evaluation and simulation results, a conclusion is drawn up in Sect. 4.

2   Related Work

Several researchers have investigated and analysed OLSR protocols for diferent aims and objectives. Nguyen et al. proposed in [6] analytical results on MPR selection based on a specific metric for a QoS purpose such as bandwidth, delay and other. We have demonstrated that the average number of neighbours selected as QoS MPRs is in $O(n^{1/3} \log n)$, with n the average number of neighbors per node. The performance evaluation shows that the number of QoS MPRs is greater than the number of MPRs by a factor of $\log(n)$.

Yi et al. [7] proposed periodic exchange of messages to maintain topology information of the networks. In at the same time, it updates the routing table in an on-demand schedule and routing the packets in multiple paths which have been decided at the source. If a link detect is weakness, the algorithm recovers the route automatically. The author improve the performance of the networks based on tow method fist, is to allows different multipath approaches on the Dijkstra algorithm. Second is the multiple routes are exploited via an original multiple description coding based on a discrete Radon transform.

Koga et al. [8] proposed selection schemes for highly efficient MPRs based on to bang a equilibrium between the two conflicting objectives. The aim is to determine a reduce set of MPRs that provide better QoS paths between any two nodes so as to maximize the QoS effect per unit maintenance cost. However, reduced set of MPRs is not always available mostly in the case of a dense network.

Dashbyamba et al. [11] propose two metrics node mobility and signal strength condition using in fuzzy logic algorithm which are not considered in OLSR for MPR selection. So, OLSR protocol cannot perfect in a highly mobile network. The authors provide a protocol that improves OLSR by considering signal strength and node mobility in the selection of MPRs. However, to better select a high quality of MPR we need more metrics which influences on the QoS of OLSR. Before presenting our improvements made to MPR selection, we interpret the basic functionality of MPR selection in the next section.

In [12], authors proposed an extension of MP-OLSR named FQ-MP-OLSR which uses fuzzy systems to find the best paths in order to improve the video streaming quality. The authors use the multipath dijikstra's algorithm to obtain the inter-twisted multiple paths that may share one more links, despite that increased significantly the routing cost when speed is higher. For this resent in our contribution we propose to adjust the value of willingness parameter node's to best perform as shown in Sect. 4.

The author in [13] proposed a new Dynamic MANET Organization Protocol (DYMO) to enhance the performance of MANET, used Fuzzy concept by taking network size and mobility as inputs metrics. DYMO uses four types of packets. A key limitation of this research is that not take into account the parameter requirement covered every routing protocol for ad hoc networks.

3 Optimized Link State Routing (OLSR) Protocol

OLSR is a proactive protocol for mobile ad hoc networks, It is an optimization over the classical link state protocol and works in a completely distributed manner and independently from other protocols. The protocol is periodically exchanging control messages to maintain topology information about network. The new thing of OLSR it is to minimize the size of control messages flooded during the route update process by employing multipoint relaying strategy. Each node in the network selects a set of 1-hop neighbour nodes as MPRs. A node which is not in MPR set can read and process control packets but does not retransmit them. All MPRs together provide connections that cover all its up-to 2-hop neighbour nodes (Fig. 1). When a 1-hop neighbour connects to any of 2-hop neighbors, it is called that the 1-hop neighbours is covering those 2-hop neighbours. For selecting the MPRs, each node periodically broadcasts a list of its 1-hop neighbour addresses using HELLO messages. The procedure of MPR selection in OLSR is described in the Algorithm 1.

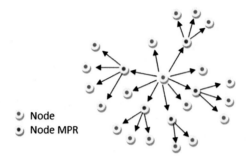

Fig. 1. A node selected as MPR (red color nodes) to flooding packets

---

Algorithm 1: MPR Selection Algorithm:

MPR(s) ← Empty
N(s) ← one-hop neighbors from node 's'
N2(s) ← two-hop neighbors reachable by N (s) nodes for each node x in N(s) do
if W(x) = WILL_ALWAYS then
Add node x to MPR(s)
Remove nodes in N2(s) that are covered by these N(s) nodes
end if
end for
for each node y in N2(s) do
if there is only one node x in N(s) with D (x, y) is defined then
Add node x to MPR(s)
Remove nodes in N2(s) that are covered by x
end if
end for
while N2(s) is not empty, do
Select node x in N(s) with non-zero reachability based on the following priority order then
Add node x to MPR(s):
(a) highest W(x)
(b) highest R(x, M)
(c) highest D(x)
end while For optimization, node M in the selected MPR(s) set can be removed only if the other nodes in the MPR(s) set still cover all nodes in N2(s).

---

4   The Improvements Made to MPR Selection

In the MPR selection phase there are several attributes nodes, which need to be considering developing QoS in OLSR. Therewith, if the probability is increase compromise various quality metrics is obtain, then to select node is more appropriate.

4.1   Fuzzy Logic and Fuzzy Set Theory

Fuzzy logic theory [14] is articulate on fuzzy set theory [15], which is proposed by Lotfi Zadeh to resolve problems that are difficult for classical set theory and logic.

Fuzzy logic theory has been commonly employed for retaining wall intelligent systems. Fuzzy set theory, permit an element x in universal set X to biased way belong to a fuzzy set A. Then, a fuzzy set can be described by a membership function U_A defined as follows: $U_A: X \rightarrow [0, 1]$ For all $x \in X$, The membership value $U_A(x)$ is the degree of truth of x in fuzzy set A, it indicates the certainty (or uncertainty) that x belongs to fuzzy set A. The fuzzy set A is completely determined by the set of tuple

$$A = \{(x, \mu A(x)) | x \in X, \ U_A(x) \in [0, 1]\}.$$

4.2 Fuzzy Logic and Fuzzy Set Theory

Our proposal Fuzzy Logic is shown in Fig. 2, it receives as input metrics SINR, Buffer Availability and Stability of a node, and returns as output the numeric value which allow sorting out the best of QMPR. The principle components of the proposed FLC are described as follows:

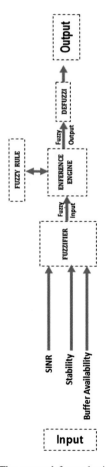

Fig. 2. The general fuzzy logic system

Fuzzifier It act based on the input membership functions, the fuzzifier transform a numerical input variable crisp into fuzzy input sets needed for the Inference Engine. Triangular and rectangular membership functions (MFs) are used here as reference because they have a lower processing metrics compared to other MFs. Figures 3, 4 and 5, show respectively, the normalized link SINR MFs, Buffer Availability MFs and Stability MFs of the proposed FLC. They have three linguistic variables Low (L), Medium (M) and High (H) (Fig. 6).

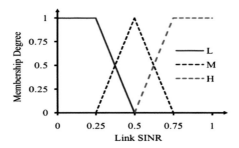

Fig. 3. Membership function for SINR

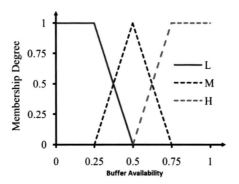

Fig. 4. Membership function for buffer availability

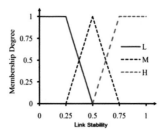

Fig. 5. Membership function for Stability

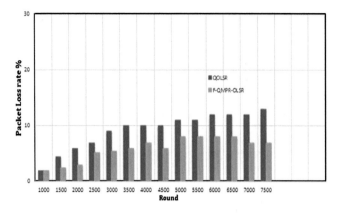

Fig. 6. Packet Loss rate varying network time

Fuzzy Rule or rule base, it contains a collection of fuzzy conditional statements (IF-THE) rules. The rule base represents the knowledge and experience of a human expert of the system. In our proposed FLC and based on the fuzzy values of SINR, Buffer Availability and Stability, node uses the IF-THEN rules to select node is more appropriate.

Below, some examples of rules are proposed shown as:

- If the SINR is high, stability is high andbuffer Availability is high then the probability of the node to be selected as MPR will high.
- If the SINR is high, stability is low and buffer Availability is medium then the probability of the node to be selected as MPR will medium.
- If the SINR is low, stability is high and buffer Availability is low then the probability of the node to be selected as MPR will low.

Defuzzifier It important process to return a numeric (crisp) value based on an already defined in output MFs. Figure 2 shows the defined output MFs for link cost. It has three linguistic variables Low (L), Medium (M) and High (H). Defuzzifier aggregates the fuzzy set into a value. In this stage we have chose Mamdani's defuzzification methods based on Center of Gravity (COG) [16]. It is used in this stage to defuzzify the fuzzy outputs sets received from Inference Engine component. The center of gravity is calculated as follows:

$$COG = \frac{\int_a^b u(x)x\,dx}{\int_a^b u(x)\,dx}$$

where μ(x) is degree of membership of element x, [a, b] is the interval of the result aggregated MF, and COG is the returned numeric value from Defuzzifier. In the implementation and experimental design, COG presents QMPR selection returned by the function FuzzyLQMPR integrate in Algorithm 2.

Algorithm 2

MPR(s) ← Empty
N(s) ← one-hop neighbors from node 's'
N2(s) ← two-hop neighbors reachable by N (s) nodes
for each node x in N(s) do
Qf= FuzzyLQMPR [SINR, ,Sn,Bn]
end for
for each node x in N(s) do
starting with greater Qf
if W(x) = WILL_ALWAYS then
    Add node x to MPR(s)
    Remove nodes in N2(s) that are covered by these N(s) nodes
end if
end for
for each node y in N2(s) do
if there is only one node x in N(s) with D (x, y) is defined then
    Add node x to MPR(s)
    Remove nodes in N2(s) that are covered by x
end if
end for
while N2(s) is not empty, do
  Select node x in N(s) with non-zero reachability based on the following priority order
then
Add node x to MPR(s):
  (a) highest W(x)
  (b) highest R(x, M)
  (c) highest D(x)
end while
For optimization, node M in the selected MPR(s) set can be removed only if the other
nodes in the MPR(s) set still cover all nodes in N2(s)

4.3   Interference Plus Noise Ratio (SINR)

The signal-to-interference-plus-noise ratio (SINR) greatest important on the impact of quantify when an amplitude constraint is placed on the radar waveform. Typically, radar waveform design techniques are based on maximizing the SINR [17] while gratifying some practical constraint(s) quantified by a suitable measure.

4.4   Buffer Availability

In this paper, we construct a multiple-metric transmission model taking into consideration the packet resequencing buffer and propose to select QMPR based on the availability of the buffer. We then mathematically analyse the model as shawn in [18].

4.5   Stability

In Ad hoc network, stability of node is amid the many factors that sensitive and important. There are no absolutely stable nodes, for this reason in this paper the concept of stability is presented by a statistic collected from the neighboring nodes that provide connection durability based on Bienaymé-Chebychev inequality. So to calculate stability is to compute the values of the received signal power from a neighboring node. In a particular case we will use variance of the signal power to estimate stability, if values are equal to zero that mean the node is strictly stable with his neighboring, the function provide the values of stability between tow nods N_1 and N_2 is calculate given in the Eq. 1 as shown in [19].

$$SNDN_1N2 = \left(\sum_i \frac{Value\_signal_{Bi}^2}{K} \right) - \left(\sum_i \frac{Value_{signalBi}}{K} \right) \qquad (1)$$

where, K is a number of observations, and $Value\_signal_{Bi}$ the values of signal power received form a neighboring node in different intervals of time.

To calculate the quality node, the algorithm use trade-off between of all the quality factors like SINR, Stability and Buffer availability. So we can implemented membership function using rules in FIS as shown in Eq. 2 that present the process of Fuzzification and Defuzzification based on Mamdani method.

$$QMPR = FuzzyLQMPR\ [SINR, Sn, Bn] \qquad (2)$$

4.6   Improvement Network Lifetime by Modification to OLSR

Our contribution on this work is at high efficient MPR selection level. As a function of OLSR standard each node has a parameter called willingness, signalize its availability to forwarding traffic through other nodes, the value of a node's willingness parameter is an integer between 0 and 7 as following:

- If 'willingness' equal to 0 must never be selected as MPR by any node.
- If 'willingness' equal to 7 must always be selected as MPR.

But in OLSR standard all willingness set to a default value equal to 3, and it is still constant along the simulation. as well, to achieve the function of algorithm 2 we have proposed to change willingness variable concept to add more metric and constraint to ensure forwarding data packets. Thus, the available residual energy of the node be taken the time of HELLO packet generated, using Eq. 3

$$willingness = round\left(\frac{E_i}{Emax} * 7 \right) \qquad (3)$$

With
E_i is the residual energy at any time
Emax   is the initial energy of the node

To this end, to select or reject a node for the transmission of packets it becomes more pertinent. The protocol does not present reliable transmission of control message. F-QMPR-OLSR is an enhancement of the OLSR routing protocol that supports multiple-metric routing criteria. However, these latest metrics dose not contains the SINR, stability and buffer availability. The aim of our contribution is consist to use these last three metrics to predict the nodes that possess the best qualities for their selection as QMPR.

4.7   Evaluation Criteria

The aim of the experiments by NS2 is to approve our proposed enhancement, by analyzing the impact of the F-QMPR-OLSR on the quality of packets transmission. Finally, we describe four QoS metrics:

- Average Energy Consumption [16]: is a measure of network energy consumption in the network given by Eq. 4.

$$E = \frac{\text{Cumulative Energy Consumption of nodes}}{\text{Total number of nodes in the network}} \tag{4}$$

- Average End-to-End Delay: Is the average difference between the time a data packet is sent by the source node and the time it is successfully received by the destination node [16].
- Packet Deliver Percentage (PDP): is computed as the percentage of the data packets delivered to the destination to those generated by the CBR souce [20].
- Routing Overheads: is the percentage between the number of dropped data packets and those sent by the sources [20].

4.8   Simulation Results and Discussion

Table 1 shows the simulation results based on four performance metrics: Averge Energ Consumption, Average End-to-End Dela, Packet Deliver Percentage (PDP) and Routing Overheads. We show that the four metrics has been improved by the protocol F-QMPR-OLSR compared to the QOLSR. We propose a mobile scenario witch nodes move in the area based on a Random Waypoint Mobility model with a speed of 20 m/s.

Table 1. Simulation parameters

Simulation time	400 s
Ad hoc network area	1000 m × 1000 m
Number of nodes	49, 69, 89, 109, 129, 149, 169
Traffic type	Constant bit rat
Mobility algorithm	Random way point
Routing protocol	OLSR
Performance parameter	SINR, stability, energy
Initial node energy	0.4 J
Network protocol	IPv4

In a particular case we will use variance of the signal power to estimate stability, if values are equal to zero that mean the node is strictly stable with his neighboring, the function provide the values of stability between tow nods

- Packet delivery percentage

Figure 7 illustrate the packet loss ratio of the data traffic in varying network time, and we observe that our modified OLSR outperform the others in the packet delivery. Thus, F-QMPR-OLSR has improve delivery percentage up to 5, 20, 30% compared to the QOLSR protocol.

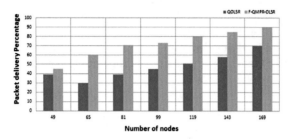

Fig. 7. Packet delivery ratio versus the number of nodes

- Packet loss rate

We present the results in Fig. 6. It's obvious fact that our modified scheme gets the less packet loss rate. Thus, F-QMPR-OLSR has reduced packet loss rate up to 10% compared to the QOLSR protocol.

The analysis of the results prove that to check compromise of SINR, stability and buffer availability using Fuzzy Logic during the phase of MPR selection is more important to avoid loss of packet.

- Energy consumption

Figure 8 illustrates and evaluated the energy consumption, and show that F-QMPR-OLSR reduce more consumption energy in different intervals of time regardless of the number of nodes.

Thus, F-QMPR-OLSR allows us to the extended lifetime network.

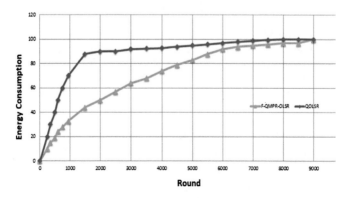

Fig. 8. Energy consumption for versus network time

5   Conclusion

In this paper, F-QMPR-OLSR protocol has been proposed as an improvement over the MPR selection in OLSR protocol. The proposed protocol use fuzzy logic and life time improvement to enhance the QoS in OLSR protocol based on independent metrics.

The aim is enhance the QoS based in new design mechanism to predict the quality nodes for the OLSR protocol, in a MANET environment, based on fuzzy logic. Simulation experiments with network simulator NS2 show that FQOLS Achieves a significant improvement of quality of packet transmission in term of QoS parameters.

As part of future work, the behavior of our proposed could be combination under other technique as cognitive radio Ad hoc routing and other performance metrics.

References

1. Royer, E.M., Toh, C.K.: A review of current routing protocols for ad hoc mobile wireless networks. IEEE Personal Commun. Mag. **1999**, 46–55 (1999)
2. Ephremides, A., Wieselthier, J.E., Baker, D.J.: A design concept for reliable mobile radio networks with frequency hopping signaling. Proc. IEEE **75**(1987), 56–73 (1987)
3. Chiang, C.-C., et al.: Routing in clustered multihop, mobile wireless networks with fading channel. In: Proceedings of IEEE SICON'97, pp. 197–211 (1997)
4. Jacquet, P., Muhlethaler, P., Clausen, T., Laouiti, A., Qayyum, A., Viennot, L.: Optimized link state routing protocol for ad hoc networks. In: Proceedings of IEEE International Multitopic Conference, pp. 62–68 (2001)
5. Mueller, S., Tsang, R.P., Ghosal, D.: Multipath Routing in Mobile Ad Hoc Networks: Issues and Challenges. Performance Tools and Applications to Networked Systems, pp. 209–234. Springer, Berlin (2004)
6. Nguyen, D.Q., Minet, P.: Analysis of MPR selection in the OLSR protocol. In: Proceedings of the 21st International Conference on Advanced Information Networking and Applications Workshops, pp. 887–892 (2007)
7. Yi, J., Cizeron, E., Hamma, S., Parrein, B.: Simulation and performance analysis of MP-OLSR for mobile ad hoc networks. In: Wireless Communications and Networking Conference, pp. 2235–2240 (2008)
8. Koga, T., Tagashira, S., Kitasuka, T., Nakanishi, T., Fukuda, A.: Highly efficient multipoint relay selections in link state qos routing protocol for multi-hop wireless networks. In: IEEE International Symposium on a World of Wireless, Mobile and Multimedia Networks & Workshops (WoWMoM 2009). IEEE (2009)
9. Abusalah, L., Khokhar, A., Guizani, M.: A survey of secure mobile ad hoc routing protocols. IEEE Commun. Surv. Tutorials **10**(4), 78–93 (2008)
10. Jacquet, P., Muhlethaler, P., Clausen, T., Laouiti, A., Qayyum, A., Viennot, L.: Optimized link state routing protocol for ad hoc networks. In: IEEE INMIC, pp. 62–68, Dec 2001
11. Dashbyamba, N., et al.: An improvement of OLSR using fuzzy logic based MPR selection. In: 15th Asia-Pacific Network Operations and Management Symposium (APNOMS) (2013)
12. Boushaba, A., Benabbou, A., Benabbou, R., Zahi, A., Oumsis, M.: An Intelligent Multipath Optimized Link State Routing Protocol for QoS and QoE Enhancement of Video Transmission in MANETs. Springer, Wien (2015)

13. Venkataramana, A., Setty, P.: Enhance the quality of service in mobile ad hoc networks by using fuzzy based NTT–DYMO. Wireless Pers. Commun. Springer Science + Business Media, New York. https://doi.org/10.1007/s11277-017-3980-2
14. Zadeh, L.A.: Fuzzy Logic. Computer **21**(4), 83–93 (1988)
15. Zadeh, L.A.: Fuzzy sets. Inf. Control **8**(3), 338–353 (1965)
16. Belkadi, M., Lalam, M., M'zoughi, A., Tamani, N., Daoui, M., Aoudjit, R.: Itelligent routing ad flow control in MAETs. J. Comput. Inform. Technol. **3**, 233–243 (2010)
17. Stoica, P., He, H., Li, J.: New algorithms for designing unimodular sequences with good correlation properties. IEEE Trans. Signal Process. **57**(4), 1415–1425 (2009). Li, J., Guerci, J.R., Xu, L.: Signal waveform's optimal under restriction design for active sensing. In: Fourth IEEE Workshop on Sensor Array and Multichannel Processing, Waltham, MA, pp. 382–386, July 2006
18. Yuta, Y., Masayoshi, S., Katsuyoshi, I.: Multipath transmission model and its route lection policy considering packet re-sequencing buffers availability. In: IEEE International Conference on Advanced Information Networking and Applications Workshops (2015)
19. Hanin, Mh., Amnai, M., Fakhri, Y.: Enhannced multi-point relay selection based on fuzzy logic. Int. Rev. Comput. Software (IRECOS) **11**(6), 462–472 (2016)
20. Aggarwal, H., Aggarwal, P.: Energy-efciency based analysis of routing protocols in mobile ad-hoc networks (MAETs). Int. J. Comput. Appl. **96**(15), 15–23 (2014)

Performance Assessment of AODV, DSR and DSDV in an Urban VANET Scenario

Khalid Kandali[✉] and Hamid Bennis

TIM Research Team, EST of Meknes, Moulay Ismail University, Meknes, Morocco
kandalikhalid@hotmail.com, hamid.bennis@gmail.com

Abstract. The wireless system of communication has recently known a considerable evolution, which has led to the appearance of a new type of networks called Vehicular Ad hoc Networks (VANET). This innovative approach is crucial for enhancing the quality of the driving experience as a whole: the safety of the drivers, traffic management and the entertainment of the passengers. Thus, the selection of an appropriate routing protocol is necessary to support high mobility, rapid changing topology and capacity of mobility prediction. In this paper, we evaluate the performance of a set of well-known routing protocols used in VANET, namely AODV, DSR and DSDV in terms of Packet Delivery Ratio (PDR), Throughput, and Normalized Routing Load (NRL), in order to find out the suitable routing protocol for high density traffic area such as Casablanca. In this paper, the real map of Casablanca is edited by Open Street Map (OSM), and the "Simulation of Urban Mobility" (SUMO) tool is used to create the mobility model, while the traffic model generation and the simulations are carried out using Network Simulator 2 (NS2).

Keywords: VANET ITS · AODV · DSR · DSDV · OSM · SUMO · NS2

1 Introduction

In recent years, the Ad hoc Vehicular Networks (VANET) have become a very interesting area of research for many researchers around the world. They are considered one of the most suitable technologies for improving safety performance and traffic conditions of intelligent transport systems (ITS) [1–3]. VANET as a sub-class of Mobile Ad hoc Networks (MANET) are characterized by its high-dynamic network connectivity and frequent change of topology. Vehicular networks are composed of vehicles and all the entities with which the vehicles can establish communications. They give three forms of communication as shown in Fig. 1: Vehicle-to-Infrastructure (V2I) where vehicles connect to fixed stations installed at the road, for the acquisition or transmission of information. Vehicle-to-Vehicle (V2V), where the communications are made only from vehicle to vehicle. This vehicle collaborates in a decentralized way, without relying on any infrastructure, and form an ad hoc network called VANET. Hybrid architecture, which combines the other two modes; In other words, the vehicle, within this architecture, could communicate with another vehicle or fixed station at the same time [3].

© Springer Nature Switzerland AG 2019
M. Ezziyyani (Ed.): AI2SD 2018, AISC 915, pp. 98–109, 2019.
https://doi.org/10.1007/978-3-030-11928-7_8

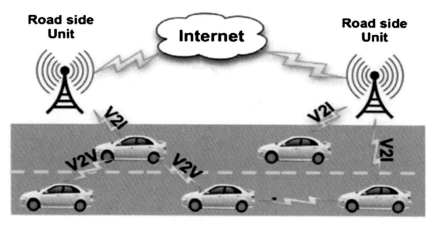

Fig. 1. Architecture of VANET [3]: vehicle-to- infrastructure network, vehicle-to-vehicle network, hybrid architecture

In V2V, all vehicles (sources and destination) behave like a router, to exchange data. If a source node fails during communication then another path can be established using any other node. This is why the choice of a routing protocol according to the situation remains a very important step. It depends on the network environment, the number of nodes that circulate and the speed of different vehicles.

In this paper, we choose AODV, DSR and DSDV as a subject of discussion since they are the most commonly used protocols. We study the performance of these three protocols for the VANET networks and for scenarios with a high density of traffic (case of the city of Casablanca). The performance is evaluated and compared in terms of Packet Delivery Ratio (PDR), average throughput and Normalized Routing Load (NRL). Furthermore, this paper has been fashioned in seven main sections. In addition to Sect. 1, Sect. 2 discusses the work already done in relation with our subject. Section 3 gives a view of the main features of VANET. Section 4 reviews the different routing protocols in VANET. Section 5 explains in details the simulation environment, the mobility and the traffic models. Section 6 presents the results analysis for different scenarios. In Sect. 7, we conclude the results of the simulation.

2 Related Works

Many efforts have been made by researchers to find the best routing protocols in VANET networks. These protocols are evaluated with VANET simulators in terms of different parameters.

In [4], the authors present the simulation results of such scenarios in order to better understand or select the optimal performing Routing protocol among DSDV, DSR and AODV against metrics selected: Packet delivery Ratio, Packet Loss Percentage and Average End to End delay. The results show that AODV out performs DSDV and DSR in unplanned areas.

In [5], authors simulated three different routing protocols and compared them in terms of PDR, average throughput, delay and total energy. From this study, AODV and DSR results in a better performance than DSDV routing protocol. In which AODV has higher performance in terms of PDR when the number of vehicles increased. In general, the results showed decreasing in average throughput and PDR when the number of vehicles is increased.

In [6], the AODV and DSR are applied on a VANET over two different scenarios, dense and sparse traffic based on cars density on the road. These protocols are evaluated on different performance metrics. The simulation found that AODV is better than DSR when we have dense mode scenario which means a large number of nodes, while DSR protocol is better than AODV when the number of nodes is not that much.

These works did not work on a real and dense mobility scenario; in addition to that, they worked on a small surface area. The results presented may be different if we consider a high density traffic area.

3   Characteristics of VANET

The main factors that characterize vehicular networks are:

High mobility: is considered the first factor in VANET. The speed and the movements of the vehicles are relatively predictable and vary according to the environment where there is the network. Consequently, its topology changes frequently. The impact of mobility on network connectivity remains one of the major difficulties in the study of vehicular networks [4].

Diversity of density: The density of vehicles in a vehicular network changes according to the urban or rural environment, the day or the night, and the hours of points or the off-peak hours. This density is not uniform with this spacio-temporal variation.

Frequent Disconnections: A direct consequence of high-speed mobility and sparse distribution of vehicles is intermittent connectivity. Because of the obstacles that prevent the propagation of signal, and the mobility that distances the communication, the links established between two entities of the network can disappear.

Features inherent to the radio channel: Because of the multiple of obstacles, especially in urban areas, the data exchanges know a serious degradation of the quality and the power of signals emitted. For the establishment of radio links, the communications are done in an unfavorable environment.

4   Routing Protocols in VANET

Routing protocols in VANET are based on multi-hop communication to transfer the packets from source to destination. These protocols are different in comparison to other protocols used in local networks. Since the VANET are characterized by high density, mobility of the nodes and frequent change of the topology [7]. Several categories of routing protocols used in VANET, such as Topology based routing protocols, that depend on the information about the network topology to perform packets forwarding

[8]. In this type of routing protocols, three main categories are classified into: Proactive, Reactive and Hybrid between proactive and reactive as shown in Fig. 2.

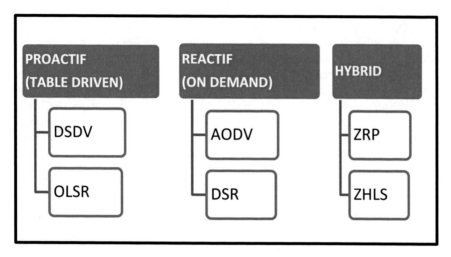

Fig. 2. Classification of routing protocols based on topology [9]

4.1 Proactive Routing Protocols

In this type of routing, the information of all associated nodes is stored in form of tables. This table is updated periodically on at each modification in topology, by an exchange of control messages. The routes are indicated based on this table. The proactive protocols don't have initial route discovery delay, but consume significant bandwidth for periodic topology updates [10].

Destination Sequenced Distance Vector (DSDV)

The Destination Sequenced Distance Vector is a table driven routing protocols based on improved version of the distributed Bellman Ford routing algorithm. The main contribution of this protocol is guarantying the loop-free routing, and reducing control overhead message. In DSDV, every node keeps up the shortest distance of each destination. It stores in its routing table the number signifying the first node on the shortest path to every destination in the network, and the number of hops for all the accessible destinations. The destination nodes generate and broadcast this number until the next updates. Whenever the network topology changes, the node update the information in its routing table and send these updates to its neighbor nodes [8].

4.2 Reactive (On-Demand) Routing Protocols

Reactive routing protocols function according to a principle called on demand, i.e. the routes between nodes of the network are established only on demand. Before the exchange of packets between a source and a destination, the node initiates a route discovery procedure by broadcasting a control packet in the network to find the shortest path to destination. Therefore, this type of protocol consumes less bandwidth by comparing with proactive protocols [8].

Ad hoc On-Demand Distance Vector Routing (AODV)

Ad hoc On-Demand Distance Vector Routing is a reactive and on demand distance vector. In this type of protocol, the nodes maintain only the information on their direct neighbor nodes that they use to determine the routes. AODV does not use periodic exchanges of network topology information, but only active communication routes are maintained. When it is necessary to send data packets from source to destination, each node searches a route by sending control packets to neighboring nodes. Each information in the table corresponds to a destination and contains several fields, essentially the recipient identifier, the next node identifier used as a relay to reach the destination, the sequence number to reach the destination and the time expiration of information [11].

Dynamic Source Routing Protocol (DSR)

Dynamic Source Routing is a reactive protocol. It works in the same way as AODV. But the difference between there is in the fact that AODV saves only the path to next hop, while DSR saves in its routing table, the whole path from source node to destination. DSR starts a route discovery only on demand. The source node determines the complete sequence of nodes to traverse that it inserts into each packet of data before it is transmitted. This sequence is used by each node in the route to determine the next relay to destination [4].

5   Simulation Setup and Performance Metrics

In this paper, we evaluate the performance of the routing protocols using NS2 simulation tool, and the SUMO tool to generate the movement of nodes and the positions of vehicles.

This process is manifested in the following diagram in Fig. 3:

5.1   Map Model

In order to implement VANET in a real environment, we have used Open Street Map (OSM) [13]. In our case, we downloaded the map model casa.osm, which is an area of high density in Casablanca. Figure 4 shows our model map:

5.2   Mobility Generation Model

Several mobility models are used in the simulation. The main purpose is to describe the movement patterns of nodes communicating in a Vehicular Ad Hoc Network. They have a great impact on performance evaluation of routing protocol [14].

In our study, we used the simulation of Urban Mobility (SUMO) as one of the main VANET Mobility simulators. Since, it is used to model the intermodal traffic systems including road vehicles, traffic transport and pedestrians [5].

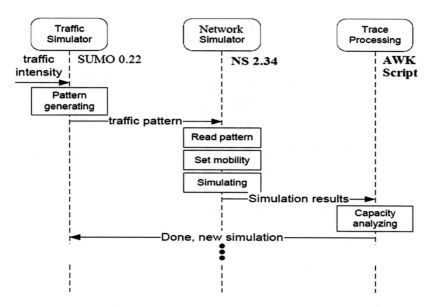

Fig. 3. Sequence diagram for simulation VANET [12]

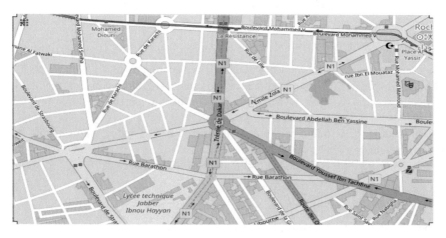

Fig. 4. Model map of Casablanca city

The commands used in this software to generate our targeted mobility model are:

Netconvert: imports road networks from the file OSM and generates roads networks in the form of .net.xml [15].

Polyconvert: imports geometrical shapes (polygons–buildings) from the file OSM and converts them to a representation supported by SUMO-GUI [15].

Ramdomtrips.Py: is used to generate random routes [15].

traceExporter.py: generating three files: activity.tcl, mobility.tcl and config.tcl.

The output of the model mobility is shown in Fig. 5.

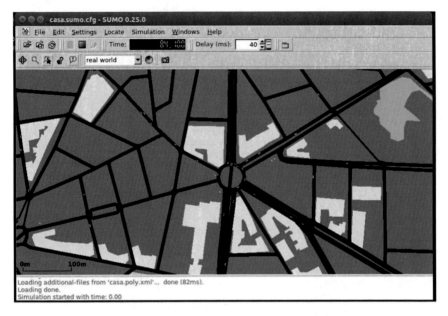

Fig. 5. Traffic mobility model file in SUMO

5.3 Traffic Genreation Model

There are many tools for network simulations, but the most frequently used are OPNET, OMNET++, Qualnet, and NS2. In this study, we selected NS2 as the network simulator which is completely free, open source tool. It supports multiple protocols, and has several features.

For creating CBR traffic connections between wireless nodes, we use script 'cbr-gen.tcl' included in NS2 [16].

Finally, NAM file is generated and the output is shown in Fig. 6.

5.4 Parameters of Simulation

In our simulation work, we evaluate the performance of original AODV, DSR and DSDV routing protocol. The VANET network has been simulated with 25, 50, 100 and 150 nodes representing moving vehicles. They are the transmitters and receivers of the information at a variety of speeds over a 1000 × 1000 m area in urban scenario, and for 200 s of simulated time. The simulation parameters are summarized in Table 1.

5.5 Performance Metrics

The performance study of three protocols is done in terms of three metrics: PDR, Throughput, and NRL. Awk scripts are used to retrieve results after the end of the simulation from the generated trace file.

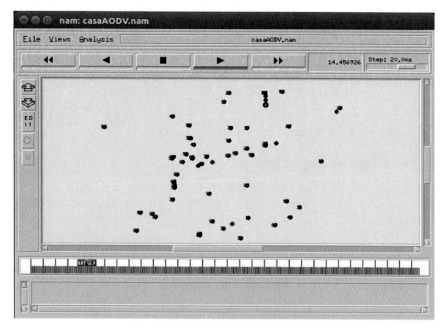

Fig. 6. NAM file generation

Table 1. Parameters of simulation

Parameter	Value
Network simulator	NS-2, 2.29.3 version
Mobility simulator	SUMO v 0.26.0
Map model	OSM (city of Casablanca)
Routing protocol	AODV, DSR and DSDV
Type of traffic/routing agent	CBR/UDP
Rate	8k
Number of vehicles	25, 50, 100, 150
Network size	1000 × 1000
Mobility model	Random trip model (RTM)
Propagation model	Two ray ground
Simulation time	200 ms
Channel type	Wireless channel
Antenna type	Omni antenna
Mac protocol	IEEE 802.11

Packet Delivery Ratio (PDR): It defines the ratio of number of packets that are successfully delivered to a destination against the number of packets that have been sent out by the source node [17].

Throughput: This metric shows the amount of data transmitted from a source to a destination per time unit over a communication link. It is measured in bits per second. [18].

Normalized Routing Load (NRL): It is calculated by dividing the number of routing packets transmitted in the network, per packet of data delivered to destination [19].

6   Results and Analysis

6.1   Packet Delivery Ratio (PDR)

Figure 7 shows the effect of increasing the number of vehicles on PDR for AODV, DSR, and DSDV. These protocols show a very low PDR. By using AODV, PDR is decreased from 55.17 to 38.25% and when the number of vehicles becomes 150, PDR becomes 10.08%. The DSR show the same evolution with a lower PDR than AODV. In the order hand, DSDV starts with a very low PDR but it becomes better than AODV and DSR when the number of vehicles become higher. Consequently, these protocols show usually a poor effect in terms of PDR. It must be over 90%.

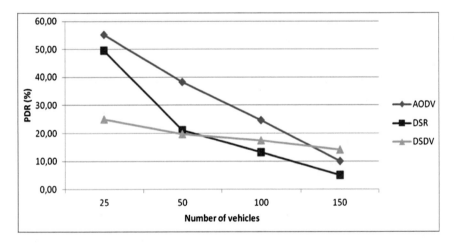

Fig. 7. Number of vehicles versus packet delivery ratio

6.2   Throughput

Figure 8 presents the average throughput in Kbps versus number of vehicle nodes for DSDV, DSR and AODV routing protocols. The maximum value of average throughput is nearly 164.19 Kbps for AODV and 141.05 Kbps for DSR, but DSDV shows a poor effect. Again, when the number of vehicles is increased, the average throughput is decreased for AODV and DSR, but it is increased for DSDV.

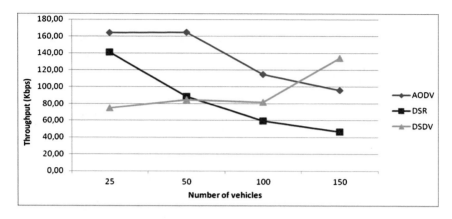

Fig. 8. Number of vehicles versus throughput

6.3 Normalized Routing Load (NRL)

Figure 9 illustrates NRL versus number of vehicle nodes for AODV, DSR and DSDV. NRL for DSDV remains low for all the number of vehicles, whereas, the NRL of AODV protocol and DSR protocol increases with increase in number of vehicles. In this scenario, DSDV protocol performs better than AODV protocol and DSR in terms of NRL.

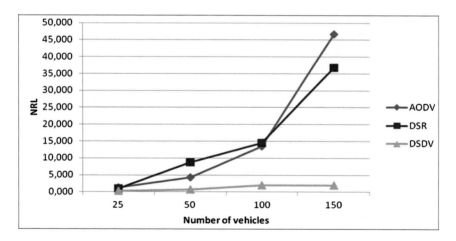

Fig. 9. Number of vehicles versus normalized routing load

7 Conclusion and Perspectives

In this paper, we studied the performance of three routing protocols (AODV, DSR and DSDV) in high density traffic (case of the city of Casablanca), in terms of Packet Delivery Ratio (PDR), Throughput, and Normalized Routing Load (NRL). The results show that AODV outperforms DSR and DSDV in terms of PDR and throughput, whereas the NRL for DSDV remains low than AODV and DSR for different number of vehicles. In other words, according to this study, we conclude that the less the number of vehicles is, the more appropriate and suitable the reactive protocols such as AODV and DSR are; and vice versa.

These routing protocols are primarily developed and implemented for use in mobile ad hoc networks. However, their direct application to VANET networks may trigger a malfunction of the network, which drives the future work to promote and adapt routing algorithms to VANET networks, especially in an urban environment.

References

1. Benamar, M., Ahnana, S., Saiyari, F.Z., Benamar, N., El Ouadghiri, M.D., Bonnin, J.-M.: Study of VDTN routing protocols performances in sparse and dense traffic in the presence of relay nodes. J. Mob. Multimed. **10**(1–2) (2014)
2. Benamar, N., Singh, K.D., Benamar, M., El Ouadghiri, D., Bonnin, J.M.: Routing protocols in vehicular delay tolerant networks: a comprehensive survey. Comput. Commun. **48**, 141–158 (2014)
3. Cunha, F., et al.: Data communication in VANETs: protocols, applications and challenges. Ad Hoc Netw. **44**, 90–103 (2016)
4. Ul-Amin, R., Nasim, F.: Performance evaluation of AODV, DSDV and DSR routing protocols in unplanned areas
5. Abdelgadir, M., Saeed, R.A., Babiker, A.: Mobility routing model for vehicular ad-hoc networks (VANETs), smart city scenarios. Veh. Commun. **9**, 154–161 (2017)
6. Shaheen, A., Gaamel, A., Bahaj, A.: Comparison and analysis study between AODV and DSR routing protocols in VANET with IEEE 802.11 b. J. Ubiquitous Syst. Pervasive Netw. **7**(1), 07–12 (2016)
7. Sharma, Y.M.: Comparative performance exploration of AODV, DSDV & DSR routing protocol in cluster based vanet environment. Int. J. Adv. Eng. Technol. (2012)
8. Rohal, P., Dahiya, R., Dahiya, P.: Study and analysis of throughput, delay and packet delivery ratio in MANET for topology based routing protocols (AODV, DSR and DSDV). Int. J. Adv. Res. Eng. Technol. **1**(2), 54–58 (2013)
9. Memon, I.R., Shah, W., Kumar, W., Mohammadani, K.H., Memon, S.A.: Performance evaluation of routing protocols in VANET on highway: police cars communication scenario (2017)
10. Sharef, B.T., Alsaqour, R.A., Ismail, M.: Vehicular communication ad hoc routing protocols: a survey. J. Netw. Comput. Appl. **40**, 363–396 (2014)
11. Rathi, D., Welekar, R.: Performance evaluation of AODV routing protocol in VANET with NS2. Int. J. Interact. Multimed. Artif. Intell. **4**(3), 23 (2017)
12. Samatha, B., Dr. Raja Kumar, K., Karyemsetty, N.: Design and simulation of vehicular adhoc network using SUMO and NS2. Adv. Wireless Mob. Commun. **10**(5), 1207–1219 (2017). ISSN 0973-6972

13. OpenStreetMap.: OpenStreetMap. [Online]. Available: https://www.openstreetmap.org/. Accessed: 04 Mar 2018
14. Mahajan, A., Potnis, N., Gopalan, K., Wang, A.: Evaluation of mobility models for vehicular ad-hoc network simulations. In: IEEE International Workshop on Next Generation Wireless Networks (WoNGeN) (2006)
15. Simulation of Urban Mobility (Sumo) For Evaluating Qos Parameters For.... [Online]. Available: https://fr.slideshare.net/iosrjce/simulation-of-urban-mobility-sumo-for-evaluating-qos-parameters-for-vehicular-adhoc-network. Accessed 04 Mar 2018
16. Kolici, V., Oda, T.: Performance evaluation of a VANET simulation system using NS-3 and SUMO. In: IEEE (2015)
17. Sataraddi, M.J., Kakkasageri, M.S.: Intelligent routing for hybrid communication in VANETs. IEEE 7th International Advance Computing Conference (IACC) (2017)
18. Sharma, R., Dr. Malhotra, J.: Performance evaluation of ADV DSR and god in VANET for city and highway scenario. Int. J. Adv. Sci. Technol. (2015)
19. Lei, D., Wang, T., Li, J.: Performance analysis and comparison of routing protocols in mobile ad hoc network. In: 2015 Fifth International Conference on Instrumentation and Measurement, Computer, Communication and Control (IMCCC), Qinhuangdao, pp. 1533–1536 (2015)

Exploiting NoSQL Document Oriented Data Using Semantic Web Tools

Nassima Soussi[(✉)] and Mohamed Bahaj

Mathematics and Computer Science Department, Faculty of Science
and Technologies, Hassan 1st University, Settat, Morocco
{nassima.soussi,mohamedbahaj}@gmail.com

Abstract. The web has experienced a quantitative explosion of digital data handled by companies manipulating numerous heterogeneous management systems that encapsulate large web sites destined for a wide audience. In fact, some web users treat this big amount of data with NoSQL databases while others prefer to use semantic web technologies, which make the communication between the web applications a very hard aim. The previous raison has motivated us to bridge the conceptual gap between them in order to make NoSQL data machine-readable and allow web applications to exchange information easily. Our main contribution is to generate RDF format from NoSQL database model with a specific focus on MongoDB as the most used document oriented database in order to make the NoSQL data available on the triplestores and to carry out some operations not supported by NoSQL systems.

Keywords: NoSQL · Document oriented database · MongoDB ·
NoSQL-to-RDF · Interoperability · Mapping system

1 Introduction

In the last decades, the volume of data (estimated that it will reach 44 Zettabytes in 2020) is increasing exponentially making the web facing the inevitable difficulty of managing intelligently this large amount of data. This problem has led to the emergence of more robust systems dedicated specifically to manage this big amount of data; among these emerging systems we quote the NoSQL and semantic web representing the main study of this paper.

The Semantic Web [1] is considered as an extension of the classic web aiming to exploit its maximum potential by attributing a meaning to data in order to ensure better human-machine cooperation and an intelligent management of the gigantic current content of the web. It is largely recognized by its ability to exchange data relying on RDF (Resource Description Framework) [2] considered as a machine readable format represented as a set of triples (subject, predicate and object). Besides of Semantic Web, NoSQL [3] was born in 2009 aiming to overcome the limitations of relational world so as to process a large amount of data on distributed hardware architectures. This system supports dynamic schema design offering to web users a high flexibility and scalability. These raisons have motivated us to elaborate an efficient Framework to map NoSQL data model to RDF format in order to make web data machine-readable, to carry out

© Springer Nature Switzerland AG 2019
M. Ezziyyani (Ed.): AI2SD 2018, AISC 915, pp. 110–117, 2019.
https://doi.org/10.1007/978-3-030-11928-7_9

some operations not supported by NoSQL systems and to unify the heterogeneous NoSQL databases model starting with document oriented databases.

The remainder of this paper is organized as follows: Section 2 exposes a brief description of some related works to the current topic. Section 3 introduces this work by presenting a grammar of MongoDB data model and RDF describing the syntax of each one. Our main contribution is presented in section 4 which explains by detail all components of the proposed framework's architecture, and then we give an example of our solution in Section 5. Finally, section 6 concludes this work and suggests some future extensions of this approach.

2 Related Works

In the last ten years, considerable efforts have been invested in the definition of tools that allow transforming several kinds of data sources into RDF format in order to make it machine-readable. Regarding the mapping of relational data to RDF [4], numerous conversion methods are defined to realize this goal such as: Triplify, Virtuoso, eD2R, D2RQ, R3 M and others. In the same light, several approaches have been developed in order to ensure the XML-to-RDF conversion: XSPARQL [5], Scissor-lift [6], Krextor library [7] and AstroGrid-D [8].

Regarding the adaptation of NoSQL systems to RDF format, all existing approaches have the same and common weakness since they don't propose a complete and detailed algorithm to ensure this interoperability; we quote for instance: the work described in [9] performs hybrid query processing by integrating both SQL and NoSQL data into a common data format (RDF); during this process, the authors have developed a very basic mapping algorithm for transforming NoSQL data (MongoDB) to RDF and they illustrate just some features supported by their solution. In addition, the authors in [10] propose a systematic attempt at characterizing and comparing NoSQL stores for RDF processing; they study just their mapping applicability but they don't trait the interoperability between these two heterogeneous systems.

Finally, to the best of our knowledge, our paper is the first work which investigates the detailed representation of NoSQL data (Document Oriented Database) using RDF format in order to contribute in the interoperability between these two different worlds and to unify their data models. In order to achieve this goal, we have established an efficient and detailed algorithm transforming each database model to its equivalent RDF components characterized by a simple and powerful structure of triples (Subject-Predicate-Object) very similar to human language (Subject-Verb-Object).

3 Overview

In this section, we describe the data model of the different components used in our transformation approach of NoSQL world to semantic web world by presenting their grammar: JSON format for MongoDB (document oriented database) and RDF format for semantic web world.

3.1 MongoDB Data Model

MongoDB is an open source database categorized as a NoSQL document-oriented database providing a high performance, availability and automatic scaling. Its architecture is based on collections of documents equivalent to tables and records in relational databases respectively; each document contains a set of {key,value} pairs representing the basic data unit in MongoDB. Like other NoSQL databases, MongoDB supports dynamic schema design, allowing the documents in a collection to have different fields and structures. The database uses a document storage and data interchangeable format called BSON, which provides a binary representation of JSON-like documents.

Collection = Document*
Document = '{' Pair (',' Pair)* '}'
Pair = Key ':' Value
Key = String
Value = SimpleValue | ComplexValue
SimpleValue = Number | String
ComplexValue = SimpleValueList | DocumentList
SimpleValueList = '[' **SimpleValue** (',' **SimpleValue**)* ']'
DocumentList = '[' Document (',' Document)* ']'

3.2 RDF Stores

The RDF (Resource Description Framework) is a graph model designed to formally describe web resources and metadata so as to enable automatic processing of such descriptions. Developed by the W3C, RDF is the basic language of the Semantic Web. Several common serialization formats are in use, we quote as example: Turtle [11], N-Triples [12], N-Quads [13], JSON-LD [14], Notation 3 (N3) [15], RDF/XML [16]. In this study, we are only interested by RDF/XML serialization syntax as described in the grammar follow:

RdfRoot = '<rdf:RDF DefaultNS SpecificNS?* >' **Node*** '</rdf:RDF>'
 DefaultNS = 'xmlns="http://www.w3.org/1999/02/22-rdf-syntax-ns#"'
SpecificNS = 'xmlns:' **NSsymbol** '=' **idPath**
NSsymbol = String
idPath = path
Node = '<rdf:Description' **IdAttr?** '>' **Property*** '</rdf:Description>'
IdAttr = 'rdf:about=' **idAttrValue**
 Property = '<'**SpecificNS**':'**PropertyName**'>' **PropertyValue**
          '</'**SpecificNS**':'**PropertyName**'>'
PropertyName = String
PropertyValue = SimpleValue | ComplexeValue
SimpleValue = Number | String
ComplexeValue = Node | Sequence | Bag
Sequence = '<rdf:Seq>' **Aggnode*** '</rdf:Seq>'
Bag = '<rdf:Bag>' **Aggnode*** '</rdf:Bag>'
Aggnode = '<rdf:li>' **AggnodeValue** '</rdf:li>'
 AggnodeValue = SimpleValue | Node

4 Architecture and Algorithms

In this stage, we present our main contribution by describing the architecture of our converter system of MongoDB data model to RDF format illustrated in Fig. 1.

Our Framework takes as input a MongoDB data as a JSON file (collection of documents) so as to return at the end the semantic equivalent RDF format.

The architecture of our Framework, as shown bellow, is composed of three basic components: JSON decomposer, Pairs Extractor and Semantic Mapping.

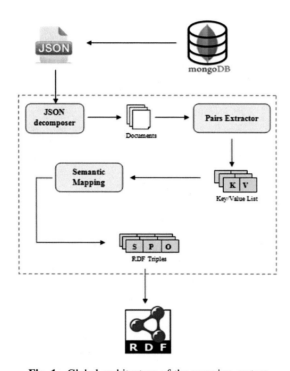

Fig. 1. Global architecture of the mapping system

4.1 JSON Decomposer

This component represents the first step in our mapping system. It takes as input a JSON file in order to decompose it and extract all documents encapsulated in this latter so as to store them in a list for ulterior use. The output list is represented as List-Doc = $\{D_1, D_2, ..., D_n\}$ (n represents a number of document).

```
Input : Collection name (Cname)
Output : List of documents (ListDoc)
Begin
 File F = NULL
 List ListDoc = NULL
 String FileName= " ", D = " "
FileName  ← Cname + ".json"
F = FileOpen(FileName , "Read")
If (F != NULL) then
       While Non EOF do
D ← FileRead("{", "}")
ListDoc.add(D)
       End While
End if
FileClose(FileName)
Return ListDoc
End Algorithm
```

4.2   Pairs Extractor

It takes as input one of the document of the previous list ListDoc, generated by JSON decomposer, in order to glance through it and extract the {key, value} pairs represented as $P_i^j = (K_i^j, V_i^j)$ of the input document $D_i = \{(K_i^1, V_i^1), (K_i^2, V_i^2),...,(K_i^m, V_i^m)\}$ with $i \in [1, n]$, $j \in [1, m]$ and m is a number of pairs in a document D_i.

```
Input : Document (D)
Output : List of pairs (ListDoc)
Begin
List Children = D.getChildren()
Entier N = Children.getLenght()
Table P[2,N]
For i ← 1 to N do
      P[i,1] ← D.getKey()
      P[i,2] ← D.getValue()
End For
Return P
End Algorithm
```

4.3   Semantic Mapping

The *SemanticMapping* is the main component of our Framework. Firstly, it converts the input MongoDB data model to a list of documents via the component *JsonDecomposer* so as to glance through it and extract for each document its pairs list using *PairsExtractor*. These pairs are used to extract the semantic correspondence between RDF and JSON format and concatenate triples so as to form the equivalent RDF store for the input MongoDB data model.

```
Input : Collection, nsLabel
Output : RDF format
Begin
String rdf  ← ' '
List ListDoc ← JsonDecomposer(Collection)
if (ListDoc.isEmpty() = False) then
rdf  += '<rdf:description'
For i ← 1 to ListDoc.getLenght() do
P ← PairsExtractor(ListDoc.get(i))
For j ← 1 to N do
   if (P[1,j] = '_id') then
        rdf += 'rdf:about = "'+ P[2,j] +'" >'
   else
        rdf += '>'
        end if

rdf+='<'+nsLabel+':'+P[1,j]+'>'+P[2,j]+'</'+nsLabel+':'+
P[1,j]+'>'
            End For
            rdf  += '</rdf:description>'
        End For
    End if
Return rdf
End Algorithm
```

5   Validation Example

In this section, we present an example that proves the validity of our approach. Firstly, we consider a JSON file illustrated in Fig. 2 containing a collection C of two documents {D₁, D₂}. The collection C encapsulates a set of {key, value} pairs for people's information (firstName, lastName, age, status, specialty and university). Starting from this JSON file, we have established the equivalent RDF file (represented in Fig. 3) based on the conversion algorithms defined previously.

```
{ _id : "http:://uhp.ac/persons/001",
     firstName : "Nassima",
     lastName: "SOUSSI",
     age : 26,
     status: "Ph.D student",
     specialty: "Computer science",
     university : "FST" }
{ _id : "http:://uhp.ac/persons/002",
     firstName : "Mohamed",
     lastName: "BAHAJ",
     status: "Teacher-researcher",
     specialty: "Computer science"
     university : "FST"  }
```

Fig. 2. Example of documents collection "Persons.json"

```
<rdf:RDF xmlns = "http://www.w3.org/1999/02/22-rdf-syntax-ns#"
xmlns:p = "http:://uhp.ac/persons/" >
   <rdf:Description    rdf:about= "http:://uhp.ac/persons/001" >
  <p:firstName>Nassima</p:firstName>
  <p:lastName>SOUSSI</p:lastName>
  <p:age>26</p:age>
  <p:status>Ph.D student</p:status>
  <p:speciality>Computer science</p:speciality>
  <p:university>FST</p:university>
   </rdf:Description>
   <rdf:Description rdf:about= "http:://uhp.ac/persons/002" >
     <p:firstName>Mohamed</p:firstName>
     <p:lastName>BAHAJ</p:lastName>
     <p:status>Teacher-researcher</p:status>
     <p:university>FST</p:university>
   </rdf:Description>
   </rdf:RDF>
```

Fig. 3. Equivalent RDF Store of JSON File "Persons.json"

6 Conclusion

Using RDF for storing NoSQL data appears a helpful method, in which NoSQL-to-RDF strategy will play a pertinent role aiming to make NoSQL data available on the semantic web and benefit from some operations not supported by NoSQL system. In this regards, we have established, to the best of our knowledge, the first approach which allow storing NoSQL Data (with a specific focus on MongoDB as the most used NoSQL database) in RDF stores considered as a powerful format for publishing and exchanging data in the web, by elaborating an efficient semantic mapping strategy for translation MongoDB data model to RDF format. One obvious extension of our work is to enhance the current mechanism by supporting more NoSQL databases types.

One obvious extension of our research regarding NoSQL-to-RDF (more precisely MongoDB database model to RDF) is to improve the performance of our approach on a real data. Another promising direction for future work is to enhance the current mechanism by supporting more NoSQL database types.

References

1. Berners-Lee, T., Hendler, J., Lassila, O.: The semantic web. Sci. Am. **284**(5), 28–37 (2001)
2. Gandon, F., Schreiber, G.:RDF 1.1 XML syntax. W3C Recommendation, 25 Feb 2014. World Wide Web Consortium (2014). http://www.w3.org/TR/rdf-syntax-grammar. Accessed October 8, 2016
3. Nayak, A., Poriya, A., Poojary, D.: Type of NOSQL databases and its comparison with relational databases. Int. J. Appl. Inform. Syst. **5**(4), 16–19 (2013)
4. Michel, F., Montagnat, J., & Faron-Zucker, C. (2014). A survey of RDB to RDF translation approaches and tools (Doctoral dissertation, I3S)
5. Bischof, S., Decker, S., Krennwallner, T., Lopes, N., Polleres, A.: Mapping between RDF and XML with XSPARQL. J. Data Seman. **1**(3), 147–185 (2012)
6. Fennell, P.: Schematron-more useful than you'd thought. XML LONDON (2014)
7. Lange, C.: Krextor—an extensible framework for contributing content math to the web of data. In: International Conference on Intelligent Computer Mathematics, pp. 304–306. Springer, Berlin (2011)
8. Breitling, F. (2009). A standard transformation from XML to RDF via XSLT.Astronomische Nachrichten, 330(7), 755-760
9. Michel, F., Djimenou, L., Faron-Zucker, C., Montagnat, J.: Translation of relational and non-relational databases into RDF with xR2RML. In 11th International Confenrence on Web Information Systems and Technologies (WEBIST'15) (2015)
10. Cudré-Mauroux, P., Enchev, I., Fundatureanu, S., Groth, P., Haque, A., Harth, A., Keppmann, L.F., Miranker, D., Sequeda, J.F., Wylot, M.: NoSQL databases for RDF: an empirical evaluation. In: International Semantic Web Conference, pp. 310–325. Springer, Berlin (2013)
11. Beckett, D., Berners-Lee, T., Prud'hommeaux, E., Carothers, G.: RDF 1.1 turtle–terse RDF triple language. W3C Recommendation. World Wide Web Consortium (Feb 2014). Available at http://www.w3.org/TR/turtle
12. Beckett, D.: RDF 1.1N-triples: a line-based syntax for an RDF graph. W3C Recommendation (2014). http://www.w3.org/TR/n-triples,25
13. Carothers, G.: RDF 1.1N-quads: a line-based syntax for RDF datasets. W3C Recommendation (2014)
14. Davis, I., Steiner, T., Hors, A.L.: RDF 1.1 JSON alternate serialization (RDF/JSON). W3C Recommendation (2013)
15. Berners-Lee, T., Connolly, D.: Notation3 (N3): a readable RDF syntax. W3C Team Submission. World Wide Web Consortium (2011). Beschikbaar op http://www.w3.org/TeamSubmission/n3
16. Gandon, F., Schreiber, G.: RDF 1.1 XML syntax: W3C Recommendation, 25 Feb 2014. World Wide Web Consortium (2014). http://www.w3.org/TR/rdf-syntax-grammar. Accessed 8 Oct 2016

Analytical Study of the Performance of Communication Systems in the Presence of Fading

Sara Riahi[1($\boxtimes$)] and Azzeddine Riahi[2]

[1] Department of Computer Science, Faculty of Sciences, Chouaib Doukkali University, PO Box 20, 24000 El Jadida, Morocco
riahisaraphd@gmail.com
[2] Department of Physics, Faculty of Sciences, IMC Laboratory, Chouaib Doukkali University, PO Box 20, 24000 El Jadida, Morocco
riahikh@gmail.com

Abstract. The environment in which a communication system emits electro-magnetic waves represents the propagation channel. The propagation of electromagnetic waves in the channel include several problems related to the propagation medium which can be intercepted, reflected or diffracted by obstacles of different nature such as buildings, buildings, trees. Depending on the nature of the path, the received signal is composed of several wave attenuated and delayed in time, causing dispersive fading. These result in a substantial degradation in performance of a communication system. So the characterization of the propagation channel is a necessary step for the development of communication system. Knowing the properties and defects that brought on a transmission, adapted techniques can be developed.

Keywords: Fading · Channel · Modelization · Noise · Rayleigh · Rice · Nakagami

1 Introduction

We live in the era of telecommunications and information. During the past two decades, digital communications have evolved. Today, information is in most cases conveyed in digital form, whether wired, radio, cellular networks or wireless local area networks or information storage systems. This has been triggered and sustained by strong demand for transmission and secure, timely and efficient information of all types. The propagation medium of electromagnetic waves often has several obstacles hindering the transmission of information. The received signal is composed of several attenuated waves and delayed in time, causing dispersive fading [1]. These results in a substantial degradation in performance of a microwave communication system. The field of statistical signal processing was still dominated by the Gaussian assumption for noise modeling. In several situations, this hypothesis is relevant and can be justified by means of the Central Limit Theorem. However, in a growing number of applications, the conventional assumption about the Gaussian nature of the noise is not verified. This is particularly the case for many communication systems, such as transmission on the

© Springer Nature Switzerland AG 2019
M. Ezziyyani (Ed.): AI2SD 2018, AISC 915, pp. 118–134, 2019.
https://doi.org/10.1007/978-3-030-11928-7_10

power grid, high-frequency communications or underwater communications. In such systems, noises with a low probability of occurrence but very high amplitudes of impulsive nature occur. Conventional models based on Gaussian distributions are insufficient to adequately represent such phenomena and the development of new more realistic models is needed. Indeed, modeling impulsive noise by a Gaussian distribution can significantly degrade the performance of transmission systems [2]. This is due mainly to the high variability of this type of noise. This variability is not compatible with Gaussian distributions but can be very well represented with non-Gaussian distributions with infinite variance. In the context of non-Gaussian distributions with infinite variance, α—stable distributions appeared. They are part of a very rich class of probability distributions which include the laws of Gauss, Cauchy and Levy and authorizing the asymmetry and heavy tails. These distributions have very interesting properties that make them very suitable for modeling impulsive processes. The encoding of the digital channel transforms the useful information sequence into a discrete coded sequence called a code word. The code word can be binary or non-binary. The challenge of coding digital information is to successfully recover the information on reception, as little as possible from the noise of the transmission channel. The receiver converts the received sequence coded into an estimated sequence of information. This sequence should ideally be the same discrete sequence transmitted, but in reality it is affected by transmission errors. The discrete sequence is then transformed into a continuous sequence and it is delivered to the output. The purpose of the theory of error correcting codes is to minimize decoding errors as much as possible, while at the same time ensuring very high transmission rates and low costs for the encoder and decoder [3]. Nowadays, there are a multitude of methods to produce good error correcting codes. The two main types of codes used are block codes and convolutional codes. Block codes can be linear or non-linear. Linear block codes can be cyclic or non-cyclic. This paper presents the different types of fading due to the effects of multipath, models of the most used in the telecommunications field channels: Rayleigh's model and Rice's model. The channels are generally modeled in the case where the order of variability is equal to two using the Gaussian law, however, if intersymbol interference (ISI) increases, the noise tends to an impulsive noise and thus the number of variability increases.

The rest of the paper is organized as follows: Sect. 2 describe the propagation phenomenon, the transmission channel is reserved to Sect. 3, Sect. 4 explain the types of fading as large-scale fading and the small scale fading, Sect. 5 detail the characteristic of fading channel, Sect. 6 present the transmission channels with fading, simulation and analysis of the results are discussed in Sect. 7, conclusions are given in Sect. 8.

2   Propagation Phenomenon

To reach the reception, the visibility between the transmitter and the receiver is not always present. Electromagnetic waves encounter obstacles. Depending on the type of obstacle encountered these waves can be reflected, diffracted, transmitted or disseminated (Fig. 1) [4].

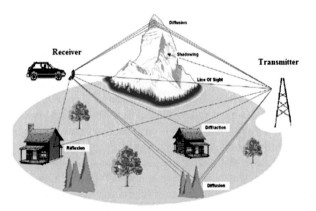

Fig. 1. The main mechanisms of propagation

Reflection: is the most familiar phenomenon. Was a reflection when an electromagnetic wave encounters an obstacle whose dimensions are large compared to the wavelength. The surface behaves as a mirror to the wave.

Refraction: occurs under the same conditions as reflection. This phenomenon enables a part of the incident wave energy to pass through the surface. The transmission is the phenomenon that allows the electromagnetic wave passed through an obstacle of a certain thickness. This is not really a basic phenomenon since to pass through the obstacle, the wave must be refracted by the incoming surface to be possibly reflected and then refracted again [2].

Diffraction: occurs when an electromagnetic wave encounters an obstacle whose dimensions are large compared to the wavelength. This is the phenomenon that allows the waves to bypass an obstacle.

Scattering: When the electromagnetic wave encounters in its path a large number of objects whose size is of the order of magnitude of the wavelength or smaller, its energy is dispersed in all directions [3].

3   The Transmission Channel

A transmission channel is a means in which electromagnetic waves propagate to transfer information between a transmitter and a receiver as shown in Fig. 2 [5].

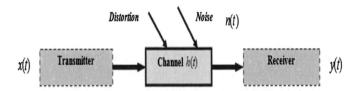

Fig. 2. Transmission channel

The characteristics of wireless signal change when moving the antenna from the transmitter to the receiver antenna. These characteristics depend on the distance between the two antennas, the path taken by the signal and the environment around the path. The received signal can be obtained from the transmitted signal if we have a model of the medium between the two. This model of the medium is called channel model [6]. In general, the power of the received signal can be obtained by converting the power of the transmitted signal by the impulse response of the channel. Note that the convolution in the time domain is equivalent to multiplication in the frequency domain. Therefore, the transmitted signal X, after propagation through the channel H becomes Y:

$$Y(f) = H(f) X(f) + N(f) \tag{1}$$

Here $H(f)$ is the channel response, and $N(f)$ is the noise.

4 Types of Fading

In practice, the received signal encounters variations in amplitude and phase. These variations represent the fading. The fading phenomena can be classified into two types [4]:

- A large scale.
- A small scale.

4.1 Large-Scale Fading

The large-scale fading due to propagation loss over long distances such as rural areas and masking effects.

4.1.1 Propagation Loss, or Path Loss

Propagation losses are defined as the ratio between the power of the received signal and the transmitted, which describes the attenuation of the average power as a function of distance. It is important to know it in order to establish an appropriate link budget for good radio coverage. Free space losses increase with frequency and with distance (Fig. 3). These path loss are shown generally in the form [7]:

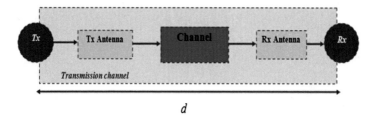

Fig. 3. Free space propagation

$$P_r = P_t P_0 \left(\frac{d_0}{d}\right)^\alpha \tag{2}$$

where P_r is the received power, P_t is the transmitted power, P_0 is the power at the distance d_0, and α represents the coefficient of the propagation loss.

$$PL(d)dB = \overline{PL}(d_0) + 10\alpha \log\left(\frac{d}{d_0}\right) \tag{3}$$

Here $\overline{PL}(d_0)$ represents the path loss at distance d_0.

We can also represent two formulas of propagation losses.

In free space where there is no object between the transmitter and the receiver and therefore the propagation loss formula is represented in the following form [8]:

$$P_r(d) = P_t \left[\frac{\sqrt{G_l}\lambda}{4\pi.d}\right]^2 \tag{4}$$

where G_l is the product of the fields of the transmitting and receiving antenna. d is the distance between the transmitter and the receiver and λ represents the wavelength $(\lambda = c/f)$. The floor presence causes some of the waves to reflect and reach the transmitter. These reflected waves may sometimes have a 180° phase shift and therefore can reduce the received power. A simple two-ray approximation for path loss can be demonstrated as follows [9]:

$$P_r = P_t \frac{G_r G_t h_t^2 h_r^2}{d^4} \tag{5}$$

Here, h_t and h_r are the antenna heights of the transmitter and the receiver, respectively.

4.1.2   The Masking Effect (The Shadowing)

Shadowing means the average power of the signal received over a large area due to the dynamic evolution of the propagation paths by which the new paths appear and the old ones disappear [5]. This effect is referred to as "shadowing". Because of the change in the immediate environment, the received power is different from the average for a given distance that affects globally propagation losses (Fig. 4).

$$PL(d)_{dB} = \overline{PL}(d_0)_{dB} + \alpha \, \log\left(\frac{d}{d_0}\right)_{dB} + X \tag{6}$$

X: represents the masking effect.

4.2   The Small Scale Fading

Small-scale power variations, known as fading, are measured over a sufficiently short time interval to neglect a large-scale change in phenomena. It concerns the rapid

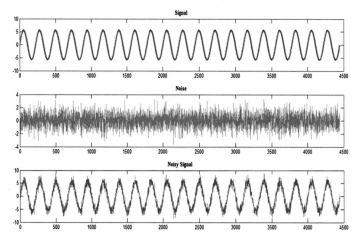

Fig. 4. The effect of noise on the transmission of a signal

variation in the signal level [10]. This variation is due to the constructive and destructive interferences of the multipaths (Fig. 5) when the mobile moves for a short distance. The delay spread of the signal Doppler shift f_d.

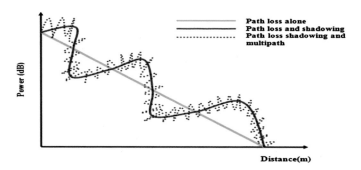

Fig. 5. Multipaths

5   Characteristic of Fading Channel

The characteristics of a fast or slow fading channel are very important for the mathematical modeling of the channel and system performance evaluation operating in these channels.

5.1   The Coherence Time

The classification of a channel in fast fading or slow fading is related to the notion of coherence time of the channel T_c which is the measure of the minimum time separation for which the impulse responses of the channel to the emission of a pure frequency are considered uncorrelated. The coherence time is inversely proportional to Doppler spread f_d [11]:

$$T_c = \frac{K_1}{\Delta f_d} \tag{7}$$

where K_1 is a constant depending on the environment. The spread is the frequency shift of the received wave, because of the displacement of the receiver or transmitter. With $f_d = f_p \cdot \frac{v}{c} \cdot \cos\theta$. Where f_d is the Doppler frequency, f_p is the carrier frequency, v is the speed of the mobile and θ is the angle between the received beam and the displacement axis [6]. Thus a channel is said to fast fade if the duration of a transmitted symbol T_s is equal to or greater than the coherence time of the $T_s \geq T_c$ channel. Otherwise the channel is said to fade slowly $(T_s \leq T_c)$.

5.2   Time Spreading

This is the difference between the longest path, also called delay spread DS and noted T_m.

$$T_m = \frac{\text{longest path} - \text{shortest path}}{c} \tag{8}$$

The latter is often used as an indicator to differentiate between broadband and narrowband channels. If the maximum propagation delay T_m of the channel is greater or equal to $T_s (T_m \geq T_s)$, the channel is called "broadband". If T_m is much smaller than $T_s (T_m \leq T_s)$, the channel is called "narrow band" [12] (Table 1).

Table 1. Delay dispersion values for different environments

Type of environment	Time spread (μs)
Free zone	<0.2
Rural area	1
Mountainous area	30
Suburban area	0.5
Urban area	3
Indoor	0.01

Note that the Doppler effect can be considered as the frequency equivalent of time spreading, and thus define a frequency spreading B_m corresponding to the difference between the largest and the smallest frequency offset inherent multipath. Also T_c is the inverse of the frequency spread $T_c \approx 1/B_m$. The coherence bandwidth is inversely proportional to the statistical delay spread of the channel T_m [13]:

$$B_c = \frac{K_2}{T_m} \qquad (9)$$

where K_2: a constant depending on the environment.

5.3   The Selective Channel and the Non-selective Frequency Channel

5.3.1   The Non-selective Frequency Channel

A channel said to be non frequency selective when $B_s \leq B_c$ or B_s is the band of the symbol. In this case, the amplitude and the phase of all the spectral components of a signal are affected in the same way by the channel, also called a flat channel [10]. The variation in the time domain is very much related to the movement of the transmitter or the receiver which introduces a spread in the frequency domain known as "Doppler Shift". If $B_s < B_c$ implies $T_s > T_c$: the signal is subject to fast fading.

5.3.2   The Frequency Selective Channel

Unlike the non-frequency selective channel, the channel is called frequency-selective when the spectral components of the signal are affected inhomogeneously by the propagation channel. The signal is subject to slow fading phenomenon if $T_s \ll T_c$ and $B_s \gg B_c$[14].

From Fig. 6 we deduce that to ensure non-selectivity, both in frequency and in time, we must simply comply with the condition [15]:

$$T_m \ll T_s \ll T_c \qquad (10)$$

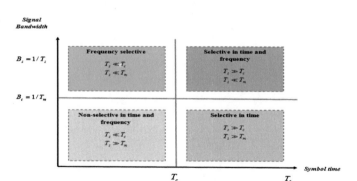

Fig. 6. Frequency and time selectivity

6   The Transmission Channels Width Fading

A channel with fading of the signal is mainly due to an echo-rich propagation environment and therefore characterized by multipath numbers, but also the relative movement of the transmitter and receiver resulting in channel time variations (Fig. 7).

A variation of a channel model with fading affecting the signal is described by the equation:

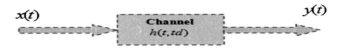

Fig. 7. Model of a fading channel

$$y(t) = h(t; td) * x(t) \tag{11}$$

where $y(t)$ is the received signal, $x(t)$ is the transmit signal, and $h(t; td)$ follows a Rice or Rayleigh distribution [9].

6.1   Rice Distribution

This model is used to characterize a fading propagation environment comprising a direct view between the transmitter and the receiver, and a multitude of incoherent paths due to the broadcasters of the environment. The probability density of the amplitude of the complex coefficient of the channel follows a law of Rice [16]:

$$f(x) = \frac{x}{\sigma^2} e - (x^2 + A^2)/2\sigma^2 \cdot I_0 \left(\frac{x \cdot A}{\sigma^2} \right) \tag{12}$$

A: The amplitude of the direct path. σ^2: Variance (the power of in-phase components and quadrature components). σ: The standard deviation. $I_0(\cdot)$: is the modified Bessel function of the first kind of order 0.

Rice's law is characterized by the Rice k factor, which represents the ratio of the main path power to the average multipath power of the scattered component. It is between 0 and $+\infty$.

$$K = \frac{\text{Direct path power}}{\text{Multipath Power}} = \frac{A^2}{2\sigma^2}$$

Rice's distribution according to the Rice K factor is [17]:

$$f(x) = \frac{x}{\sigma^2} e^{-\left(\frac{x^2}{2\sigma^2} + k \right)} \cdot I_0 \left(\frac{x}{\sigma} \sqrt{2K} \right) \quad \text{for } x > 0 \tag{13}$$

The average of Rice's distribution is given by:

$$E(x) = e^{-k/2} \sqrt{\left(\frac{\pi.x}{2k+2} \right)} \left[(1+k) \cdot I_0 \left(\frac{k}{2} \right) + k \cdot I_1 \left(\frac{k}{2} \right) \right] \tag{14}$$

I_1 represents the modified Bessel function of the first order.

The power is defined by: $P = \frac{1}{2} E(x^2)$, The moment of order 2 is given by:

$$E(x^2) = 2\sigma^2 + b_0^2 \tag{15}$$

With: $b_0^2 = \frac{k \cdot E(x^2)}{k+1}$ And: $\sigma^2 = \frac{E(\sigma^2)}{2k+2}$.

Therefore:

$$f(x) = (k+1) \cdot e^{-\frac{xk}{p}} e^{\frac{(k+1)x^2}{2p}} \cdot I_0\sqrt{x \cdot \frac{2k^2+2k}{p}} \quad \text{For } p \geq 0 \tag{16}$$

By posing: $r = \frac{R\sqrt{2}}{E_0}$ and $a = \frac{A\sqrt{2}}{E_0}$.

Where R is the amplitude of the total field. Therefore:

$$p(r) = r \exp\left(-\frac{r^2+a^2}{2}\right) \cdot I_0(ar) \tag{17}$$

The calculations for this expression were made by Rice who plotted the curves for different values of a (Fig. 8).

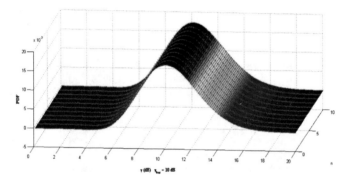

Fig. 8. Rician PDF with Average SNR = 10 dB

When the mobile is well clear, which corresponds to a very large, the field received is essentially due to the direct wave [12]. Note that when $K = 0$ the distribution of Rice becomes a Rayleigh distribution, and reflects the fading of the specular component. Conversely, if K tends to infinity, the channel becomes without fading and the transmission is just on additive white Gaussian noise [18].

6.2 Rayleigh Distribution

This is the distribution used to model the fading due to incoherent multipath when the transmitter and the receiver are not in direct view. It is one of the most common propagation channels in dense urban environments [14]. Since $h(\tau;t)$ can be modeled by complex Gaussian random processes, this implies that envelope $|h(\tau,t)|$ follows a

Rayleigh distribution and phase $\arg(h(\tau,t))$ follows a uniform distribution over $[0, 2\pi]$. The channel modeled by a Rayleigh distribution is given by [19]:

$$f(x) = \frac{x}{\sigma^2} e^{-\left(\frac{x^2}{2\sigma^2}\right)} \quad x \geq 0 \tag{18}$$

The first and second order moments of a Rayleigh variable are given by [13]:

$$E(x) = \sqrt{\frac{\pi}{2}} \cdot \sigma \quad E(x^2) = 2 \cdot \sigma \cdot S^2 \tag{19}$$

This model leads to deeper than the observed reality fadings, except in the most severe conditions of the urban environment. In these conditions, $E_z = E_r = E_c \cos 2\pi ft - E_s \sin 2\pi ft$; E_c and E_s are Gaussian processes with zero mean value (assuming the φ_i-distributed $[0, 2\pi]$). The E_i contributions are independent, and the mean squared Value of E_c and E_s is equal to $1/2\,E_0^2$. The power is (Fig. 9):

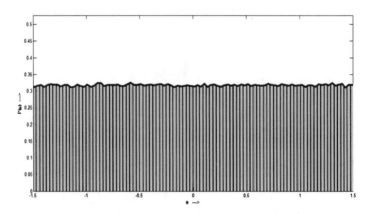

Fig. 9. Simulated PDF of phase of Rayleigh distribution

$$p(x) = E(x^2) = 2\sigma^2 = 1 \tag{20}$$

The probability of error at fixed average power is much higher because of the probability of fading [20]:

$$P_{err} = \int_0^\infty p(\gamma) \cdot p(\gamma)d\gamma = \frac{1}{2}\left[1 - \sqrt{\frac{\Gamma}{1-\Gamma}}\right] \tag{21}$$

And $\Gamma = E(\gamma(t)) = E\left(|\alpha(t)|^2\right)\frac{E_b}{N_0} = \frac{E_b}{N_0}$.

6.3 Distribution of Nakagami-M

In most cases, the Rayleigh and Rice distributions are sufficient to characterize the fading distribution of the signals received in a mobile radio channel [17]. For example, if the channel is characterized by two paths of comparable powers and stronger than the others, the statistical expression of the received signal can no longer be approximated by the Rice distribution [21] (Fig. 10).

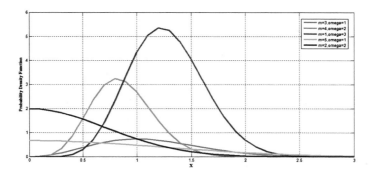

Fig. 10. Density of probability of fading of a Nakagami channel

This distribution is referred to as "Nakagami-m distribution" whose probability density is given by [22]:

$$p(r) = \frac{2}{\Gamma(m)} \left(\frac{m}{\Omega}\right)^m r^{2m-1} \exp\left(-\frac{m}{\Omega} r^2\right), \quad r \geq 0.5 \tag{22}$$

where $\Gamma(m)$ is the gamma function, $\Omega = E\{r^2\}$ is the root mean square value and m is the fade parameter.

$$m = \frac{E^2\{r^2\}}{Var\{r^2\}} \tag{23}$$

7 Simulation and Analysis of the Results

The realistic description of the propagation channel in complex environment requires the use of appropriate modeling. Channel modeling methods can be divided into types: statistical modeling and deterministic modeling. Statistical modeling of the radio propagation channel consists of extracting the average behavior of the channel, based on signals generally derived from measurement campaigns. It thus reflects the influence of the channel on a link, using statistical tools (Fig. 11).

It is considered more often than the time variation of the channel in the case of flat type fading follows a Rayleigh distribution. On the other hand, Rice's distribution can

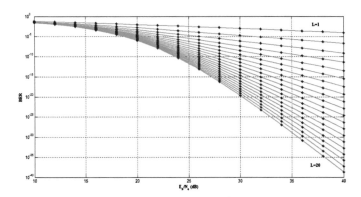

Fig. 11. Quadrature amplitude modulation through a fading channel with a diversity order ranging from 1 to 20

describe small-scale fading on the signal level. The validity of a statistical model depends on the quantity and especially the reliability of the initial data used to establish it. A statistical model is all the more reliable as a large number of initial data will have been used to obtain it (Fig. 12).

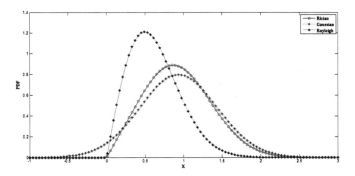

Fig. 12. Probability density function of a Gaussian, Rice and Rayleigh channel–medium SNR

Deterministic modeling is most often likened to the use of a simulation tool that can predict the signal received for a given link. The modeling done is specific to the simulated environment. Sometimes the signals used for statistical modeling come from deterministic modeling (Fig. 13).

Indeed, the simulation tools must be validated to ensure the relevance of the signals generated and the results obtained. The validation is made from measurement campaigns. Conversely, the measures constitute globalization of a set of phenomena modifying the signal as it passes through the channel. Deterministic modeling tools can therefore be used to better extract the different phenomena involved in the case of a measurement (Fig. 14).

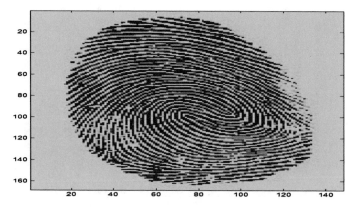

Fig. 13. Original input image

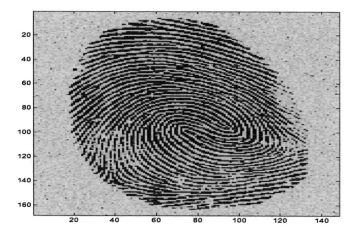

Fig. 14. Gaussian noise/Rayleigh noise

If in some cases, channels without similar, we note that depending on the transmission channel model used and the type of modulation used the performance vary considerably. All tend towards a channel without fading when their parameters increase. For M-ary modulations, for any channel model, the probability of error per symbol increases when the modulation used requires a lot of state (Fig. 15).

At the reception level, maximum likelihood and maximum after-effects are equivalent when the symbols are equiprobable. These techniques are then combined and the choice on the detection of a symbol is based on its probability of appearance in the respond of the different other symbols (Fig. 16).

The most frequently used channel model in digital transmissions, which is also one of the easiest to generate and analyze, is the additive white Gaussian noise channel. This noise models both noises of internal origin and noise from external sources. This model is however rather associated with a wired transmission, since it represents an almost perfect transmission from the transmitter to the receiver (Fig. 17).

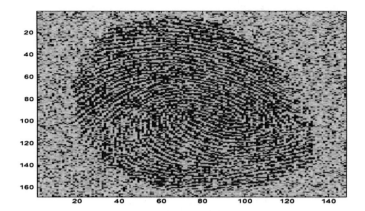

Fig. 15. Rician noise

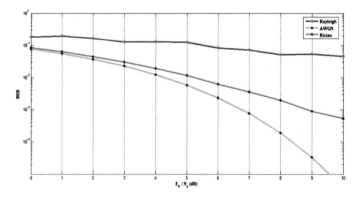

Fig. 16. Denoised Signal

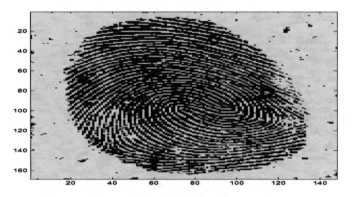

Fig. 17. Bit error rate in a Gaussian channel, Rayleigh channel and Rice channel

The model of the white Gaussian noise channel (AWGN) is compound according to the principle of Fig. 2 of a white Gaussian noise added to the modulated wave. The specificity of a white noise lies in the uniformity of its spectral power density over the entire frequency band. Due to its bandwidth theoretically infinite, it is difficult to express the white noise, so it is assumed that the noise summed with the receiver input signal has been filtered by an ideal filter, width great band to the useful band. The white Gaussian noise is a function whose frequency components have the same magnitude, while the amplitude of the function itself at each moment is distributed according to a normal distribution. Figure 12 represents the probability density of white Gaussian noise with a zero mean value.

8 Conclusion

This paper aims to study the link performance in environments with both the fast fading and shadowing. Among the many works dealing with the performance evaluation of digital communications, there are few that take into account the short-term effects of the channel and the long-term effects. We were mainly interested in fast fading channels and in the presence of shadowing. Fading directly impacts the system's short-term performance and changes the probability of error. Indeed, over a relatively short period of time compared to the duration of a whole communication, the average power received at the receiver will not vary significantly. In this case, the link performance is characterized by the average error probability.

Acknowledgements. We would like to thank the CNRST of Morocco (I 012/004) for support.

References

1. Cotton, S.L., Scanlon, S.G.: Characterization and modeling of the indoor radio cannel at 868 MHz for a mobile body worn wireless personal area network (2007)
2. Gorcin, A., Arslan, H.: Identification of OFDM signals under multipath fading channels. In: IEEE Military Communications Conference, Orlando (2012)
3. Dixit, S., Katiyar, H.: Performance of OFDM in time selective multipath fading channel in 4G systems (2015)
4. Chin, W.L., Kao, C.W., Qian, Y.: Spectrum sensing of OFDM signals over multipath fading channels and practical considerations for cognitive radios. IEEE Sens. J. (2016)
5. Magableh, A.M., Matalgah, M.M.: Accurate closed-form approximations for the BER of multi-branch amplify-and-forward cooperative systems with MRC in Rayleigh fading channel. WSEAS Trans. Commun. **12** (2013)
6. Kumar, S., Sharma, S.: Error probability of different modulation schemes for OFDM based WLAN standard IEEE. Int. J. Eng. (2010)
7. Li, Y.: Pilot-symbol-aided channel estimation for OFDM in wireless systems. IEEE Trans. Veh. Technol. (2000)
8. Gupta, A.: Improving channel estimation in OFDM system using time domain channel estimation for time correlated Rayleigh fading channel model. Int. J. Eng. Sci. Invent. (2013)
9. Prasad, R.: OFDM for wireless communication system (2004)

10. Manhas, P., Soni, M.K.: Comparison of OFDM system in terms of BER using different transform and channel coding. Eng. Manuf. (2016)
11. Zhang, X., Yu, H., Wei, G.: J. Wireless Commun. Network (2010)
12. Inlays, A., Ansari, E.A., Akhtar, S.: Accurate BER analysis and performance of different modulation schemes over wireless fading channels (2013)
13. Babich, F., Lombardi, G.: Statistical analysis and characterization of the indoor propagation channel. IEEE Trans. Commun. (2000)
14. Pavlović, D.C., Sekulović, N.M., Milovanović, G.V., Panajotović, A.S., Stefanović, M.C.: Statistics for ratios of Rayleigh, Rician, Nakagami-, and Weibull Distributed random variables (2013)
15. Pop, M.F., Beaulieu, N.C.: Limitations of sum-of Sinusoids fading channel simulators. IEEE Trans. Commun. (2001)
16. Wang, W., Ottosson, T., Sternad, M., Ahlén, A., Svensson, A: Impact of multiuser diversity and channel variability on adaptive OFDM. In: Proceedings of the IEEE Vehicular Technology Conference (2003)
17. Sofotasios, P.C., Fikadu, M.K., Muhaidat, S., Cui, Q., George, K.: Full-duplex regenerative relaying and energy-efficiency optimization over generalized asymmetric fading channels (2017)
18. Ryu, J., Lee, J.K., Lee, S.-J., Kwon, T.: Revamping the IEEE 802.11a PHY simulation models (2008)
19. Mohammed, A.A., Yu, L., Al-Kali, M., Adam, E.E.B.: BER analysis and evaluated for different channel models in wireless cooperation networks based OFDM system. In: Fourth International Conference on Communication Systems and Network Technologies, Bhopal (2014)
20. Laleh, N., Chintha, T.: BER analysis of arbitrary QAM for MRC diversity with imperfect channel estimation in generalized Rician fading channels, July 2006
21. Schlenker, J., Cheng, J., Schober, R.: Asymptotically tight error rate bounds for EGC in correlated generalized Rician fading. In: IEEE International Conference on Communications (2013)
22. Salahat, E., Saleh, H.: Novel average bit error rate analysis of generalized fading channels subject to additive white generalized Gaussian noise. In: IEEE Global Conference on Signal and Information Processing (2014)

Novel Configuration of Radio over Fiber System Using a Hybrid SAC-OCDMA/OFDM Technique

K. S. Alaoui[1(✉)], Y. Zouine[2], and J. Foshi[1]

[1] LEIMP: Laboratory Electronics, Instrumentation and Measurement Physics, Faculty of Science and Technology, Errachidia, Morocco
kaoutarsaidi@gmail.com
[2] ISET Laboratory, National School of Applied Sciences, ENSA of Kenitra, Ibn Tofail University Kenitra, Kenitra, Morocco

Abstract. Radio over fiber technology will play an important role in solving problems facing wireless technology. Envisaging a global village, people could transmit and receive "anytime, anywhere, and anything". In addition, the explosive growth in internet applications such as the World Wide Web, demonstrates the tremendous increase in bandwidth and low power that the coming world of multimedia interactive applications will require from future networks. ROF technology uses multicarrier modulation like orthogonal frequency division multiplexing (OFDM), which provides an opportunity of having an increased in bandwidth together with an affordable cost and this idea has recently become a suitable topic for many research works. On the other hand, SAC-OCDMA (Spectral Amplitude Coding Optical Code Division Multiple Access) technique is able to enhance the data rate of system and increase the number of user. In this paper we introduce a ROF link using a hybrid OFDM/SAC-OCDMA technique.

Keywords: Radio over fiber · SAC-OCDMA · OFDM · Access network

1 Introduction

The next generation of cellular mobile phone systems will make extensive use of microcells. This will permit a large increase in the numbers of users and will also allow a significant increase in the available channel bandwidth, so that broadband services can be offered, in addition to the voiceband services offered with current systems. The introduction of large numbers of microcells will result in the need to interconnect huge numbers of cells and microcells, and this can be carried out effectively using optical fiber, which offers a high transmission capacity at low cost [1]. Radio over fiber systems have many advantages and applications such as:

© Springer Nature Switzerland AG 2019
M. Ezziyyani (Ed.): AI2SD 2018, AISC 915, pp. 135–144, 2019.
https://doi.org/10.1007/978-3-030-11928-7_12

Advantages	Applications	
	Indoor	Outdoor
• Enhanced microcellular coverage • Higher capacity • Lower cost • Lower power • Easier installation	• Airport terminals • Shopping centers • Large offices,	• Underground • Tunnels • Narrow streets • Highways

ROF technology uses multicarrier modulation like orthogonal frequency division multiplexing (OFDM), which offers an opportunity of increasing a bandwidth together with an reasonable cost and this idea has recently become a suitable topic for many research works [2, 3]. Due to its less Inter Symbol Interference (ISI), computational complexity and more robustness as compared to other multiplexing schemes and Orthogonal Frequency Division Multiplexing (OFDM) has been extensively used in wireless communication. OFDM dominated in wireless broadcast system such as Wi-Fi and WiMAX because of its robustness to multipath fading and high sub-carrier density through the digital FFT and IFFT [4]. Optical code-division multiple-access (OCDMA) techniques are also suggested to be a more flexible solution in optical local area networks because multiple users are able to access the network asynchronously and simultaneously.

In recent years, spectral amplitude coding(SAC) scheme of optical CDMA has been introduced to eliminate the MAI effect and preserve the orthogonality between the users in the system. Several quasi-orthogonal code families are used in such spectral amplitude coded optical CDMA (SAC-OCDMA) systems.

In this paper we introduce a ROF link using a hybrid OFDM/SAC-OCDMA technique to achieve a high- speed data rate and large bandwidth.

2 Radio over Fiber Technology

Radio-over-Fiber (RoF) technology entails the use of optical fiber links to distribute radio frequency signals from a central location (headend) to Remote Antenna Units (RAUs). In narrowband communication systems and WLANs, RF signal processing functions such as frequency up-conversion, carrier modulation, and multiplexing, are performed at the BS or the RAP, and immediately fed into the antenna. RoF makes it possible to centralize the RF signal processing functions in one shared location (headend), and then to use optical fiber, which offers low signal loss (0.3 dB/km for 1550 nm, and 0.5 dB/km for 1310 nm wavelengths) to distribute the RF signals to the RAUs, as shown in Fig. 1. The centralization of RF signal processing functions enables equipment sharing, dynamic allocation of resources, and simplified system operation and maintenance. These benefits can translate into major system installation and operational savings [1], especially in wide-coverage broadband wireless communication systems, where a high density of BS/RAPs is necessary as discussed above.

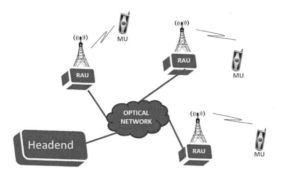

Fig. 1. The radio over fiber system concept (RAU: Remote Antenna Units, MU: Mobile Units)

3 OFDM

OFDM is used extensively in broadband wired and wireless communication systems because it is an effective solution to inter Symbol interference (ISI) caused by a dispersive channel. Very recently, a number of papers have described the use of OFDM in a range of optical systems including optical wireless, multimode fiber and single mode fiber.

In practice, OFDM systems are applied using a combination of Fast Fourier Transform (FFT) and Inverse Fast Fourier Transform (IFFT) blocks as shown in Fig. 2.

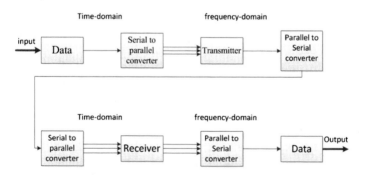

Fig. 2. Block diagram of a simple OFDM system

An OFDM system considers the source symbols at the transmitter side (e.g. QAM or PSK symbols that can be presented in a single carrier system) to be in the frequency-domain. These symbols are used as inputs to an IFFT block that transfers the signal into time-domain. If the number of subcarriers used in the system is N then the IFFT takes in N symbols as an input at a time with a time period T second. The basic functions for an IFFT are N orthogonal sinusoids. These sinusoids each have a different frequency. Each of those input symbol behaves like a complex value for the corresponding sinusoidal basis function. And the output of the IFFT is the summation of all N sinusoids. After that the output of the IFFT block passed through a digital-to-analog (D/A) converter and employed to modulate the carrier which results in the ODFM signal. And this process can be expected as an easy way to modulate data onto N orthogonal subcarriers. And at the receiver, an FFT block is used to bring the received signal it back into the frequency domain. The received signal is initially down converted to the baseband signal and then passed through an analog-to-digital (A/D) converter in order to get the digitized values. The digital values is again portioned into blocks of length N and demodulated block by block by the FFT. Thus the original symbols are generated that were sent as inputs to the transmitter IFFT block. When the FFT output samples are plotted in the complex plane, they will from a constellation (such as QPSK, QAM, etc.) [5].

4   SAC-OCDMA

In OCDMA systems, each user is given one code word for distinctness. The main factor of performance degradation in optical code-division multiple-access (CDMA) systems is the multiuser access interference (MAI). In spectral-amplitude- coding (SAC) systems, MAI is solely a function of the in-phase cross correlations among the address sequences (also known as signature sequences or spreading sequence or simply code sequences). If the in-phase cross correlation among the address sequences is fixed, then the balanced detection receiver is able to suppress MAI completely.

In SAC-OCDMA systems, each user is assigned with a sequence code that serves as its address. A user modulates its code with each data bit and asynchronously initiates transmission. Thus, this modifies its spectrum appearance, in a way recognizable only by the intended receiver Fig. 3. Let $\lambda = \sum_{i=1}^{N} x_i y_i$ as the in-phase cross correlation of two different sequences $X = (x_1, x_2, \ldots, x_N)$ and $(Y = y_1, y_2, \ldots, y_N)$. A code with length N, weight w and in-phase cross correlation λ can be denoted by (N,w,λ) [6]. The code is considered possess an ideal in-phase cross correlation when $\lambda = 1$.

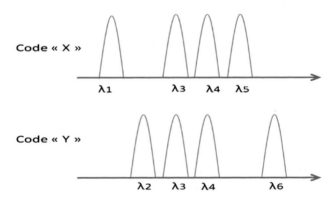

Fig. 3. Codes example for SAC-OCDMA

The balanced detection receiver is able to suppress MAI completely, provided that the family of codes used satisfies the following property: $\lambda_{XY} = \lambda_{\overline{X}Y}$, λ_{XY} is the in-phase cross-correlation function between the codes of the desired user X and that of an undesired user Y. $\overline{X}$ is a sequence complementary to X.

5 System Design

The system design consists of three main parts which are the transmission part, the transmission link and the receiver part.

Figure 4 shows the block diagram of the Radio over Fiber link using hybrid OFDM/SAC-OCDMA system.

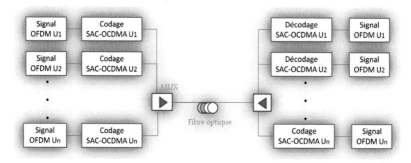

Fig. 4. The block diagram of the RoF link using hybrid OFDM/SAC-OCDMA

The proposed configuration combines SAC-OCDMA technology and OFDM. For the transmission part the OFDM signal based on 16-QAM is generated. The OFDM subcarriers with independent unipolar digital signal are optically modulated onto the code sequence using an optical modulator. The data streams are orthogonal to each other in both code chips and subcarriers, which cannot only eliminate the crosstalk between the sub-channels, but also ensure the security of the data. In RoF link using hybrid OFDM/SAC-OCDMA system, each user is allocated with one sub-channel including one specific code chip and one or more subcarriers. The subcarriers can be used for different services, such as voice/video signal, point to point (P2P) and WiMax signals. Then the modulated code sequences are combined together and transmitted through the optical fiber link.

At the receiver, an optical splitter is used to separate the different modulated code sequences to different optical network users. Then, the resulting signal is detected by the photodetector to convert optical signal to electrical signal, OFDM receiver module which decodes an electrical QAM- OFDM signal as generated by transmitter block (Fig. 5).

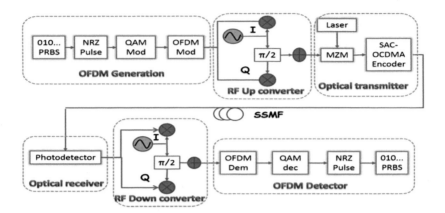

Fig. 5. The proposed configuration combines SAC-OCDMA and OFDM

The proposed configuration contains the Optical transmitter situated at the Headend or Central Office (CO) and several Remote Antenna Units, comprises an Optical Network Units (ONUs) and antennas, located at some particular distant location. Here the Optical transmitter comprises the fundamental blocks of RF OFDM transmitter and a RF-to-Optical (RTO) up-converter. And after passing through the optical link each ONU includes an optical-to-RF (OTR) down-converter and a RF OFDM receiver.

In the RF OFDM transmitter, the input digital data are first converted from serial to parallel block of bits consisting of information symbol where each symbol comprise multiple bits of M-ary coding. And, in our proposed model we used M-ary QAM for constellation. The time domain OFDM signal is obtained through Inverse Fast Fourier Transform (IFFT). The baseband OFDM signal can be up-converted to a RF passband through a RF IQ mixer. The subsequent RTO up-converter transforms the baseband signal to the optical domain using an optical IQ modulator comprising a Mach-Zehnder-modulator (MZM) with a 90-degree phase offset. Then finally the optical signal is transmitted through a standard single mode fiber (SSMF).

At the receiving end the optical signal travelling through the SSMF is converted back to RF OFDM signal by the OTR down-converter. The received RF signal is detected by a PIN photodetector which converts the optical signal to an electrical one. Besides the PIN photodetector the ONU also contains a digital I-Q demux, followed by an FFT (Figs. 6, 7 and 8).

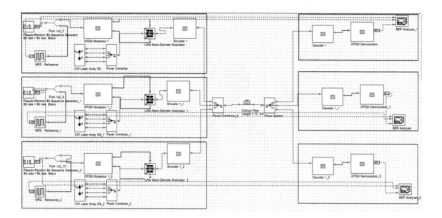

Fig. 6. The propose system architecture

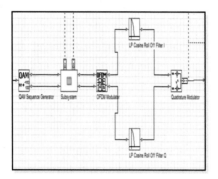

Fig. 7. OFDM modulator

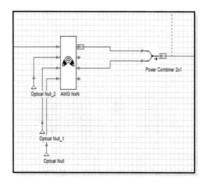

Fig. 8. Encoder SAC-OCDMA

RF signal at the output of the OFDM modulator.

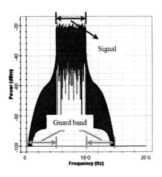

Table 1 show the Bipolar Walsh Hadamard code with a code length of 4 and showing which wavelength should be chosen.

Table 1. Walsh Hadamard codes

Walsh Hadamard codes for 3 users	Chosen wavelength
1010	$\lambda_1\lambda_3$
1100	$\lambda_1\lambda_2$
1001	$\lambda_1\lambda_4$

Knowing that: $\lambda 1 = 193.1$ Thz, $\lambda 2 = 193.2$ Thz, $\lambda 3 = 193.3$ Thz, $\lambda 4 = 193.4$ Thz. Figures 9 and 10 show the different optical carriers emitted by the lasers.

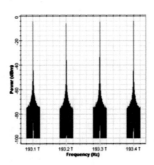

Fig. 9. The different optical carriers

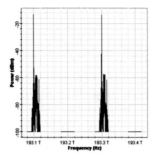

Fig. 10. The first user SAC-OCDMA optical signal

On reception, the photodetector detects the light and transforms it into an electrical signal before demodulating the signal. The low-pass filter has been set up to eliminate the high frequencies. Thereafter the amplifier limited in gain for the purpose of amplifying the signal, finally down to a baseband signal but it is noisy, the latter comes from the electronic and optoelectronic components. To reduce the impact of this noise, another low-pass filter is used.

The received OFDM signal after decoding (Figs. 11 and 12).

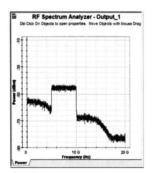

Fig. 11. The received OFDM signal after decoding

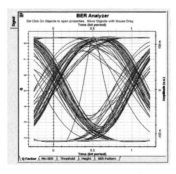

Fig. 12. Diagram of the eye user 1

6   Conclusion

In this paper we proposed a hybrid radio over fiber link based on various modulation schemes and simulated through a fiber optic. Previous research works related to PON derived bit error rate (BER) from the measured vector magnitude and compared the performance among different modulation techniques but never showed the performance for both OFDM and SAC-OCDMA together. But in our paper we investigate the performances of ROF link using a hybrid OFDM/SAC- OCDMA technique.

References

1. Wake, D.: Radio over fiber systems for mobile applications. In: Al-Raweshidy, H., Komaki, S. (eds.) Radio over Fiber Technologies for Mobile Communications Networks. Artech House, Inc., USA (2002)
2. Lin, Y.M.: Demonstration and design of high spectral efficiency 4 Gb/s OFDM system in passive optical networks. In: Proceedings of OFC, Anaheim, USA, Paper OThD7 (2007)
3. Duong, T., Genay, N., Pizzinat, A., Charbonnier, B., Chanclou, P., Kazmierski, C.: Low cost multi band-OFDM for remote modulation of colourless ONU in hybrid WDM/TDM-PON architecture. In: Proceedings of ECOC, Berlin, Germany, Paper 5.4.2   (2007)
4. Hara, S.: Multicarrier Techniques for 4G Mobile Communications. Artech House, Norwood, MA, Incorporated (2003)
5. Nowshin, N., Arifuzzman, A.K.M., Tarique, M.: Demonstration and performance analysis of ROF based OFDM-PON system for next generation fiber optic communication. Int. J Comput. Netw. Commun. (IJCNC) 4(1), 193 (2012). https://doi.org/10.5121/ijcnc.2012.4114
6. Zouine, Y., Madini, Z.: Analyse des performances de plusieurs codes pour un système W-OCDMA d'un reseau EPON

A Hybrid Multilingual Sentiment Classification Using Fuzzy Logic and Semantic Similarity

Youness Madani[(✉)], Mohammed Erritali, and Jamaa Bengourram

Faculty of Sciences and Technics, Sultan Moulay Slimane University,
Beni Mellal, Morocco
younesmadani9@gmail.com, m.erritali@usms.ma, bengoram@yahoo.fr

Abstract. Classifying tweets into classes (Positive, Negative or neutral) or extracting their sentiments know in recent years a great development, and researchers try to find new methods and approaches that give good results. In this paper, we propose a new hybrid approach based on the semantic similarity using the WordNet dictionary and the fuzzy logic with its three important steps (Fuzzification, Rule Inference/aggregation and Defuzzification) for classifying tweets into three classes: positive, negative or neutral. The experimental results show that our approach outperforms some other methods from the literature.

Keywords: Opinion mining · Sentiment analysis · Twitter · Fuzzy logic · Information retrieval systems · Semantic similarity · Wordnet · Big data · Hadoop

1 Introduction

Nowadays, many people post feedbacks about a product or services on the Internet (Social Networks, Forums, e-commerce website ... etc.). These customer feedbacks contain a lot of information. By extracting information, companies can improve quality of products or services or even can launch new products or services. To extract information from feedbacks, it first needed to classify according to sentiments it contains which commonly known as sentiment classification or sentiment analysis.

Sentiment Analysis (SA) sometimes called opinion mining is a process that consists of analysing a text to extract opinions, emotions, attitudes and assign a relevant sentiment usually positive, negative or neutral, sometimes it tries to give to a document or a sentence (review) a degree of importance (polarity). This process can use the natural language processing through a combination of pre-processing steps, the statistical methods (Lexicon-based approach, corpus-based approach ...) and also the machine learning classification techniques. Sentiment classification is performed at three levels: document level, sentence level and feature level, and in each one of this three levels, SA makes either a subjectivity classification or an objectivity classification.

© Springer Nature Switzerland AG 2019
M. Ezziyyani (Ed.): AI2SD 2018, AISC 915, pp. 145–158, 2019.
https://doi.org/10.1007/978-3-030-11928-7_13

Among variety of social media networks Twitter (which launched in 2006) is the popular microblogging website with over 328 millions of active users per month and about 500 million tweets per day in over 40 languages, messages are limited to 140 characters and are known under the name tweets and may include text, URLs, other user mentions and hashtag metadata to messages, these tweets represent the users opinions and thoughts expressed in short and simple messages. Twitter gives everyone the power to create and share ideas and information instantly and without hindrance.[1]

Many works from the literature use the machine learning algorithms and also some statistical techniques, and all these methods treat the classification of sentiment in a "black-and-white" manner, while in reality sentiments are rarely clear-cut and contain imprecise data, ambiguity or vagueness and may belong to multiple classes, from that we use in our work the Fuzzy Logic with its different steps (fuzzification, fuzzy rules inference, Defuzzification). Fuzzy logic can well deal with vagueness and ambiguity and it is similar to natural language and natural thinking, which is close to human brains.

Fuzzy logic idea is similar to the human being's feeling and inference process, Fuzzy logic is an approach of computing based on "degrees of truth" rather than the usual "true or false" (1 or 0) Boolean logic on which the modern computer is based. The theory of fuzzy logic is mainly aimed at turning a black and white problem into a grey problem, in the context of set theory, deterministic logic is corresponding to crisp sets, the idea of fuzzy logic was invented by Professor L. A. Zadeh of the University of California at Berkeley in 1965.

In this paper we propose a new approach to classify tweets into three classes (positive, negative and neutral) using a proposed hybrid approach based on Fuzzy logic and the concepts of information retrieval systems with the use of the semantic similarity.

Our work will be divided into a number of parts, the first concerning the extraction of the tweets from Twitter using a Twitter API and storing them in database. And after the storage step the second one concern the application of Natural Language Processing (NLP) Methods and the extraction of the opinion words. And finally, the classification of the stored tweets into three classes: positive, negative and neutral, by applying our proposed approach.

The rest of this paper is organised as follows: Sect. 2 presents literature review, in Sect. 3 we will describe our Research methodology (the different text preprocessing methods exist in the litterature, how we collect the tweet, how we classify tweets using our proposed method). Section 4 presents the experimental results and finally, in Sect. 5 it is the conclusion and the perspectives.

2   Literature Review

The classifiers based on ML techniques treat the classification of sentiment in a "black-and-white" manner, while in reality sentiment is rarely clear-cut, most of the previous works focus on the methods of deterministic algorithms without

---

[1] https://about.twitter.com/fr/company.

considering fuzziness of the sentiments. Reality is always far from optimistic. Firstly, sentiment terms are fuzzy. The same word can explain different sentiment orientations even in the same domain. Secondly, sentiments of human are many times fuzzy. For instance, one may use one word to express more than one feeling at the same time.

In recent years, fuzzy approaches have started to emerge for text processing and sentiment analysis, although that the number of papers lies to fuzzy logic still until today a little compared to the papers that use ML techniques or statistical approaches, in the literature, we find some works that use Fuzzy logic in the sentiment analysis.

Authors in [1] proposed a fuzzy computing model to identify the polarity of Chinese sentiment words. This paper is mainly embodied in three aspects, the first consist of computing the sentiment intensity of sentiment morphemes and sentiment words using three existing Chinese sentiment lexicons, secondly authors of this article constructed a fuzzy sentiment classifier and a corresponding classification function of the fuzzy classifier by virtue of fuzzy sets theory and the principle of maximum membership degree, and Thirdly they constructed four sentiment words datasets to demonstrate the performance of their model.

Another work that uses fuzzy sets in sentiment analysis is that presented in [2], in this article the authors introduced a new fuzzy logic based approach for the text classification especially the classification of Twitter's message, inputs used in the proposed fuzzy logic-based model are multiple useful features extracted from each Twitter's message. The output is its degree of relevance for each message to an event called "Sandy", for that, they used a number of fuzzy rules and the different defuzzification methods existing in the literature and for the fuzzification, they selected the trapezoidal-shaped membership function because it is simple and commonly used. The proposed fuzzy system in this work has as inputs 7 linguistic variables and as outputs 1 linguistic variable wich is the relevance of the tweet with sandy. As experimental results, they compared five commonly used defuzzification methods, and they conclude that the centroid method is more effective and efficient than the other methods. Additionally, they conducted a comparison with the well-known keyword search method and the results reveal that the proposed fuzzy logic-based approach is more suitable to classify the relevant and irrelevant Twitter's messages.

Dragoni and Petrucci [3] proposed a method that integrates fuzzy logic for the representation of the polarity associated with linguistic features belonging to a particular domain. This paper discussed how linguistic overlaps between domains can be exploited for computing document polarity in a multi-domain environment using Fuzzy models.

Authors of [4] present a hybrid approach to the sentiment analysis problem at the sentence level. This new method uses natural language processing (NLP) as essential techniques, a sentiment lexicon enhanced with the assistance of SentiWordNet, and fuzzy sets to estimate the semantic orientation polarity and its intensity for sentences, which provides a foundation for computing with sentiments. For demonstrating the use of a hybrid approach authors compared their work with two supervised machine learning algorithms: Naive Bayes (NB) and Maximum Entropy (ME). The Experimental Results show that the proposed hybrid method using sentiment lexicons, NLP essential techniques and fuzzy sets, significantly improved the results obtained using Naive Bayes (NB) and Maximum Entropy (ME), with a high level of accuracy (88.02%) and precision (84.24%).

Researchers in the article presented in [5] used Neural Network and Fuzzy sets to improve the quality of sentiment classification. This classification method uses advantages of both fuzzy logic and Neural Network NN to build a classifier. Authors proposed to fuzzify the input reviews to classify using Gaussian Membership function, and they used MAX principle for defuzzification, and for the classification, they used A Multi-layer perceptron back propagation network (MLPBPN).

3   Research Methodology

In this section we going to present the different steps of our work and the methodology of our proposed approach, as we have presented earlier the aim of our work is to classify tweets (sentiment analysis) linked to a domain, product, movie reviews ... etc., we classify each tweet according to three classes: positive, negative and neutral(subjectivity and objectivity classification) using the fuzzy logic system and the semantic similarity (the notions of information retrieval systems). To make our proposed approach we have to implement different steps either in the collection of tweets, the preparation of the tweets (text preprocessing methods) for the classification or in the step of the classification with our proposed hybrid approach.

3.1   Collection of Tweets

The first step of our work that is very important is the step of the collection of the tweets to classify, for that we use a twitter API called Twitter4j[2] that gives us the possibility to retrieve tweets according/linked to a product, a hachtag or a movie review in a specefied time (for example between june 2015 and june 2017), the retrived tweets was after stored in a relational database such as Mysql and after we transform them to HDFS directly using Hadoop Sqoop. Our work can also use the Apache Flume[3] to extract and store the tweets directly in HDFS.

---

[2] Twitter4J (twitter4j.org/) is an unofficial Java library for the Twitter API. With Twitter4J, you can easily integrate your Java application with the Twitter service. Twitter4J is an unofficial library.

[3] https://flume.apache.org/, Flume is a distributed, reliable, and available service for efficiently collecting, aggregating, and moving large amounts of log data. It has a simple and flexible architecture based on streaming data flows. It is robust and fault tolerant with tunable reliability mechanisms and many failover and recovery mechanisms. It uses a simple extensible data model that allows for online analytic application.

For using the Twitter4j API or the Apache Flume we need to create a twitter application [6] that gives as 4 parameters wich is very important for retrieving tweets (Consumer Key, Consumer Secret, Access Token and Access Token Secret).

After we create the twitter application we get parameters such as Access Token, Access Token Secret, Consumer Key (API Key) and Consumer Secret (API Secret), these parameters will be used after by the Twitter4j API or the Apache Flume to collect and to build a dataset of tweets for the analysis (classification step).

3.2   Text Preprocessing Method

After the steps of the collection of tweets and translate those written in another language than English, we have constructed our Multilingual dataset, but before the classification and the application of our proposal, we must make some text pre-processing methods to prepare the tweets for the classification and to delete the noise exist in them. Several works from the literature demonstrate that the application of the text preprocessing methods on the tweets improve the quality of the classification [7], in our work we apply some text preprocessing methods such as:

- Tokenization: Which is the phase of splitting the tweet into terms or tokens by removing white spaces, commas and other symbols etc. This step is very important in our work because we focus on individual words.
- Removing numbers: that not express any emotions or attitudes. In general, numbers are no use when measuring sentiment and are removed from tweets to refine the tweet content.
- Removing Stopword: There is a kind of word called stopword. They are words of common function in a sentence, such as 'a', 'the', ',', 'to', 'at', etc. These words seem useless for the analysis of the Feeling, therefore they should be deleted.
- Removing Punctuations: We dont need pits as characteristics, this are only symbols for separate sentences and words so we delete them from tweets.
- Stemming: Stemming is another very important process. In our work and because we focus on English language we use the Porter stemming [8].
- Effect of negation: we use a list of words which express the negation such as: not, do not, will not, never, cannot, does not ... etc., after classification if the tweet is positive or negative Then we use this type of pre-processing text, the idea is that if the tweet, for example, is positive but contains a negation then it will be negative and vice versa.
- Extraction of opinion words: The important step in the text pre-processing methods in our work is the step of Part-Of-Speech (POS) tags, it is a step that gives us the type of each word in the tweets (Verb, Noun, Adjective, Adverb ...). In this step we use the hypothesis that says that only verb, adverb and adjective can express opinions in a tweet. From this hypothesis,

we decide to delete each word of the tweet that is not a verb, adjective or adverb. In this step, we use the Apache OpenNLP library.[4]

3.3   Semantic Similarity and Our Proposed Method

In this subsection, we will present how we use the semantic similarity in our work to make a hybrid approach with the fuzzy logic concepts. For that, we use the notions of the information retrieval systems (IRS) and some semantic similarity measures.

Our proposed method consists of defining for each tweet to classify two measures: **positivity** and **negativity** by calculating the semantic similarity between the tweet and two opinion documents Dp (positive document) and Dn (negative document), the document Dp contains positive opinion words such as happy, good, exciting, fabulous ... etc., and the document Dn contains negative opinion words such as anger, sadness, fear ... etc.

If we want to compare our work with the concepts of the IRS, the tweet to classify will play the role of the query and the two documents Dp and Dn will play the role of the research's database (corpus), so if we want to classify a tweet it is like we make a query in an IRS to have the desired information from the database. In our work and because we want to make a hybrid approach between the semantic similarity and the fuzzy logic concepts we need to calculate for each tweet the initial crisp values of the input variables that we have named **positivity** and **negativity**.

For calculating the positivity measure of a tweet, we calculate the average of the sum of the semantic similarity between each opinion word of the tweet and each word from the positive document Dp, and because the value of the similarity semantic is between 0 and 1 the positivity of the tweet will be also between 0 and 1.

In the same way, for the negativity measure of a tweet, we calculate the average of the sum of the semantic similarity between each opinion word of the tweet and each word from the negative document Dn, and because the value of the similarity semantic is between 0 and 1 the negativity of the tweet will be also between 0 and 1.

In the literature we find a lot of approaches to calculate the semantic similarity, Wu and Palmer [9] proposed a similarity measure that is based on the following principle: Given an ontology W formed by a set of nodes and a root node R.X and Y is two words of the ontology that we want calculate their similarity. The principle of the similarity calculation is based on two distances (N1 and N2) which separate the nodes X and Y from the root node (R) and the distance between the subsuming concept (CS) or most specific concept (CPS) of X and Y from the node R. Resnik [10] has used the notion of semantic distance in the following way: two concepts are more similar if the value of the semantic distance between them is small. Another method to calculate the semantic

---

[4] The Apache OpenNLP library is a machine learning based toolkit for the processing of natural language text.

similarity is that proposed by Leacock and Chodorow [11] which is based On the length of the shortest path between two synsets of Wordnet. In [12] authors proposed a new measure of semantic similarity, The basic idea of this measure is that if two concepts are linked together by a very short path and which "does not change the direction" then the two concepts are similar.

The choice of the approach from those exists in the literature is very important in our work because it plays an important role when classifying tweets. To facilitate the choice of an approach than another, we try to calculate the semantic similarity between two identical documents and choosing the approach or approaches that give good results. Table 1 illustrates the results obtained. And to implement each approach from those presented earlier we use the semantic dictionnary **WordNet**.

Table 1. Similarity and execution time in msec with different approaches

Approaches	Measurement	
	Similarity	Execution time (ms)
Leacock and Chodorow	0.14	1016
Wu and Palmer	0.13	1297
Resnik	0.04	1360
Jiang Conrath	0.04	1391
Lin	0.02	1344

From Table 1 we remark that the best approach is the Leacock and Chodorow approach which gives the greatest similarity with minimal execution time, also the approach of Wu and Palmer gives good results. So from these results, we decide to calculate the semantic similarity between the tweet and the documents Dp and Dn using the approach of Leacock and Chodorow.

Figure 1 shows how we calculate the positivity and the negativity of a tweet to classify using our proposal.

From Fig. 1, the first thing we need to do is the creation of the two opinion documents Dp and Dn(Dp contains the positive opinion words and Dn contains the negative opinion words) and after the application of the different text pre-processing methods on the tweet to classify (and translate it if it is not written in English) and the extraction of the opinion words, we calculate the semantic similarity using Leacock and Chodorow approach between each opinion word of the tweet and each word of Dp to calculate the positivity measure, and between each opinion word of the tweet and each word of Dn to calculate the negativity measure.

3.4   Proposed Fuzzy Logic System

in this subsection we describe our hybrid sentiment analysis approach based on semantic similarity and the fuzzy logic system (FLS), as presented before,

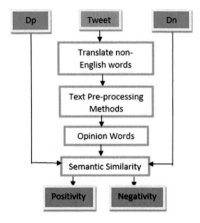

Fig. 1. Calculation of positivity and negativity

the fuzzy logic system begins with a crisp value and after we fuzzify it using different steps (fuzzification, Rules inference) and finally return a crisp value in the output using the defuzzification methods (centroid, Mean/Max...). Figure 2 presents the general structure of a fuzzy logic system.

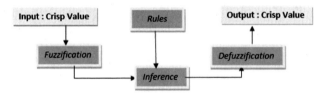

Fig. 2. Fuzzy logic system

From Fig. 2 and as comparaison with our proposed approach, the input (crisp value) of the fuzzy logic system is the two measures (positivity and negativity) calculated using the semantic similarity between the tweet and the two opinion documents, and the output (crisp value) is the class of the tweet (positive, negative or neutral).

So as presented and said earlier the first step in an FLS is the definition of the inputs and the outputs, that is to say, the definition of the linguistic variables in the input and in the output for our proposed FLS. In our case and because we want to classify the tweets according to three classes (positive, negative and neutral), we define two input variables that are the **positivity** and the **negativity** of the tweets, and one output variable which is the class (sentiment) of the tweet to classify.

In an FLS each variable either in the input or in the output is called linguistic variable, and each linguistic variable has a number of values that can take, this values called linguistic terms or the fuzzy sets. So for example in our case we have two linguistic variables in the input that are the positivity and the negativity and each one has three linguistic terms that are **low, moderate and high**, this means that the positivity and the negativity variables can take three possible values (low, moderate and high) or in other words can belong to three different fuzzy sets. In the same way, in the output, we have a linguistic variable that is the class of the tweet and it can also take three different linguistic terms that are positive, negative and neutral.

After we have defined the linguistic variables and their linguistic terms in the input and the output. The next step of our FLS is the definition of the crisp values of the inputs with which we going to begin our approach, for that and as explained in Sect. 4.3, we use the semantic similarity, the notions of the information retrieval system and the different text preprocessing methods to calculate the positivity and the negativity of the tweet that will play the role of input's crisp values.

Fuzzification Step after we calculate the crisp value of each input, the next step is the fuzzification step in which we fuzzify the input variables using the membership function (MF) of each linguistic term, that is calculating the degree of belonging of the input to each fuzzy set (linguistic term), in this work we use two membership functions that are: trapezoidal-shaped MF and the triangular MF.

The trapezoidal-shaped MF is a function that depends on four scalar parameters a, b, c and d, as given by the formula 1:

$$f(x) = \begin{cases} 0 & \text{si } x \leqslant a \\ \dfrac{x-a}{b-a} & \text{si } a \leqslant x \leqslant b \\ 1 & \text{si } b \leqslant x \leqslant c \\ \dfrac{d-x}{d-c} & \text{si } c \leqslant x \leqslant d \\ 0 & \text{si } d \leqslant x \end{cases} \tag{1}$$

On the other hand, the triangular MF is a function that depends on three scalar parameters a, b and c, as given by the formula 2:

$$f(x) = \begin{cases} 0 & \text{si } x \leqslant a \\ \dfrac{x-a}{b-a} & \text{si } a \leqslant x \leqslant b \\ \dfrac{c-x}{c-b} & \text{si } b \leqslant x \leqslant c \\ 0 & \text{si } c \leqslant x \end{cases} \tag{2}$$

In our case, we need to fuzzify the inputs variables using one of the MFs presented earlier, for that we have to define the MF of each linguistic term of the inputs. The linguistic variables "positivity" and "negativity" have three linguistic terms (three fuzzy sets) so we need to define three MFs, one for the fuzzy set "low", one for "moderate" and also another one for "high". The next step to calculate the MFs is the definition of the parameters a, b, c and d for each linguistic term. The choice of these parameters depends on the domain of the application of the FLS and also needs an expert in this domain that has the experiences and the materials to define these parameters, for example in our case and because the inputs "positivity" and "negativity" have values between 0 and 1, the values a, b, c and d will also be in the range [0;1].

After the membership functions were defined for both input and output, the next step is to define the fuzzy control rules.

Rules Inference The next step after the fuzzification of the inputs is the step of the definition and the application of the different rules for our problem, that is to say, combine membership functions with the control rules to derive the fuzzy output. In our work and because we have two inputs and one output with three linguistic terms, we have defined nine fuzzy rules using the IF-THEN model with the AND logic operation between the value of the inputs. The nine rules of our FLS are the following:

- **IF** Positivity is low **AND** Negativity is low **THEN** Class is Neutral.
- **IF** Positivity is moderate **AND** Negativity is moderate **THEN** Class is Neutral.
- **IF** Positivity is high **AND** Negativity is high **THEN** Class is Neutral.
- **IF** Positivity is low **AND** Negativity is moderate **THEN** Class is Negative.
- **IF** Positivity is low **AND** Negativity is high **THEN** Class is Negative.
- **IF** Positivity is moderate **AND** Negativity is high **THEN** Class is Negative.
- **IF** Positivity is moderate **AND** Negativity is low **THEN** Class is Positive.
- **IF** Positivity is high **AND** Negativity is moderate **THEN** Class is Positive.
- **IF** Positivity is high **AND** Negativity is low **THEN** Class is Positive.

After the application of the different rules of our system, the next step is the implication of them to generate the value of the output of each one. In our case and because we use the AND operation between the inputs, the outputs take the minimum value between the inputs. The last step in the rules inference is the aggregation of the results obtained for each output to find one value for each one, for example for the output **neutral** we will find three different values by applying three rules and for finding the final value of the output "neutral" we calculate the maximum of these three values.

Defuzzification After the fuzzification of the inputs and the application of the nine rules of our FLS, we find the degree of belonging of our output (class of the tweet) to each output fuzzy set (positive, negative and neutral) and to find the final result of our FLS that have to be in the form of a crisp value we need to apply the defuzzification step.

The defuzzification process is meant to convert the fuzzy output back to the crisp or classical output to the control objective. The fuzzy conclusion or output is still a linguistic variable, and this linguistic variable needs to be converted to the crisp variable via the defuzzification process.

In this work we use 4 defuzzification techniques that are commonly used, which are:

- **Max-Membership principle**: this method calculates the maximum between the value of belonging of the output to each fuzzy set.
- **Centroid Method**: sometimes called Centre of area or centre of gravity, The Center of Gravity method (COG) is the most popular defuzzification technique and is widely utilized in actual applications. This method is similar to the formula for calculating the center of gravity in physics.
- **Weighted average Method** This method is only valid for symmetrical output membership functions.
- **Mean-Max Method**: This method (also called middle-of-maxima) is closely related to the first method, except that the locations of the maximum membership can be non-unique (i.e., the maximum membership can be a plateau rather than a single point).

After we find the final crisp value of the output (CVO), the final step is to compare the result obtained with three range: tweet is negative if CVO is between 0 and 0.4, it is neutral if CVO is strictly greater than 0.4 and strictly less than 0.6 and it is positive if CVO is between 0.6 and 1.

4   Experimental Results

In this section we going to present some experimental results of our work. As presented earlier the first step consist of conctructing the dataset of tweets (the collection of tweets) using the Twitter4j API and Apache Flume. For that our dataset contains the tweets published between january 2016 and january 2017 and contain the word "Iphone" that is to say we will classify tweets related to the iphone product.

As presented earlier our FLS contains two input variables (positivity and negativity) and one output variable (class of the tweet), the range of each variable is between 0 and 1 and each one has three linguistic terms(linguistic values or fuzzy sets): low, moderate and high for the input variables, and negative, neutral and positive for the output variable.

For calculating the initial values(crisp values) for the inputs we use our proposed approach based on semantic similarity and the notions of information retrieval systems as presented previously. In our FLS we use two membership functions for the fuzzification that are: **Trapezoidal MF** and **Triangular MF**, nine IF-THEN rules and four defuzzification methods(Max-Membership, Centroid, Weighted average, Mean-Max). From that we have eight combination possible for making a choice to which fuzzification/defuzzification methods using in the process of the classification. Table 2 shows the results obtained for the error rate after the classification of the tweets using eight possible combination: Trapezoidal MF/Max-Membership, Trapezoidal MF/Centroid, Trapezoidal MF/Weighted average, Trapezoidal MF/Mean-Max, Triangular MF/Max-Membership, Triangular MF/Centroid, Triangular MF/Weighted average, Triangular MF/Mean-Max.

Table 2. Error rate using differents fuzzification/defuzzification combinations

Fuzzification	Defuzzification	ER (%)
Trapezoidal MF	Max-Membership	23
	Centroid	14
	Weighted average	32
	Mean-Max	23
Triangular MF	Max-Membership	32
	Centroid	25
	Weighted average	23
	Mean-Max	21

From Table 2 the best fuzzification/defuzzification combination is the one in which we have used the Trapezoidal MF for the fuzzification and the Centroid method for the defuzzification with a high classification rate (86%) and a error rate equal to 14%. From these results we use in our proposed FLS the Trapezoidal-shaped MF for fuzzify the inputs and the centroid method for finding the final crisp value of our system.

To demonstrate the results obtained using our proposed approach (A), we compare our method with some other techniques from the litterature such as: a lexicon based approach method based on AFINN dictionnary (B) and Word-Net[?], an approach based on semantic similarity that calculate the degree of the relevance between the tweet to classify and three opinion documents (Approach 1 (C)), an approach that calulate the semantic similarity between each word of the tweet and the words **negative** and **positive** (Approach 2 (D)), an approach based on SentiWordNet dictionnary (E), and finally an hybrid approach based on SentiWordNet and fuzzy logic (F).

Figure 3 shows the results obtained.

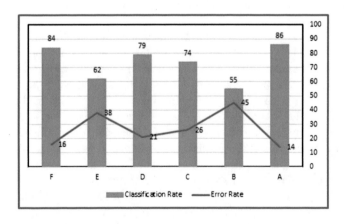

Fig. 3. Comparison results

According to Fig. 3, our approach based on fuzzy logic and the semantic similarity between the tweet to classify and the two opinion documents outperforms the other approaches with a classification rate equal to 86% and with 14% for the error rate, all that demonstrates how the fuzzy logic can improve the quality of the classification.

5 Conclusion

In this article we have presented a proposed approach based on fuzzy logic and the semantic similarity using WordNet dictionnary for classifiying the tweets into three classes (positive, negative or neutral), this work gives us the opportunity to familarise with the concepts of the suzzy logic and also how we can calculate the positivity and the negativity of tweets based on semantic similarity between the tweet to classify and two opinion documents, and how we can combine between the results obtained after we apply the semantic similarity and the fuzzy logic system.

Our fuzzy logic system uses the results obtained after the calculation of the positivity and the negativity of the tweet, to give at the end its sentiment (positive, negative or neutral).

The proposed sentiment analysis methods is multingual and it is developed in a parralel way using the hadoop framework with the Hadoop Distributed File System (HDFS) and the MapReduce programming model.

The experimental results show that using the fuzzy logic in the classfication of tweets improve the quality of our method, and that our proposed approach outperforms some other methods from the litterature.

As perspectives of this work, our next article will be in the same way, that is to say the classification of the social networks (Facebook, Twitter ...) data using fuzzy logic but this time using the notion of information retrieval systems.

References

1. Wang, B., Huang, Y., Wu, X., Li, X. : A fuzzy computing model for identifying polarity of Chinese Sentiment Words. Comput. Intell. Neurosci. (2015). [En ligne]. Disponible sur: https://www.hindawi.com/journals/cin/2015/525437/
2. Wu, K., Zhou, M., Lu, X.S., Huang, L.: A fuzzy logic-based text classification method for social media data. In: 2017 IEEE International Conference on Systems, Man, and Cybernetics (SMC), Banff Center, Banff, Canada, 5–8 Oct 2017
3. Dragoni, M., Petrucci, G.: A fuzzy-based strategy for multi-domain sentiment analysis. Int. J. Approx. Reason. **93**, 59–73 (2018). https://doi.org/10.1016/j.ijar.2017.10.021
4. Appel, O., Chiclana, F., Carter, J., Fujita, H.: A hybrid approach to the sentiment analysis problem at the sentence level. Knowl. Based Syst. (2016). https://doi.org/10.1016/j.knosys.2016.05.040
5. Sathe, J.B., Mali, M.P.: A hybrid sentiment classification method using neural network and fuzzy logic. In: 2017 11th International Conference on Intelligent Systems and Control (ISCO), pp. 93–96, Jan 2017. https://doi.org/10.1109/ISCO.2017.7855960

6. Madani, Y., Bengourram, J., Erritali, M.: Social login and data storage in the big data file system HDFS. In: Proceedings of the International Conference on Compute and Data Analysis, New York, NY, USA, pp. 91–97 (2017)
7. Madani, Y., Bengourram, J., Erritali, M.: A parallel Semantic sentiment analysis. In: Proceedings of the 3rd International Conference on Cloud Computing Technologies and Applications (CloudTech'17), Rabat, Morocco, 24–26 Oct 2017
8. Madani, Y., Erritali, M., Bengourram, J.: Arabic stemmer based big data. J. Electron. Comm. Organ. (JECO) **16**(1), 17–8 (2018). https://doi.org/10.4018/JECO.2018010102
9. Wu, Z., Palmer, M.: Verb semantics and lexical selection. In Proceedings of the 32nd Annual Meeting of the Associations for Computational Linguistics, pp. 133–138 (1994)
10. Resnik, P.: Using information content to evaluate semantic similarity in a taxonomy. In: IJCAI, pp. 448–53 (1995)
11. Leacock, C., Chodorow, M.: Combining local context and WordNet similarity for word sense identification. In: Fellbaum, C. (ed.) WordNet: An Electronic Lexical Database. MIT Press, Cambridge (1998)
12. Hirst, G., St. Onge, D.: Lexical chains as representation of context for the detection and correction malapropisms. In: Fellbaum, C. (ed.) WordNet: An Electronic Lexical Database, pp. 305–332. The MIT Press, Cambridge (1998)

Fuzzy Semantic-Based Similarity and Big Data for Detecting Multilingual Plagiarism in Arabic Documents

Hanane Ezzikouri[1(✉)], Mohamed Oukessou[1], Madani Youness[2], and Mohamed Erritali[2]

[1] LMACS Laboratory, Mathematics Department, Faculty of Sciences and Techniques, Sultan Moulay Slimane University, BP: 523 Beni-Mellal, Morocco
ezzikourihanane@gmail.com
[2] TIAD Laboratory, Computer Sciences Department, Faculty of Sciences and Techniques, Sultan Moulay Slimane University, BP: 523 Beni-Mellal, Morocco

Abstract. Plagiarism (intelligent-monolingual) is a complicated fuzzy process, adding translation and making it a cross language problem turn thing to be more obfuscated, what pose difficulties to current plagiarism detection methods. Multilingual plagiarism nature could be more complicated than simple copy + translate and paste, it is defined as the unacknowledged reuse of a text involving its translation from one natural language to another without proper referencing to the original source. Before the detecting process several NLP techniques were used to characterize input texts (tokenization, stop words removal, post-tagging, and text segmentation). In this paper, fuzzy semantic similarity between words is studied using WordNet-based similarity measures Wu & Palmer and Lin. In any data processing system the common problem is efficient large-scale text comparison, especially fuzzy-based semantic similarity to reveal dishonest practices in Arabic documents, first due to the complexity of the Arabic language and the increase in the number of publications and the rate of suspicious documents sources of plagiarism. To remedy this, vague concepts and fuzzy techniques in a big data environment will be used. The work is done in a parallel way using Apache Hadoop with its distributed file system HDFS and the MapReduce programming model. The proposed approach was evaluated on 400 English and Arabic cases of different sources (news, articles, tweets, and academic works), including 25% machine based translated plagiarism cases, and 75% translated (machine and human based) with a percentage of obfuscated plagiarism e.g. handmade paraphrases and back-translation. We effectuate some experimental verifications and comparisons showing that results and running time of Fuzzy-WuP are better than Fuzzy-Lin. Results are evaluated based on three testing parameters: precision, recall and F-measure.

Keywords: CLPD · Fuzzy sets · Semantic similarity · Hadoop · HDFS · MapReduce

© Springer Nature Switzerland AG 2019
M. Ezziyyani (Ed.): AI2SD 2018, AISC 915, pp. 159–169, 2019.
https://doi.org/10.1007/978-3-030-11928-7_14

1 Introduction

By dint of the rise of computer science and the development of information technologies, information is easily within everyone's reach, which facilitate generating more and more data and information what lead to an explosive growth in the amount of data and the increase of plagiarism issues. Big data has reached critical mass in every sector and continues on an exponential progress, broadcasting of digital information technologies have intensified its growth that makes an already hard fuzzy task even harder, detecting plagiarism in such huge amount of data seems to be impossible from the first sight, even after applying an information retrieval system that may reduce the number of candidates but still generating thousands of candidate documents that should be processed especially when dealing with cross language plagiarism detection (CLPD), because any document may be one of the suspects sources for the document query, this number is continually growing, which poses difficult challenges in the field of information retrieval and plagiarism detection as well.

Cross-Language Plagiarism refers to the unacknowledged reuse of a text involving its translation from one natural language to another without proper referencing to the original source, it's a sort of plagiarism idea, because texts are totally changed but ideas in the original texts remain unchanged; Such a change in the syntax and semantics of texts requires a deep and concentrated processing, then we confront two major factors, the management of large mass of data in all candidate documents and the number of operations required for this kind of plagiarism detection process. The nature of Cross-Language Plagiarism practices could be more complicated than simple copy translate and paste, in CLPD languages from source and suspicious documents differ, thus the process exposes the need for a vague concept and fuzzy sets techniques to reveal dishonest practices in Arabic documents.

In this paper, we propose an itemized fuzzy semantic based similarity approach for analyzing and comparing texts in CLP cases based on Big Data, in accordance with the WordNet lexical database [1], to detect plagiarism in documents translated from/to Arabic. Arabic is known as one of the richest human languages in terms of words constructions and meanings diversity. We focus in our work on obfuscated plagiarism cases where texts are translated and rephrased from one language to another with no reference to the original source.

So as we said earlier, the number of documents published every day increases explosively, and to detect plagiarism for a document there is a lot of treatment to be done, therefore we need a large storage volume for storing all this data and also it is the problem of the time needed for having the results of the detection. To remedy this problem our proposal consists of parallelizing our method by working in a Big Data system with the Apache Hadoop using the HDFS (Hadoop Distributed File System) and the Hadoop MapReduce. Preliminary operations and text preprocessing of inputs such as tokenization, part-of-speech (POS) tagging, lemmatization and stop words removal for deleting meaningless words and reducing the noise exist in the text. Text segmentation is done using word 3-gram. A fuzzy semantic-based approach is obtained based on the fact that words from two translated compared texts have in general, Strong fuzzy similarity words of the meaning from the second language.

2   Why Big Data for PD?

These days the quantity of data generated on the web is unimaginable, the amount of data and the frequency generated by, produced the 'big data' term, defined by Gartner [2] as "high volume, velocity and variety of data that demand cost-effective, innovative forms of processing for enhanced insight and decision making" and the recently added Veracity and Value based on the fact that accurate analysis could be affected by the quality of captured data. In any plagiarism detection system, a big common problem in data processing is efficient large-scale text comparison, especially semantic based similarity. The increase in the number of publications directly implies an increase in the number of suspicious documents sources of plagiarism, most research works in this area have used big data in the information retrieval phase [3, 4]. Zhang et al. [5] Presented a sequence-based method to detect the partial similarity of web pages using MapReduce, composed of two sub-tasks, sentence level near-duplicate detection and sequence matching. Erritali et al. [6] proposed an approach of semantic similarity measures using WordNet as an external network semantic resource and a new MapReduce algorithm. The proposed approach was compared with other approaches, experimental results review that the proposed approach gives better results on running time performance and increases the measurement of semantic similarity. Dwivedi et al. [7] introduced a SCAM (Standard Copy Analysis Mechanism) plagiarism detection algorithm, the proposed detection process is based on natural language processing by comparing documents and a modified Map-Reduce based SCAM algorithm for processing big data using Hadoop and detect plagiarism in big data.

Information Retrieval of documents in a Big Data environment get lately so much attention since detecting similar documents becomes a basic and important problem and a preliminary stage of many research topics like in the plagiarism detection for reducing the number of candidate documents as usually the documents collections are huge corpuses or sometimes the web (i.e. If we are talking about plagiarism detection, the selection of candidate documents stage). However, the number of candidates remain enormous for a highly deep analysis such a fuzzy semantic similarity process.

3   Fuzzy Semantic Similarity and Big Data for CLPD

One of the most important problems in plagiarism detection is the huge masse of information and data generated especially when the source collection is a voluminous corpuses as in the Web, a solution that is still young and growing is the use of Big Data technologies to parallelize the work (i.e. Fuzzy CLPD process in [8]), i.e. distributing and sharing it between several machines (Big Data cluster), using Apache Hadoop framework with Hadoop distributed file system HDFS for distributing the storage of the documents to analyze and also for storing the result after the application of our CLPD method, and MapReduce programming model for the parallelization and the development of our proposal.

In a cross-language semantic based similarity detection process where words borders are not clear and the intersection of meanings of words are fuzzy, the fuzzy set theory seems to be the right way to treat such case. Fuzzy set theory introduced by

Lofti Zadeh in 1965 based on his mathematical theory of fuzzy sets, which is a generalization of the theory of classical sets, it permits the gradual assessment of the membership of elements in a set with the aid of a membership function valued in the real unit interval [0, 1]. Fuzzy set theory could be used in a wide range of domains especially for handling uncertain and imprecise data that linked with CLPD.

Cross-Language Plagiarism is a fuzzy complex operation. Each word in a document is associated with a fuzzy set that contains words with the same meaning with a degree of similarity (commonly less than 1) (Fig. 1); so the use of fuzzy sets theory in CLPD looks to be an obvious way to solve the problem. Fuzzy set theory and CLPD turn up to be the perfect couple, however, the important number of operations and the running time implies to search for a solution to improve performance and results, this solution is to use the Big Data technologies.

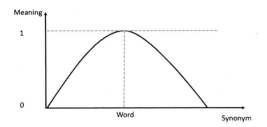

Fig. 1. A word's fuzzy set synonyms

4 The Proposed Method

4.1 Preprocessing

The work presented in this paper is based on work done in [8], it handles intelligent multilingual plagiarism detection using fuzzy semantic-based similarity methods and big data technologies (Hadoop, HDFS and MapReduce). Input text and candidates are from two distant languages Arabic and English, the creation of a suitable target data of each document is elementary, various text preprocessing methods based on NLP techniques are implemented (Fig. 2) and described in details in [8].

Semantic Similarity is the similarity between two concepts in a taxonomy (e.g. WordNet [1]), where synonymous words are joined together to form synonyms sets called also synsets; synsets that share a common property are linked with more general words called hypernyms, and most specific words called hyponyms. Several similarity measures have been proposed in the last few years, LCH, WuP, RES, LIN, LESK, and HSO [9–14].

Our proposed algorithm in this paper is based on two semantic similarity approaches (Wu & Palmer and Lin), which use WordNet to automatically evaluate semantic relations between words, in WordNet, a word may be polysemous which means a word may occurs in one to many synsets, each corresponding to a different meaning.

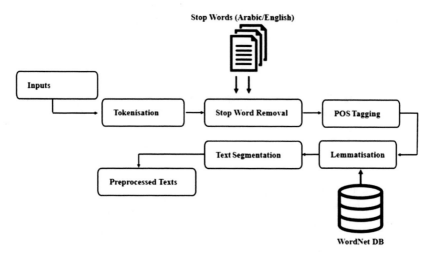

Fig. 2. Texts preprocessing for CLPD [8]

4.2   Used Metrics: Wu & Palmer and Lin

WuP [10] measure is:

$$SIM_{WuP} = 2 \times \frac{depth(LCS(C1, C2))}{depth(C1) + depth(C2)} \qquad (1)$$

where C1, C2 are two concepts (in the form of synsets), depth(x) is the total number of edges from the root of the WordNet DAG (Fig. 3) to the concept x.

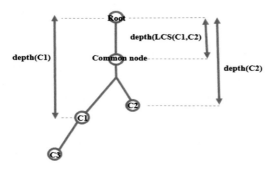

Fig. 3. Directed-acyclic-graph (DAG) for WordNet

The LIN similarity [12, 14] is defined by:

$$SIM_{LIN}(C1, C2) = 2 \times \frac{\log(P(CS(C1, C2)))}{\log P(C1) + Log P(C2)} \qquad (2)$$

where CS(C1, C2): represents the most specific concept (which maximizes the similarity value) between C1 and C2 in the taxonomy. LIN similarity verify $0 \leq SIM_{LIN} \leq 1$.

4.3 Fuzzification

Fuzzy semantic-based approach is obtained based on the fact that words from two translated compared texts have in general a strong fuzzy similarity words of the meaning from the second language [4]. Several research focuses on the importance of the text preprocessing methods especially at Part-Of-Speech (POS) level and its integration with fuzzy based methods for an efficient identification of similar documents [15].

In Fuzzy inference systems, Fuzzification is an essential component. In the fuzzifier process, relationship between inputs and linguistic variables is defined by a fuzzy membership function. In this work to fuzzify the relationship of word pairs (from text pairs), we propose to work with the Lin's semantic similarity approach as a fuzzy memberships function, comparing it with the Wu and Palmer method proposed in [8]. The Lin and WuP fuzzy membership functions [expressed bellow Eq. (3)] are used to fuzzify the semantic similarity of word pairs (from input texts):

$$\mu_{1a_i b_j} = Lin(a_i, b_j) \text{ and } \mu_{2a_i b_j} = Wup(a_i, b_j) \qquad (3)$$

The membership functions accept all the intermediate values between 0 and 1. The values of a membership function, called membership degrees or grades of membership, precisely specify to what extent an element belongs to a fuzzy set [16], i.e. for identical words or synonyms (totally similar) membership degree is 1, and 0 for dissimilar words (i.e. do not have any semantic relationship).

A fuzzy inference system was constructed to evaluate the similarity of two texts and infer about plagiarism. For the evaluation of relationships of a word in first text with regard to words in the other text, we used the fuzzy PROD operator as presented in the following formulas: $\mu_{a_1, B} = 1 - \prod_{b_j \in B, j \in [1, m]} \left(1 - Wup(a_1, b_j)\right)$

$$\mu_{a_n, B} = 1 - \prod_{b_j \in B, j \in [1, m]} \left(1 - Wup(a_n, b_j)\right) \qquad (4)$$

Then the average sum is calculated:

$$\mu_{A, B} = \left(\sum_{i=1}^{n} \mu_{a, B}\right) \Big/ n \qquad (5)$$

4.4 Research Methodology and Algorithm

Our main contribution in this article is to fuzzify the method of detecting the plagiarism using two fuzzy semantic similarity approaches (fuzzy WuPalmer and fuzzy Lin) in a parallel manner using the Apache Hadoop (HDFS + MapReduce).

The idea is to store the inputs of our work (the candidate documents and the text for which we want to verify the plagiarism: Arabic text in our work) and also the results of the proposed methods in HDFS for distributing the storage between several machines (Hadoop Cluster). Moreover, for the development of our proposal, we use the MapReduce programming model to give back our method parallel (a parallel plagiarism's detection).

Inputs are from two different languages, an Arabic text and a corpus of potential candidate source of plagiarism in English. Before we apply our method we need to prepare the inputs for the phase of plagiarism's detection, for that there are various steps before getting the final result.

The first step is the text preprocessing methods, which contain several NLP processes (tokenization, stop words removal, post-tagging [17] ...) and word 3-grams (W3G) segmentation, this step is pivotal since Arabic has a complex morphology and one of the most difficult languages to treat. After that, the second step we prepare the inputs is the storage of them in HDFS (distributing the storage). The resulting text (Arabic text) and every single text from the corpus (the English texts one by one) are used as inputs for the fuzzy inference system, then Wu and Palmer and Lin semantic similarity measurement are modelled as membership functions. The output is a similarity score between the Arabic text and each input text from the corpus. Figure 4 shows the different steps of our work.

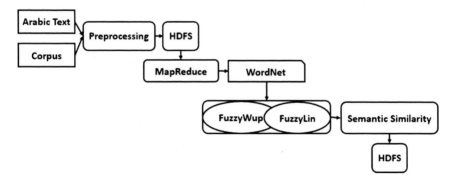

Fig. 4. Parallel cross language plagiarism detection system

Algorithm : MapReduce Programming Model for the proposed method

---

Inputs : Arabic Text, English text from the corpus
Require : Semantic Similarity between inputs
S_Wup ← 0; S_Lin ← 0; C ← 0;
AR ← *Text Preprocessing*(Arabic Text); EN ← *Text Preprocessing*(English Text);
Segmentation1[] ← *W3G*(AR); Segmentation2[] ← *W3G*(EN);
For all word In Segmentation1
   For all term In Segmentation2
      If word In WordNet
         Then word ← *WordNet*(word);
      Else   word ← *Translate*(word);
      End If
      Fuzzy_Wup ← 1 - *Wup*(word, term); Fuzzy_Lin ← 1 - *Lin*(word, term);
      S_Wup ← S_Wup + Fuzzy_Wup; S_Lin ← S_Lin + Fuzzy_Lin;
      C ← C + 1;
   End For
End For
Sim_Wup=S_Wup/C; Sim_Lin=S_Lin/C;
Write(Arabic Text || English text, Sim_Wup or Sim_Lin)

As presented earlier and shown in the algorithm above, each input of the MapReduce algorithm contains two texts: Arabic and English to calculate the semantic similarity (detecting plagiarism).

To distribute the storage of inputs and parallelize the work of the plagiarism's detection, we construct a Hadoop cluster that contains three machines Hadoop Nodes, this cluster has a master machine and two slave machines. Each node is an Ubuntu 15.04 machine. The figure below shows the configuration of our cluster (Fig. 5).

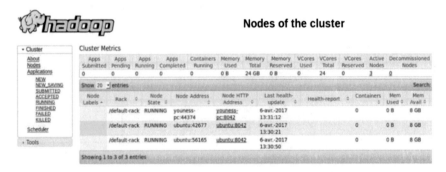

Fig. 5. Clusters configuration

5   Experimental Results and Discussion

Testing corpus is built up from 400 English and Arabic documents from different sources (news, articles, tweets, and academic works). In order to detect the cross language plagiarism, 100 are simply translated (machine based) with no change, and 300 documents are translated from English to Arabic with a percentage of obfuscated plagiarism after translation (paraphrasing, back-translation, etc.).

Two fuzzy semantic metrics implemented in the system are compared: Fuzzy Wu & Palmer and Lin. Results of the fuzzy CLPD are evaluated based on three testing parameters: precision, recall and F-Measure. Results presented in Figs. 6 and 7 are some of the experimental tests that demonstrate that the Fuzzy Wu & Palmer have high performance than Fuzzy Lin.

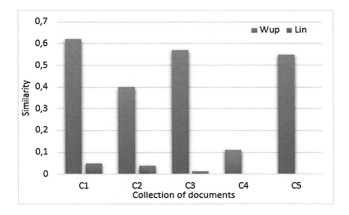

Fig. 6. Comparison of similarity of Fuzzy-WuP and Fuzzy-Lin

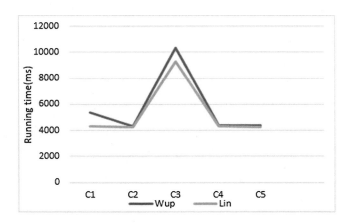

Fig. 7. Comparison of running time of WuP and Lin similarity measures

6   Discussion

Based on the evaluation results and the previous results in [8], Fuzzy WuP achieves better performance compared to Fuzzy Lin in all tests using different parameters (precision, recall and F-measure) Table 1. As said before our testing corpus contains several form of plagiarism ranging from simple translation to other one that make

Table 1. Precision, recall and F-measure for parallel fuzzy CLPD

	Fuzzy-WuP	Fuzzy-Lin
Precision	0.54	0.27
Recall	0.66	0.37
F-measure	0.594	0.312

serious changing in the text. While testing, we noticed that the fuzzy Lin is not effective in detecting the plagiarized documents in a big mass of data, however, it gave average performance dealing with plagiarism in small texts. Therefore Fuzzy Lin is not suitable for detection plagiarism in high volumes of information. Indeed, Fuzzy WuP maintain to be the best semantic similarity measure for detection obfuscated plagiarism in a big data environment. Hence, no matter how the translated plagiarized text is modified and the structure changed, such serious changing is the principal reason to involve fuzzy theory in plagiarism detection then similarity can still be detected.

The Parallel fuzzy-based Cross Language Plagiarism Detection using the lexical taxonomies such as WordNet in a big data environment presented in this paper achieves good results in comparison with some existing models and approaches namely fuzzy IR method in [18] such as word correlation factors obtained from large corpora that require allocation of disk space to save the word-to-word correlation factor tables.

The processing time required to search for words and retrieve their correlation value is one of the main problems of former models and becomes a major issue for extending the use of parallel fuzzy-based CLPD approach, which have widely been reduced in our proposed model.

7 Conclusion

In this paper we have presented our Parallel fuzzy-based Cross Language Plagiarism Detection using WordNet and big data. Nowadays, most of the current plagiarism detection tools are not suitable for detection the most important kind of plagiarism, plagiarists are pushing plagiarism to a very high level using translation (human or machine based), paraphrasing, back-translation and a lots of manipulation to avoid to be caught with plagiarism detection systems, obfuscated semantic plagiarism is a substantial issue and concern especially in academic works.

Different pre-processing methods based on NLP techniques were used (lemmatization, stop word removal and POS tagging), texts were segmented to 3-gram. Two fuzzy semantic measure WuP and Lin similarity measure were evaluated to judge the similarity in compared texts. Using a testing corpus of 400 handmade (rewording, paraphrasing, back-translation, idea adoption, etc.) and artificial plagiarism cases, the fuzzy plagiarism detecting method using two fuzzy semantic similarity approaches (fuzzy-WuP and fuzzy-Lin) in a parallel manner using Apache Hadoop (HDFS + MapReduce), hadoop was used for performance enhancement and time reducing, data were distributed across the cluster of machines (master and two slaves); processing time doesn't increase in comparison of the important number of operations needed for such process. The results were evaluated using three testing parameters: precision, recall and F-Measure which led to conclude that the proposed model obtained a reliable and significant performance with the WuP similarity measure.

References

1. Miller, G.A.: WordNet: a lexical database for English. Commun. ACM **38**(11), 39–41 (1995)
2. Beyer, M.A., Laney, D.: The Importance of 'Big Data': A Definition, pp. 2014–2018. Stamford CT Gart. (2012)
3. Najafabadi, M.M., Villanustre, F., Khoshgoftaar, T.M., Seliya, N., Wald, R., Muharemagic, E.: Deep learning applications and challenges in big data analytics. J. Big Data **2**, 1 (2015)
4. Parhami, B.: A highly parallel computing system for information retrieval. In: Proceedings of the 5–7 Dec 1972, Fall Joint Computer Conference, Part II, pp. 681–690. New York, NY, USA (1972)
5. Zhang, Q., Zhang, Y., Yu, H., Huang, X.: Efficient partial-duplicate detection based on sequence matching. In: Proceedings of the 33rd International ACM SIGIR Conference on Research and Development in Information Retrieval, pp. 675–682 (2010)
6. Erritali, M., Beni-Hssane, A., Birjali, M., Madani, Y.: An approach of semantic similarity measure between documents based on big data. Int. J. Electr. Comput. Eng. **6**(5), 2454 (2016)
7. Dwivedi, J., Tiwary, A.: Plagiarism detection on bigdata using modified map-reduced based SCAM algorithm. In: 2017 International Conference on Innovative Mechanisms for Industry Applications (ICIMIA), pp. 608–610 (2017)
8. Ezzikouri, H., Erritali, M., Oukessou, M.: Fuzzy-semantic similarity for automatic multilingual plagiarism detection. Int. J. Adv. Comput. Sci. Appl. **8**(9), 86–90 (2017)
9. Leacock, C., Chodorow, M.: Combining local context and WordNet similarity for word sense identification. WordNet Electron. Lex. Database **49**(2), 265–283 (1998)
10. Wu, Z., Palmer, M.: Verbs semantics and lexical selection. In: Proceedings of the 32nd Annual Meeting on Association for Computational Linguistics, pp. 133–138 (1994)
11. P. Rensik, "Using information content to evaluate semantic similarity," in Proceedings of the 14th International Joint Conference on Artificial Intelligence, 1995, pp. 448–453
12. Lin, D.: An information-theoretic definition of similarity. Icml **98**, 296–304 (1998)
13. Hirst, G., St-Onge, D.: Lexical chains as representations of context for the detection and correction of malapropisms. WordNet Electron. Lex. Database **305**, 305–332 (1998)
14. Lin, D.: Principle-based parsing without overgeneration. In: Proceedings of the 31st Annual Meeting on Association for Computational Linguistics, pp. 112–120 (1993)
15. Gupta, D., Vani, K., Singh, C.K.: Using natural language processing techniques and fuzzy-semantic similarity for automatic external plagiarism detection. In: 2014 International Conference on Advances in Computing, Communications and Informatics (ICACCI), pp. 2694–2699 (2014)
16. Werro, N.: Fuzzy Classification of Online Customers, Fuzzy Management Methods
17. Manning, C., Surdeanu, M., Bauer, J., Finkel, J., Bethard, S., McClosky, D.: The Stanford CoreNLP natural language processing toolkit. In: Proceedings of 52nd Annual Meeting of the Association for Computational Linguistics: System Demonstrations, pp. 55–60 (2014)
18. Yerra, R., Ng, Y.-K.: A sentence-based copy detection approach for web documents. In: International Conference on Fuzzy Systems and Knowledge Discovery, pp. 557–570 (2005)

Contribution to the Improvement of the Quality of Service Over Vehicular Ad-Hoc Network

Ansam Ennaciri[1]([✉]), Rania Khadim[2], Mohammed Erritali[2], Mustapha Mabrouki[1], and Jamaa Bengourram[1]

[1] Department of Industrial Engineering, Faculty of Sciences and Techniques, Sultan Moulay Slimane University, Beni Mellal, Morocco
ennaciri.ansam@gmail.com,
{mus_mabrouki,bengoram}@yahoo.fr
[2] TIAD Laboratory, Department of Computer Sciences, Faculty of Sciences and Techniques, Sutan Moulay Slimane University, Beni Mellal, Morocco
khadimrania@gmail.com, m.erritali@usms.ma

Abstract. Nowadays Vehicular Ad hoc Network represents an interesting part of intelligent transportation system (ITS). This latter attempt to answer the question of how to improve road safety, to maintain best-effort-of service, and to provide better conditions for drivers and passengers. Indeed, connected vehicles will operate in a connected/smart city. It then becomes necessary to implement solutions to manage urban traffic while responding as accurately as possible to road traffic and congestion problems. However, the Quality of service is an important consideration in vehicular ad hoc networks because of rapid development in network technology and real time applications like multimedia, voice, video streaming, etc. In this paper, we propose a new approach for road traffic management in smart cities, which maintain shortest paths, based on graph theory in order to facilitate traffic management, through using a specific algorithm. In order to improve the quality of service over vehicular ad hoc network, a new method is then presented, which ensures vehicle safety by minimizing the number of interchange between vehicles, minimize energy and lifetime of the sensors.

Keywords: Graph theory · Video streaming · Ad-hoc network · VANET · QOS

1 Introduction

In recent decades, vehicles have become more and more important in our daily lives. Car traffic has become a daily occurrence in some cities due to the traffic jams. An even bigger problem is that of safety, the WHO (World Health Organization) statistics show that there are on average 1.2 million deaths and between 20 and 50 million serious injuries caused by road accidents. To overcome the problems of safety and road traffic, many initiatives have been taken by the governments, associations and car

© Springer Nature Switzerland AG 2019
M. Ezziyyani (Ed.): AI2SD 2018, AISC 915, pp. 170–190, 2019.
https://doi.org/10.1007/978-3-030-11928-7_15

manufacturers. Among these initiatives, we have the awareness campaigns, the introduction of a strict highway code and the improvement of public transit.

The field of ad hoc networks is a very promising field since it allows spontaneous creation of a network without any infrastructure.

An ad hoc network is simply made up of multiple vehicles able to exchange information for the purpose of improving road safety or allowing passenger's access to the Internet.

However, an intuitive and simple way of designing ad hoc networks is to consider that they correspond to the ultimate generalization of wireless networks because they limit the role of the fixed infrastructure as much as possible. This generalization is achieved by improving the connectivity capabilities of wireless network [1]. The limited range of terminals requires the presence of a routing protocol to establish communication between two distant entities. Several routing protocols have been proposed in the VANET group. They allow to find shortest paths in terms of number of hops.

Routing constraints depend on both: the mobility of the networks and the type of information to be routed. Indeed some networks are more mobile than others, and we know how the disconnections are expensive. The nature of the information depends on the applications that we are trying to execute. These are more or less sensitive to latency in communications.

The most difficult type of service to support is video streaming applications, that involve sending a data flow from a server to the customer [2]. The volume of data is very large and the flow of data-sent does not support to be interrupted. Nevertheless the flow constraint refers to the concept of the quality of service [3, 4]. It is known, for example, that the various IEEE 802.11 standards cannot ensure the quality of service because of the probabilistic implementation of the physical layer [5]. Moreover, the Scatternets would make it possible to envisage this service in multi-hops. Regarding Wi-Fi, despite the problems of quality of service, several proposals are made by dealing with the problem in various ways. In [6], the authors propose a mechanism of adaptation of the flow rate according to the rate of loss of perceived information. They carry out a simulation to verify their assumptions. Routing and mobility are not treated in this proposal. In [7], the authors propose a routing algorithm for a vehicular ad hoc network. Simulations are made and the algorithm is compared with AODV (routing protocol that is dedicated to VANETs). Finally, in [8], the authors evaluate three approaches for assessing QoE(Quality of Experience) in video streaming application over wireless networks.

In summary, audio and video streaming applications are difficult to adapt to the constraints of ad hoc wireless networks and especially since stations are mobile.

The transmission of video packets must consider the main parameters that characterize ad-hoc networks, namely throughput, packet loss, end-to-end delay and jitter. In recent years, several techniques have been used by multimedia applications to overcome variations in these factors and to minimize their effects on the quality of the video perceived by the receiver. It is about: Transcoding [9, 10], SVC(Sclable Video Coding) [11, 12], MDC (Multiple Description Coding) [13], ARQ (Automatic Repeat Request) [14], UEP (Unequal Error Protection) [15] and Errors concealment [16].

The main objectives of the vehicular networks are to disseminate information related to road traffic and all other kinds of information [17, 18]. The nature of road traffic information is limited to the specific geographical area such as accident information. In [19] the author proposed a new routing mechanism allowing the transmission of a message optimally. Thus, the applications that are usable in these networks collect information in sensor networks, which may have significant connection delays [20].

The shortest path's problems [21, 22] between two vertices in weighted graphs are well known for a long time, and polynomial algorithms are available for different types of graphs: Dijkstra in the case of positive weights, Bellman in the general case [23, 24].

Due to the collisions arising and the network's topology, the catwalk can pick on various relays for each newly generated packet, and any relay node picks on its next hop nodes based on the current state of its neighborhood.

In this article, we address these issues by interesting to the vehicle network corresponding to the modern requirements and more specifically to the optimization of the itineraries via different criteria of quality of service, using adapted methods derived from the operational research.

In this project, we propose effective solutions to overcome this problem. Firstly, we propose to design and develop optimization techniques to plan an efficient and effective vehicular network infrastructure. Secondly, we propose to design and develop the quality of service (QoS) based on adaptive management mechanisms to ensure real-time, robust and efficient communications.

Remainder of this paper is organized as follows: In Sect. 2 we present a generic design of our algorithms for multi constrained routing. Then our own proposed of quality of service will be discussed in Sect. 3. Section 4 talks about our experimentations and the obtained results. The paper is concluded in Sect. 5.

2   Interconnections and Graphs

We present the network interconnection by a simple graph, which edges are the links, and the nodes are the equipments. The links are assigned to one or more positive weight functions. These weights can represent the distance between the end's node, the data transmission delay on the link, the throughput, the cost, and so on [25].

We assume that the network is connected. However, transiently, network components may become temporarily isolated due to the mobility, the failure, etc.

Indeed, we consider that the values of the weights on the two arcs between the two equipment of the network can be different;

The edge weights are used by the routing table calculation algorithms to determine the best route between any two nodes of the graph. We assume that each weight function is homogeneously distributed on the graph and gives positive values in R +.

We recall here the usual notions of the theory of graphs which will allow us to describe as closely as possible the characteristics of a topological graph [26, 27].

Let $G = (V; E; \Omega)$ be the weighted topological graph (Fig. 1), where V is the set of nodes, E is the set of arcs and Ω is the set of weight functions associated with each arc. The weighted topological graph is defined by:

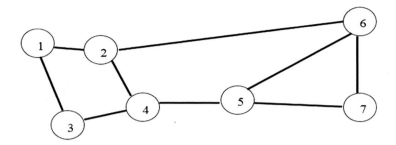

Fig. 1. Representation of graph G

$$E \subset V \times V$$
$$\forall f \in \Omega : V \times V \to R + \qquad (1)$$
$$\forall u \in V, \forall v \in V, si(u, v) \in V : f(u, v) \text{finite}$$

We extend the set of weight functions, defined on E, to any pair of nodes of graph:

$$\forall u \in V, \forall f \in \Omega : f(u, u) = 0$$
$$\forall (u, v) \notin E, \forall f \in \Omega : u \neq v \Leftrightarrow f(u, v) = \propto \qquad (2)$$

We denote the neighborhood of distance k of node u in a graph G:

$$\Gamma_k(u) = \{v \in G : dist(u, v) = k\} \qquad (3)$$

where <dist> the function of the number of hops between two nodes.

- The constraint composition rules:

Let (G; V; E;) be the topological graph weighted with $|V| = n$ nodes and $|E| = m$ arcs. Each arc $(v_i; v_j) \in E$ is associated with one or more metrics (weight functions).

Let $f(v_i; v_j)$ be one of these metrics. The value of f on the path $p = (v_0; v_1;...v_k)$ can follow one of the rules of Compositions:

- Additive metric: a metric f is additive if

$$f(p) = \sum_{i=1}^{k} f(v_{i-1}, v_i) \qquad (4)$$

It is clear that delay (Del), jitter (Gig), number of hops, and cost (C) are additive metrics.

- Multiplicative metric: a metric f is multiplicative if

$$f(p) = \prod_{i=1}^{k} f(v_{i-1}, v_i) \qquad (5)$$

2.1   The Quality of Service

For a good quality of service, no driver has any benefit in waiting in the vehicle when he is pulling up before leaving the vehicle. Since the Quality of Service (QoS) is an important point in all networks, it seems interesting to study the ways of introduction this notion in the ad hoc networks (VANETs) where the nodes are in movement [28].

The purpose of a calculation of the routing table is to determine the path (i.e., a set of links to be traversed), to establish a connection from a source node to a destination node. This calculation is included in the routing protocol, which allows the dissemination of the information necessary for this calculation.

Actually, QoS that can be offered to the connection is directly linked to the choice of the path. The different constraints imposed by the connection (rate, delay, rate of loss, etc.) must be taken into consideration in the route calculation. These parameters may vary according to the links borrowed. Therefore, it is necessary to implement a routing algorithm whose function is to find the best possible path between the source and the recipient in order to satisfy the different quality criteria imposed. The calculation must also divide the resources of the network as homogeneously as possible. Besides, the route calculation should be as simple as possible in order to avoid complexities in terms of execution time.

An algorithm for calculating a route with QoS consists on finding a path between a source and a destination that satisfies QoS requirements (bandwidth, delay, etc.) while efficiently using the resources of the network (cost, load balance, etc.).

The shortest path algorithms proposed in this article aim to the ensure the quality of service management in dynamic networks without any central entity. Thus, the routing tables must be adaptive (dynamic) and distributed between the nodes of the network. The calculations are done on a topological graph, which represents the state of the network.

The Quality Of service criteria: In this section, we propose to precisely determine a certain number of QoS indicators for a vehicular network. The term of quality of service is used in a very broad sense that include all system actors' interests: passengers, drivers, transporters, local authorities.

- Absurd waiting times

Figure 2 shows that it should not be any waiting time; In other terms whatever the objective function of the optimization, the solutions that presenting this type of waiting time, will always have a quality of service that is too low for the passengers.

The top diagram represents a situation with absurd waiting times represented by ellipses, and the diagram below shows the corresponding situation without these waiting times.

This case indicates that the deletions of the expectations are done by a delay and/or advancement. This only reflects the fact that people do not wait for the stop just after going up or just before going down whatever their desired service completion date.

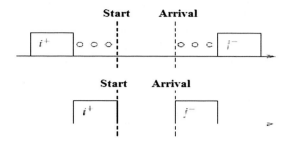

Fig. 2. Absurd waiting time

- Distance covered

This criterion is the most classic in the network of vehicles. The distance is an attribute associated to each arc (section) (vi,vj).

To obtain the distance, we need just sum the distance of each arc concerned.

Nevertheless, it may be more relevant to model the network by a p-graph, to making this case more complex.

- Duration

It is exactly the same calculation as the distance covered, the only difference is to add the service durations and the waiting times to the arcs. The only minimal paths in terms of duration are sufficient to obtain an optimal solution.

If a constraint is imposed on the total distance covered, it then becomes pertinent to consider the alternative tracers as the criterion of the distance traveled.

- Sensitivity to disturbances

Disturbances in a network can be modification of the network, delay of a vehicle, modification of the set of requests to be served.

The sensitivity of the system to these disturbances can be measured in different ways: by the ability to find a new acceptable solution within a reasonable time, or by the difference between the old solution and the new one.

The quality of service is then associated with notions of robustness, the method of calculation of rounds and that of solutions.

The spatio-temporal distribution of the vehicles is a criterion for reducing the sensitivity of the system to the arrival of new requests. If at any time, all the vehicles are distributed rationally face to the distribution of the appearance of new requests on the territory, the system will be able to receive new requests.

2.2 The Main Issue

As we have already seen, the architecture of an ad hoc vehicular network is characterized by the absence of a pre-existing fixed infrastructure, unlike conventional telecommunication networks. An automotive ad hoc network must be organized automatically, so that it can be quickly deployed and adapted to the conditions of propagation, traffic and the different movements that may occur within mobile units [29].

The problem for a network is to determine optimal data routing (messages, images, etc.) in the sense of a certain performance criterion.

These problems in vehicular networks [30] are linked to their unpredictable nature. The proposed algorithms must take account of certain constraints:

- The absence of an infrastructure that prevents centralized control and imposes a distributed resolution;
- The dynamics of the network and the rapid loss of validity of roads that impose appropriate updating mechanisms [31]. That is, the roads constructed must comply with the constraints of the VANETs.

Indeed, the shortest path in number of hops is likely to be the fastest in transmission time. Moreover, the path that uses the least number of nodes is presumably, the most energy efficient.

However, latency issues should also be considered when connecting and reconnecting. Not without mentioning the problem of the flooding of the broadcast of the frames during the transmission of the data. Indeed the data transmitted between two different nodes is received several times, while it is beneficial to be received only once [32].

Hence, the need to have a single path or a way to find a sub-graph that crosses all the nodes.

3 Proposed Approaches and Results

The implementation of the modeling of a system could be based on well-known and mastered objects, which are graphs with its cortege. Indeed, there is a simple analogy between networks and graphs. The entities of a system are associated with the nodes of a graph and the interactions between entities are associated with the edges.

It is desired to send packets on a vehicular network between input nodes and output nodes connected to each other by an ad-hoc network responsible for dispatching packets over the network. The network can be represented by a graph $G = (M, N)$ of which m is a set of vertices and n is the set of arcs such that each arc is identified by an ordered pair of vertices (u, v).

$$[|a, b|] = \{a, a + 1, a + 2, \ldots b - 1, b\}$$

$$G = \{Ui/i \in 1, \} \qquad (6)$$

/n: number of edges of the whole graph

$$A = \{Uij/j \in [|1, m - 1|]\} \qquad (7)$$

/m: number of vertices

$$d(A) = \sum_{j=1}^{n-1} d(Uij) \tag{8}$$

/d(A): the global distance
We must found

$$A* = d(A*) = \min d(A) \tag{9}$$

3.1   Used Method

Our work will proceed in three steps:

As a first step, we will configure the nodes according to our protocol (Algorithm 1). And as result we will have a routing table of each graph node.

In the next Step (Algorithm 2), we will calculate the Shortest path. When a frame is received, it will be decided at which node one will transmit the information.

In the end and this is the most important part of our work, that of amelioration of the quality of Service (Algorithm 3).

Algorithm 1:

Description
In the Algorithm 1(Fig. 3), we suppose that there are two types of frames:

- Information frames
- Frames that inform the appearance of a new node or change of routing table.

Description

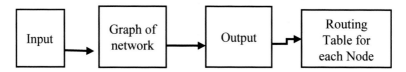

Fig. 3. Schematic presentation of Algorithm 1

At the beginning, the routing table is empty
Each node (x) has two cases:

1. If it receives a frame from another node y:

   - Receiving the routing table of the node (y).
   - Verification, if this table contains new information.
   - Updating its own routing table and returning its new routing table to all nodes directly connected to it.

2. Detection of a new node (z) that does not belong to its routing table:

- Adding a new box associated with this new node (z).
- It sends its own table to the new node (z) and asks it to return its routing table.
- Updating after receiving the new table.
- Sending the new table to the other nodes.

Then, by applying the Algorithm 1-based approach and using the adjacency matrix (Table 1) on the graph (Fig. 4), the routing matrix (Table 2) was constructed.

Table 1. Adjency matrix

	1	2	3	4	5	6	7
1	0	0	1	1	0	1	1
2	0	0	0	1	0	1	0
3	1	0	0	0	1	1	1
4	1	1	0	0	0	1	1
5	0	0	1	0	0	0	1
6	1	1	1	1	0	0	0
7	1	0	1	1	1	0	0

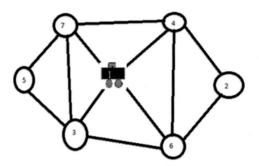

Fig. 4. Modeling of Vanet network

Table 2. Routing matrix

	1	2	3	4	5	6	7
1	1	4	3	4	3	6	7
2	4	2	4	4	4	6	4
3	1	1	3	1	5	6	7
4	1	2	1	4	1	6	7
5	3	3	3	3	5	3	7
6	1	2	3	4	1	6	1
7	1	1	3	4	5	1	7

Algorithm 1:

```
G a connected graph of n vertices
Let M be its adjacent matrix (of size n x n)
M (i, j) = 1 if there is a stop between i and j
M (i, j) = 0 otherwise
Let A be the routing matrix (of size n x n)
A (i, i) = i
A (i, j) = k if i # j and there exists a path from i to
j passing through k and there is a between i and k
Input: M
Output: A
Function f: ---> Routing table update.
Input : i,j

  h = 0
  For k=1 to n do
    If k#i and k#j and A(i,k)=0 et A(j,k)#0
      A(i,k) = j
      h = h + 1
          End If
  End For

  if h#0
    For k=1 to n do
    if k#i et k#j and A(i,k)#0
        f(A(i,k),i)
  End If
  End For
  End If
End Function

Debut
  For i=1 to n do
    For j=1 to n do
      A(i,j) = 0
    End For
  End For

For i=1 to n do
    A(i,i) = i
For j=1 to i-1 do
    If M(i,j)=1
IF A(i,j)#0
```

```
    A(i,j) = j
    A(j,i) = i
Else
                    A(i,j) = j
A(j,i) = i
f(i,j)
                    f(j,i)
End If
End If
End For
End For
End

Return A
```

Algorithm 2:

Description:
By applying the Algorithm 2 as shown in Fig. 5 on the input graph (Fig. 6), and using the adjacency matrix (Table 3), the optimal path was constructed from routing matrix (Table 4).

Description:

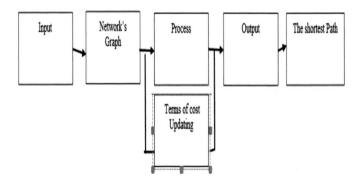

Fig. 5. Schematic diagram of Algorithm 2

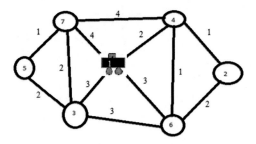

Fig. 6. Graph connectivity in VANETs

Table 3. Adjency matrix for Algorithm 2

	1	2	3	4	5	6	7
1	−1	−1	3	2	−1	3	4
2	−1	−1	−1	1	−1	2	−1
3	3	−1	−1	−1	2	3	2
4	2	1	−1	−1	−1	1	4
5	−1	−1	2	−1	−1	−1	1
6	3	2	3	1	−1	−1	−1
7	4	−1	2	4	1	−1	−1

Table 4. ROUTING matrix for Algorithm 2

	1	2	3	4	5	6	7
1	(1,0)	(4,3)	(3,3)	(4,2)	(3,5)	(4,3)	(7,4)
2	(4,3)	(2,0)	(6,5)	(4,1)	(4,6)	(6,2)	(4,5)
3	(1,3)	(6,5)	(3,0)	(6,4)	(5,2)	(6,3)	(7,2)
4	(1,2)	(2,1)	(6,4)	(4,0)	(7,5)	(6,1)	(7,4)
5	(3,5)	(7,6)	(3,2)	(7,5)	(5,0)	(3,5)	(7,1)
6	(1,3)	(2,2)	(3,3)	(4,1)	(3,5)	(6,0)	(3,5)
7	(1,4)	(4,5)	(3,2)	(4,4)	(5,1)	(3,5)	(7,0)

Algorithm 2:

```
G a connected graph of n vertices
Let M be its adjacent matrix (of size n x n) (with the
cost of each edge)
M (i, j) # -1 if there is a stop between i and j M (i,
j) represents the cost of the edge between i and j
M (i, j) = -1 otherwise
Let A be the routing matrix (sizeof  n x n x 2)
  A(i,i,1) = i
  A(i,i,2) = 0
                A (i, j, 1) = k if i # j and there exists
an optimal cost path from i to j passing through k and
there is an edge between i and k
              A (i, j, 2) ---> Represents the cost of
the optimal path from i to j

  Input  : M
  Output : A

  Fonction f : ---> Routing table update
     Input : i,j
                                         --
>Routing table update of vertex I, from vertex routing
table j
     h = 0
     For k=1 to n do
       If (A(j,k,1)#-1)
         If ((A(i,k,1)=-1) or (A(j,k,2)+M(j,i)<A(i,k,2)))
           A(i,k,1) = j
          A(i,k,2) = A(j,k,2) + M(j,i)
            h = h + 1
         End If
       End If
     End For

     If h#0
       For k=1 to max(i,j) do
       If ((k#i) and (k#j) et (M(i,k)#-1))
          f(k,i)
       End If
       End For
     End If
   End Function
```

```
Debut
  For i=1 to n do
    For j=1 to n do
      A(i,j,1) = -1
      A(i,j,2) = -1
    End For
  End For

  For i=1 to n do
    A(i,i,1) = i
    A(i,i,2) = 0
    For j=1 to i-1 do
      If M(i,j)#-1
      If ((A(i,j,1)=-1) or (M(i,j)<A(i,j,2)))
          f(i,j)
          f(j,i)
        End If
      End If
    End For
  End For
End

Return A
```

Amelioration of Quality of service Method:

Description:

The following Schema (Fig. 7) consists of the following elements:

Firstly, each node is specified by a limited internal memory and a queue.

Besides, each frame is specified by a wait time. In addition, each frame is characterized by an index that represents the number of collisions.

In the initial case, we assign an initial time to wait which equals: time max = max of waiting time.

However, when transmitting several frames at the same time and at the same destination, we will have a collision. For each collision, we consider two classes of frame representing important frame and usual frame.

The first type of collision is when single important frames collide with other usual frames, which allow to the transmission of the important frame and penalization of the other usual ones.

The second type is when several important frames or usual frames are collided with each other, both of them will be penalized.

Nevertheless, each user in a collision has a random number, which represents the number of cycles to wait in order to try his communication. This random number grows as the number of collisions increases. In the case of the number of collisions exceeding a threshold, the frames will be abandoned.

Otherwise, each frame has its own contention window CW that will be initialized at 1 when a new node enters.

If the frame is in a collision, we multiply CW by two. And, we choose the cycle number

$$x_{cycle} \in [0, 2CWmax] \tag{10}$$

If this frame is important, it will wait for x cycle before the next transmission, and if it is usual, it will wait for x cycle + A, such as A is constant which will be fixed at the beginning, in order to favor the important frames with respect to the other usual frames.

4 Approach Illustration and Results

Our work is aim to improve the performance of Ad Hoc networks by using the quality of service in terms of losses in the case of widespread video transmissions as well as minimize transmission delay.

The performance of the quality of service was measured with respect to metrics like Packet Loss Ratio and Mean Sojourn time in two different scenarios: number of packets per node and no of node.

However, the different scenarios were made with Eclipse.

In our scenarios, number of packets per node, and number of nodes connected in a network at a time is varied, through which the comparison graphs of Algorithm 1, Algorithm 2 and Algorithm 3 is obtained. We called the mean sojourn time Tm, the random time interval between its input and its output from the system. The mean sojourn time Tm is obtained by analyzing what happens for a given frame.

Packet loss ratio is a very important ratio to measure the performance of routing protocol. The packet loss ratio can be obtained from the total number of packets that never reached the destination divided by the total data packets sent from sources. Mathematically it can be shown as Eq. (10).

$$Packet\ Loss\ Ratio = (nbr\ Sent\ Packet - nbr\ Received\ Packet)/nbr\ Sent\ Packet * 100 \tag{11}$$

where:

Nbr Sent Packets = Number of sent packets.

Nbr Received Packets = Number of received packets.

The results are fairly constant with respect to mean sojourn time, only increasing slightly in the case of increasing the number of packet and also the number of nodes (Fig. 8).

However, Algorithm 2 performance well in all conditions even if the number of nodes increases because nodes become more stationary will lead to more stable path from source to destination.

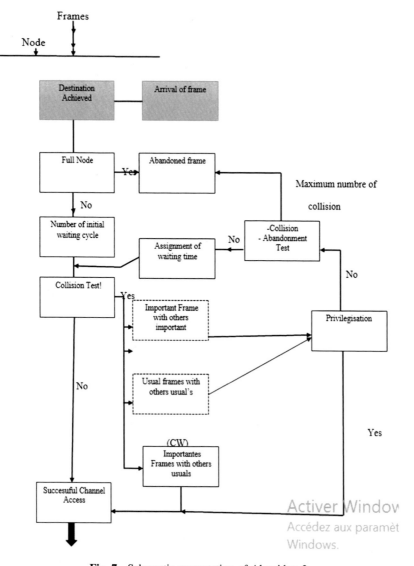

Fig. 7. Schematic presentation of Algorithm 3

The Packet Loss Ratio versus the number of packers per node is depicted in Fig. 9. With increasing number of nodes, Algorithm 2 show worst-performance, It remains same for all less number of nodes, but with increasing the number of nodes, Algorithm 2 show maximum packet loss.

When looking at the number of packets dropped from a network-size perspective, it can be seen from Fig. 3 that the difference in performance increases with the total number of nodes in the network.

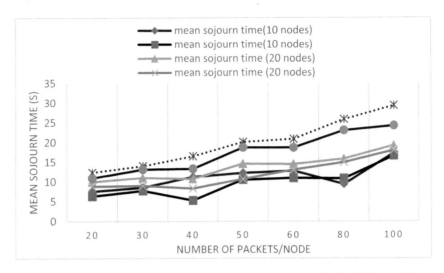

Fig. 8. Mean sojourn time versus the number of packet per node for different nodes

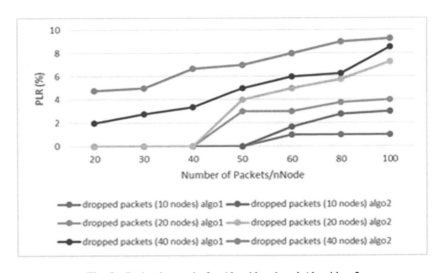

Fig. 9. Packet loss ratio for Algorithm 1 and Algorithm 2

Figure 10 shows the mean sojourn time versus the number of packets/node for different algorithm.

In particular, the Performance of Algorithm 2 remains constant for increasing number of packets, whereas his performance is more better than Algorithm 1.

It is also observed that the performance of Algorithm 3 outperforms to the Algorithm 1 and Algorithm 2 in all conditions.

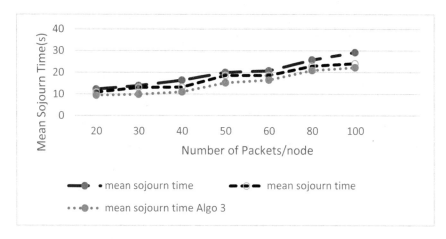

Fig. 10. Mean sojourn time for different algorithms

Now, we assume that we know how to divide the information between the usual frames and the urgent frames by using the information of the nodes. In this case, it imposes a quality of service on the sojourn time.

Based on the Fig. 11, it is shown that Algorithm 3 is even better than both algorithm (Algorithm 1 and Algorithm 2) in all conditions.

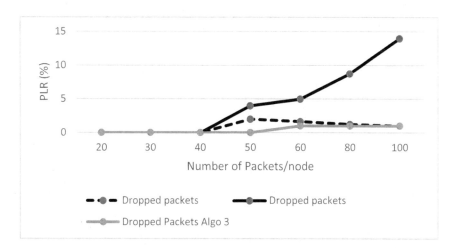

Fig. 11. Packet loss ratio for different algorithms

Furthermore, It remains same for all less number of packets, but with increasing of the number of packet, Algorithm 2 show maximum packet loss.

It is also observed that Algorithm 2 is even better than Algorithm 1, but lower than Algorithm 3 in packet loss ratio.

As consequence, it can be concluded that these graphs are found very helpful in the statistical analysis of these quality of service performance.

5   Conclusion

The use of wireless links for streaming video on the Internet becomes more common today. One of the key issues facing Vehicular Ad Hoc Networks (VANETs) is the lack of robust and cost-effective ongoing connectivity and Quality of Service (QoS) support.

In particular, as the network complexity increases, our proposed algorithm is able to improve the performance in dynamic network.

In this paper, we focused on routing solutions to ensure a certain quality of service in vehicular ad hoc networks at the real-time management, and a better packet loss performance, which are often a great goal for drivers.

The results indicate that the performance of our method (Algorithm 3) shows the best performance for VANET network in all conditions.

However, simulation results show that Algorithm 2 performs best in case of mean sojourn time compared with Algorithm 1, but still can't compete with Algorithm 3. Furthermore, Algorithm 1 performs well in case of packet loss ratio compared with the Algorithm 2. It is clearly seen that the Algorithm 1 increases the mean sojourn time, so automatically a large part of the packets will go through the longest paths or the longest edges, which implies that the packets are not too crowded in the nodes and then they can't be lost.

Our protocol will prove to be essential to serve the drivers, to have a reliable service that allows them to make a trip as quickly as possible with a minimum of space and time. And so contribute to a better life by protecting our beautiful planet.

Acknowledgements. The authors would like to express their sincere gratitude to the Department of Industrial Engineering at the Faculty of Sciences and Techniques of Beni Mellal, and TIAD laboratory, Department of Computer Sciences at the University of Sultan Moulay Sliman for their supervision and guidance throughout the period of research.

References

1. Daniel, A., Paul, A., Ahmad, A., Rho, S.: Cooperative intelligence of vehicles for intelligent transportation systems (ITS). Wireless Pers. Commun. **87**(2), 461–484 (2016)
2. Ennaciri, A., Erritali, M., Mabrouki, M., et al.: Performance analysis of streaming video over vehicular ad-hoc. In: 2016 13th International Conference on Computer Graphics, Imaging and Visualization (CGiV), IEEE, pp. 375–380 (2016)
3. Wahab, O.A., Otrok, H., Mourad, A.: VANET QoS-OLSR: QoS-based clustering protocol for vehicular ad hoc networks. Comput. Commun. **36**(13), 1422–1435 (2013)
4. Ash, G.R.: Traffic Engineering and QoS Optimization of Integrated Voice and Data Networks. Morgan Kaufmann (2006)
5. Gehrsitz, T., Kellerer, W.: QoS and robustness of priority-based MAC protocols for the in-car power line communication. Veh. Commun. (2017)

6. Kazantzidis, M.I., Wang, L., Gerla, M.: On fairness and efficiency of adaptive audio application layers for multihop wireless networks. In 1999 IEEE International Workshop on Mobile Multimedia Communications, (MoMuC '99), pp. 357–362, 15–17 Nov 1999
7. Sharma, P., Kaul, A., Garg, M.L.: Performance analysis of video streaming applications over VANETs. Int. J. Comput. Appl. **112**(14) (2015)
8. Piamrat, K., Viho, C., Bonnin, J.-M. et al.: Quality of experience measurements for video streaming over wireless networks. In: Sixth International Conference on Information Technology: New Generations, ITNG'09, pp. 1184–1189. IEEE (2009)
9. Xin, J., Lin, C.-W., Sun, M.-T.: Digital video transcoding. Proc. IEEE **93**(1), On page(s): 84–97 (Jan. 2005)
10. Ahmad, I., Wei, X., Sun, Y., Zhang, Y.-Q.: Video transcoding: an overview of various techniques and research issues. IEEE Trans. Multimedia **7**(5), 793–804 (Oct 2005)
11. Avramova, Z., De Vleeschauwer, D., Spaey, K., Wittevrongel, S., Bruneel, H., Blondia, C.: Comparison of simulcast and scalable video coding in terms of the required capacity in an IPTV network. Packet Video **2007**, 113–122 (2007)
12. Wien, M., Cazoulat, R., Graffunder, A., Hutter, A., Amon, P.: Real-time system for adaptive video streaming based on SVC. IEEE Trans. Circuits Syst. Video Technol. **17**(9), 1227–1237 (2007)
13. Wei, Z., Cai, C., Ma, K.-K.: A novel H.264-based multiple description video coding via polyphase transform and partial prediction. In: International Symposium on Intelligent Signal Processing and Communications (ISPACS '06), pp. 151–154 (Dec 2006)
14. Loguinov, D., Radha, H.: On retransmission schemes for real-time streaming in the internet. In: Proceedings In IEEE INFOCOM 2001, Twentieth Annual Joint Conference of the IEEE Computer and Communications Societies, vol. 3, pp. 1310–1319 (2001)
15. Bouazizi, I., Gunes, M.: Distortion-optimized FEC for unequal error protection in MPEG-4 video delivery. In: Proceedings of Ninth International Symposium on Computers and Communications (ISCC 2004), vol. 2, pp. 615–620 (June–July 2004)
16. Chen, T.P., Chen, T.: Second-generation error concealment for video transport over error prone channels. In: Proceedings of International Conference on Image Processing, vol. 1, pp. I-25–I-28 (2002)
17. Hasrouny, H., Samhat, A.E., Bassil, C., Laouiti, A.: VANet security challenges and solutions: a survey. Veh. Commun. **7**, 7–20 (2017)
18. Mageid, S.A.: Connectivity based positioning system for underground vehicular ad hoc networks. Int. J. Comput. Netw. Appl. (IJCNA) **4**(1), 1–14 (2017)
19. Nekovee, M.: Epidemic algorithms for reliable and efficient information dissemination in vehicular. Intell. Transp. Syst. IET **3**, 104–110 (2009)
20. Pathirana, P.N.: Node localization using mobile robots in delaytolerant sensor networks. IEEE Trans. Mob. Comput. **4**(3), 285–296 (2005)
21. Rahem, A.T., Ismail, M., Abdullah, N.F., et al.: New mathematical model to find the shortest path based on Boolean algebra operations for networks. In: 2016 IEEE 3rd International Symposium on Telecommunication Technologies (ISTT), pp. 112–114. IEEE (2016)
22. Steinbock, C., Biham, O., Katzav, E.: Distribution of shortest path lengths in a class of node duplication network models. Phys. Rev. E **96**(3), 032301 (2017)
23. Makariye, N: Towards shortest path computation using Dijkstra algorithm. In: 2017 International Conference on IoT and Application (ICIOT), pp. 1–3. IEEE (2017)
24. Broumi, S., Talea, M., Bakali, A.,et al.: Application of Dijkstra algorithm for solving interval valued neutrosophic shortest path problem. In: 2016 IEEE Symposium Series on Computational Intelligence (SSCI), pp. 1–6. IEEE (2016)
25. Eiza, M.H., Ni, Q.: An evolving graph-based reliable routing scheme for VANETs. IEEE Trans. Veh. Technol. **62**(4), 1493–1504 (2013)

26. Patel Pragnesh, V., Baxi, M.A.: Improved graph-based reliable routing scheme for VANETs. Int. J. Sci. Eng. Res. **5**(5) (2014)
27. Bittner, S., Raffel, W.-U., Scholz, M.: The area graph-based mobility model and its impact on data dissemination. In: Proceedings of the Third IEEE International Conference on Pervasive Computing and Communications Workshops, PERCOMW '05, pp. 268–272 (2005)
28. Gu, D., Zhang, J.: QoS enhancement in IEEE 802.11 wireless area networks. IEEE Commmu Mag. **41**(6), 120–124 (2003)
29. Golestan, K., Jundi, A., Nassar, L., Sattar, F., Karray, F., Kamel, M. et al.: Vehicular ad-hoc networks (VANETs): capabilities, challenges in information gathering and data fusion. In: Autonomous and Intelligent Systems, pp. 34–41. Springer (2012)
30. Sattari, M.R.J., Noor, R.M., Ghahremani, S.: Dynamic congestion control algorithm for vehicular ad hoc networks. Int. J. Softw. Eng. Appl. **7**, 95–108 (2013)
31. Mohammed, N.H., El-Moafy, H.N., Abdel-Mageid, S.M., Marie, M.I.: Mobility management scheme based on smart buffering for vehicular networks. Int. J. Comput. Netw. Appl. (IJCNA). **4**(2), 35–46 (2017)
32. Hadded, M., Zagrouba, R., Laouiti, A., et al.: An optimal strategy for collision-free slots allocations in vehicular ad-hoc networks. In: Vehicular Ad-hoc Networks for Smart Cities, pp. 15–30. Springer, Singapore (2015)

Sustainable Development: Clustering Moroccan Population Based on ICT and Education

Zineb El Asraoui[(✉)] and Abdelilah Maach

Mohammadia School of Engineers-LRIE Team, Mohammed V University,
Rabat, Morocco
{zinebelasraoui,amaach}@gmail.com

Abstract. ICT and education relationship is increasingly recognized as important enablers of sustainable development growth. However, the validity of this theory still ambiguous in countries under development: as the case of morocco. The present study focused on determining the correlation between education (university degree as factor) and ICT (Internet access as factor). Data was extracted from public census 2014. A procedure combining tabular data and machine learning algorithms (K-means) was used to determine clusters of population accordingly to their access to Internet and level of education. The results showed that using K-means algorithm four clusters were identified for both rural and urban domains. This identification was verified by a level deepening starting with the regions then municipalities. This profound allows us to make a comparison between the regions and the municipalities clusters in the same territory (rural or urban), then an analysis based on resemblance between rural and urban population. The following conclusions are drown. For both urban and rural territories, the population of the cluster with the highest level of ICT and education, does not completely match with its counterpart in the municipalities. The same conclusion is applied for the lowest clusters. The comparison between the urban and rural clusters proves the incoherence between the two. The regions (or municipalities) that are in the cluster with the highest levels in the urban domain figure in the cluster with the lowest levels, and vice versa.

Keywords: Sustainable development · ICT · Education · Clustering · K-means

1 Introduction

In order to equilibrate the balance between the three axes of sustainable development (economic, social and environmental), the United Nations adapted a resolution after the General Assembly of 25 [1], summarized in 17 goals and 167 targets [2]. These objectives include education: facilitate access to education at all levels, improve its quality and increase schooling rate. Moreover, as the world is moving towards technology, many voices rise to combine education and ICT. Germany, Netherlands, Iceland and United Kingdom have conducted an investigation commissioned by the European Commission in autumn 2011, entitled "European Survey of Schools:

© Springer Nature Switzerland AG 2019
M. Ezziyani (Ed.): AI2SD 2018, AISC 915, pp. 191–204, 2019.
https://doi.org/10.1007/978-3-030-11928-7_16

ICT and Education—ESSIE". The report of the committee emphasizes "Students and teachers in Europe are keen to 'go digital', computer numbers have doubled since 2006 and most schools are now 'connected', but use of ICTs (Information and Communication Technologies) and digital skill levels are very uneven" [3].

In Africa, wanting to achieve the same objectives, a study financed by the International Research Development Centre (IDRC) of Canada used data from a transnational study (Pioneer ICT-Schools Project in Africa). The results showed that "multiple uses of ICT in the participating schools, albeit centered on teaching ICT basic skills. A biaxial model with four quadrants is used to visualize the range of ICT usages in the schools. The analysis reveals a limited pedagogical use of ICT to teach academic subjects in most of the schools. Approximately 80% of the reported uses involved teaching ICT basic skills, while barely 17% involved subject-specific ICT integration for teaching and learning purposes" [4].

Particularly in Morocco, the integration of ICT in education identifies numerous obstacles that have showed their sensitivity to geographical localization: urban or rural [5] (a study based on the interview of 33 principals of primary and secondary schools and 4 departmental and regional officials responsible for the implementation of the government's ICT mainstreaming strategy). Another study based on the importance of integrating ICT into higher education (established on teachers' experience using ICT in teaching university students, and the opinion of students in the use of ICTs) exhibits the contribution of ICT in the provision of enriching and variants educational models. "These models share features of a technology-based training also emphasizes self-directed, independent, flexible and interactive learning" [6]. It should be noted that there is a remarkable lack of studies on education and ICT in Morocco, which really touches on these two axes based on large data that can provide reliable results, hence the need for present study.

Our intention in this paper is to introduce ICT and education as two factors to understand Morocco's population distribution based on geographical division. In addition, it is our aim to explore the difference between urban and rural classification results to conclude on the sensibility of ICT and education to the geographical placement.

Several studies use clustering in various domains to understand the distribution of a population in relation to a specific issue, the example of Crete, a clustering of the habitants to understand the attitude of urban residents towards the development of tourism has produced "Three clusters: the 'Advocates' (identified by their high appreciation of tourism benefits); the 'Socially and Environmentally Concerned' (characterized by a consensus towards the environmental and social costs of tourism expansion); and the 'Economic Skeptics' (who showed lower appreciation of tourism's economic benefits)" [7]. In the medical field, a clustering was used to separate cancerous from noncancerous tissues and cell lines [8]. Clustering Analysis has also revealed its importance in the computer sphere to analyze Network Traffic for Protocol- and Structure-Independent Botnet Detection to detect the hosts that share both similar communication patterns [9].

The present study investigates how Morocco's population are clustered based on internet access and university degree (the first symbolizes ICT, and second represents education) for both urban and rural domain. This paper is organized as follow: in the second section, we explained the methodology and material used in our study, then the third section we represented results of clustering urban population: regions and municipalities ones based on k-means algorithm and using R studio. The forth section includes the same clustering for rural population (for both regions and municipalities individuals). Finally, in the fifth section we end up by extricate the differences between the two results.

2 Methodology and Material

2.1 Statistical Data

Our analysis is based primarily on the 2014 census statistical data of the Moroccan population. This information are directly accessible on the official website of the High Commission of the Plan [10]. The census data is collected in each territory by direct door-to-door interviews.

The information gathered is presented in a tabular form; the first four columns contains geographical data, each municipality has a code that refers to its prefecture and region. The rest of the tables include socio-demographical and household data each one apart. We then combined data from the Individual table with the Household table in order to access it from one table source. The parameters we exploit in our analysis are ICT (Internet access) and educational level (university degree).

2.2 Data Analysis Method

Clustering analysis is divided on two types: hierarchical clustering and partitional clustering that contain K-means, K-Medoids and CLARA clustering.

In our study, we employed the K-means [11] algorithm using R (version 3.4.2) [12].

K-means algorithm is an unsupervised classification method for determining clusters of a given population based on predetermined factors. The number of classes, K, is set in advance.

Having initialized the k centers of classes, all individuals are assigned, after many iterations, to the cluster whose center is the closest according to the distance chosen.

Our case we used Euclidean distance whose formula:

$$\text{deuc}(x, \ y) = \sqrt{\sum_{i=1}^{n} (y_i - x_i)^2} \tag{1}$$

To explain K-means principle, let $X = \{x_i\}$, $i = 1; \ldots; n$ be the set of n d-dimensional points to be clustered into a set of K clusters, $C = \{c_k; \ k = 1; \ldots; K\}$. K-means algorithm finds a partition such that the squared error between the empirical mean of a cluster and the points in the cluster is minimized. Let μ_k be the mean of cluster c_k. The squared error between μ_k and the points in cluster c_k is defined as

$$J(c_k) = \sum_{x_i \in c_k} ||x_i - \mu_k||^2 \tag{2}$$

The goal of K-means is to minimize the sum of the squared error over all K clusters (within-cluster sum of square WSS),

$$J(C) = \sum_{k=1}^{K} \sum_{x_i \in c_k} ||x_i - \mu_k||^2 \tag{3}$$

K-means starts with an initial partition with K clusters and assign patterns to clusters so as to reduce the squared error. Since the squared error always decreases with an increase in the number of clusters K (with $J(C) = 0$ when $K = n$), it can be minimized only for a fixed number of clusters. The main steps of K-means algorithm are as follows:

1. Select an initial partition with K clusters; repeat steps 2 and 3 until cluster membership stabilizes.
2. Generate a new partition by assigning each pattern to its closest cluster center.
3. Compute new cluster centers [13].

To select number of clusters we used the Elbow method that looks at the total WSS as a function of the number of clusters:

One should choose a number of clusters so that adding another cluster does not improve much better the total WSS.

The optimal number of clusters can be defined as follow:

1. Compute clustering algorithm (e.g., k-means clustering) for different values of k.
2. For instance, by varying k from 1 to 10 clusters.
3. For each k, calculate the total within-cluster sum of square (WSS).
4. Plot the curve of WSS according to the number of clusters k.
5. The location of a bend (knee) in the plot is generally considered as an indicator of the appropriate number of clusters [11].

3   Data Analysis Results for Urban Population

This section summarizes the result of the clustering for the urban domain, based on depth by level: region, prefecture, and commune.

The first step to implement K-means is to determine the number K of clusters. To do so, we applied the elbow method [14]. The results are shown in Fig. 1.

This outcome shows that we can set four classes, for both levels (regions and municipalities). Having the identical class number for the two levels enabled us to perform a comparison between levels (regions and municipalities) on one side, and between domains (urban and rural) on the other side.

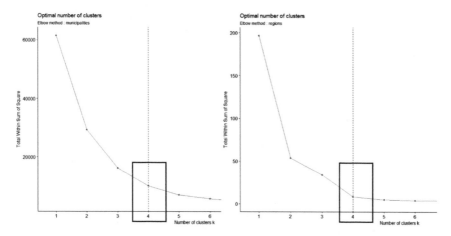

Fig. 1. Number of clusters for regions (right) and municipalities (left)

3.1   K-Means for Region's Population

In this section, we realized the first clustering of the urban population by regions. The input factors are Internet Access and University degree. The results are shown in Fig. 2 and Table 1.

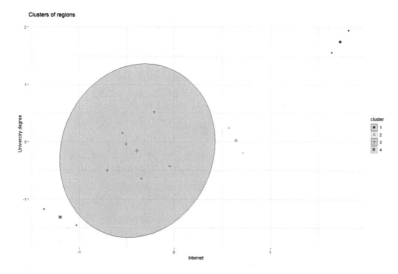

Fig. 2. Urban regions' cluster plot

Results show that "04: Rabat-Salé-Kenitra" and "06: Grand Casablanca-Settat" are placed in the same cluster [UR1-centroid (31.78, 10.91%)] with the highest percentage of Internet access and University degree.

Table 1. Urban regions' cluster geographical placement and centroids

Geographical placement	Administrative subdivisions of the Kingdom	Internet access (%)	University degree (%)	Clusters	Centroid Internet (%)	University degree (%)
04.	Rabat-Salé-Kénitra	32.1	11.2	1	31.78	10.91
06.	Grand Casablanca-Settat	31.4	10.6			
01.	Tanger-Tetouan-AlHoceima	24.7	7.7	2	27.46	8.33
02.	Oriental	23.6	7.3			
03.	Fès-Meknès	24.1	9.1			
08.	Drâa-Tafilalet	22.9	8.2			
10.	Guelmim-Oued Noun	22.8	8.5			
11.	Laayoune-Sakia El Hamra	22.1	7.5			
07.	Marrakech-Safi	27.2	8.7	3	23.38	8.06
09.	Souss-Massa	27.7	8			
05.	Béni Mellal-Khénifra	19.5	6.5	4	20.20	6.33
12.	Eddakhla-Oued Eddahab	20.9	6.1			

On the other hand, cluster UR4 (that includes "05: Beni Mellal-Khenifra" and "12: Dakhla-Oued Eddahab") is characterized by the lowest rates with a centroid (20.20, 6.33%). Cluster UR2 whose centroid (27.46, 8.33%) is located between the two extreme clusters, it contains "07: Marrakech-Safi" and "09: Souss-Massa".

Finally, cluster UR3 (23.38, 8.06%) involves the remaining regions.

3.2   K-Means for Municipalities' Population

The same approach is employed for the clustering by municipalities (considering 4 as number of clusters). The results are shown in Fig. 3 and Table 2.

Figure 3 contains the four clusters of urban municipalities. It gives an idea on the clusters form and their densities.

Table 2 includes the distribution of municipalities on each cluster as well as their centroids. Cluster UM1 (58.07, 25.03%) contains 2% of urban municipalities, cluster UM2 (30.78, 9.83%) contains 16%, cluster UM3 (19.35, 6.30%) contains 42% and cluster UM4 (10.18, 4.20%) contains 40%.

4   Data Analysis Result for Rural Population

The objective of this part is to reveal the clusters of the rural domain. Still based on a development by scale: region and municipalities.

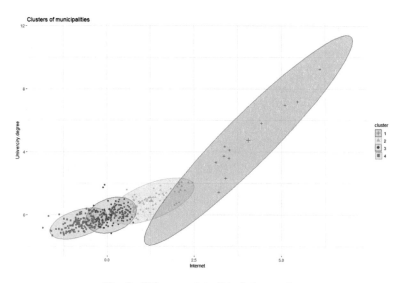

Fig. 3. Urban municipalities' cluster plot

Table 2. Urban municipalities' distribution and centroids

	Number of municipalities	Percentage (%)	Centroid	
			Internet (%)	University degree (%)
Cluster UM1	11	2	58.07	25.03
Cluster UM2	86	16	30.78	9.83
Cluster UM3	233	42	19.35	6.30
Cluster UM4	220	40	10.18	4.20

We started by identifying the number of clusters for rural regions and municipalities using the elbow method. As shown in Fig. 4, for both (regions and municipalities) the optimal number of clusters is four.

4.1 K-Means for Regions' Population

In this regard, we will generate clusters of rural areas based on ICT and Educations factors. The results are shown in Fig. 5 and Table 3.

The exploration of this clustering, places of the regions of "10: Guelmim-Oued Noun" and "11: Laayoune-Sakia El Hamra" in the same cluster RR1 (6.47, 3.41%), with the highest rate of internet access and university degree. Cluster RR4 (2.88, 1.18%) that includes regions "01: Tangier-Tetouan-Al Hoceima", "03: Fes-Meknes", "04: Rabat-Salé-Kenitra", "06: Grand Casablanca-Settat", "07: Marrakech-Safi") is characterized by the territories that have the lowest percentages. The RR2 (6.28, 1.95%) is placed between two extreme clusters, contains "12: Eddakhla-Oued Eddahab" and "09: Souss-Massa". And finally, cluster RR3 (4.31, 1.89%) that contains the resting regions.

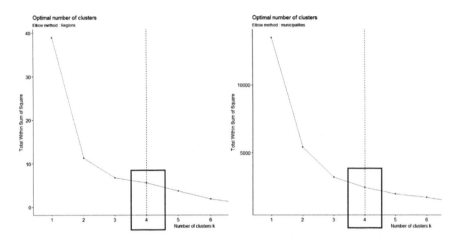

Fig. 4. Number of clusters for regions (left) and municipalities (right)

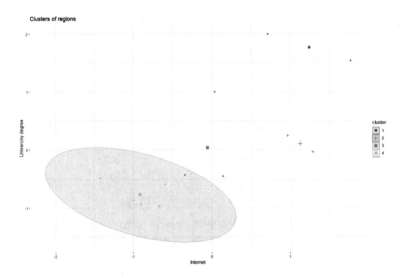

Fig. 5. Rural regions' cluster plot

4.2   K-Means for Municipalities" Population

By following the same method of analysis, we produced the clusters of municipalities as showing in Fig. 6 and synthesizes their distribution on each cluster in Table 4.

The results showed that cluster RM4 (1.17, 0.99%) contains 54% of rural municipalities with the lowest centroid followed by cluster RM3 (3.52, 1.59%), cluster RM2 (6.84, 2.61%) and cluster RM1(12.76, 3.60%) in decreasing order of the distribution of these municipalities 29, 12 and 5%.

Table 3. Rural regions' cluster geographical placement and centroids

Geographical placement	Administrative subdivisions of the Kingdom	Internet access	University degree	Cluster	Centroid Internet access	University degree
10.	Guelmim-Oued Noun	5.6	3.6	RR1	6.47	3.41
11.	Laayoune-Sakia El Hamra	7.4	3.2			
09.	Souss-Massa	6	2.1	RR2	6.28	1.95
12.	Eddakhla-Oued Eddahab	6.5	1.8			
02.	Oriental	4.6	1.5	RR3	4.31	1.90
05.	Béni Mellal-Khénifra	3.8	1.5			
08.	Drâa-Tafilalet	4.5	2.7			
01.	Tanger-Tetouan-Al Hoceima	2.7	1.1	RR4	2.88	1.18
03.	Fès-Meknès	2	1.4			
04.	Rabat-Salé-Kénitra	2.9	1			
06.	Grand Casablanca-Settat	3.4	1.3			
07.	Marrakech-Safi	3.3	1			

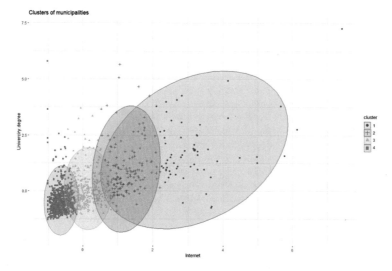

Fig. 6. Rural municipalities' cluster plot

Table 4. Rural municipalities' distribution and centroids

	Number of municipalities	Percentage (%)	Centroid	
			Internet (%)	University degree (%)
Cluster RM1	60	5	12.76	3.60
Cluster RM2	154	12	6.84	2.61
Cluster RM3	372	29	3.52	1.59
Cluster RM4	693	54	1.17	0.99

5   Comparison Between Urban and Rural Results

5.1   Intra-comparison

To better understand the distribution of the population according to the two classifications (by region and by municipality), we proceeded by a fusion of the two results.

The two Tables 5 and 6 describe the result of the following classification: for each region, we develop the distribution of its sub-communes on UM1, UM2, UM3 and UM4 clusters.

Table 5. Urban regions distribution on municipalities clusters

			Urban municipalities			
			Cluster 1 (%)	Cluster 2 (%)	Cluster 3 (%)	Cluster 4 (%)
Urban Regions	Cluster 1	R4	8	17	33	42
		R6	6	30	40	24
	Cluster 2	R7	1	13	51	35
		R9	0	26	57	17
	Cluster 3	R1	0	19	48	33
		R2	0	9	60	31
		R3	1	9	27	63
		R8	0	22	39	39
		R10	0	33	50	17
		R11	0	0	80	20
	cluster 4	R5	0	3	33	64
		R12	0	0	100	0

The analysis of the homogeneity between the regions and its sub- municipalities (Table 5) shows that region 11 ranks first, belonging to UR3 and 80% of its subcommunes are in UM3. Followed by Regions 02 and 10 with a respective percentage of 60 and 50% of their sub-municipalities that are in the same cluster level as their regions. Lastly, Region 12 is part of UR4 while none of its sub-municipalities is in UM4. Regions 04 and 06 are in UR1, only 8 and 6% (respectively) of their submunicipalities that are included in UM1.

Table 6. Rural regions distribution on municipalities clusters

			Rural municipalities			
			Cluster 1 (%)	Cluster 2 (%)	Cluster 3 (%)	Cluster 4 (%)
Rural regions	Cluster 1	R10	13	33	13	40
		R11	20	13	7	60
	Cluster 2	R9	11	19	26	44
		R12	25	0	13	63
	Cluster 3	R2	9	20	26	45
		R5	3	19	27	51
		R8	9	19	38	34
	Cluster 4	R1	1	9	36	54
		R3	1	4	25	70
		R4	1	5	33	60
		R6	3	5	30	62
		R7	2	7	31	61

We did the same calculation for the rural case and the results are shown in the Table 6.

The same conclusions are made for the rural domain. Regions 03, 06 and 07 that belong to RR4 have respective percentages of 70, 62 and 61% of their sub-municipalities that register under RM4. While for 12, 10 and 09 only 0, 13 and 19% of their sub-municipalities that belongs to the same degree of cluster.

For both rural and urban domains. The difference between the clusters of regions and municipalities is explained by the difference between the centroids of the two clusters (as Table 7 shows, the centroids of the regions are smaller than those of the communes).

Table 7. Difference between urban and rural regions' centroids

Difference between URX and RRX	Internet access (%)	University degree (%)
X = 1	25.31	7.50
X = 2	21.19	6.38
X = 3	19.06	6.17
X = 4	17.32	5.15

The figure above (Fig. 7) summarizes the results of the two urban and rural clustering, knowing that especially in this figure URX means urban region X, and RRX means rural region X.

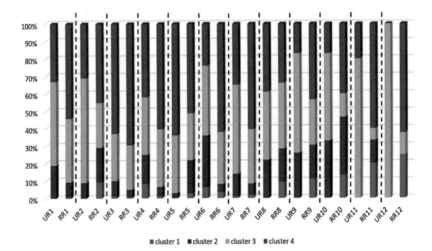

Fig. 7. Urban and Rural regions distribution on municipalities clusters

5.2   Inter-comparison

The comparison between the classification of the urban and rural domains shows that there are differences on multiple levels.

First, the difference between centroids. The results obtained contradict the assumption that the centroids of the rural domain must be close as showed Table 7.

Firstly, the difference between the UR1 and RR1 cluster is the highest with 25.31% for the internet access factor and 7.5% for the university degree factor. While, UR4 and RR4 characterized with the least difference (17.32% for internet access, 5.15% for university degree).

Secondly, the urban classification is totally different from the rural one. The assumption that the urban and rural domain of the same region must belong to the same level of classification is rejected by analyzing the results of our study.

Table 8 summarizes the difference between the internet access and university degree of the urban and rural domain of the same region. Then a classification in ascending order is made based on the Euclidean distance of the result data (we calculated it so that we could develop one classification instead of tow if we take ICT as factor and education as another factor).

The balance sheet treatment puts Region 12 in first place since it has the lowest distance, this difference is due to the fact that its urban domain is in level 4 and the rural one in level 2. However, the regions 04 and 06 which were ranked last with the greatest Euclidean difference (25.60 and 30.50% respectively).

This comes back to their urban population which is in the first cluster UR1, while inhabitants of the rural domain are at the bottom of the clustering (cluster RR4).

Table 8. Difference between Urban and Rural municipalities' centroids

Region	Cluster urban	Custer rural	Difference		Euclidian distance (%)
			Internet accessc	University degree (%)	
12	UR4	RR2	13.92	4.38	14.59
5	UR4	RR3	15.89	6.13	17.03
10	UR3	RR1	16.91	4.65	17.54
11					
2	UR3	RR3	19.07	4.43	19.58
8					
1	UR3	RR4	20.5	6.88	21.63
3					
9	UR2	RR2	21.18	6.38	22.12
7	UR2	RR4	24.58	7.15	25.60
4	UR1	RR4	28.9	9.73	30.50

6 Conclusion

The present study focused on the clustering of Morocco's population based on two factors ICT (Internet access) and Education (University degree). First, we combined between two databases (individual database and household database) from 2014 census to generate one table source for rural and urban population. For both domains, we used k-means clustering to build clusters for regions and municipalities (we adapt the elbow method to determinate number of clusters) in order to determinate resemblance between them. Moreover, a cross-comparison and intra-comparison was made to examine Morocco's population morphology.

The following conclusions were drown:

- For both urban and rural territories, four clusters are fined.
- In both urban and rural territories, regions' centroids are lower than municipalities' centroids. Indeed, for the same level of clustering (for example UR3 and UM3) the municipalities clusters does not contain sub-municipalities of regions that were clustered in the same level.
- The urban and rural clustering are different: For the same region, rural and urban domain does not fit in the same level. That is shows the gap between tow populations in the same territory.

Regarding the importance of using ICT in education for sustainable development, worldwide countries are racing to combine them in a way to improve educational system by using new approaches and methods. The main contribution of our study, is that we can define barriers to integration of ICT in education to localize problems in a way to be effective in determine solutions.

Generally, these results have shown another facet of the relationship between ICT and education according to the distribution of the Moroccan population, which will help the state in its approach of merging the two factors for improving the quality of the education. The clustering of the Moroccan population obtained will allow treating each class according to its characteristics and the challenges that revealed to have best results.

References

1. United Nations: Transforming our world: the 2030 Agenda for (2015)
2. https://www.un.org/sustainabledevelopment/sustainable-development-goals/
3. Buda, A.: ICT in Education. In Information and Communication Technologies in Education Overview in Visegrad countries, University of Ostrava, Ostrava, pp. 15–32 (2014)
4. Karsenti, T., Ngamo, S.T.: Qualité de l'éducation en Afrique: le rôle potentiel des TIC. Int. Rev. Educ. **53**(5–6), 665–686 (2007)
5. Mastafi, M.: Obstacles à l'intégration des technologies de l'information et de la communication (TIC) dans le système éducatif marocain. CARISM and IREC, University Panthéon Assas Paris **2**, 50–65 (2014)
6. Naciri, H.: Using ICT to improve higher education in Morocco. In: Conference Proceedings. ICT for language learning. libreriauniversitaria. it Edizioni, p. 467 (2015)
7. Andriotis, K., Vaughan, R.D.: Urban residents' attitudes toward tourism development: the case of Crete. J. Travel Res. **42**(12), 172–185 (2003)
8. Alon, U., Barkai, N., Notterman, D.A., Gish, K., Ybarra, S., Mack, D., Levine, A.J.: Broad patterns of gene expression revealed by clustering analysis of tumor and normal colon tissues probed by oligonucleotide arrays. Proc. Nat. Acad. Sci. **96**(112), 6745–6750 (1999)
9. Gu, G., Perdisci, R., Zhang, J., Lee, W.: BotMiner: clustering analysis of network traffic for protocol-and structure-independent botnet detection. In: USENIX Security Symposium, vol. 5, n° %12, pp. 139–154 (2008)
10. https://www.hcp.ma
11. Kassambara, A.: Practical Guide to Cluster Analysis in R, sthda.com, p. 2017 (2017)
12. https://www.rstudio.com/products/rstudio/download/
13. Jain, A.K.: Data clustering: 50 years beyond K-means. Pattern Recognit. Lett. **31**(8), 651–666 (2010)
14. Kodinariya, T.M., Makwana, P.R.: Review on determining number of cluster in K-means clustering. Int. J. **1**(6), 90–95 (2013)

Datamining for Fraud Detecting, State of the Art

Imane Bouazza[1(✉)], El Bachir Ameur[1], and Farid Ameur[2]

[1] LaRIT Laboratory, Faculty of Science, Ibn Tofail University,
Kenitra, Morocco
Imanebouazza18@gmail.com, ameurelbachir@yahoo.fr
[2] Tax Department, Ministry of Economy and Finance, Rabat, Morocco
ameur_farid@yahoo.fr

Abstract. Fraud detection is a rapidly developing field; several technologies have been used to prevent fraud such as data mining (DM). The use of data mining applications have shown their utility in different fields and have attracted increasing attention and popularity in the financial world. Data mining plays an important role in the field of fraud because it is often applied to extract and discover the truths hidden behind very large amounts of data. For this purpose, our contribution explores the applications of data mining techniques to fraud detection, and groups the various researches carried out in this field from 1966 to 2017. The result of this study will support and guide future research in this field.

Keywords: Datamining · Fraud detection · Intelligent system

1 Introduction

Fraud detection is the most complex task for differents domains; as an example, fraud detection is the most important mission of a tax administration which have to ensure that all taxpayers respect their tax obligations in terms of declarations and payments. With the evolution of the number of taxpayers, the diversification and the complexity of fraud techniques, conventional methods of fiscal control have shown their limits. The use of data management applications has shown their utility in different areas; such as fraud by credit card, money laundering, fraud in telecommunications, fraud in e-commerce transactions, fraud insurance and subscription fraud etc. [1–5] (Derrig 2002; Cortes et al. 1999).

DATAMINING technique allows the processing of large volumes of data. It has become a central area of application for the knowledge discovery in database. An important task in the detection of fraud is the construction of models, profiles, or fraudulent behaviours. They can be used as decision support tools for planning strategies of tax audit. It comes to rely on the historical verification data to plan effectively for future audits.

The tax audit planning is usually a difficult task, because of the constraints of the human and financial resources necessary to conduct monitoring missions. It faces two contradictory issues:

© Springer Nature Switzerland AG 2019
M. Ezziyyani (Ed.): AI2SD 2018, AISC 915, pp. 205–219, 2019.
https://doi.org/10.1007/978-3-030-11928-7_17

- Maximize revenue: identify taxpayers who will be selected for the defrauded tax collection is maximized.
- Reduce the costs of control: choose the taxpayers for the audit so as to reduce the resources needed to carry out the control.

Ngai et al. [6] concludes that the most urgent challenge in detecting fraud is "to bridge the gap between practitioners and researchers" and that "research should direct its attention to finding more practical principles and Practitioners to help them design, develop and implement data mining and business intelligence systems".

In this contribution, we provided examples from different domain. We introduced recent research that applies a variety of data mining techniques to the control and fraud context. We presented and compared the key techniques of data analysis, data extraction.

The structure of the document is as follows: we start with the history of fraud, definition and properties, we cited the different types of fraud. This is followed by the definitions of DATA Mining (DM); We show its characteristics, properties and applications. After presenting the techniques of DM. Then we quoted the various searches by techniques through time.

2 Literature Review

The effective detection of accounting fraud has always been important complex task for accounting professionals. The examination of financial fraud is in fact one of the most important questions that the economic and social spin-offs of fraud can be massive [7].

The techniques of fraud are developing and internationalizing, the detection of tax fraud becomes a complex problem (see the example of Spathis et al. [7]), which makes the fight against this phenomenon more important than ever. Despite the strengthening of action plans by the various agencies involved, fraud is costly for the treasury. The difficulty for the administration is that it is a matter of isolating some cases of fraud from thousands of possible cases.

Traditionally, auditors are responsible for detecting fraud on the financial statements. With the emergence of a growing number of companies, auditors have become overburdened with the task of detecting fraud. As a result, various data mining techniques are used to reduce the workload of listeners.

Data mining (DM) plays an important role in the detection of financial fraud because it is often used to extract and discover the truths hidden behind very large amounts of data. Several authors have treated this subject based on the different methods of DM. The following six data mining methods are most commonly used (classification, regression, grouping, prediction, boundary detection, and visualization).

3 Fraud

More than 49 papers on the subject published between 1997 and 2008 have been analysed and classified into four categories of financial fraud (bank fraud, insurance fraud, securities fraud and Commodity and other related financial fraud). This means that financial fraud is a serious problem worldwide and even more so in fast-growing countries [8].

The Oxford English Dictionary [9] defines fraud as "criminal or criminal deceit intended to result in financial or personal gain". According to Kirkos et al. [10] fraud can be defined as deliberate fraud committed by management that causes damage to investors and creditors through material misleading financial statements. During Audit Process, auditors must estimate the possibility of management fraud.

Phua et al. [2] also describe fraud as leading to abuse of a profit organization's system without necessarily having direct legal consequences. Wang et al. [11] define it as "a deliberate act that is contrary to the law, rule or policy aimed at obtaining unauthorized financial benefits". On (2012) Lin et al. [12] identified five main fraud factors, including "Low Performance", "Need for External Financing", "Financial Distress", "Insufficient Board Control" and "Competition or Market Saturation" by Sequence. However, the experts' judgments were simply based on their own experience and expertise.

Fraud is becoming an increasingly serious problem, and as a result, effective fraud detection has always been an important but complex task for accounting professionals [6, 13] (Pai et al. 2011).

The detection of fraud is a difficult problem because fraudsters make their best efforts to make their behavior legitimate. Another difficulty is that the number of legitimate files is much higher than the number of fraudulent cases. For this purpose the detection of fraud has become one of the best established applications of data mining in industry and government [2]. Several data mining techniques have been applied in financial fraud, such as neural networks [10, 14–17], the logistic regression models (2002) [18–20], the Bayes naïve method [10, 21–23].

4 Data Mining

According to Turban et al. (2007) [24], data mining is a semi-automatic process that uses statistical, mathematical, artificial intelligence and machine-learning techniques to extract and identify potential and Useful information stored in a large database. There are several definitions of data mining.

On (2007), Turban et al. (2007) define data mining as a process that uses statistical, mathematical, artificial and machine-learning techniques to extract and identify useful information, and acquire knowledge from a large database. Data Mining (DM) is an iterative process in which progress is defined by discovery, either by automatic or manual methods [10].

According to Han and Kamber [25] Data mining (DM), also known as "discovery of knowledge in databases" (KDD), is the process of discovering significant models in large Plus, it is also an application that can bring important competitive advantages to make the right decision [26]. DM is an exploratory and complex process involving several iterations. We will call data mining all the techniques that make it possible to transform data into knowledge. It could be defined as an attempt to discover new and meaningful relationships and facts on large data sets [27]. Exploration is done at the initiative of the system, by a business user, and its purpose is to fulfil one of the following tasks: Classification, Estimation, Prediction, Grouping by similarities, Segmentation (or clustering), Description, Optimization.

According to Glen et al. [28] the quality of grading data extraction techniques can be measured by precision classification, robustness and ability to interpret the results of the classification [25]. Classification techniques include the induction of decision trees [29], the Bayesian belief networks [11, 30], neural networks [31–33], support vector machines [34] and genetic algorithms [35].

The classification: was the most popular and the only way used to identify fraudulent financial statements (Dianmin et al. 2007).

Regression: is the most widely used method for detecting financial problems Report Fraud [18, 20]. Variable transformations in regression models have also been studied in the context of Detection fraud.

A neural network: is another popular data mining technique that has been successfully used to detect fraud of financial statements [15, 36]. The neural network does not assume the independence of an attribute and is able to extract inter-correlated data and is an appropriate Alternative for problems where some of the assumptions associated with the regression are invalid.

Decision trees: the objective of decision trees is classification by dividing observations into mutually exclusive and exhaustive subgroups by correctly selecting the attributes that best separate the sample. Koh and Low [37] constructs a decision tree to predict hidden problems in the financial statements by examining the following six variables: Fast Assets in Current Liabilities, Market Value of Total Assets, Total assets, interest payments to earnings before interest and taxes, net income for total assets and retained earnings out of total assets

Forecasting: Classification and estimation are data mining techniques used to reveal the characteristics of previously identified variables in a data set. Data mining authors often differentiate "prediction" techniques from classification and estimation [38].

Clustering: Similarly, clusters of journal entries can be identified that do not fall under an established or known Pattern [35, 39]. Self-organized maps based on neural networks [40] and density-based techniques [39]. An important subset of clustering for fraud detection is the out-of-scope data mining. Techniques to Identify Outliers include algorithms based on distance and density [38].

Frawley et al. [41] indicate that the goal of data mining is to obtain useful and non-explicit information from data stored in large repositories. On the basis of data mining techniques, a response model can be constructed as a decision model for the prediction or classification of a domain problem potentially as expert systems [42].

4.1 Application of Data Mining Techniques to Fraud

Data mining techniques used in many applications. DM has successfully applied to several areas of financial problems. Recent examples are as follows. Huang, Hsu and

Wang (2007) [43] adopted the mining approach of the time series to simulate human intelligence and automatically discover financial database models. Kirkos et al. [10] used the extraction classification to identify fraudulent financial statements [10, 29]. Chun and Park [44] incorporated regression analysis and case-based reasoning to predict the stock market index [44]. However, few of these studies focused on the data cluster approach and even fewer empirical investigations were topics related to the prediction of financial distress. Therefore, Chen et al. [36], used data clustering to improve the accuracy of Predicting bankruptcy in a capital market.

Data mining is most useful in an exploration scenario analysis in which there is no predetermined notion about what will be an "interesting" result [45].

On (2011) Zhou and Kapoor [46], mentioned that most financial fraud based on data mining, detection techniques are mainly based on classification, which is the process of explanation and differentiation of data classes in order to predict the class of data, Objects whose class label is unknown

Building classifiers based on decision trees requires no domain knowledge or parameterization and is therefore suitable for the exploratory discovery of knowledge [25, 37].

Breiman et al. [47] developed the decision tree classification and regression tree (CTD) algorithms which is a nonparametric statistical method used to construct a decision tree to choose from a large number of explanatory variables that are Very critical for determining the response variable [31].

Zhang and Zhou [5] argue that classification and prediction are the process of identifying a set of common characteristics and patterns that describe and distinguish classes or concepts of data.

Lin et al. [48] used data mining techniques to sort fraud factors and rank the importance of fraud factors. Among the methods used are logistic regression, decision trees (CART) and RNA (artificial neural networks).

The techniques used by Nuno et al. [49] are supervised learning methods for the classification problem, as it is common for fraud detection applications have marked data for training. We chose to test three different models that were used: Logistic regression due to its popularity, and random forests and vector support machines.

Several detection methods were examined by Zhou and Kapoor [46] such as classification, regression, neural network and decision trees.

Whitrow et al. [50] also worked on a credit card fraud detection with data from a bank. They studied the use of transaction aggregation when using random forests, vector support machines, and logistic regression and nearest K neighbourhood techniques, which has proved that transaction aggregation has improved performance in some situations, with the aggregation period being an important parameter.

Lee and Yeh [51] applied binary logistic regression to generate dichotomous prediction models.

Chen and Du [36]: Several classification techniques have been suggested to predict financial distress using ratios and data from these financial statements, for example, univariate approaches (Beaver 1966), multivariate approaches, linear multiple Discriminant approaches [52], logistic regression [53–55], Factor analysis [56] and by stages [57].

Shin and Lee [58] and Tsai [59] reported that stepwise regression is a common traditional statistical technique used to perform function selection.

Bhattacharyya et al. [60] compared the performance of random forests, vector machine supports and logistic regression to detect fraud of credit card transactions in an international financial institution framework.

Chen et al. [36] empirically show that a neural network provides not only promising predictive accuracy, but may also have better detection power and lower cost of erroneous classification compared to a logit model and assay auditor judgements. They suggest that an artificial intelligence technique proves very well in identifying a fraud presence, and therefore it can be a support tool for practitioners.

Feroz et al. [61] observed that the relative success of neural network models was due to their ability to "learn" what was important. Financial fraud writers have had incentives to appear prosperous, as evidenced by high profitability.

Pacheco et al. [62] developed an intelligent hybrid system composed of NN (neural network) and a fuzzy expert system to diagnose financial problems.

Brooks [9] also applied various models of neural networks to detect the fraud of financial declarations with great success.

Fanning and Cogger [15] used neural networks to detect management fraud. The study provided an in-depth examination of key public predictors of fraudulent financial statements.

Koskivaara [63] examined the impact of various pre-processing models on NN's predicted capacity during the audit of the financial accounts.

Busta and Weinberg [64] used neural networks to distinguish between "normal" and "manipulated" financial data. They examined the numerical distribution of numbers in the underlying financial information.

Sohl and Venkatachalam [65] used the retro-propagating neural networks for prediction of financial statement fraud.

Cerullo and Cerullo [16] explained the nature of fraud and financial statement fraud as well as the characteristics of Neural Networks (NN) and their applications. They illustrated how NN packages could be used by various companies to predict the occurrence of fraud.

Lin et al. [48] uses technical data mining to sort out fraud factors and rank the importance of fraud factors. The methods on which it based logistic regression, decision trees (CART) and RNA (artificial neural networks).

Calderon and Cheh [66] examined the effectiveness of neural networks as a potential risk factor for enterprise risk-based auditing.

Ravisankar et al. [8] used data mining techniques such as Multilayer Transmission Neural Network (MLFF), Support Vector Machines (SVM), Genetic Programming (GP), Data Management Method (GMDH), logistic regression (LR) and the PNN probabilistic neural network) to identify companies that resort to financial statement fraud. He showed that the PNN outperformed all the techniques without feature selection, and GP and PNN outperformed the others with feature selection and with slightly equal accuracy.

According to Lin et al. [48] a neural network system works quite well and could be a support tool for practitioners. It also implies that continuous innovation in artificial intelligence is needed and could be used to facilitate the evaluation of audit evidence.

Sugumaran et al. [67] reported that decision trees are also one of the popular methods for selecting features.

Kirkos et al. [10] used the ID3 decision tree and the Bayesian belief network to successfully detect fraud on financial statements.

The purpose of the study adapted by Kirkos [10] was to study the utility and compare the performance of three Data Mining techniques by detecting fraudulent financial statements using published financial data. The methods used were decision trees, neural networks and Bayesian beliefs.

Olszewski [68] proposed a fraud detection method based on viewing user accounts to conduct threshold type detection.

The K-means algorithm is a well-known and commonly used clustering algorithm [25].

A good clustering method will produce high quality clusters with strong intra-class similarity and low inter-class similarity [69].

Chen et al. [36] studied the prediction performance for the clustering approach is more aggressively influenced compared to the BPN (A back-propagation network) model. Finally, the BPN (A back-propagation network) approach gets better prediction accuracy than the DM grouping approach in the development of financial distress Prediction model,

Whitrow et al. [50] also worked on a credit card fraud detection with data from a bank. They studied the use of transaction aggregation when using random forests, vector support machines, logistic regression and nearest K neighborhood techniques. Proven that transaction aggregation has improved performance in certain situations, with the aggregation period being an important parameter

Srivastava et al. [70], built a model based on a hidden Markov model, focusing on fraud detection for credit card issuing banks.

Ameur and Tkiouat [27] used the prediction task to predict fraudulent taxpayers and non-fraudulent taxpayers in light of the historical overlap following tax audits previously conducted.

4.2   Distribution of Articles by Data Mining Techniques to Fraud

In this step we examine the distribution of different methods of the DM technique used between (1997) and (2017) for the detection of fraud in different domains (see Table 1).

Table 1. Distribution of articles by data mining techniques

Fraudulent domain	Data mining application class	Data mining techniques	References
Credit card fraud	Classification	Ada boost algorithm, decision trees, CART, RIPPER, Bayesian belief network	[27]
		Neural networks, discriminant analysis	[71]
		K-nearest neighbor, logistic model, discriminant analysis, Naïve Bayes, neural	[24, 25]
		CART	[31]
		Network decision trees	[29, 67]
		Support vector machine, evolutionary algorithms	[72]
		Supervised learning method	[49]
	Clustering	Hidden Markov model	[70]
		Self-organizing map	[21, 40, 73]
Money laundering	Classification	Network analysis	[74]
Crop insurance fraud	Regression	Yield-switching model	[75]
		Logistic model, probit model	[30, 76]
Healthcare insurance fraud	Classification	Association rule	[30]
		Polymorphous (M-of-N) logic	[77]
		Self-organizing map	[68, 78]
	Visualization	Visualization	[79]
	Outlier detection	Discounting learning algorithm	[80]
Automobile insurance fraud	Classification	Logistic model	[81]
		Neural networks	[14]
		Principal component analysis of RIDIT (PRIDIT)	[81]
		Logistic model, decision trees, neural networks, support vector machine,	[82]
		Fuzzy logic	[82–84]
		Logistic model	[18, 19, 53, 80, 84–89]
		Logistic model, Bayesian belief network	[20]
		Self-organizing map	[90]
		Naïve Bayes	[91]
	Prediction	Evolutionary algorithms	[92]
		Logistic model	[89]
	Regression	Probit model	[92]
		Logistic model	[93, 94]

(*continued*)

Table 1. (*continued*)

Fraudulent domain	Data mining application class	Data mining techniques	References
Corporate fraud	Classification	Neural networks, decision trees, Bayesian belief network	[10]
		Decision trees	[27]
		Regression trees	
		CART	[27]
		Regression	[58]
Financial fraud		Multicriteria decision aid (MCDA), UTilite's Additives DIScriminantes (UTADIS)	[7]
		Evolutionary algorithms	[95]
		Fuzzy logic	[88, 96]
		Neural networks	[17]
		Logistic model	[19]
		CART	[12, 48, 97]
		Neural networks, logistic model	[98]
		Decision trees, neural networks, Bayesian belief network, K-nearest neighbor	[22]
	Clustering	Naïve Bayes	[39, 99]
	Prediction	Neural networks (NN)	[15, 16, 63–66, 53, 32, 33, 62, 100, 101]
		Regression logistique	[54]
	Regression	Logistic model	[18, 53]
	Classification	Prediction	[5, 51]
		Decision trees	[25, 28, 102]
		Neural networks	[46]
		Regression	[46]
		Discriminant analysis	[55, 103]

5   Conclusion

This article present the state of the art for the detection of fraud using DM techniques. We have clearly presented its definitions, its properties, its applications and the various scientific currents related to the detection of the fraud using the techniques date Mining from (1966) to (2017). We provide an annotated bibliography of resources for those deepening DM techniques for fraud detection of financial fraud, insurance fraud, securities and commodities fraud and other related financial frauds). The main data mining techniques used are logistic models, neural networks, the Bayesian belief network, and decision trees, all of which solutions to the problems inherent in the detection and classification of fraudulent data.

We also recalled that the traditional methods of tax auditing are limited as the evolution of the number of taxpayers, and the diversification and complexity of fraud techniques, complex systems.

We conclude that the use of data-mining applications has shown utility in different domains. The use of datamining techniques and tools can help in detecting and anticipating the acts of fraud and take immediate measures to limit their financial impacts. After this descriptive contribution, our target is to focus our study for a specific problem of fraud. (tax fraud) and try to establish a new model as a decision making tool for tax fraud detecting.

References

1. Bolton, R. J., Hand, D.J. Statistical fraud detection: a review. Stat. Sci. **17**(3), 35–255 (2002)
2. Phua, C., Lee, V., Smith, K., Gayler, R.: A comprehensive survey of data mining-based fraud detection research. Artif. Intell. Rev. **2005**, 1–14 (2005)
3. Yue, X., Wu, Y., Wang, Y. L., Chu, C.: A review of data mining-based financial fraud detection research. In: International Conference on Wireless Communications, Networking and Mobile Computing, pp. 5519–5522 (2007)
4. Fawcett, T., Provost, F.: Adaptive fraud detection. Data Min. Knowl. Disc. **1**(3), 91–316 (1997)
5. Zhang, D., Zhou, L.: Discovering golden nuggets: data mining in financial application. IEEE Trans. Syst. Man Cybern. **34**(4) (Nov 2004)
6. Ngai, E., Hu, Y., Wong, Y., Chen, Y., Sun, X.: The application of data mining techniques in financial fraud detection: a classification framework and an academic review of literature. Decis. Support Syst. **50**(3), 559–569 (2011)
7. Spathis, C.T., Doumpos, M., Zopounidis, C.: Detecting falsified financial statements: a comparative study using multicriteria analysis and multivariate statistical techniques. Eur. Account. Rev. **11**(3), 509–535 (2002)
8. Ravisankar, P., Ravi, V., Raghava Rao, G., Bose, I.: Detection of financial statement fraud and feature selection using data mining techniques (2011)
9. Oxford Concise English Dictionary, 10th edn. Publisher (1999)
10. Kirkos, E., Spathis, C., Manolopoulos, Y.: Data mining techniques for the detection of fraudulent financial statements. Expert Syst. Appl. **32**(4), 995–1003 (2007)
11. Bashir, A., Khan, L., Awad, M.: Bayesian networks. In: Wang, J. (ed.) Encyclopedia of Data Warehousing and Mining: I-Z, pp. 89–92. Idea Group Inc., Hershey, PA (2006)
12. Lin, C.C., Huang, S.Y., Chiu, A.A.: Fraud detection using fraud triangle risk factors with analytic hierarchy process. In: 2012 Annual Meeting of the American Accounting Association (2012)
13. Goode, S., Lacey, D.: Detecting complex account fraud in the enterprise: the role of technical and non-technical controls. Decis. Support Syst. **50**(4), 702–714 (2011)
14. Viaene, S., Dedene, G., Derrig, R.A.: Auto claim fraud detection using bayesian learning neural networks. Expert Syst. Appl. **29**(3) [41], 653–666 (2005)

15. Fanning, K.M., Cogger, K.O.: Neural network detection of management fraud using published financial data. Int. J. Intell. Syst. Account. Financ. Manag. **7**(1), 21–41 (1998)
16. Cerullo, M.J., Cerullo, V.: Using neural networks to predict financial reporting fraud. Comput. Fraud Secur., 14–17 (May/June 1999)
17. Green, P., Choi, J.H.: Assessing the risk of management fraud through neural network technology. Auditing: J. Pract. Theor. **16**(1), 14–28 (1997)
18. Yuan, J., Yuan, C., Deng, X., Yuan, C.: The effects of manager compensation and market competition on financial fraud in public companies: an empirical study in China. Int. J. Manag. **25**(2), 322–335 (2008)
19. Bell, T.B., Carcello, J.V.: A decision aid for assessing the likelihood of fraudulent financial reporting. Auditing: J. Pract. Theor. **19**(1), 169–174 (2000)
20. Bermúdez, L., Pérez, J.M., Ayuso, M., Gómez, E., Vázquez, F.J.: A Bayesian dichotomous, model with asymmetric link for fraud in insurance. Insur.: Math. Econ. **42**(2), 779–786 (2008)
21. Quah, J.T.S., Sriganesh, M.: Real-time credit card fraud detection using computational intelligence. Expert Syst. Appl. **35**(4) (2008)
22. Kotsiantis, S., Koumanakos, E., Tzelepis, D., Tampakas, V.: Forecasting fraudulent financial statements using data mining. Int. J. Comput. Intell. **3**(2), 104–110 (2006)
23. Caudill, S.B., Ayuso, M., Guillén, M.: Fraud detection using a multinominal logit model with missing information. J. Risk Insur. **72**(4), 539–550 (2005)
24. Yeh, I.C., Lien, C.: The comparisons of data mining techniques for the predictive accuracy of probability of default of credit card clients. Expert Syst. Appl. **36**(2), 2473–2480 (2008)
25. Han, J., Kamber, M.: Data Mining: Concepts and Techniques. Morgan Kaufmann, San Francisco, CA, USA (2001)
26. Huang, M.J., Chen, M.Y., Lee, S.C.: Integrating data mining with casebased reasoning for chronic diseases prognosis and diagnosis. Expert Syst. Appl. **32**(3), 856–867 (2007)
27. Ameur, F., Tkiouat, M.: Taxpayers Fraudulent behavior modeling the use of datamining in fiscal fraud detecting Moroccan case. Appl. Math. **3**(10), 1207–1213 (2012). https://doi.org/10.4236/am.2012.310176
28. Gray, G.L., Debreceny, R.S. (2014)
29. Siciliano, R., Conversano, C.: Decision tree induction. In: Wang, J. (ed.) Encyclopedia of Data Warehousing and Mining: I-Z, pp. 353–358. Idea Group Inc., Hershey, PA (2006)
30. Yang, W., Hwang, S.: A process-mining framework for the detection of healthcare fraud and abuse. Expert Syst. Appl. **31**(1), 56–68 (2006)
31. Lee, T.S., Chiu, C.C., Chou, Y.C., Lu, C.J.: Mining the customer credit using classification and regression tree and multivariate adaptive regression splines. Comput. Stat. Data Anal. **50**(4), 1113–1130 (2006)
32. Smith, K.A.: Neural networks for prediction and classification. In: Wang J. (ed.) Encyclopedia of Data Warehousing and Mining: I–Z. Idea Group Inc., Hershey, PA, pp. 865–869 (2006)
33. Zhang, G.P.: Neural networks for classification: a survey. IEEE Trans. Syst. Man Cybern. **30**(4), 451–462 (2000)
34. Steinwart, I., Christmann, A.: Support Vector Machines. Springer Science, New York, NY (2008)
35. Cox, E.: Fuzzy Modeling and Genetic Algorithms for Data Mining and Exploration. Morgan Kaufmann, San Francisco (2005)
36. Chen, W.-S., Du, Y.-K.: Using neural networks and data mining techniques for the financial distress prediction model (2009)
37. Koh, H.C., Low, C.K.: Going concern prediction using data mining techniques. Manag. Auditing J. **19**(3), 462–476 (2004)

38. Han, J., Kamber, M.: Data Mining: Concepts and Techniques, 2nd edn. Morgan Kaufmann, San Francisco (2006)
39. Berkhin, P.: A survey of clustering data mining techniques. In: Kogan, J., Nicholas, C., Teboulle, M. (eds.) Grouping Multidimensional Data: Recent Advances in Clustering, pp. 25–71. Springer, Heidelberg (2006)
40. Kohonen, T.: Self-Organizing Maps, 3rd edn. Springer, Heidelberg (2000)
41. Frawley, W.J., Paitetsjy-Shapiro, G., Matheus, C.J.: Knowledge discovery in databases: an overview. AI Mag. 13, 57–70 (1992)
42. Lu, C.L., Chen, T.C.: A study of applying data mining approach to the information disclosure for Taiwan's stock market investors. Expert Syst. Appl. 36(2), 3536–3542 (2009)
43. Yue, D., Wu, X., Wang, Y., Li, Y., Chu, C.H.: A Review of Data Mining-Based Financial Fraud Detection Research, International Conference on Wireless Communications, Networking and Mobile Computing, pp. 5519–5522 (2007)
44. Chun, S.H., Park, Y.J.: A new hybrid data mining technique using a regression case based reasoning: application to financial forecasting. Expert Syst. Appl. 31(2), 329–336 (2006)
45. Kantardzic, M.: Data Mining: Concepts, Models, Methods, and Algorithms'. Wiley, IEEE Press (2002)
46. Zhou, W., Kapoor, G.: Detecting Evolutionary Financial Statement Fraud (2011)
47. Breiman, L., Friedman, J., Olshen, R., Stone, S.: Classification and Regression Trees. Chapman and Hall/CRC Press, Boca Raton, FL (1984)
48. Lin, C.-C., Chiu, A.-A., Huang, S.Y., Yen, D.C.: Detecting the financial statement fraud: the analysis of the differences between data mining techniques and experts' judgments (2015)
49. Carneiroa, N., Figueiraa, G., Costac, M.: A data mining based system for credit-card fraud detection in e-tail (2017)
50. Whitrow, C., Hand, D.J., Juszczak, P., Weston, D., Adams, N.M.: Transaction aggregation as a strategy for credit card fraud detection. Data Min. Knowl. Disc. 18(1) 30–55 (2009). http://www.springerlink.com/index/10.1007/s10618-008-0116-z, http://dx.doi.org/10.1007/s10618-008-0116-z
51. Lee, T.S., Yeh, Y.H.: Corporate governance and financial distress: evidence from Taiwan. Corp. Gov. Int. Rev. 12(3), 378–388 (2004)
52. Meyer, P.A., Pifer, H.: Prediction of bank failures. J. Financ. 25, 853–868 (1970)
53. Spathis, C.T.: Detecting false financial statements using published data: some evidence from Greece. Manag. Auditing J. 17(4), 179–191 (2002)
54. Dimitras, A.I., Zanakis, S.H., Zopounidis, C.: A survey of business failure with an emphasis on prediction methods and industrial applications. Eur. J. Oper. Res. 90(3), 487–513 (1996)
55. Altman, E.L., Edward, I., Haldeman, R., Narayanan, P.: A new model to identify bankruptcy risk of corporations. J. Banking Financ. 1, 29–54 (1977)
56. Blum, M.: Failing company discriminant analysis. J. Account. Res., 1–25 (1974)
57. Laitinen, E.K., Laitinen, T.: Bankruptcy prediction application of the Taylor's expansion in logistic regression. Int. Rev. Financ. Anal. 9, 327–349 (2000)
58. Shin, K.S., Lee, Y.J.: A genetic algorithm application in bankruptcy prediction modeling. Expert Syst. Appl. 23(3), 321–328 (2002)
59. Tsai, C.F.: Feature selection in bankruptcy prediction. Knowl.-Based Syst. 22(2), 120–127 (2009)
60. Bhattacharyya, S., Jha, S., Tharakunnel, K., Westland, J.C.: Data mining for credit card fraud: a comparative study. Decis. Support Syst. 50(3), 602–613 (2011)

61. Feroz, E.H., Kwon, T.M., Pastena, V., Park, K.J.: The efficacy of red flags in predicting the SEC's targets: an artificial neural networks approach. Int. J. Intell. Syst. Account. Financ. Manag. **9**(3), 145–157 (2000)

62. Pacheco, R., Martins, A., Barcia, R.M., Khator, S.: A hybrid intelligent system applied to financial statement analysis. In: Proceedings of the 5th IEEE Conference on Fuzzy Systems, vol. 2, pp. 1007–10128, New Orleans, LA, USA (1996)

63. Koskivaara, E.: Different pre-processing models for financial accounts when using neural networks for auditing. In: Proceedings of the 8th European Conference on Information Systems, vol. 1, pp. 326–3328, Vienna, Austria (2000)

64. Busta, B., Weinberg, R.: Using Benford's law and neural networks as a review procedure. Manag. Auditing J. **13**(6), 356–366 (1998)

65. Sohl, J.E., Venkatachalam, A.R.: A neural network approach to forecasting model selection. Inf. Manag. **29**(6), 297–303 (1995)

66. Calderon, T.G., Cheh, J.J.: A roadmap for future neural networks research in auditing and risk assessment. Int. J. Account. Inf. Syst. **3**(4), 203–236 (2002)

67. Sugumaran, V., Muralidharan, V., Ramachandran, K.I.: Feature selection using decision tree and classification through proximal support vector machine for fault diagnostics of roller bearing. Mech. Syst. Signal Process. **21**(2), 930–942 (2007)

68. Olszewski, D.: Fraud detection using self-organizing map visualizing the user profiles. Knowl.-Based Syst. **70**, 324–334 (2014)

69. Chen, A.P., Chen, C.C.: A new efficient approach for data clustering in electronic library using ant colony clustering algorithm. Electron. Libr. **24**(4), 548–559 (2006)

70. Srivastava, A., Kundu, A., Sural, S., Majumdar, A.: Credit card fraud detection using hidden Markov model. IEEE Trans. Dependable Secur. Comput. **5**(1), 37–48 (2008)

71. Dorronsoro, J.R., Ginel, F., Sánchez, C., Cruz, C.S.: Neural fraud detection in credit card operations. IEEE Trans. Neural Netw. **8**(4), 827–834 (1997)

72. Chen, R., Chen, T., Lin, C.: A new binary support vector system for increasing detection rate of credit card fraud. Int. J. Pattern Recogn. Artif. Intell. **20**(2), 227–239 (2006)

73. Zaslavsky, V., Strizhak, A.: Credit card fraud detection using self-organizing maps. Inf. Secur. **18**, 48–63 (2006)

74. Gao, Z., Ye, M.: A framework for data mining-based anti-money laundering research. J. Money Laundering Control **10**(2), 170–179 (2007)

75. Atwood, J.A., Robinson-Cox, J.F., Shaik, S.: Estimating the prevalence and cost of yield-switching fraud in the federal crop insurance program. Am. J. Agric. Econ. **88**(2), 365–381 (2006)

76. Jin, Y., Rejesus, R.M., Little, B.B.: Binary choice models for rare events data: a crop insurance fraud application. Appl. Econ. **37**(7), 841–848 (2005)

77. Major, J.A., Riedinger, D.R.: EFD: a hybrid knowledge/statistical-based system for the detection of fraud. J. Risk Insur. **69**(3), 309–324 (2002)

78. He, H., Wang, J., Graco, W., Hawkins, S.: Application of neural networks to detection of medical fraud. Expert Syst. Appl. **13**(4), 329–336 (1997)

79. Sokol, L., Garcia, B., Rodriguez, J., West, M., Johnson, K.: Using data mining to find fraud in HCFA health care claims. Top. Health Inf. Manag. **22**(1), 1–13 (2001)

80. Yamanishi, K., Takeuchi, J., Williams, G., Milne, P.: On-line unsupervised outlier detection using finite mixtures with discounting learning algorithms. Data Min. Knowl. Discov. **8**(3), 275–300 (2004).[47]

81. Brockett, P.L., Derrig, R.A., Golden, L.L.: Fraud classification using principal component analysis of RIDITS. J. Risk Insur. **69**(3), 341–371 (2002)

82. Viaene, S., Derrig, R.A., Baesens, B., Dedene, G.: A comparison of state-of-the-art classification techniques for expert automobile insurance claim fraud detection. J. Risk Insur. **69**(3), 373–421 (2002) [50]

83. Pathak, J., Vidyarthi, N., Summers, S.L.: A fuzzy-based algorithm for auditors to detect elements of fraud in settled insurance claims. Manag. Auditing J. **20**(6), 632–644 (2005)

84. Tennyson, S., Salsas-Forn, P.: Claims auditing in automobile insurance: fraud detection and deterrence objectives. J. Risk Insur. **69**(3), 289–308 (2002)

85. Artís, M., Ayuso, M., Guillén, M.: Modelling different types of automobile insurance fraud behaviour in the Spanish market. Insur. Math. Econ. **24**(1), 67–81 (1999)

86. Artís, M., Ayuso, M., Guillén, M.: Detection of automobile insurance fraud with discrete choice models and misclassified claims. J. Risk Insur. **69**(3), 325–340 (2002)

87. Viaene, S., Ayuso, M., Guillén, M., Van Gheel, D., Dedene, G.: Strategies for detecting fraudulent claims in the automobile insurance industry. Eur. J. Oper. Res. **176**(1), 565–583 (2007)

88. Deshmukh, A., Romine, J., Siegel, P.H.: Measurement and combination of red flags to assess the risk of management fraud: a fuzzy set approach. Manag. Financ. **23**(6), 35–48 (1997)

89. Weisberg, H.I., Derrig, R.A.: Quantitative methods for detecting fraudulent automobile bodily injury claims. Risques **35**, 75–101 (1998)

90. Brockett, P.L., Xia, X., Derrig, R.A.: Using Kononen's self-organizing feature map to uncover automobile bodily injury claims fraud. J. Risk Insur. **65**(2), 245–274 (1998)

91. Viaene, S., Derrig, R.A., Dedene, G.: A case study of applying boosting naive Bayes to claim fraud diagnosis. IEEE Trans. Knowl. Data Eng. **16**(5), 612–620 (2004)

92. Sternberg, M., Reynolds, R.G.: Using cultural algorithms to support re-engineering of rule-based expert systems, in dynamic performance environments: a case study in fraud detection. IEEE Trans. Evol. Comput. **1**(4), 225–243 (1997)

93. Crocker, K.J., Tennyson, S.: Insurance fraud and optimal claims settlement strategies. J. Law Econ. **45**, 469–507 (2002)

94. Belhadji, E.B., Dionne, G., Tarkhani, F.: A model for the detection of insurance fraud. Geneva Papers Risk Insur. **25**(4), 517–538 (2000)

95. Welch, J., Reeves, T.E., Welch, S.T.: Using a genetic algorithm-based classifier system for modeling auditor decision behavior in a fraud setting. Int. J. Intell. Syst. Account. Financ. Manag. **7**(3), 173–186 (1998)

96. Deshmukh, A., Deshmukh, Talluru: A rule-based fuzzy reasoning system for assessing the risk of management fraud. Int. J. Intell. Syst. Account. Financ. Manag. **7**(4), 223–241 (1998)

97. Bai, B., Yen, J., Yang, X.: False financial statements: characteristics of China's listed companies and CART detecting approach. Int. J. Inf. Technol. Decis. Making **7**(2), 339–359 (2008)

98. Lin, J.W., Hwang, M.I., Becker, J.D.: A fuzzy neural network for assessing the risk of fraudulent financial reporting. Manag. Auditing J. **18**(8), 657–665 (2003)

99. Holton, C.: Identifying disgruntled employee systems fraud risk through text mining: a simple solution for a multi-billion dollar problem. Decis. Support Syst. **46**(4), 853–864 (2009)

100. Koskivaara, E.: Artificial neural networks in auditing: state of the art. ICFAI J. Audit Pract. **1**(4), 12–33 (2004)

101. Chen, H.J., Huang, S.Y., Shih, Y.N., Hsiao, C.T.: Discussing the financial fraud factor detection. Chin. Manage. Rev. **12**(4), 1–22 (2009)

102. Huang, S.Y., Lin, C.C., Chiu, A.A.: Using data mining techniques to identify and rank the fraud factors. In: American Accounting Association Annual Meeting and Conference on Teaching and Learning in Accounting (2014)
103. Altman, E.L.: Financial ratios, discriminant analysis and the prediction of corporate bankruptcy. J. Financ. **23**(3), 589–609 (1968)

Deep Learning Technology for Identifying a Person of Interest in Real World

Hamid Ouanan[(⊠)], Mohammed Ouanan, and Brahim Aksasse

Department of Computer Science, ASIA Team, M2I Laboratory,
Faculty of Science and Techniques, Moulay Ismail University,
BP 509 Boutalamine, 52000 Errachidia, Morocco
ham.ouanan@gmail.com, ouanan_mohammed@yahoo.fr,
baksasse@yahoo.com

Abstract. In this paper, we will propose a new embedded system prototype called PubFace, which uses the CNN model trained from scratch on facial celebrity images [1], to identify a "Person of Interest" in public space. This is done by tuning this model on new dataset comprising 5000 real images of 1000 different identity collected from social networks as Facebook and Instagram. After I got permission of collected images persons to use their facial images in this scientific research project. Then, we have investigated some ways for compressing the number of parameters of the resulting model to reduce the memory needed for both storing and performing a forward pass while simultaneously preserving acceptable good accuracy.

Keywords: Face recognition · Artificial intelligence · Deep learning · Person of interest

1 Introduction

The Face Recognition is growing as a major research area because of the broad choice of applications in the fields of commercial and law enforcement. Traditional FR algorithmic solutions are facing challenges like object illumination, pose variation, expression changes, and facial disguises. Unfortunately these limitations decrease the performance in object identification and verification. To overcome all these limitations, deep learning based techniques [2], are actively being used in many areas. These techniques perform an assumption that by collecting massive training sets, deep networks will have sufficient examples of both inter-subject and intra-subject appearance variations. From these variations, artificial neural networks can learn to generate discriminative features, which amplify subject identity and suppress other, confounding appearance variations. So, to train face recognition systems based on deep convolutional neural networks (CNNs), very large training sets are needed with millions of labeled images. Recently, the number of face images has been growing exponentially on social network such as Facebook and Twitter. As an example, the director of Facebook AI Research Yann LeCun has said, "almost 1 billion new photos were uploaded each day on Facebook in 2016". However, large training datasets are not publicly available and very difficult to collect. In addition, to build large dataset by

© Springer Nature Switzerland AG 2019
M. Ezziyyani (Ed.): AI2SD 2018, AISC 915, pp. 220–227, 2019.
https://doi.org/10.1007/978-3-030-11928-7_19

downloading the images from search engine is very difficult, time consuming, data filtering, most financially challenging. One way to get around a lack of large face datasets is to augment face datasets by synthesizing new possible views of the face images they contain. Thereby, an existing face set is expanded to many times its size by introducing supplementary intra-subject appearance variations such as pose variations.

2 Related Works

In this section, we draw up a state-of-the-art review of data augmentation algorithms and the face recognition methods giving good results.

CNNs are a class of deep, feed-forward artificial neural networks that has successfully been applied to analyzing visual imagery. A CNN is a type of feed-forward artificial neural network where the individual neurons are tiled in such a way that they respond to overlapping regions in the visual field; and have their design based around the biological visual mechanism in living organisms [3]. Individual cortical neurons respond to stimuli only in a restricted region of the visual field known as the receptive field. The receptive fields of different neurons partially overlap such that they cover the entire visual field. CNNs use relatively little pre-processing compared to other image classification algorithms. This means that the network learns the filters that in traditional algorithms were hand-engineered. This independence from prior knowledge and human effort in feature design is a major advantage. They have applications in image and video recognition, recommender systems [4].

Deep CNN feature extractor obtained by concatenating several linear and nonlinear operators replaced conventional features extractors. These features demonstrated their potential by producing promising face recognition rates in the wild. A popular approach of this class of methods is proposed by Facebook AI group named DeepFace [5], which using an 8-layer CNN architecture, the first three layers are conventional convolution-pooling-convolution layers. The subsequent three layers are locally connected, followed by two fully connected layers. Pooling layers make learned features robust to local transformations but result in missing local texture details. DeepFace is trained on a dataset of four million images spanning 4000 subjects. This approach achieve excellent recognition accuracy near human visual system in the LFW benchmark [6]. This work is extended by the [7], Unlike DeepFace [5] whose features are learned by one single big CNN, DeepID is learned by training an ensemble of small CNNs, used for network fusion. Another face recognition approach has been proposed named WebFace [8] trains a 17-layer CNN that includes 10 convolutional layers, 5 pooling layers and 2 fully connected layers.

3 The Proposed Method

We will propose a new embedded system prototype called PubFace, which uses the CNN model proposed in [1] trained from scratch on facial celebrity images to identify a "Person of Interest" in public space. This is done by tuning [9] this model on new dataset comprising 5000 real images of 1000 different identity collected from social networks as Facebook and Instagram. After getting the permission to use the collected images of some people for their facial images in this scientific research project, we have investigated some ways for compressing [10, 11] the number of parameters of the resulting model to reduce the memory needed for both storing and performing a forward pass while simultaneously preserving acceptable good accuracy. Finally, we used this model on the Raspberry Pi 3 ARM based core using the OpenCv_DNN module (OpenCV 3.3) [12] to reach the real-time Artificial Intelligence (AI) performance.

3.1   Data Embedded Platform

The Raspberry Pi 3 B Model was selected to be an embedded platform target because of its high performance/low cost ratio. This model is characterized by the following technical specifications:

- Quad Core 1.2 GHz Broadcom BCM2837 64bit CPU
- 1 GB RAM
- BCM43438 wireless LAN and Bluetooth Low Energy (BLE) on board
- 40-pin extended GPIO
- 4 USB 2 ports
- 4 Pole stereo output and composite video port
- Full size HDMI
- CSI camera port for connecting a Raspberry Pi camera
- DSI display port for connecting a Raspberry Pi touchscreen display
- Micro SD port for loading your operating system and storing data
- Upgraded switched Micro USB power source up to 2.5A (Fig. 1).

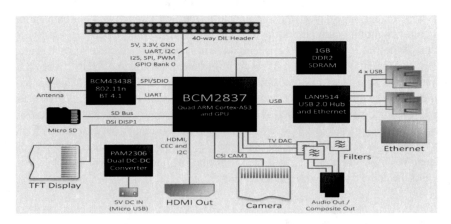

Fig. 1. Main stages of the dataset building process

In order to capture the real time images flux on our platform, we must insert a camera, which is an important part of our application. The better the facial image quality provided by the camera is, the better is data the target model have to work with to produce impressive results. This is likely to improve the detection and recognition rates. The immediate choice was the Raspberry Pi official camera module [13]. This is a small camera module connected to the raspberry board (Fig. 2), through Mobile Industry Processor Interface (MIPI).

Some points in favors of this module lie in its connectivity: since it connects to a dedicated interface in the Raspberry Pi without any USB ports needed and possibly with less power consumption.

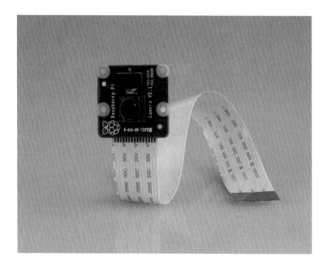

Fig. 2. Illustration of camera module

3.2 Fine-tuning Using the Pre-trained Model

Training deep CNNs from scratch requires a lot of computation power and large amounts of training data. CNNs are comprised of several layers, which are different feature extractors, trained to find the differentiating features of a given dataset. Related studies have shown that the first layers of CNNs trained on images usually react to general low-level visual features such as oriented edges and corners. In contrast, the later layers learn more complex features like eyes. Due to the generality of the initial features, the first part of a CNN trained for facial images can generate features that are of interest for other facial images of different identity. One way to overcome these issues is to take benefit of the generality of features, and to transfer them from the pre-trained model to the target model.

The deep CNN model proposed in [1] (the base model) was trained on five millions of facial celebrity images with the purpose to identify 4000 different public figures and that ambition remains. The majority of layers in this model can be kept they are.

However, since the last fully connected layer of this model contains 4000 figure as outputs, that layer has to be adjusted in size and retrained to fit the new 1000 identities. This enables us to get the benefits of training the trained CNN model from scratch with large facial images dataset, without having to perform it all. Therefore, the amount of parameters that require learning are reduced, which leads to faster training. Figure 3 illustrate the architecture of this CNN model.

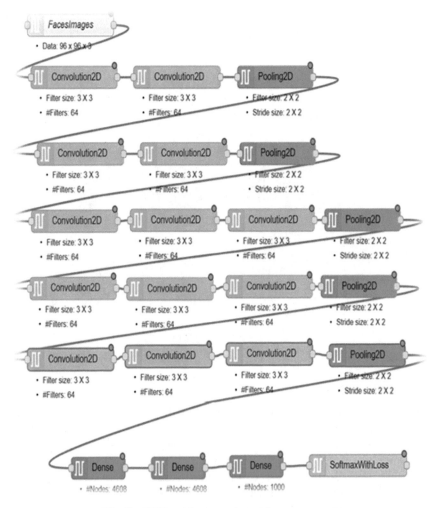

Fig. 3. CNN architecture adopted in our approach

A decision was made to copy the pre-trained weights of all convolutional layers, fc6 and fc7 from the base model to the target model. Then, we freeze these weights by setting the rates to zero. Moreover, we retrain only the last layer, fc8, initialized with a

Gaussian distribution with mean $\mu = 0$ and standard deviation $\sigma = 0.01$. The result model (the target model) will be referred to as the frozen model.

The layers in the base model are designed to receive data of a certain size. Thus, some pre-processing on the data is often required. The base model accepts RGB images of size 96×96. Accordingly, before feeding the input to the target model, resizing is performed on facial images whose sizes differ from 96×96. After that, pixel-wise mean is applied as mean-subtraction to (on average) center the pixel values around zero, by subtracting the mean calculated from the dataset currently used for training. The pixel-wise mean is calculated separately for each pixel and channel.

3.3   Compressing the Target CNN Model

The model resulted from the transfer learning achieved by using the new dataset has reached a high level of accuracy on real facial images. However, this model contains hundreds of millions of parameters including the weights and biases. It is closely related to the offline storage, which is referred to as the memory requisite for representing the parameters of this model when saved on the hard drive, and the memory footprint, which is the amount of run-time memory requisite to deploy and run this model. This allows using this model on server with large graphical processing units (GPU). Still, problems like data privacy and internet connectivity need usage of embedded deep learning devices. Usually, when considering the use of a CNN model on an embedded platform, three major factors must be taken into account: limited compute power, limited memory, and limited bandwidth. These factors place limitations on the amount of parameters in this network model. In this regard, enormous efforts from researches all around the world are geared towards accelerating the runtime and decreasing the size of these deep CNNs. Hence, decreasing the run-time memory requirement, which can make their use deployment in real time applications on embedded platforms with memory and limited computing power similar to Raspberry PI and TI DM3730 etc.

Reducing the size of a CNN model does not only involve the problem of how to compress it, but also the problem of how to preserve the accuracy level. Both the size of the model stored on the hard drive and the memory needed to perform a forward pass are of concern. The major chunk of time in a CNN model is spent on convolutional layers, while most of the storage is spent on FC layers. For example, in the result CNN model, 90: of the computation time is spent on convolutional layers and 90: of the model size is from the weights of FC layers. The main reason behind this high excessive computation is the use of floating point operations which is the number of operations concerning floating point numbers that are executed during different phases of this CNN model. To make up for these shortcomings, we propose using the floating-point numbers only for representing the weights and using the fixed-point numbers for representing the activations because the minimum needed data precision of fixed-point weights change through different layers of this CNN model.

4 The Experiments and Tests

The operating system (OS) used in our implementation is Raspbian. It is a GNU/Linux operating system, especially designed and optimized for Raspberry Pi platforms. Its current version is based on the latest version of the Debian distribution. This operating system is used through a micro SD card of 32 GB class 10 u 3. This kind of SD cards is chosen because of its high debit, 90 mb/s. When the operating system completes the loading step, we deploy the target CNN model using the module DNN of the OpenCV library to the hardware system to run the face recognition in real time on static or dynamic images flux (video) or the multimedia data transmitted from a connected camera (Fig. 4).

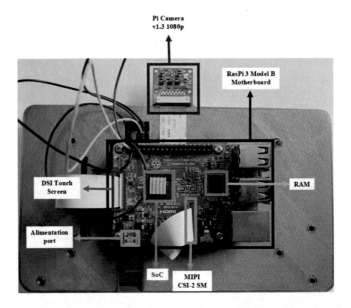

Fig. 4. Illustration of our RasPi 3 model B embedded board based project

The entire CNN model was implemented in python using the deep-learning framework Keras [14]. The use of the pre-processing and the alignment procedures prior to the classification increased the recognition rate from 90 to 98%. This was used as a benchmark we compare the proposed approach to an OpenCV classifier was that achieved the highest performance known as Fisherface (Table 1).

Table 1. Accuracy of different methods on the LFW dataset

Method	Accuracy rate (%)	Classification time (ms)
Fisherface	96	420
Our proposed model	98	90

5 Conclusion

In this paper, we have proposed our deep-learning based approach called Pubface that leads to an impressive combination between the hardware and the software results, with respect to both speed and accuracy compared to traditional the OpenCV classifier known as Fisherface that achieved the highest performance, even when the resources are limited. Pubface can recognize faces with 98% accuracy in real time, which is pretty much as good as humans can do. It is an amazing technology.

References

1. Ouanan, H., Ouanan, M., Aksasse, B.: Face recognition using deep features. Lect. Notes Netw. Syst. **25**, 78–85 (2017)
2. Ouanan, H., Ouanan, M., Aksasse, B.: Non-linear dictionary representation of deep features for face recognition from a single sample per person. Procedia Comput. Sci. **127**, 114–122 (2018)
3. Masakazu, M., Mori, K., Mitari, Y., Kaneda, Y.: Subject independent facial expression recognition with robust face detection using a convolutional neural network. Neural Netw. **5**, 555–559 (2003)
4. Portugal, I., Alencar, P., Cowan, D.: The use of machine learning algorithms in recommender systems: a systematic review. Expert Syst. Appl. (2017)
5. Yaniv, T., Ming, Y., Marc'Aurelio, R., Lior, W.: DeepFace: closing the gap to human-level performance in face verification. In: Proceedings of the IEEE Conference on Computer Vision and Pattern Recognition, pp. 1701–1708. (2014)
6. Huang, G.B., Ramesh, M., Berg, T., Learned-Miller, E.: Labeled faces in the wild: A database for studying face recognition in unconstrained environments, University of Massachusetts, Amherst, Technical Report, pp. 07–49. (2007)
7. Sun, Y., Liang, D., Wang, X., Tang, X.: Deepid3: face recognition with very deep neural networks, arXiv preprint arXiv:1502.00873 (2015)
8. Yi, D., Lei, Z., Liao, S., Li, S.Z.: Learning face representation from scratch. arXiv preprint arXiv:1411.7923. (2014)
9. Pan, S.J., Yang, Q.: A survey on transfer learning. IEEE Trans. Knowl. Data Eng. **22**(10), 1345–1359 (2010)
10. Han, S., Mao, H., Dally, W.J.: eep compression: compressing deep neural networks with pruning, trained quantization and huffman coding. arXiv preprint arXiv:1510.00149 (2015)
11. Lin, D., Talathi, S., Annapureddy, S.: Fixed point quantization of deep convolutional networks. In: International Conference on Machine Learning, pp. 2849–2858. (2016)
12. OpenCV.: [Online]. Available: https://docs.opencv.org/3.2.0/de/d25/tutorial_dnn_build.html . Accessed 30 April 2018
13. Raspberry Pi Foundation: Raspberry Pi Camera Module Product Page. URL: http://www.raspberrypi.org/products/camera-module/. Accessed 24 Mar 2018
14. Keras: The Python Deep Learning library. [Online]. Available: https://keras.io/. 30 April 2018

The Discrete Swallow Swarm Optimization for Flow-Shop Scheduling Problem

Safaa Bouzidi[1]([⊠]), Mohammed Essaid Riffi[1], Morad Bouzidi[1], and Mohammed Moucouf[2]

[1] LAROSERI Laboratory, Department of Computer Science,
Chouaib Doukkali University, El Jadida, Morocco
sfbouzidi@gmail.com
[2] Department of Mathematics, Chouaib Doukkali University,
El Jadida, Morocco

Abstract. The flow-shop scheduling problem is a well-known problem in production system. The objective is minimizing the total time it takes to process the entire job called makespan. In order to solve this NP-hard problem, we approve a new adaptation approach based on the intelligent behaviors of swallows, it is the discrete swallow swarm optimization algorithm (DSSO) present a recent metaheuristic method used to solve a combinatorial problem. The proposed algorithm is tested on different benchmarks instances and compared with different proposed algorithms. The results demonstrate that the proposed algorithm is more efficient than the other compared algorithms. It can be used to solve large instances of flow shop scheduling problem effectively.

Keywords: Swallow swarm optimization algorithm · Combinatorial problem · Metaheuristic · Flow-shop scheduling problem · Makespan

1 Introduction

Scheduling a set of tasks (e.g. jobs) means scheduling their processing by assigning them the required resources (e.g. machines), in the objective to minimize the production costs and time. The theory of scheduling deals with mathematical models but also analyzes very complex real situations, for example in production workshops and logistical problems.

Single machine scheduling, parallel machine scheduling, flow-shop scheduling, job-shop scheduling, open shop scheduling are the different types of scheduling problems where classify in the literature with different constraint and performance measures [1].

© Springer Nature Switzerland AG 2019
M. Ezziyyani (Ed.): AI2SD 2018, AISC 915, pp. 228–236, 2019.
https://doi.org/10.1007/978-3-030-11928-7_20

The flow-shop scheduling problem is a NP-hard type combinatorial problems [16] simulated the first by Johnson in 1954 [6]. To resolve this problem we should find the optimum makespan by processing set of tasks (e.g. jobs) in set of resource (e.g. machine). In this paper, we approved the new approach of discrete swallow swarm optimization for solving the flow-shop scheduling problem.

In the literature, the researchers have given many different approaches for solving the flow-shop scheduling problem. In addition the three important approaches are exact solution methods, heuristics and metaheuristics [8] such as the branch and bound algorithm [2], genetic algorithm [12–14], ant colony optimization [18], particle swarm optimization [19], cuckoo search algorithm [11], bee colony algorithm [10].

The rest of this paper is organized as follows: The first section present the description of the Swallow Swarm Optimization Algorithm. In the second section, the Flow-shop scheduling problem is explained. The third section devote the proposed adaptation to solve the Flow-shop scheduling problem, and next section presents a set of experimental results obtained by using some benchmarks instances from OR-library [17].

2 Swallow Swarm Optimization Algorithm

The swallow swarm algorithm [13] was inspired by the collective movement of swarm and the interaction between particles has attained good position to find food. It is metaheuristic algorithm based on the special characteristic of swallow, including intelligent social life relation, hunting skills, and speedy flight.

The SSO has common characteristics with PSO but also several important differences [7], like the use of three kinds of particles: leader, explorer and aimless particles. Each of which has some responsibility in the colony, that thought doing it guides the colony toward a good position.

The largest part of the colony is represent as explorer particle (e_i). Their primary role is searching in the problem space, if this particle find the best place in the problem space, it can plays role as a head leader (HL_i) but if it is in good place, not the best in analogy with its neighboring particles, it is chosen as a local leader (LL_i). This particle performs the exploration behavior under the influence of some parameters:

- The position of the head leader.
- The position of the local leader.
- The best individual experience along the path.
- The previous path.

The main updating equations are as follows:

$$e_{i+1} = e_i + V_{i+1} \tag{1}$$

$$V_{i+1} = V_{HL_{i+1}} + V_{LL_{i+1}} \tag{2}$$

$$V_{HL_{i+1}} = V_{HL_i} + \alpha_{HL}\text{rand}()(e_{best} - e_i) + \beta_{HL}\text{rand}()(HL_i - e_i) \tag{3}$$

$$V_{LL_{i+1}} = V_{LL_i} + \alpha_{LL}\text{rand}()(e_{best} - e_i) + \beta_{LL}\text{rand}()(LL_i - e_i) \tag{4}$$

where:

- $\alpha_{HL}, \beta_{HL}, \alpha_{LL}$ and β_{LL} are acceleration control coefficients adaptively defined [6].
- V_{HL} = Velocity of lead leader,
- V_{LL} = Velocity of leader local,
- e_{best} = best position of the explorer particle,
- e_i = current position of the explorer particle.

The aimless particle (o_i) of colony moves randomly in the problem space without reaching the specific object, and shares the results with other members of the colony. Their responsibility is the exploration; they have nothing to do with the header leader and local leader. They simply move with respect to their previous positions. Mathematically the main equation to update position is:

$$O_{i+1} = O_i + \left[rand(\{-1, 1\}) * \frac{rand(\min_S, \max_S)}{1 + rand()} \right] \tag{5}$$

The colony is divided into groups, so there are two types of Leader particle (l_i): local and header leader. The best position in the group is favored as the local leader, and the best position among the local leader is chosen as a header leader. The particles change their direction and converge according to the position of these particles.

The following pseudo-code represents the steps of the SSO algorithm:

Algorithm1. Pseudo-code of SSO algorithm

```
Begin
Generate randomly population of n particle
t=1
While (t<max number of iteration) do
for each particle of swarm do
evaluate fitness f(eᵢ) of all particle
end for
```
Sort objective function from min to max and form HL_i, LL_i et O_i
```
if(f(eᵢ) > f(e_best)) then
```
$e_{best} = e_i$
```
end if
if(f(eᵢ) > f(LLᵢ)) then
```
$LL_i = e_i$
```
end if
if(eᵢ = 0 || e_best = 0)
```
$\alpha_{LL} = \beta_{LL} = 2$
```
else
determinate  αLL  and  βLL
end if
updating velocities V_{LL_{i+1}} [equation (3)]
if(f(eᵢ) > f(HLᵢ))
```
$HL_i = e_i$
```
end if
if( eᵢ = 0 || e_best = 0)
```
$\alpha_{HL} = \beta_{HL} = 1.5$
```
else
determinate  αHL  and  βHL
end if
updating velocities V_{HL_{i+1}} with equation (3)
updating position eᵢ and velocities Vᵢof particle with equations
(2) and (4)
updating aimless particle O_{i+1} with equation (5)
if(f(Oᵢ) > f(HLᵢ))
```
$HL_i = O_i$
```
end if
if(f(LLᵢ) > f(HLᵢ))
```
$HL_i = LL_i$
```
end if
t=t+1
end while
return best of HL
End
```

---

3   Flow-Shop Scheduling Problem

The flow-shop scheduling problem is the one of the most important issues in the area of production system [3]. It is described as a scheduling of a set of jobs by a set of different machines in series. Where each job visits each machine exactly once with respecting the same order of routing. In addition, a job can not begin processing on the second machine until it has completed processing on the first one. However, the goal is to have the continuity of the flow of the jobs during the processing by the machines. This can be get by reducing the delays between two consequent jobs; thus, reducing the overall makespan.

Mathematically, the job is described as set of J of n jobs $J = \{J_1, \ldots, J_n | (n \geq 1)\}$, and the machine is represented as a set of M of m machines $M = \{M_1, \ldots , M_m | (m \geq 1)\}$. In additional, each job characterized by a sequence of operations, $O = \{O_1, \ldots, O_m | (m \geq 1)\}$. Then every operation is represented by a pair m_{O_K} and $t_{O_K} (k \in [1, (n * m)])$, where m_{O_K} indicates the machine M_K on which the operation O_K must be executed, and t_{O_K} corresponds to the period taking for process the operation O_K, however $C_{\max}$ defined the total time taken to execute all the operations machines for all the n jobs.

4   The Proposed Adaptation to Solve Flow-Shop Scheduling Problem

Discrete Swallow Swarm Optimization (DSSO) is an adapted version of SSO, in the aim to solve the discrete combinatorial problems. In this paper, we will take as a model DSSO algorithm, performed by BOUZIDI [5], but we applied novel operators [4].

4.1   Algorithm Parameters

In this section, we present the adaptation of different main parameters used to resolve the FSSP is:

- Position is a schedule.
- Velocity is defined as a set of permutation between two jobs.

4.2   Operator and Method

To update the velocity and the position, we used new operators representing as follow:

a. *Addition operator*: The addition between the position and velocity is a position, which velocity translates the order of item the position. The addition between two velocities present a new velocity.
b. *The multiplication operator*: The multiplication between the velocity and coefficient is given by random swaps in velocity if random number between 0 and 1 is less than the coefficient, else it does nothing.
c. *Subtraction operator*: The subtraction between two positions is presented as a velocity.

For searching a new solution, we use the 2-opt method. That is a local search method in the aim to compare each possible combination of the swapping mechanism.

4.3   DSSO Steps

Respecting the general process of SSO proposed by Neshat et al. [13], the different steps of proposed to resolve the FSSP can be described as following:

- **Step 1**: Generate randomly a set of n starting schedule.
- **Step 2**: Initialize all parameters.
- **Step 3**: Verify if the maximum iteration is obtained, if this is true go to step 10 else go to step 4.
- **Step 4**: Divided the solution in m groups.
- **Step 5**: For each solution in the group calculate the makespan and sort it from minimum to maximum solution.
- **Step 6**: Select the Leaders (best schedule) and the aimless (bad schedule) particles.
- **Step 7**: For every explorer particles updating velocities and position by using the Eqs. (1) and (2).
- **Step 8**: Generate a new solution by using the 2-opt method.
- **Step 9**: Update the aimless particles by using Eq. (5).
- **Step 10**: Return the global best schedule.

5   Computational Results and Disscution

To validate this adaptation, it was interpreted under the C++ language and run under an Intel® Core ™ i5-4300 M CPU @ 2.60 GHz machine with 4 GB of RAM. The results obtained from 10 executions of this adaptation on these instances are presented in Table 1, the first column of which indicates the name of the instance, the second column indicates the number of jobs and machine, and the third BKS is the best value of the known optimum. The Best and Worst columns indicate respectively the best and the bad solution found. The next column Average presents the result means, The SD column displays the standard deviation of the solutions. The ErrBest column, and ErrAvr shows respectively the percentage error of the best and average result. This value is calculated according to Eq. 6; which presents the formula to retrieve the percentage error value of a solution S. C1% indicates the number of solutions where relative error is less than 1, and Copt is the number of solutions equal to optimum known solution, that means the number of iteration which its relative error is null. The last column time which presents the average execution time in seconds.

$$Err_S = \frac{Cost\ of\ solution\ S - BKV\ of\ instance}{BKV\ of\ instance} \tag{6}$$

From these results, we notice that this adaptation reaches the optimum for the majority of instances. In an average time of 37 s, to measure its performance compared to the other methods that are hybrid backtracking search algorithm(HBSA) [9] and

Table 1. Results obtained by DSSO in 10 executions

Instance	n × m	BKS	Best	Worst	Average	SD	Errbest	Erravr	$C_{1\%}/C_{Opt}$	Time
Car1	11 × 5	7038	7038	7038	7038	0.00	0.00	0.00	10/10	0.00
Car2	13 × 4	7166	7166	7166	7166	0.00	0.00	0.00	10/10	0.00
Car3	12 × 5	7312	7312	7312	7312	0.00	0.00	0.00	10/10	0.00
Car4	14 × 4	8003	8003	8003	8003	0.00	0.00	0.00	10/10	0.00
Car5	10 × 6	7720	7720	7720	7720	0.00	0.00	0.00	10/10	0.00
Car6	8 × 9	8505	8505	8505	8505	0.00	0.00	0.00	10/10	0.00
Car7	7 × 7	6590	6590	6590	6590	0.00	0.00	0.00	10/10	0.00
Car8	8 × 8	8366	8366	8366	8366	0.00	0.00	0.00	10/10	0.00
Hel1	100 × 10	516	515	516	515.7	0.46	−0.19	−0.06	10/07	104.40
Hel2	20 × 10	136	135	136	135.9	0.30	−0.74	−0.07	10/09	5.30
ReC01	20 × 5	1247	1247	1247	1247.0	0.00	0.00	0.00	10/10	1.55
ReC03	20 × 5	1109	1109	1109	1109.0	0.00	0.00	0.00	10/10	1.12
ReC05	20 × 5	1242	1242	1245	1244.7	0.90	0.00	0.22	10/01	0.59
ReC07	20 × 10	1566	1566	1566	1566.0	0.00	0.00	0.00	10/10	1.52
ReC09	20 × 10	1537	1537	1537	1537.0	0.00	0.00	0.00	10/10	3.27
ReC11	20 × 10	1431	1431	1431	1431.0	0.00	0.00	0.00	10/10	2.58
ReC13	20 × 15	1930	1930	1936	1934.2	1.99	0.00	0.2	10/01	52.26
ReC15	20 × 15	1950	1951	1963	1958.0	4.31	0.05	0.41	10/00	24.81
ReC17	20 × 15	1902	1902	1914	1906.5	4.70	0.00	0.24	10/05	38.67
ReC19	30 × 10	2093	2099	2111	2106.4	3.95	0.29	0.64	10/00	86.62
ReC21	30 × 10	2017	2026	2046	2037.7	6.39	0.45	1.03	04/00	97.91
ReC23	30 × 10	2011	2021	2028	2023.0	2.24	0.50	0.60	10/00	102.31

golden ball algorithm(GBA) [15]. The Fig. 1 shows the difference compared to the relative error of the best solution of these three methods. The Fig. 2 shows the difference of the methods compared to the relative error of the solution means, we see a comparison between HBSA and DSSO in the first Errbest with a small advantage of the

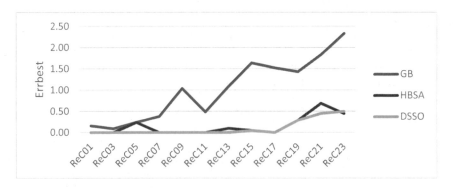

Fig. 1. Comparison of Errbest methods GBA, HBSA and DSSO

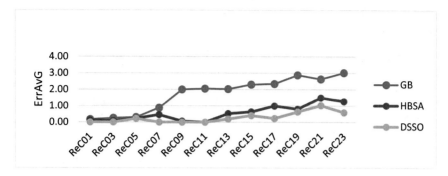

Fig. 2. Comparison of ErrAvg methods GBA, HBSA and DSSO

proposed method, and compared to ErrAvg we see that the proposed method returns the good results compared to other methods.

6 Conclusion

This paper give a new adaptation of discrete swallow swarm optimization to solve the flow-shop scheduling problem by using the new operators. Based on the special characteristic of the swallow swarm, that consist on divided the swarm on three important particle for the objective to research the optimum schedule in the minimum total time for executing all the operation. The obtained results proved that the proposed algorithm is able to find the solution in the minimum time with negligible percentage error, and the comparison shows the performance of the DSSO than others meta-heuristic. It can be also applied directly for solving all variants of scheduling problem.

References

1. Allahverdi, A., Gupta, J.N.D., Aldowaisan, T.: A review of scheduling research involving setup considerations. Omega **27**, 219–239 (1999). https://doi.org/10.1016/S0305-0483(98)00042-5
2. Allaoui, H., Artiba, A.: Scheduling two-stage hybrid flow shop with availability constraints. Comput. Oper. Res. **33**, 1399–1419 (2006). https://doi.org/10.1016/j.cor.2004.09.034
3. Błażewicz, J., Ecker, K.H., Pesch, E., Schmidt, G., Weglarz, J.: Scheduling Computer and Manufacturing Processes. Springer-Verlag, Berlin Heidelberg (1996)
4. Bouzidi, M., Riffi, M.E., Serhir, A.: Discrete particle swarm optimization for travelling salesman problems: new combinatorial operators. In: Proceedings of the Ninth International Conference on Soft Computing and Pattern Recognition (SoCPaR 2017), pp. 141–150. Springer, Cham (2017)
5. Bouzidi, S., Riffi, M.E.: Discrete swallow swarm optimization algorithm for travelling salesman problem. In: Proceedings of the 2017 International Conference on Smart Digital Environment, pp. 80–84. ACM, New York, NY, USA (2017)
6. Johnson, S.M.: Optimal two- and three-stage production schedules with setup times included. Nav. Res. Logist. Q. **1**, 61–68 (1954). https://doi.org/10.1002/nav.3800010110

7. Kaveh, A., Bakhshpoori, T., Afshari, E.: An efficient hybrid particle swarm and swallow swarm optimization algorithm. Comput. Struct. **143**, 40–59 (2014). https://doi.org/10.1016/j.compstruc.2014.07.012

8. Liao, C.-J., Tjandradjaja, E., Chung, T.-P.: An approach using particle swarm optimization and bottleneck heuristic to solve hybrid flow shop scheduling problem. Appl. Soft Comput. **12**, 1755–1764 (2012). https://doi.org/10.1016/j.asoc.2012.01.011

9. Lin, Q., Gao, L., Li, X., Zhang, C.: A hybrid backtracking search algorithm for permutation flow-shop scheduling problem. Comput. Ind. Eng. **85**, 437–446 (2015). https://doi.org/10.1016/j.cie.2015.04.009

10. Liu, Y.-F., Liu, S.-Y.: A hybrid discrete artificial bee colony algorithm for permutation flowshop scheduling problem. Appl. Soft Comput. **13**, 1459–1463 (2013). https://doi.org/10.1016/j.asoc.2011.10.024

11. Marichelvam, M.K., Prabaharan, T., Yang, X.S.: Improved cuckoo search algorithm for hybrid flow shop scheduling problems to minimize makespan. Appl. Soft Comput. **19**, 93–101 (2014). https://doi.org/10.1016/j.asoc.2014.02.005

12. Murata, T., Ishibuchi, H., Tanaka, H.: Genetic algorithms for flowshop scheduling problems. Comput. Ind. Eng. **30**, 1061–1071 (1996). https://doi.org/10.1016/0360-8352(96)00053-8

13. Neshat, M., Sepidnam, G., Sargolzaei, M.: Swallow swarm optimization algorithm: a new method to optimization. Neural Comput. Appl. **23**, 429–454 (2013). https://doi.org/10.1007/s00521-012-0939-9

14. Reeves, C.R.: A genetic algorithm for flowshop sequencing. Comput. Oper. Res. **22**, 5–13 (1995). https://doi.org/10.1016/0305-0548(93)E0014-K

15. Sayoti, F.: Golden Ball Algorithm for solving Flow Shop Scheduling Problem. Int. J. Interact. Multimedia Artif. Intell. **4**, 15–18 (2016)

16. Sotskov, Y.N., Shakhlevich, N.V.: NP-hardness of shop-scheduling problems with three jobs. Discrete Appl Math **59**, 237–266 (1995). https://doi.org/10.1016/0166-218X(95)80004-N

17. Taillard, E.: Benchmarks for basic scheduling problems. Eur. J. Oper. Res. **64**, 278–285 (1993). https://doi.org/10.1016/0377-2217(93)90182-M

18. Yagmahan, B., Yenisey, M.M.: Ant colony optimization for multi-objective flow shop scheduling problem. Comput. Ind. Eng. **54**, 411–420 (2008). https://doi.org/10.1016/j.cie.2007.08.003

19. Zhang, C., Sun, J., Zhu, X., Yang, Q.: An improved particle swarm optimization algorithm for flowshop scheduling problem. Inf. Process. Lett. **108**, 204–209 (2008). https://doi.org/10.1016/j.ipl.2008.05.010

An Overview of Big Data and Machine Learning Paradigms

Imad Sassi[(✉)], Samir Anter, and Abdelkrim Bekkhoucha

Laboratoire Informatique de Mohammedia (LIM), FSTM, Hassan II University
of Casablanca, Casablanca, Morocco
{imadsassi7,antersamir}@gmail.com,
abekkhoucha@hotmail.com

Abstract. Big Data is one of the most famous concepts in the world of new technology and decision making nowadays. It refers to a huge mass of varied and complex data that is gathered from different sources and exceeds the storage and processing capacity of traditional applications and whose analysis and exploitation must increasingly be done in real time. The value of information in Big Data is very important because it offers many benefits in forecasting accuracy, assisting in the design of new strategies and decision making. Thus, one of the major challenges is data analysis which requires new techniques and algorithms to search for hidden information, correlations and relationships in large amount of data. In this context, Machine Learning allows the use of Big Data full potential. In the first part of this paper, we will present an overview of Big Data, its characteristics and sources as well as its application areas. Then, we will discuss some of problems and challenges related to this concept. Examples of Big Data technologies and platforms will also be presented. In the second part, we will highlight some of the most promising Big Data Analytics methods, mainly Machine Learning. We conclude by proposing a taxonomy of Machine Learning techniques and algorithms in the context of Big Data.

Keywords: Big data · IoT · Data analytics · Machine learning · Hadoop · MapReduce

1 Introduction

We are living in an era which is marked by technical progress thanks to the rise of information and communication technologies that are having a great impact on the way our society functions [1]. Today, in our world there is a huge volume of information that is generated and manipulated, and which continues to grow dramatically [2].

For years, Big Data has been influencing global growth because of its significant impact on decision-making and the development of business strategies and models in several industry sectors such as mobile telephony, social networks, media and medicine. It is clear that this large amount of data requires a great deal of work to be able to collect, manage and process it in order to extract valuable information. Obviously, this work is painful to do manually, hence the need of automation of this task [3].

© Springer Nature Switzerland AG 2019
M. Ezziyyani (Ed.): AI2SD 2018, AISC 915, pp. 237–251, 2019.
https://doi.org/10.1007/978-3-030-11928-7_21

The evolution of the Internet of Things (IoT) domain generates an exponential increase of data on the network. The volume of data, their heterogeneity, their speed of production and changing over time, their distributions on multiple databases, the huge number of parameters of these data and full of other complexity factors, make operations of gathering, storage, processing, analysis, exploration and visualization tedious tasks especially with the lack of current capacities of databases, software engineering and traditional applications.

A large number of platforms are being developed to handle this huge amount of heterogeneous data. Big Data and analytics are at the forefront of high volume data processing technologies with very complex, multi-dimensional characteristics. Among these, Hadoop, an open source platform able to distribute data simultaneously on multiple servers and MapReduce that allows to perform parallel calculations on distributed data.

One of the major challenges of Big Data is the management, analysis and research of interesting hidden information from a large amount of data which requires new techniques such as Machine Learning which is one of the most promising Big Data Analytics [4, 5].

Machine Learning is the science of creating algorithms and programs which learn on their own [6]. Once designed, they do not need a human to become better. The term Machine Learning is self-explanatory. Machines learn to perform tasks that aren't specifically programmed to do [7]. Some of the common applications of Machine Learning include following: Web search, spam filters, recommender systems, advertising placement, credit scoring, fraud detection, stock trading, computer vision, security and drug design. Many techniques are put into practice like supervised clustering, regression, naive Bayes, etc.

2   Big Data

In the literature, there is no general agreement on the meaning of the term Big Data. Several definitions were given to Big Data. In 2011, the International Data Corporation (IDC) defines Big Data as "A new generation of technologies and architectures designed to economically extract value from very large volumes of a wide variety of data by enabling high-velocity capture, discovery, and/or analysis" [8].

Another definition was given by Gartner: "Big Data is high-volume, high-velocity and high-variety information assets that demand cost-effective, innovative forms of information processing for enhanced insight and decision making" [9].

But, although these definitions and many others may differ, generally speaking, Big Data is: a large volume of structured and unstructured data that comes from a variety of sources and is often produced and manipulated in real time. With these complex features, this data exceeds the capabilities of traditional applications in terms of storage and processing.

2.1   Characteristics of Big Data: The 3v Model (from 3 to 42v)

The concept of Big Data is defined through the theory of 3V (Volume, Variety and Velocity of data) (see Fig. 1) [9].

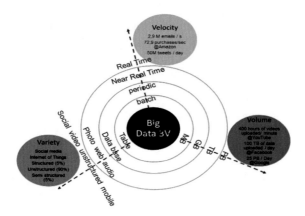

Fig. 1. Big Data 3V model

The best-known definition is Gartner's 3V: The origin of the Gartner's interpretation or 3Vs dates back to February 2001 by Douglas Laney in his white paper published by Meta Group, which Gartner subsequently acquired in 2004. Laney noted that because of the development of e-commerce activities, data is developed in three dimensions, namely: Volume, Velocity, and Variety [10–13].

1. Volume: The amount of data that is generated, stored or used continues to explode exponentially day by day. Just look at the units of measurement for this large amount of data that has changed from the Gigabyte era to Terabytes (10^{12} bytes) passing Petabytes (10^{15} bytes) to Exabytes (10^{18} bytes), Zettabytes (10^{21} bytes) or even Yottabytes (10^{24} bytes) [14].
2. Velocity: Speed refers to streaming data and those in interaction due to the very high rate of data generation, gathering and sharing. This characteristic is therefore related to the time of data updating and analyzing. Processing can be done in real time (or near real time) or offline. In some cases, data is no longer stored but must be streamed [15].
3. Variety: Big Data come from several sources which explains the heterogeneity of these. Big Data can be text, images, multimedia content, digital traces, connected objects, etc. There are different formats and different structures of Big Data. We are talking about structured, semi-structured and unstructured data [12].

   - Structured data are the basic data types such as integers, characters, and arrays of integers or characters. They are used in relational databases [10].
   - Unstructured data refers to information that either does not have a pre-defined data model and/or does not fit well into relational tables. It refers to any data that

has no identifiable structure. Unstructured data have no predefined format: email, books, journals, documents, videos, photos [10].

- Semi-structured data are a combination of the two previous types of data, they are generally represented using XML. It's a form of structured data that does not conform to an explicit and fixed schema (e.g., weblogs, social media feeds) [16].

Most of produced data are unstructured and so traditional database management tools are unable to handle it [12].

It's clear that the Douglas Laney's 3Vs definition has been widely regarded as the "common" attributes of Big Data, but there are many Big Data models like 4, 5 and 6V:

- IBM 4V (4Vs definition of Zikopoulos): IBM added another attribute or "V" for "Veracity" on the Laney's 3Vs notation, which is known as the 4Vs of Big Data [2]. It defines each "V" as following:
  - Volume stands for the scale of data
  - Velocity denotes the analysis of streaming data
  - Variety indicates different forms of data
  - Veracity implies the uncertainty of data.
- Demchenko 5V: Yuri Demchenko added the value dimension along with the IBM 4Vs' definition [16].
- Microsoft 6V: For the sake of maximizing the business value, Microsoft extended Douglas Laney's 3Vs attributes to 6Vs, which it added Variability, Veracity, and Visibility.
  - Variability: refers to the complexity of data set. In comparison with "Variety" (or different data format), it means the number of variables in data sets.
  - Veracity: focuses on trustworthiness of data sources.
  - Visibility: emphasizes the need to have a full picture of data in order to make informative decision.

Other features are widely discussed in several Big Data papers like: Validity, Venue, Vocabulary, Vagueness, etc.

Of course, the inflation of the studied characteristics of Big Data continues its inexorable march, and through two decades, we had the 7V's, the 8V's, then 10V and even the 42V's of Big Data.

2.2   Big Data Sources

The diversity of formats and structures of Big Data is a consequence of the different sources from which these data prove (see Fig. 2). Big Data can be created by: social Media, the Internet of Things, telecommunications and mobile devices (data generated by GPS devices, smart cars, mobile computing devices, PDAs, mobile phones), financial transactions, marketing and advertising, biological and environmental sensors, meteorology, scientific simulations, healthcare, facilities, equipment, transportation, energy, also from other activities which derive from new technologies such as: website links, emails, twitter responses, product reviews, pictures/images, written text on various platforms and many other new applications that have all the characteristics of volume, velocity and variety [17].

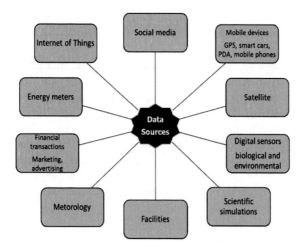

Fig. 2. Big Data sources

2.3   Big Data Applications

Today, Big Data invades many sectors of our life (See Fig. 3) [18–20]. Offering many benefits such as phenomenal computing capacity, improved customer experience, good understanding of customer behavior, anticipation of needs, increasing revenue and productivity and decision-making support, several fields are promising as areas of application of Big Data. In particular, agriculture, energy, health and medicine, environment, tourism, services, finance, education, politics, etc. For example, in:

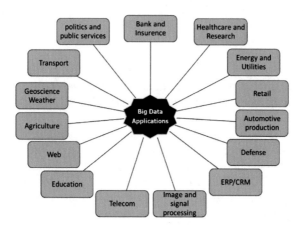

Fig. 3. Big Data applications

- Agriculture: Big Data makes it possible to exploit weather data, plant and animal species data, seed data and livestock history to reduce losses, predict crop costs, livestock health status, or the amount of pesticides needed.

- Energy: The use of Big Data in this sector allows us to design strategies to deliver energy efficiently, reduce costs, predict energy demand in real time, and make huge savings in terms of consumption.
- Health and medicine: Accumulated data collected from each patient's medical history, hospital admissions, physician visits, or emergency department visits, if stored and analyzed, provide a complete and detailed view of patients or populations and can therefore contribute to predictive modeling, clinical decision-making, risk prevention and therefore public health.
- Environment: In the field of environment, Big Data allows with the collection of millions of meteorological data, geological maps and information on lands or seas to refine strategies in relation with agriculture for example. The use of Big Data makes it possible to predict what will be the environmental situation in the future and therefore to anticipate climate change, aridness and water shortages which will be of great benefit to humanity.
- Marketing: With Big Data, we can get to know customers better through their purchases in store and online, their preferences broadcast on social networks, their browsing habits on the Internet. By analyzing consumer behavior and using Big Data, we can refine customer targeting and improve the effectiveness of advertising campaigns, online or offline.
- Science and research: These are the original application fields of Big Data. The contribution of this one is quite obvious: by allowing the processing of different types of data, it allows the science to make significant advances in the exploration of large complex data, quite varied and often produced in real time.
- Telecommunications: This industry, in the process of transformation thanks to Big Data, benefits more from much more speed and efficiency. With the use of Big Data, phone operators can index thousands of documents in just a few minutes. The ability to locate users has opened up many opportunities for advertisers. It also enables customers to be targeted and therefore creates personalized offers and packages based on historical data to distinguish themselves from the competition, achieving high returns and significant savings.
- Tourism: In the tourism industry, Big Data utilize data collected from customers through travel history, food preferences, the most searched destinations on the Internet and applies predictive techniques to provide a fully personalized service to optimize prices, reduce costs and maximize profits.
- Government: Big Data enables governments to make accurate decisions and conduct effective economic, social and environmental policies, thereby improving the services provided to citizens.
- Media and information: With Big Data, you can access a lot of information about people. For example, tweeting analysis has become a common source of information for understanding the behavior or tastes of a population. In addition, social networks are proving to be an effective communication tool for conveying messages to the public.
- Transport: In the transport sector, the analysis of large data (data of passages, geolocation of people and cars, etc.) can be used to model population movements in order to adapt infrastructures and services (timetables, frequency of trains).

2.4   Big Data Technologies

Big Data analysis and processing requires specific tools. Among these applications, that have largely developed, most of which are based on the open source concept, we quote:

- Massively Parallel Processing (MPP): Big Data is based on data processing systems organized on several nodes or parallel clusters. This type of processing makes it possible to generate very high-performance computations on reduced infrastructures (processors, servers). Multiple data processing tasks are executed directly on the nodes where are the data concerned in order to avoid congestion of the network and to ensure a fast processing.
- Hadoop: Hadoop is a database-specific architecture developed in 2008 by Yahoo to better generalize the use of massively parallel storage and processing of MapReduce. It can handle multiple types of data (including unstructured data) in large quantities. The two main features of Hadoop are the MapReduce framework and the Hadoop Distributed File System (HDFS). HDFS allows to distribute data and perform powerful processing on this data through MapReduce by distributing an operation on several nodes to parallelize it [21–24].
- MapReduce: a parallel programming model for very large amounts of data processing developed by Google in 2003. It is composed of two main functions executed sequentially: Map and Reduce. coupled with Hadoop (which is actually its main implementation), MapReduce is the calculation mode for processing Big Data. It presents a Map function (data distribution on several parallel clusters where the intermediate calculations will be performed) and a Reduce function (the results of the distributed intermediate calculations are reentered for the final calculation) [25].
- NoSQL: SQL databases require a well-defined data structure and have limited storage capacity. However, Big Data brings huge unstructured or semi-structured data streams of different formats. This makes the SQL databases inadequate for Big Data use cases. NoSQL databases (e.g., HBase, Cassandra, DynamoDB, Couchbase) offer more flexibility to adapt with different non-relational data structures. They support one or more flexible data models including: key-value, documents, graph and columns [26].
- HDFS (Hadoop Distributed File System): a file system that makes it possible to store very important data on a cluster by disregarding the capabilities of the machines, or their state. HDFS benefits from cluster scalability. This means that, theoretically, the storage space can expand as needed by simply adding low-cost machines into the cluster. The data is secure, and the system is fault-tolerant [27].
- IN-Memory: In-memory processing is used to describe the processes that are performed in the RAM of the computer equipment, rather than on external servers.
- Spark: a Big Data processing framework that supports a wide range of applications successfully [28]. Spark introduces a new abstraction, Resilient Distributed Datasets (RDDs). As Hadoop, Spark relies on a distributed storage system (e.g., HDFS) to store the input and output data of the jobs submitted by users. Spark consists of seven elements: Spark core of data engine, Spark cluster manager (includes Hadoop, Apache Mesos, and built-in Standalone cluster manger), Spark SQL, Spark streaming, Spark Machine Learning Library, Spark GraphX, and Spark programming tools.

Beyond these basic tools, Big Data must be put into practice and offer services related to the direct needs of the company and the researcher. This is the whole purpose of the Hadoop ecosystem in which we find among the best known:

- Yarn: Yarn (Yet Another Resource Negotiator) is a main component of Hadoop. It has two roles: cluster resource management and application management. Yarn is responsible for allocating system resources to the various applications running in a Hadoop cluster and scheduling tasks to be executed on different cluster nodes [29].
- Pig: a platform for analyzing large data sets that consists of a high-level language for expressing data analysis programs. It aims to increase the performance of Hadoop/MapReduce by proposing a programming language allowing faster processing [30].
- Hive: a framework for querying and analysis of data that is stored in HDFS. Hive is an open source-software that lets programmers analyze large data sets on Hadoop. It allows to perform queries on a Hadoop cluster directly in SQL. Beside these complementary bricks that make Hadoop easier to access and faster, there are corollary database structures to Hadoop [31].
- HBase: a NoSQL-type column-oriented database that runs on top of Hadoop as a distributed and scalable big data store. HBase is based on the distributed file system (HDFS) allowing high fault tolerance and fast data access. It is a file system suitable for applications managing large data sets. HBase is particularly well suited for storing very large volumes of data and has outstanding performance for massive reads and writes of data [32].
- Cassandra: an open source, distributed, scalable and fault-tolerant NoSQL-type column-oriented database created at Facebook. Cassandra has been designed and built to be completely decentralized, transparently manage the loss of a part of the cluster and to run between several datacenters [33].
- Sqoop: a tool designed to transfer data between Hadoop and relational data-bases or mainframes (i.e., import data from a relational database management system (RDBMS) into the Hadoop Distributed File System (HDFS)) [34].
- ZooKeeper: a distributed, open source coordination service for distributed applications [35].
- Ambari: an open source product which offers software tools for provisioning and managing Hadoop data clusters [36].

2.5   Big Data Challenges and Issues

The complex characteristics of Big Data make their gathering and storage then management and processing, for the extraction of valuable information or the search for models, very painful. Indeed, many challenges and problems, in relation to platforms, systems, machines and also algorithms arise. These are directly related to the volume, variety, velocity, veracity and value of Big Data [37–43].

The following table (see Table 1) presents the most important challenges and problems of Big Data:

Table 1. Issues and challenges of Big Data

Issues and challenges	
Related to platforms, systems and machines	Related to algorithms
— Storage, Heterogeneity, Noise, outliers, incomplete, and inconsistent data, imbalanced dataset — Real-time analysis of data flows from different sources, Multidimensional queries on large datasets — Semantics of data — Energy consumption, bandwidth for data transmission, Data transfer optimization, communication and synchronization between systems — Fault tolerance — The cost — Data movement and management — Security and Privacy issues	– Problems of traditional algorithms to process data of different types — Most of the traditional machine learning algorithms are not designed for parallel computing — Information exchange (synchronization) between different machine learning procedures may incur bottlenecks — Further reduce the computation time — Features of the database — Imbalanced dataset

3 Big Data and Machine Learning

The capabilities of today's traditional applications and current software engineering are insufficient for a very fast, accurate and highly responsive analysis of Big Data. The volume of data is too large for comprehensive analysis, and the correlations and relationships between these data are too important for analysts to test all the assumptions to derive a value from these data. Machine Learning is ideal for exploiting the hidden opportunities of Big Data [44]. Big Data is the essence of Machine Learning which is the technology that makes full use of the potential of it to extract value from massive and varied data sources without having to rely on a human [45].

Machine Learning is an Artificial Intelligence technology that seeks to develop programs that allow machines to learn and make decisions without human intervention. To learn and grow, however, machines need data to analyze and to train on [5, 46, 47].

Machine Learning techniques allow automatic and scalable ways in which insights from large, multi-dimensional data can be gleaned. Machine Learning is therefore learning, drawing operational or behavioral predictions from the data. Broadly, Machine Learning is the ability for computers to automatically learn patterns and make inferences from data [48–51].

Learning methods for Machine Learning can be categorized as supervised learning, unsupervised learning, semi-supervised learning and reinforcement learning.

– Supervised Learning: all data are labeled and the algorithms learn to predict the output from the input data [5, 7, 52]. The system learns to classify its data according to what the expert (the human) indicates to him beforehand. Examples of Supervised Learning: Regression, Decision Tree, KNN, etc.

- Unsupervised Learning: all data are unlabeled and the algorithms learn to inherent structure from the input data [5, 7, 52]. The system will have to detect the similarities in the data it receives and organize them according to these into different homogeneous groups. Examples of Unsupervised Learning: K-means, Expectation-maximization, etc.
- Semi Supervised Learning: Some data are labeled but most of them are unlabeled [53]. It is often used when the structure of the data needs to be understood and categorized in addition to allowing predictions to be made.
- Reinforcement Learning: Reinforcement learning is the case where the algorithm learns behavior given an observation. The action of the algorithm on the environment produces a return value that guides the learning algorithm [7, 47, 54]. Example of Reinforcement Learning: Markov Decision Process.

Machine Learning algorithms can be classified along many different tasks. Some of the most common Machine Learning tasks:

- Classification: a predictive technique that assigns the objects of a database to one of the predefined classes according to a predefined classification model. Their distribution is based on different specificities that overlap. The most common method of classifying data automatically is to use decision trees [5, 7, 44, 52].
- Regression: predict numeric target label of a data point. The prediction will be based on learning from a known data set. It's a learning a function that maps a data item to a variable real-valued prediction [7, 44, 52].
- Clustering: also called unsupervised clustering or classification, seeks to identify and create homogeneous subsets of objects, categories, or groups (i.e., clusters) to describe data, from a heterogeneous total set of objects in the database. The idea is to determine classes that must be at once as homogeneous as possible while at the same time distinguishing between each other at best [55–57].
- Dimensionality reduction: aims to exploit the inherent structure of data in an unsupervised way by summarizing or describing data using less information [52, 58].
- Association rule: An association rule learning problem seeks to discover rules that describe large parts of data. For instance, people who buy a product p1 also tend to buy a product p2 [52, 59].
- Anomaly detection: it's the prediction and identification of elements or events that do not conform to an expected model or other elements present in a dataset [60].

There are many different techniques used to perform Machine Learning tasks such as: Decision Trees [61], Bayesian Algorithms [52, 62, 63], Artificial Neural Networks [64] and Deep Learning [65, 66].

The following table (see Table 2) gives a summary of Machine Learning tasks and techniques in the context of Big Data. Here, we propose a taxonomy of Machine Learning using two ways to classify algorithms. The first is a grouping of algorithms by learning style (e.g., supervised, unsupervised), the second is a grouping of algorithms by from or function similarity:

Table 2. Machine learning taxonomy

	By learning Style		By algorithm similarity	
Machine Learning	Supervised	Classification	Regression algorithms	Ordinary Least Squares Regression (OLSR)-Linear Regression-Logistic Regression-Stepwise Regression-Multivariate Adaptive Regression Splines (MARS)-Locally Estimated Scatterplot Smoothing (LOESS)-Standard regression-Lasso regression-Polynomial
		Regression	Decision trees	Classification and Regression Tree (CART)-Iterative Dichotomiser 3 (ID3)-C4.5-C5.0-Chi squared Automatic Interaction Detection (CHAID)-Decision Stump-M5-Conditional Decision Trees-Random Forest-Multivariate Adaptive Regression Splines (MARS)-Gradient Boosting Machines (GBM)
	Unsupervised	Clustering	Bayesian algorithms	Naïve Bayes-Gaussian Naive Bayes-Multinomial Naive Bayes-Averaged One Dependence Estimators (AODE)-Bayesian Belief Network (BBN)-Bayesian Network (BN)
		Dimensionality reduction	Instance-based algorithms	Nearest Neighbor-k Nearest Neighbor (kNN)-Learning Vector Quantization (LVQ)-Self Organizing Map (SOM)-Locally Weighted Learning (LWL)
			Regularization algorithms	Ridge Regression - Least Absolute Shrinkage and Selection Operator - (LASSO)-Elastic Net-Least Angle Regression (LARS)
		Association rule	Kernel methods	Support Vector Machines (SVM)-Radial Basis Function (RBF)-Linear Discriminant Analysis (LDA)
			Ensemble methods	Boosting-Bootstrapped Aggregation-AdaBoost-Stacked Generalization-Gradient Boosting Machines-Gradient Boosted Regression Trees (GBRT)-Random Forest
		Anomaly detection	Deep learning	No drop Deep Learning-drop out Deep Learning-drop connect Deep Learning-Restricted Boltzmann Machine (RBM)-Deep Belief Networks (DBN)-Deep Convolutional neural Network-Stacked Auto encoders-Deep Recurrent neural networks
	Semisupervised	Classification	Artificial Neural Networks	Perceptron-Back Propagation-Hopfield Network-Radial Basis Function Network (RBFN)-Adaptive Resonance Theory (ART) networks-Logic learning machine-Self Organizing Map-Learning Vector Quantization (LVQ)
		Regression	Clustering Algorithms	K means-Gaussian mixtures-C means-K Medians - Fuzzy C Means-Expectation Maximisation (EM)-Hierarchical Clustering-Neural Networks-Hidden Markov Model-Adaptive resonance theory-one class support vector machine-Birch-Dbscan-Mean shift-Optics
	Re-inforcement		Dimensionality reduction algorithms	Principle component analysis-Principal Component Analysis (PCA)-Principal Component Regression (PCR)-Partial Least Squares Regression (PLSR)-Sammon Mapping-Multidimensional Scaling (MDS)-Projection Pursuit-Linear Discriminant Analysis (LDA)-Mixture Discriminant Analysis (MDA)-Quadratic Discriminant Analysis (QDA)-Flexible Discriminant Analysis (FDA)-Feature hashing-Sammon Mapping-Projection Pursuit
			Association rule algorithms	Apriori algorithm-Eclat algorithm-FP growth algorithm
			Semisupervised algorithms	Self training-Co training-Multiview Learning-Self paced Co training (SPaCo)-transductive inference-Active-Generative models-Low density separation-Graph based methods-Transduction
			Re-inforcement algorithms	Marcov decision process-Q functions-Q learning-Q iteration-Cost Sensitive Learning (CSL)-State action reward state action (SARSA)-Temporal Difference learning (TD)-Learning Automata

4 Conclusion and Future Work

Throughout this paper, we have attempted to provide a detailed overview of Big Data and Machine Learning paradigms. Going through Big Data characteristics and ending with the description of Big Data tools and technologies mainly Hadoop and MapReduce. We then treated the Machine Learning paradigm by proposing a taxonomy that is neither unique nor exhaustive and that leaves the door open to the reader to choose the desired technique and algorithm since there is no compromise on the superiority of one algorithm over another or even on the criteria of quality measurement of algorithms that remains an open debate. We've tried to focus on the main challenges and problems of Big Data, whether those related to data, systems and platforms or those related to algorithms (e.g., communication between systems, outliers, incomplete and inconsistent data, security and privacy issues).

In the past, data mining techniques were used to uncover unknown models and relationships of interest from structured, homogeneous and small datasets. At present, the complex characteristics of Big Data, require a sufficiently high scalability of management and mining tools. The ability to store and manage a large volume of data, the ability to process data from different formats of different structures and the ability to quickly access and retrieve large data, especially for data flows, has become a requirement.

The collection of Big Data and the expansion of the Internet of Things (IoT) have created a perfect environment for the growth of new applications and services of Artificial Intelligence. According to several players in the field of Big Data, Machine Learning is one of the main strategic technological trends in the future. Artificial intelligence and advanced Machine Learning which is composed of many technologies and techniques (e.g., deep learning, neural networks, natural language processing (NLP)) are areas of constant innovation and continuous development that allow going beyond traditional algorithms to create systems that understand, learn, make predictions or decisions autonomously.

Given the current state of Machine Learning tools and algorithms, it is not easy to perform sophisticated analysis when data is very large. Thus, to perform such analyzes, it is necessary to devote a major effort to the adaptation of existing methods to make them robust against large volumes of data. It is in this context that MapReduce's variations of Machine Learning algorithms appeared, such as those allowing the extraction of association rules or clustering. In this direction, many libraries and frameworks (e.g., Mahout library, WEKA, MLlib (Spark's machine learning library), TensorFlow (Deep Learning Framework)) was built to provides a variety of data mining, Machine Learning, and information retrieval algorithms to handle very large data.

From the point of view of data mining problem, in this paper, we have given a brief introduction to the concept of Machine Learning. Several researches are focused on the exploration of Machine Learning techniques, especially Deep Learning, in greater depth in order to better frame and improve them or adapt them to the Big Data context to deal with the different problems that arise from Big Data's characteristics (3V). Current research is trying to run Machine Learning algorithms on parallel platforms and distributed system to improve the performance and efficiency of existing algorithms in the context of Big Data (e.g., Radoop) which means that there is still need to develop new powerful and effective algorithms and to design new technologies to access massive data and react in real time.

Open source applications dedicated to Big Data like Apache Hadoop, Spark, In-Memory, NoSQL and others will dominate the Big Data space, and this trend seems likely to continue. So, there is a lot of work to be done to expand the use of its technologies and look for ways to speed up their processing of large data.

In order to meet future challenges, businesses, companies and organizations need to move and invest more and more in the parallel processing and distributed storage of their Big Data resources which is no longer an option but a necessity.

Big Data and Machine Learning represent the next computer revolution. And like every revolution, it will transform the way we live, work and think.

References

1. Gantz, J., Reinsel, D.: The digital universe in 2020: Big data, bigger digital shadows, and biggest growth in the far east. IDC iView IDC Anal. Future **2007**, 1–16 (2012)
2. Buyya, R., Calheiros, R.N., Dastjerdi, A.V. (ed.): Big data: Principles and Paradigms. Morgan Kaufmann (2016)
3. Fayyad, U., Piatetsky-Shapiro, G., Smyth, P.: From data mining to knowledge discovery in databases. AI magazine **17**(3), 37 (1996)
4. Chen, M., Mao, S., Liu, Y.: Big data: a survey. Mob. Netw. Appl. **19**(2), 171–209 (2014)
5. Suthaharan, S.: Machine Learning Models and Algorithms for Big Data Classification. Springer, Boston (2016)
6. Samuel, A.L.: Some studies in machine learning using the game of checkers. IBM J. Res. Dev. **3**(3), 210–229 (1959)
7. Mitchell, T.M., et al.: Machine learning, vol. 45, pp. 870–877. Burr Ridge, IL: McGraw Hill (1997)
8. Gantz, J., Reinsel, D.: Extracting value from chaos. IDC iview **1142**(2011), 1–12 (2011)
9. Sicular, S.: Gartner's big data definition consists of three parts, not to be confused with three "v" s. Gartner, Inc 27 (2013)
10. Erl, T., Khattak, W., Buhler, P.: Big Data Fundamentals: Concepts, Drivers & Techniques. Prentice Hall, Upper Saddle River, NJ, USA (2016)
11. Russom, P.: Big Data Analytics. TDWI Best Practices Report, Fourth Quarter, 19(4), pp. 1–34 (2011)
12. Mahalakshmi, S., Saiashwini, C., Meghana, S.: Research study of big data clustering techniques. Int. J. Innov. Res. Sci. Eng. 80–84 (2001)
13. Yang, C., Huang, Q., Li, Z., Liu, K.: Big Data and cloud computing: innovation opportunities and challenges. Int. J. Digit. Earth **10**(1), 13–53 (2017)
14. Ericsson, L.: More than 50 billion connected devices. White Paper **14**, 124 (2011)
15. Kudyba, S.: Big Data, Mining, and Analytics: Components of Strategic Decision Making. CRC Press (2014)
16. Demchenko, Y., De Laat, C., Membrey, P.: Defining architecture components of the Big Data Ecosystem. In: International Conference on Collaboration Technologies and Systems, pp. 104–112. (CTS), IEEE (2014)

17. Hashem, I.A.T., Chang, V., Anuar, N.B., Adewole, K., Yaqoob, I., Gani, A., et al.: The role of big data in smart city. Int. J. Inf. Manage. **36**(5), 748–758 (2016)
18. Chen, H., Chiang, R.H.L., Storey, V.C.: Business Intelligence and Analytics: From Big Data to Big Impact, pp. 1165–1188. MIS quarterly, (2012)
19. Herland, M., Khoshgoftaar, T.M., Wald, R.: A review of data mining using big data in health informatics. J. Big Data **1**(1), 2 (2014)
20. Chen, M., Mao, S., Zhang, Y., Leung, V.C., et al.: Big Data: Related Technologies, Challenges and Future Prospects. Springer, Heidelberg (2014)
21. Eadline, D.: Hadoop 2 Quick-Start Guide: Learn the Essentials of Big Data Computing in the Apache Hadoop 2 Ecosystem. Addison-Wesley Professional (2015)
22. Oussous, A., Benjelloun, F.Z., Lahcen, A.A., Belfkih, S.: Big data technologies: a survey. J. King Saud Univ.Comput. Inf. Sci. (2017)
23. Singh, D., Reddy, C.K.: A survey on platforms for big data analytics. J. Big Data **2**(1), 8 (2015)
24. Landset, S., Khoshgoftaar, T.M., Richter, A.N., Hasanin, T.: A survey of open source tools for machine learning with big data in the Hadoop ecosystem. J. Big Data **2**(1), 24 (2015)
25. Dean, J., Ghemawat, S.: MapReduce: simplified data processing on large clusters. Commun. ACM **51**(1), 107–113 (2008)
26. Pokorny, J.: NoSQL databases: a step to database scalability in web environment. Int. J. Web Inf. Syst. **9**(1), 69–82 (2013)
27. Shvachko, K., Kuang, H., Radia, S., Chansler, R.: The hadoop distributed file system. In: IEEE 26th symposium on Mass storage systems and technologies (MSST), 2010, pp. 1–10. IEEE (2010)
28. Zaharia, M., Chowdhury, M., Franklin, M.J., Shenker, S., Stoica, I.: Spark: cluster computing with working sets. HotCloud **10**(10–10), 95 (2010)
29. Vavilapalli, V. K., Murthy, A. C., Douglas, C., Agarwal, S., Konar, M., Evans, R. et al.: Apache hadoop yarn: Yet another resource negotiator. In: Proceedings of the 4th annual Symposium on Cloud Computing, pp. 5. ACM (2013)
30. Gates, A., Dai, D.: Programming Pig: Dataflow Scripting with Hadoop. O'Reilly Media, Inc. (2016)
31. Shaw, S., Vermeulen, A., Gupta, A., Kjerrumgaard, D.: Hive architecture. In: Practical Hive, pp. 37–48. Apress, Berkeley, CA (2016)
32. George, L.: HBase: The Definitive Guide: Random Access to your Planet-size Data. O'Reilly Media, Inc. (2011)
33. Carpenter, J. Eben, H.: Cassandra: The Definitive Guide: Distributed Data at Web Scale. O'Reilly Media, Inc (2016)
34. Vohra, D.: Using apache sqoop. In: Pro Docker, pp. 151–183. Apress, Berkeley, CA (2016)
35. Junqueira, F., Reed, B.: ZooKeeper: distributed process coordination. O'Reilly Media, Inc. (2013)
36. Wadkar, S., Siddalingaiah, M.: Apache ambari. In Pro Apache Hadoop, pp. 399–401. Apress, Berkeley, CA. (2014)
37. Tsai, C.W., Lai, C.F., Chao, H.C., Vasilakos, A.V.: Big data analytics: a survey. J. Big Data **2**(1), 21 (2015)
38. Fahad, A., Alshatri, N., Tari, Z., Alamri, A., Khalil, I., Zomaya, A.Y., et al.: A survey of clustering algorithms for big data: taxonomy and empirical analysis. IEEE Trans. Emerg. Topics Comput. **2**(3), 267–279 (2014)
39. L'heureux, A., Grolinger, K., Elyamany, H.F., Capretz, M.A.: Machine learning with big data: challenges and approaches. IEEE Access, **5**(5), 777–797 (2017)
40. Bolón-Canedo, V., Remeseiro, B., Sechidis, K., Martinez-Rego, D., Alonso-Betanzos, A.: Algorithmic challenges in Big Data analytics. In: ESANN 2017 Proceedings, European

Symposium on Artificial Neural Networks, Computational Intelligence and Machine Learning, pp. 519–528 (2017)

41. García, S., Ramírez-Gallego, S., Luengo, J., Benítez, J.M., Herrera, F.: Big data preprocessing: methods and prospects. Big Data Anal. **1**(1), 9 (2016)

42. Chu, W.W.: Data mining and knowledge discovery for Big Data. Stud. Big Data, 1 (2014)

43. Che, D., Safran, M. Peng, Z.: From big data to big data mining: challenges, issues, and opportunities. In: International Conference on Database Systems for Advanced Applications, pp. 1–15. Springer, Berlin, Heidelberg (2013)

44. Alpaydin, E.: Introduction to Machine Learning. MIT press (2014)

45. Liu, T. Y., Chen, W., Wang, T.: Distributed machine learning: Foundations, trends, and practices. In: Proceedings of the 26th International Conference on World Wide Web Companion, pp. 913–915. International World Wide Web Conferences Steering Committee (2017)

46. Dean, J.: Big data, Data Mining, and Machine Learning: Value Creation for Business Leaders and Practitioners. Wiley (2014)

47. Qiu, J., Wu, Q., Ding, G., Xu, Y., Feng, S.: A survey of machine learning for big data processing. EURASIP J. Adv. Signal Process. **2016**(1), 67 (2016)

48. Chen, C.P., Zhang, C.Y.: Data-intensive applications, challenges, techniques and technologies: a survey on big data. Inf. Sci. **275**, 314–347 (2014)

49. Kotu, V., Deshpande, B.: Predictive analytics and data mining: concepts and practice with rapidminer. Morgan Kaufmann (2014)

50. Han, J., Pei, J., Kamber, M.: Data Mining: Concepts and Techniques. Elsevier (2011)

51. Kelleher, J. D., Mac Namee, B., D'arcy, A.: Fundamentals of Machine Learning for Predictive Data Analytics: Algorithms, Worked Examples, and Case Studies. MIT Press (2015)

52. Friedman, J., Hastie, T., Tibshirani, R.: The elements of statistical learning (Vol. 1, No. 10). New York, NY, USA: Springer series in statistics (2001)

53. Zhu, X.: Semi-supervised learning literature survey. Comput. Sci. Univ. Wisconsin-Madison **2**(3), 4 (2006)

54. Sutton, R.S., Barto, A.G.: Reinforcement Learning: An Introduction. MIT press, Cambridge (1998)

55. Jain, A.K.: Data clustering: 50 years beyond K-means. Patt. Recogn. Lett. **31**(8), 651–666 (2010)

56. Sajana, T., Rani, C.S., Narayana, K.V.: A survey on clustering techniques for big data mining. Indian J. Sci. Technol. **9**(3) (2016)

57. Aggarwal, C.C., Reddy, C.K. (ed.).: Data Clustering: Algorithms and Applications. CRC press (2013)

58. Ghodsi, A.: Dimensionality reduction a short tutorial. Department of Statistics and Actuarial Science, Univ. of Waterloo, Ontario, Canada, 37, pp. 38 (2006)

59. Bishop, C.M.: Pattern Recognition and Machine Learning, vol. 60, p. 78. Springer, New York (2006)

60. Chandola, V., Banerjee, A., Kumar, V.: Anomaly detection: a survey. ACM Comput. Surv. (CSUR) **41**(3), 15 (2009)

61. Quinlan, J.R.: Induction of decision trees. Mach. Learn. **1**(1), 81–106 (1986)

62. Neal, R.M.: Bayesian Methods for Machine Learning. NIPS tutorial, 13 (2004)

63. Murphy, K. P.: Machine Learning: A Probabilistic Perspective. MIT Press (2012)

64. Schalkoff, R. J.: Artificial Neural Networks, vol. 1. New York: McGraw-Hill (1997)

65. Lecun, Y., Bengio, Y., Hinton, G.: Deep learning. Nature, **521**(7553), 436 (2015)

66. Goodfellow, I., Bengio, Y., Courville, A. et al.: Deep Learning, vol. 1, Cambridge: MIT press (2016)

Improved CSO to Solve the TSP

Abdelhamid Bouzidi[1,2(✉)] and Mohammed Essaid Riffi[2]

[1] LIMIE (Laboratoire d'Innovation en Management et Ingénierie pour l'Entreprise), Centre El Jadida, Groupe ISGA, El Jadida, Morocco
mr.abdelhamid.bouzidi@gmail.com
[2] LAROSERI Lab, Faculty of Science, El Jadida, Morocco
said@riffi.fr

Abstract. The Travelling Salesman Problem (TSP) is a known optimization problem by the important number of its applications and its complexity (classified as NP-hard combinatorial optimization). That explains the important to propose some novel methods to solve it. The Cat Swarm Optimization (CSO). metaheuristic is a nature-inspired behavior of real life of the cats that was adapted in 2013 to solve the TSP, to improve its efficiency, this paper aims propose a novel improved CSO characterized by a dynamic Mixture Ratio used to exchange the mode of the cat (Seeking or tracing mode), add a novel parameter that consider the best position the selected cat and other improvement. The results by the application of the proposed methods to solve some benchmark instances of TSPLIB; show that the novel proposal method is more efficient.

Keywords: TSP · Cat swarm optimization · Computational intelligence · Combinatorial optimization · Mixture ration

1 Introduction

The motivation to use the computational intelligent is the needs to benefit of time, money etc.... in the aims to increase the quality of the human life. After the introduction of computer, the researcher, engineer and others had try to use it and improve it in order to reach solving an important number of problem in different areas as industry, medicine, finance, marketing, and transportation. So, to solve any problem, it should be formulated. In the case of the combinatorial optimization the graph theory was introduced for that, and the first model, which is the basic one is the Travelling salesman problem.

The travelling salesman problem [1] is a combinatorial optimization problem that can be described as a salesman who would like distribute its merchandise to a set of cities, for that he should start by its depot to travel all cities and return to the depot, by visiting each cities at once. This problem was formulated to a Hamiltonian graph, each city is presented by a node, each path is presented by an edge, where the edge cost present the distance. So, solving the TSP problem is finding the Hamiltonian graph with the optimal (minimal) cost.

© Springer Nature Switzerland AG 2019
M. Ezziyyani (Ed.): AI2SD 2018, AISC 915, pp. 252–260, 2019.
https://doi.org/10.1007/978-3-030-11928-7_22

The TSP problem was simple to formulate, but hard to solve it, given that this problem complexity as NP-Hard. The need interested to solve is the important number of its application as data transmission in computer networks, transport, logistics, scheduling.

In order to reach the suboptimal solution within a reasonable execution time, the researchers proposed various methods classified into two categories are: exact methods (that give solution in a small problem size) and approximate methods. The second category is divided into two class, are the heuristic algorithm that defined to by apply to a determined problem, and the metaheuristic that can be applied to solve a different problems type, and give a solution in a reasonable execution time. The researcher's had proposed many metaheuristics such as the genetic algorithm [2], Ant colony Optimization(ACO) [3], Particle Swarm Optimization [4, 5], cat Swarm optimization [6], penguins search optimization [7], Swallow Swarm Optimization [8], Bat Swarm Optimization [9], invasive weed optimization [10], symbiotic organisms search algorithm [11], and hybrid methods such as, hybrid ACO and 3-opt algorithm [12]; glowworm swarm optimization and complete 2-opt algorithm [13].

This paper aims propose a novel improvement to the Cat Swarm Optimization (CSO) algorithm, to increase its efficiency to solve the TSP. So the present paper is organized as follow, the Sect. 2; is a presentation of the studied metaheuristic, by presented the real nature behavior of cat, and it's formulation. Section 3; the proposal improvement to the CSO to solve combinatorial optimization problem. After that, the Sect. 4 present the result of the application of proposed improved CSO to solve the some benchmark instances of TSPLIB [14], and a discussion. Finally, a conclusion and some perspectives.

2   Cat Swarm Optimization

2.1   Nature Inspired

The Cat Swarm optimization algorithm, is bio-inspired nature behavior of any feline that have the same behavior even it had a different environment of life, as the cat, tiger, lion …

The feline creatures are known by its velocity, and it past a majority of its time in rest (2/3 of its life), and the other part in purchasing a prey or any moving object. This is concept considered by the researcher's to be modeled.

2.2   Literature

In the first, the CSO was proposed to solve the mono objective continued optimization problem [15]. Giving the efficiency of this metaheuristic results; some researchers had focus its interest to apply it to solve some theoretical or real application problems such as [16, 17], or improve it by respecting the modeled real life of cats such as [6, 18, 19], in the aims increase its performance or extends its applications area.

In literature there is an important number of CSO application such as, improved meta-heuristic techniques for simultaneous capacitor and DG allocation in radial distribution networks by Kawtar et al. [20], Optimizing least-significant-bit substitution by Wang et al. [21], optimal placement of multiple UPFC's in voltage stability enhancement under contingency by Gálvez et al. [22], Single bitmap block truncation coding of color images by Cui [23], linear antenna array synthesis by Pappula et al. [24].

2.3   Formulation

The behavior of cats was modeled in 2016 by Tsai et al. [15], as a set of cat, living in the same swarm. Each cat had two modes, are:

- The Seeking Mode (SM): present the cat when it's at rest.
- The Tracing Mode (TM): present the cat when it trace it path according its velocity to hunt a prey or any moving object.

In cat real life, there exist a numerous properties, but only some the important one are chosen. The chosen one are used it was used to hunt a pray or in the rest position to observe its prey, the considered properties in this methods are:

- The position: present the solution
- The velocity: present the velocity to move to a novel position.
- The flag: Present the cats mode (TM or SM)

Also, the best position in the swarm is registered in the Gbest parameter.

2.4   CSO Process Description

The process of the CSO algorithm can be described as follow:

Step 1. Generation of population
Step 2. Initialization of each cat

- Positions:
    - This contribution use a random generation of solution (position).
- Velocity
    - Each cat's velocity is initialized by a null value.
- Flag
    - Each cat's Flag is initialized by a null value.

Step 3. Update the flag
Step 4. Process

The CSO will execute the process until achieve the stopping criterion. The process is composed by two mode, which are Seeking Mode that the cat can execute one of them according to the value of the flag. In the end of each iteration, the flag of each cat is updated.

The Seeking Mode

In the seeking mode (SM) the cat use four parameters:

SMP: Number of chats in **SM**

CDC: Dimension selected to carry the mutation

SRD: the first position to choose randomly

SPC: a Boolean value indicating whether a cat can be selected for the trace mode

The process of the can be described as follow:

```
Begin
        j=SMP
    For   k →   1 to SMP
        if(SPC==true)
            Begin
                j=j-1
                SRD = random() ;
                Pi = |FSi − FSmax|
                     ───────────
                     FSmax−FSmin
                Alpha = random()
                If(pi<alpha)
                        mutation(cat k , SRD, CDC)
            EndIf
        EndFor
END
```

The Tracing Mode

This is the hunting, where every cat $_k$ moves quickly by it's velocity V_i to trace his path. The description of the process is as follows

```
Begin
    For i →  1 to SMP
      if(SPC==false)
      //update_velocity
```

$$V_i = w*V_i + r * c * (X_{best} − X_i)$$

```
      //update_position
```

$$X_i = X_i + V_i$$

```
      EndIf
    EndFor
    END
```

With :

r : is a random value in [0,1]

c : a constant values

w : Inertie value

Update the flag

Update the flag by respecting the mixture ratio values.

3 Improved CSO to Solve Tsp

The CSO was proposed in the first to solve the continued optimization problem and extended in the first to solve the combinatorial optimization problem in 2013 by A. Bouzidi et al., and to test and prove its efficiency, this method was applied to solve the TSP problem [6]. After that, the CSO was applied to solve some of TSP applications, such as the quadratic assignment problem [25], the Job Shop scheduling Problem (JSSP) [26], and the Flow Shop Scheduling Problem (FSSP) [27], for simultaneous capacitor and DG allocation in radial distribution networks [28], Solving the high school timetabling [29].

The first version of discrete CSO, had propose some modification of operation and operator, because the type of the solution in combinatorial optimization (a vector/schedule) is not as in continued optimization problem (a number). The result by the application the first discrete CSO, had demonstrate that this methods can reach the best optimal solution got by other metaheuristics, but it had an important average error. In the aim's improve its performance, the quality of the solution and minimize the execution time, some improvement was proposed by respecting the real life of the cats. So, some improvement had been proposed, are:

3.1 Generation Improvement

In the aims improve the execution time, after the generation. The local search; simple descent metaheuristic is applied to each generate cat position.

3.2 Edge Exchange Solution in Seeking Mode

As any metaheuristic, the CSO algorithm start by the generation and initialization of the population, after that it start the process by combining two type of solution search, that are the intensification and diversification. In the first version of CSO the tracing mode present the intensification, and the seeking mode present the diversification. In the two modes of research, the method use only a simple permutation of nodes.

To increase the diversification in the SM, this contribution had propose in the first use exchange of edges instead of exchange the vertex, after selecting two vertices, the method swap the two edges that starting by the selected vertices.

3.3 Improved Exchange Mode

This improvement concerns the method of cat's mode choice. The proposed improvement closed the already proposed by Wang [30] in continued optimization problem. Giving that in real life of cats, it's possible that all the swarm can be in the seeking or tracing mode, it not depend the population number. By this last idea, the proposed CSO project the real life of the cats by proposing an improvement which is that the flag parameter will be a probability value randomly generated between zero and one. If the probability is minus or equals to 1/3, the cat process is the tracing mode, else the cat's process will be the seeking mode. By this improvement the cat's mode is autonomous changed as in the nature behavior, it not depend the swarm. It mean that our proposed improved CSO version, will not use the mixture ration parameter.

3.4 Keep the Best Position of Each of Each Cat

In real life of cat's, the cat's mark their territory by leaving small amounts of urine. To memories I's best position. And indicate to others that it's its personal place.

This idea was used in this version of CSO, by adding a novel parameter called Cbest that keep the best position of a selected cat. This parameter will be considered in the update of the velocity in the Tracing mode. So the equation to update the velocity will be:

$$v_k = w \times v_k + r_1 \times c_1 \times (x_{best} - x_k) + r_2 \times c_2 \times (x_{cbest} - x_k) \qquad (1)$$

3.5 CSO Process

The general process of the CSO was not changed, as it was described in the following pseudocode.

Begin:

(1) Generate N cats
(2) Initialize flag, velocity, position every cat.
(3) apply local search to cats position
(4) update Cbest of each cat
(5) Initialize gbest with the lowest fitness cat in swarm.
(6) for each cat in swarm
        If the flag of the selected cats TM
    Apply selected cat into TM process
      Else
       Apply selected cat into TM process
      EndIf
    Update gbest
    End for
(7) Update the Cbest of each cats
(8) Update Gbest
(9) Re-pick number of cats and set a novel flag value.
    If the condition is to terminate yes then complete the program
    Else repeat **(6), (7), (8)** and **(9)**.

End.

---

4   Results & Discussion

After describing the proposal improved CSO algorithm, this part present the results by the application of the proposal improved CSO to solve some benchmark instances proposed in TSPLIB [14]. In order to verify the efficiency of the improved CSO, the average percentage error (AVG) of the the obtained results are compared to the AVG of the existing CSO in the literature. The instance choice to solve was randomly.

The proposed improved CSO algorithm was implemented in C++ language, which run on an Ultrabook characteristic's 2.1 GHz ,2.59 GHz Intel Core i7 PC with 8G of RAM. For each instances, the best and worst result obtained in ten executions are collected, and the number of the cat is one hundred.

For each instance, the average percentage error is calculated by the following formula:

$$\%avg\_err = \frac{\frac{BEST + Worst}{2} - \textbf{BKS}}{\textbf{BKS}} \times 100 \tag{2}$$

(The BKS present the best known solution found by other methods)
The used constant parameters values are: (Table 1)

Table 1.   Used parameters values

SMP	CDC	MR	c_1, c_2	r_1, r_2	W
5	0.8	0.3	2.05	[0,1]	0.729

4.1   Table of Results

The result by the application of the proposal methods is collected in the following table composed by a set columns that are:

- *instance*: The instance name.
- *size*: Number of nodes.
- *bks*: best known solution found by others methods
- *AVG*: Average percentage Error. (Table 2)

Table 2.   Result by the application of the improved CSO to TSP instances

Instance	Size	Best known solution	AVG	
			CSO [6]	Improved CSO
a280	280	2579	3.96	0.23
Berlin52	52	7542	1	0.00
Ch130	130	6110	2.32	0.12
Ch150	150	6528	2.09	0.07
eil51	51	426	0.08	0.00
gil262	262	2378	6.16	0.26

4.2   Discussion

The comparison of the AVG of the obtained results by the application of the improved and the old version of the CSO algorithm to solve some benchmark instances, show that the AVG of the proposed method is lower than the old one, which prove that the proposal improvement CSO increase efficiency of the cat swarm optimization.

5   Conclusion

This research paper had proposed a new improved Cat swarm optimization to solve the traveling salesman problem to improve its efficiency for solving the combinatorial optimization problem. The obtained result by the application of the proposal improved CSO algorithm to solve some benchmark instances of the TSPLIB had demonstrate that this paper had reach its aims. The future work is more improve the CSO to reduce its average error and also extend the CSO algorithm to solve some real applications based the TSP.

References

1. Hoffman, K.L., Padberg, M., Rinaldi, G.: Traveling salesman problem In: Encyclopedia of Operations Research and Management Science, pp. 1573–1578 (2013)
2. Larranaga, P., Kuijpers, C.M.H., Murga, R.H., Inza, I., Dizdarevic, S.: Genetic algorithms for the travelling salesman problem: a review of representations and operators. Artif. Intell. Rev. 13(2), 129–170 (1999)
3. Pang, S., Ma, T., Liu, T.: An improved ant colony optimization with optimal search library for solving the traveling salesman problem. J. Comput. Theor. Nanosci. 12(7), 1440–1444 (2015)
4. M. Clerc.: Discrete particle swarm optimization, illustrated by the traveling salesman problem. In: New Optimization Techniques in Engineering, pp. 219–239 (2004)
5. M. Bouzidi, Riffi, M.E., Serhir, A.: Discrete Particle Swarm Optimization for Travelling Salesman Problems: New Combinatorial Operators. In: International Conference on Soft Computing and Pattern Recognition, pp. 141–150 (2017)
6. Bouzidi, A., Riffi, M.E.: Discrete cat swarm optimization to resolve the traveling salesman problem. Int. J. Adv. Res. Comput. Sci. Softw. Eng. (IJARCSSE) 3(9), 13–18 (2013)
7. Mzili, I., Riffi, M.E.: Discrete penguins search optimization algorithm to solve the traveling salesman problem. J. Theor. Appl. Inf. Technol. 72(3), 331–336 (2015)
8. Bouzidi, S., Riffi, M.E.: Discrete swallow swarm optimization algorithm for travelling salesman problem. In: Proceedings of the 2017 International Conference on Smart Digital Environment, pp. 80–84 (2017)
9. Osaba, E., Yang, X.-S., Diaz, F., Lopez-Garcia, P., Carballedo, R.: An improved discrete bat algorithm for symmetric and asymmetric traveling salesman problems. Eng. Appl. Artif. Intell. 48, 59–71 (2016)
10. Zhou, Y., Luo, Q., Chen, H., He, A., Wu, J.: A discrete invasive weed optimization algorithm for solving traveling salesman problem. Neurocomputing 151, 1227–1236 (2015)
11. Ezugwu, A.E.-S., Adewumi, A.O.: Discrete symbiotic organisms search algorithm for travelling salesman problem. Expert Syst. Appl. 87, 70–78 (2017)

12. GÜLCÜ, Ş., MAHI, M., BAYKAN, Ö.K., Kodaz, H.: A parallel cooperative hybrid method based on ant colony optimization and 3-Opt algorithm for solving traveling salesman problem. Soft Comput. **22**(5), 1669–168 (2018)
13. Chen, X., Zhou, Y., Tang, Z., Luo, Q.: A hybrid algorithm combining glowworm swarm optimization and complete 2-opt algorithm for spherical travelling salesman problems. Appl. Soft Comput. **58**, 104–114 (2017)
14. G. Reinelt.: http://comopt.ifi.uni-heidelberg.de/software/TSPLIB95/. [Online]
15. Chu, S-C., Tsai, P-W., Pan, J-S.: Cat swarm optimization. In: Pacific Rim International Conference on Artificial Intelligence, pp. 854–858 (2006)
16. Panda, G., Pradhan, P.M., Majhi, B.: IIR system identification using cat swarm optimization. Expert Syst. Appl. **38**(10), 12671–12683 (2011)
17. Panda, G., Pradhan, P.M., Majhi, B.: Direct and inverse modeling of plants using cat swarm optimization. Handbook of Swarm Intelligence, pp. 469–485 (2011)
18. Orouskhani, M., Mansouri, M., Teshnehlab, M.: Average-inertia weighted cat swarm optimization. In: International Conference in Swarm Intelligence, pp. 321–328 (2011)
19. Razzaq, S., Maqbool, F., Hussain, A.: Modified cat swarm optimization for clustering. In: International Conference on Brain Inspired Cognitive Systems, pp. 161–170 (2016)
20. Kanwar, N., Gupta, N., Niazi, K.R., Swarnkar, A.: Improved meta-heuristic techniques for simultaneous capacitor and DG allocation in radial distribution networks. Int. J. Electr. Power Energy Syst. **73**, 653–664 (2015)
21. Wang, Z-H., Chang, C-C, Li, M-C.: Optimizing least-significant-bit substitution using cat swarm optimization strategy. Inf. Sci. **192**, 98–108 (2012)
22. Kumar, G.N., Kalavathi, M.S.: At swarm optimization for optimal placement of multiple UPFC's in voltage stability enhancement under contingency. Int. J. Electr. Power Energy Syst. **57**, 97–104 (2014)
23. Cui, S-Y., Wang, Z-H., Tsai, P-W., Chang, C-C., Yue, S.: Single bitmap block truncation coding of color images using cat swarm optimization. In: Recent Advances in Information Hiding and Applications, pp. 119–138. Springer, Berlin (2013)
24. Pappula, L., Ghosh, D.: Linear antenna array synthesis using cat swarm optimization. AEU-Int. J. Electr. Commun. **68**(16), 540–549 (2014)
25. Riffi, M.E., Bouzidi, A.: Discrete cat swarm optimization for solving the quadratic assignment problem. Int. J. Soft Comput. Softw. Eng. [JSCSE] **4**(6), 85–92 (2014)
26. Bouzidi, A., Riffi, M.E.: Cat swarm optimization to solve job shop scheduling problem. Information Science and Technology (CIST), 2014 In: Third IEEE International Colloquium in Information, pp. 202–205 (2014)
27. Bouzidi, A., Riffi, M.E.: Cat swarm optimization to solve flow shop scheduling problem. J. Theor. Appl. Inf. Technol. **72**(2), 239–243 (2015)
28. Kanwar, N., Gupta, N., Niazi, K., Swarnkar, A. A.: Improved meta-heuristic techniques for simultaneous capacitor and DG allocation in radial distribution network. Int. J. Electr. Power Energy Syst. **73**, 653–664 (2015)
29. Skoullis, V.I., Tassopoulos, I.X., Beligiannis, G.N.: Solving the high school timetabling problem using a hybrid cat swarm optimization based algorithm. Appl. Soft Comput. **52**, 277–289 (2017)
30. Wang, J.: A new cat swarm optimization with adaptive parameter control. Genetic and Evolutionary Computing, pp. 69–78. Springer, Cham, (2015)

Fast and Stable Computation of the Tchebichef's Moments Using Image Block Representation and Clenshaw's Formula

Hicham Karmouni[1(✉)], Tarik Jahid[1], Mhamed Sayyouri[2], Abdeslam Hmimid[1], Anass El-affar[1], and Hassan Qjidaa[1]

[1] CED-STIC, LESSI, Faculty of Sciences Dhar El-Mehraz, Sidi Mohamed Ben Abdellah University, Fez, Morocco
hicham.karmouni@usmba.ac.ma
[2] LabSIPE, National School of Applied Sciences, Chouaib Doukkali University, El Jadida, Morocco

Abstract. In this paper, we propose a new method of stable computation of the discrete orthogonal moments of Tchebichef and its inverse. In this method, we have combined two main concepts. The first concept is Clenshaw's recurrence formula to accelerate the calculation process of the Tchebichef moments. The second concept is the partitioning of the image into a set of blocks of fixed sizes where each block is processed independently. This method is meant to accelerate the computation time and improve the quality of images reconstruction. In order to demonstrate the efficiency, the stability and the precision of the proposed method compared to the direct method based of Clenshaw's recurrence formula, some simulations have been performed on different types of images.

Keywords: Tchebichef's moments · Clenshaw's recurrence formula · Image reconstruction · Lapped block-based method

1 Introduction

The image moments have been largely used for different functions such as such as pattern recognition and image analysis [1–8, 10–20]. Teague [3] introduced the moments with or-thogonal basis functions, then Mukundan et al. [8] announced the Tchebichef moments as a novel set of orthogonal moments, since its are discrete, it represents an image with minimum amount of information redundancy. They also compare it to Zernike and Legendre moments [3, 4] to ensure superior feature representation capability of Tchebichef moments. However, many algorithms have been edited for the calculation of orthogonal moments and its inverse [12, 17], but still not that efficient as we hope. Mukundan et al. [8] set a straightforward method which needs quite excessive operations for the computation of basis Tchebichef polynomials of various orders, but it costs a lot of time to do the job.

Then, Wang [20] introduced a Clenshaw recursion formula to transform the kernels of the Tchebichef moments and its inverses, and proposed a new algorithm for the rapid computation of the Tchebichef moment and its inverses. But, one can not apply this

© Springer Nature Switzerland AG 2019
M. Ezziyyani (Ed.): AI2SD 2018, AISC 915, pp. 261–273, 2019.
https://doi.org/10.1007/978-3-030-11928-7_23

algorithm for the images of big sizes for two problems: the cost of the computation that is high and the numerical instability of the values of the polynomials of Tchebichef which influences the quality of reconstruction of the image.

In this paper, we will present a novel algorithm that provides a fast and stable method for calculating Tchebichef moments. This algorithm is based on two fundamental notions: the first is Clenshaw's formula of recurrence to accelerate the process of calculating Tchebichef moments. The second concept is the partitioning of the image into a set of fixed size blocks where each block will be processed independently. This method is purely local and intended to accelerate the computation time and improve the quality of image reconstruction.

Thus, the reduction of the image space allows the use of the Tchebichef's discrete orthogonal moments of low order during the calculation process [20–25]. The calculation of the Tchebichef moments of the image blocks provides a better representation of the image. Thus, to reconstruct large images, we need to calculate Tchebichef moments for high orders. During this calculation, very large (unstable) numerical values are obtained which can not be supported by the machine, resulting in a loss of information. To overcome this problem, we propose to decompose the image in blocks to ensure the numerical stability of moment values. In order to demonstrate the effectiveness of this proposal compared to other existing methods in terms of numerical stability, computation time and reconstruction quality and noise robustness, simulations have been carried out.

The paper is organized as follows. In the Sect. 2, we introduce the polynomes and the moments of Tchebichef. In Sect. 3, we define Clenshaw's recurrence and it application on Tchebichef moments and its inverse computation. In Sect. 4, the reconstruction method based on Lapped blocks (LBBRM) is presented. In Sect. 5, we will demonstrate the effectiveness of our approach in terms of time computation and in terms of image reconstruction for binary and grayscale images. Finally, we conclude the work.

2   Tchebichef's Moments and its Inverses

The pth order Tchebichef's moments T_p of 1D N points signal $f(x)$, is defined as:

$$T_p = \frac{1}{\widetilde{\rho}(p,N)} \sum_{x=0}^{N-1} \widetilde{t}_p(x) f(x) \tag{1}$$

where $p = 0, 1, 2, \ldots$, $\widetilde{t}_p(x)$ denotes the pth order scaled Tchebichef polynomials and $\widetilde{\rho}(p,N)$ is the squared-norm of the scaled polynomials [8]. They are given by:

$$\widetilde{t}_p(x) = \frac{p!}{N^p} \sum_{k=0}^{p} (-1)^{p-k} \binom{N-1-k}{p-k} \binom{p+k}{p} \binom{x}{k} \tag{2}$$

and:

$$\widetilde{\rho}(p,N) = \frac{N(1 - (1/N^2))(1 - (2/N^2))\ldots(1 - (p^2/N^2))}{2p+1} \tag{3}$$

The scaled Tchebichef polynomials obey a general three-term recursive relation [20]:

$$\widetilde{t}_n(x) = \frac{(2n-1)}{n}\widetilde{t}_{n-1}(x) - \frac{(n-1)}{n} \times \left(1 - \frac{(n-1)^2}{N^2}\right)\widetilde{t}_{n-2}(x) \tag{4}$$

where $n = 2, 3, \ldots, N-1$

The $(p+q)$th order Tchebichef moments T_{pq} of a 2D image function $f(x,y)$ on the discrete domain of $[0, N-1] \times [0, M-1]$, is defined as:

$$T_{pq} = \frac{1}{\widetilde{\rho}(p,N)\widetilde{\rho}(q,M)} \sum_{x=0}^{N-1}\sum_{y=0}^{M-1} \widetilde{t}_p(x)\widetilde{t}_q(y)f(x,y) \tag{5}$$

Then for a digital signal $f(x)$ and/or an image $f(x,y)$, their reconstruction from Tchebichef moments is defined respectively as:

$$f(x) = \sum_{p=0}^{N-1} T_p\widetilde{t}_p(x) \tag{6}$$

and

$$f(x,y) = \sum_{p=0}^{N-1}\sum_{q=0}^{M-1} T_{pq}\widetilde{t}_p(x)\widetilde{t}_q(y) \tag{7}$$

So, the straightforward algorithm is divided into three steps, calculate the moments and then reconstruct from those moments.

3   Clenshaw's Recurrence Formula Applied on Tchebichef Basis

3.1   Clenshaw's Recurrence Formula

Clenshaw's recurrence formula is a way to evaluate a sum of products of indexed coefficients by functions that obey a recurrence relation [24].

The sum must fit as follows:

$$I(x) = \sum_{n=0}^{k} c_n F_n(x) \tag{8}$$

$F_n(x)$ can be represented as a recurrence relation:

$$F_{n+1}(x) = \alpha(n,x)F_n(x) + \beta(n,x)F_{n-1}(x) \tag{9}$$

For a certain functions $\alpha(n,x)$ and $\beta(n,x)$.

Then the sum $I(x)$ can be represented as follows:

$$I(x) = \beta(1,x)F_0(x)\psi_2 + F_1(x)\psi_1 + c_0F_0(x) \tag{10}$$

To get ψ_1 and ψ_2 we must solve backwards for $n = K, K-1, \ldots, 1$ the following recurrence:

$$\begin{aligned}\psi_{k+2} &= \psi_{k+1} = 0 \\ \psi_n &= \alpha(n,x)\psi_{n+1} + \beta(n+1,x)\psi_{n+2} + c_n\end{aligned} \tag{11}$$

Clenshaw's recurrence formula has been used with the inverse discrete polynomial transform [20], and for the discrete cosine transform (DCT) [25].

3.2   Computation of Tchebichef Moments

The transformation can be executed on two steps, 1D case already defined and the 2D case, this is possible during to the separability of 2D Tchebichef polynomials [8].

The scaled Tchebichef polynomials $\tilde{t}_p(x)$ can be derived from a three-term recurrence (8), with the respect to the variable x:

$$\begin{aligned}(N-x)x\tilde{t}_p(x) &= (-p(p+1) - (2x-1)(x-N-1) - x)\tilde{t}_p(x-1) \\ &\quad + (x-1)(x-N-1)\tilde{t}_p(x-2)\end{aligned} \tag{12}$$

For $x = 2, \ldots, N-1$

With:

$$\begin{aligned}\tilde{t}_p(0) &= \frac{(1-N)(2-N)(3-N)\ldots(p-N)}{N^p} \\ \tilde{t}_p(1) &= \tilde{t}_p(0)\left(1 + \frac{p(p+1)}{1-N}\right)\end{aligned} \tag{13}$$

Let us define:

$$F_x(p) = \tilde{t}_p(x) \tag{14}$$

From the relation (12) about $\tilde{t}_p, \tilde{t}_{p-1}, \tilde{t}_{p-2}$ as an equivalent three term recursive relation about $\tilde{t}_{p+1}, \tilde{t}_p, \tilde{t}_{p-1}$ for matching the description of the form (9), we can define the following equation for $x = 0, \ldots, N-2$._

$$\alpha_a(x,p) = -\frac{p(p+1)+2(x+1)(x-N)+x+1}{(x+1)(N-x-1)}$$

$$\beta_a(x,p) = \beta_a(x) = \frac{x(x-N)}{(x+1)(N-x-1)}$$

(15)

$$\alpha_a(N-1,p) = 0$$

(16)

$$\beta_a(N-1) = 0, \quad \beta_a(N) = 0$$

We define also for $x = N-1,\ldots,0$

$$\psi_{N+1} = \psi_N = 0$$

$$\psi_x = \alpha_a(x,p)\psi_{x+1} + \beta_a(x+1)\psi_{x+2} + f(x)$$

(17)

Then we can express Eq. (10)

$$T_p = \frac{1}{\widetilde{\rho}(p,N)} \left[f(0)F_0(p) + F_1(p)\psi_1 + \beta_a(1)F_0(p)\psi_2 \right]$$

$$= \frac{1}{\widetilde{\rho}(p,N)} \left[f(0)\widetilde{t}_p(0) + \widetilde{t}_p(1)\psi_1 + \beta_a(1)\widetilde{t}_p(0)\psi_2 \right]$$

(18)

$$= \frac{1}{\widetilde{\rho}(p,N)} \left[f(0) + \frac{N-1-p(p+1)}{N-1}\psi_1 + \frac{1-N}{2(N-2)}\psi_2 \right]$$

From the two precedent equations we conclude

$$T_p = \frac{\widetilde{t}_p(0)}{\widetilde{\rho}(p,N)} \psi_0$$

(19)

The algorithm can be extended to 2D Tchebichef moment. We rewrite Eq. (5) as:

$$T_{pq} = \frac{1}{\widetilde{\rho}(p,N)} \sum_{x=0}^{N-1} \widetilde{t}_p(x)\omega_x(q)$$

(20)

With

$$\omega_x(q) = \frac{1}{\widetilde{\rho}(q,M)} \sum_{y=0}^{M-1} \widetilde{t}_q(y)f(x,y)$$

(21)

Thus the coefficients $\omega_x(q)$ defined by Eq. (21) are first evaluated for each $x = N-1,\ldots,0$

$$\psi_{M+1} = \psi_M = 0$$

$$\psi_y = \alpha_a(y,q)\psi_{y+1} + \beta_a(y+1)\psi_{y+2} + f(x,y)$$

(22)

for $y = M-1,\ldots,1,0$

$$\omega_x(q) = \psi_0 \tilde{t}_q(0)/\tilde{\rho}(q,M) \tag{23}$$

Then $\omega_x(q)$ are applied to evaluate T_{pq} defined in Eq. (5):

$$\begin{aligned}\varphi_{N+1} &= \varphi_N = 0\\\varphi_x &= \alpha_a(x,p)\varphi_{x+1} + \beta_a(x+1)\varphi_{x+2} + \omega_x(q)\end{aligned} \tag{24}$$

for $x = N-1, .., 1, 0$

$$T_{pq} = \varphi_0 \cdot \tilde{t}_p(0)/\tilde{\rho}(p,N) \tag{25}$$

We can easily extend the derivation of this algorithm similarly to n-dimensional Tchebichef moments computing.

3.3   Reconstruction from Tchebichef Moments

Wang et al. [20], demonstrate that the recursive relation (4) can be reedited as an equivalent of three-term recurrence from:

$$\begin{aligned}\tilde{t}_{n+1}(x) &= \frac{(2n+1)}{n+1}\tilde{t}_n(x) - \frac{n\left(1-\frac{n^2}{N^2}\right)}{n+1}\tilde{t}_{n-1}(x)\\n &= 1, 2, \ldots., N-1\end{aligned} \tag{26}$$

With

$$\begin{aligned}\tilde{t}_0(x) &= 1,\\\tilde{t}(x) &= \frac{2x-N+1}{N}\end{aligned} \tag{27}$$

Define:

$$F_n(x) = \tilde{t}_n(x) \tag{28}$$

Then from the precedent (9) equation we get:

$$\alpha_b(n,x) = \frac{(2n+1)(2x-N+1)}{(n+1)N} \tag{29}$$

$$\beta_b(n,x) = \beta_b(n) = -\frac{n(N^2-n^2)}{(n+1)N^2} \tag{30}$$

Applying Clenshaw's recurrence formula on Eq. (6), we get:

$$f(x) = T_0 \tilde{t}_0(x) + \tilde{t}_1(x)\psi_1 - \frac{N^2 - 1}{2}\tilde{t}_0(x)\psi_2$$
$$= T_0 + \frac{(2x - N + 1)}{N}\psi_1 - \frac{N^2 - 1}{2N^2}\psi_2 \tag{31}$$

Where ψ_1 and ψ_2 are recursively obtained from:

$$\psi_{N+1} = \psi_N = 0$$
$$\psi_p = \alpha_b(p, x)\psi_{p+1} + \beta_b(p + 1)\psi_{p+2} + T_p \tag{32}$$

for $p = N - 1, \ldots, 0$

So ψ_0 reached, and can be used to rewrite (31) as:

$$f(x) = \psi_0 \tag{33}$$

For the 2D case, the inverse moment transform (7) can be rewritten as:

$$f(x, y) = \sum_{p=0}^{N-1} \omega_p(y)\tilde{t}_p(x) \tag{34}$$

Where

$$\omega_p(y) = \sum_{q=0}^{M-1} T_{pq}\tilde{t}_q(y) \tag{35}$$

The coefficients $\omega_x(q)$ defined by (35) are evaluated for each $p = N - 1, \ldots, 0$

$$\psi_{M+1} = \psi_M = 0$$
$$\psi_q = \alpha_b(q, y)\psi_{q+1} + \beta_b(q + 1)\psi_{q+2} + T_{pq} \tag{36}$$

for $q = M - 1, \ldots, 0$

$$\omega_p(y) = \psi_0 \tag{37}$$

Then $\omega_x(q)$ are used to recursively evaluate the function $f(x, y)$ defined in (34):

$$\varphi_{N+1} = \varphi_N = 0$$
$$\varphi_p = \alpha_b(p, x)\varphi_{p+1} + \beta_b(p + 1)\varphi_{p+2} + \omega_p(y) \tag{38}$$

for $p = N - 1, \ldots, 0$

$$f(x, y) = \varphi_0 \tag{39}$$

Using Clenshaw's recurrence formula allow to considerably reduce the computation time of Tchebichef's moments and its inverses. Further, we need to reduce the error of reconstruction. So, in the next section we describe two algorithms based on image partitioning.

4 Lapped Block-Based Image Analysis Method by Tchebichef's Moments

In this section, we present the Lapped Block Image Analysis [22, 23, 26] method to compute the Tchebichef's moments of each block and to reconstruct the image from these blocks instead of the global reconstruction. Indeed, let (M, N) be the image size by pixels and let (k, l) represent the block size as shown in (Fig. 1a), by introducing the variables:

$$s_1 = \frac{M}{k}, s_2 = \frac{N}{l} \tag{40}$$

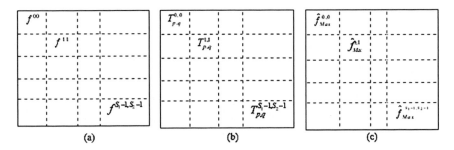

Fig. 1. Illustration of the LBBRM. **a** Division of the input image into Nb subimages, **b** moment extraction for each block, and **c** reconstruction and merging the Nb blocks

We can deduce the total number of image blocks that can be set as $N_b = s_1 \times s_2$.

Then, let the image function be associated to each f^{p_1,p_2} as shown in (Fig. 1a), thus, each subset will be defined as follows:

$$f^{p_1,p_2}(x, y) = \{f(i, j) / i, j \in f^{p_1,p_2}\} \tag{41}$$

From that, we can get a reconstructed image as shown in (Fig. 1c):

$$\widehat{f}(x, y) = \bigcup_{p_1=0}^{(s_1-1)} \bigcup_{p_2=0}^{(s_2-1)} \widehat{f}^{p_1,p_2}(x, y) \tag{42}$$

According to these definitions, we introduce the Tchebichef's moments using a digital filter related to each image block as shown in (Fig. 1b), we obtain:

$$T_{pq}^{p_1,p_2} = \frac{1}{\widetilde{\rho}(p,N)\widetilde{\rho}(q,M)} \sum_{x=p_1k}^{(p_1+1)k} \sum_{y=p_2l}^{(p_2+1)l} \widetilde{t}_p(x)\widetilde{t}_q(y)f^{p_1,p_2}(x,y) \tag{43}$$

where

$$T_{pq}^{p_1,p_2} = \frac{1}{\widetilde{\rho}(p,N)} \sum_{x=p_1k}^{(p_1+1)k} \widetilde{t}_p(x)\omega_x^{p_1,p_2}(q) \tag{44}$$

with

$$\omega_x^{p_1,p_2}(q) = \frac{1}{\widetilde{\rho}(q,M)} \sum_{y=p_2l}^{(p_2+1)l} \widetilde{t}_q(y)f^{p_1,p_2}(x,y) \tag{45}$$

The (Fig. 2) Summarises the block diagram of Tchebichef's based on Clenshaw's recurrence formula. The significant reduction of the image space during partitioning makes it possible to represent the minute details of the image with only low orders of Tchebichef's discrete orthogonal moments, which ensures the digital stability during the processing of the image.

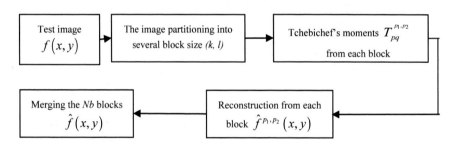

Fig. 2. Image reconstruction process diagram

5 Results and Simulations

In this section, we give experimental results to validate the theoretical results developed in the previous sections. This section is divided into two sub-sections. In the first sub-section, we will compare the time computation of Tchebichef's moments by the direct based on Clenshaw's recurrence formula and the proposed methods based on Clenshaw's recurrence formula with the block image representation for binary and gray-scale images. In the second part, we will test the ability of Tchebichef's moments using the suggested method for the reconstruction of binary and gray-scale images.

5.1 The Computational Time of Tchebichef's Moments

In this sub-section, we will compare the computational time of Tchebichef's moments by two methods: the direct method based on Eq. (20) and the proposed method based on LBBRM usage Eq. (42).

In the first example, a set of four binary images with size 128×128 pixels (Fig. 3) selected from the well-known MPEG-7 CE-shape-1 Part B database [27] were used as test images. In the second example, a set of four gray-scale images with a size of 128×128 pixels, shown in (Fig. 4), are used.

Fig. 3. Binary images: Bat, Beetle, Camel and Rat

Fig. 4. Gray-scale images: Cameraman, House, Livingroom and Lake

The process of calculating discrete orthogonal moments Tchebichef is carried out using: The method of partitioning the image to blocks: each of the four images contains 2048 blocks of size $[4 \times 4]$ and 512 blocks of size $[8 \times 8]$. The moments are calculated for orders ranging from 0 to 4 for blocks of size $[4 \times 4]$ and from 0 to 8 for blocks of size $[8 \times 8]$.

Tables 1 and 2 represents the average time of calculation of Tchebichef's moments for the four binary images and the four gray-scale images using the two methods located earlier. Note that the algorithm was implemented on a PC Dual Core 2.10 GHz, 2 GB of RAM.

Table 1. Average computation time in second of binary images using two methods

Method	Direct method	LBBRM size $[8 \times 8]$	LBBRM size $[4 \times 4]$
Average time (s)	0.055	6.0242e-003	3.2145e-003

The two tables show that the proposed methods are faster than the direct one because the computation of Tchebichef moments by two proposed methods depends only on the number of blocks instead of the image's size.

Tab 2. Average computation time in second for gray-scale images using two methods

Method	Direct method	LBBRM size [8 × 8]	LBBRM size [4 × 4]
Average time (s)	0.114	9.1452e-003	5.2714e-003

5.2 Image Reconstruction Using Tchebichef's Moments

In this sub-section, we will discuss the ability of Tchebichef's moments for the reconstruction using the proposed methods.

The difference between the original image $f(x, y)$ and the reconstructed images $\hat{f}(x, y)$ is measured using the mean squared error (MSE) defined as follows:

$$MSE = \frac{1}{M \times N} \sum_{x=0}^{M-1} \sum_{y=0}^{N-1} \left(f(x, y) - \hat{f}(x, y)\right)^2 \qquad (46)$$

To illustrate the performance of the proposed approach in terms of reconstruction quality, our algorithm is tested on two types of images (Figs. 3 and 4).

The image reconstruction test by blocks of sizes $[4 \times 4]$ and $[8 \times 8]$ is performed using the discrete orthogonal moments of Tchebichef by the two methods:

- The direct method based on Eq. (20).
- The proposed method based on LBBRM on Eq. (42).

The two figures show that the reconstruction errors by the method in question are smaller using the Tchebichef's moments. This shows that the proposed approach is effective in terms of reconstruction quality for binary and gray-scale images.

The two figures (Figs. 5 and 6) represent the mean square errors between the reconstructed images and the original images as a function of the orders. The order varies between 0 and 8 for blocks of size $[4 \times 4]$, and between 0 and 12 for blocks $[8 \times 8]$.

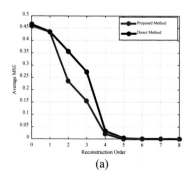 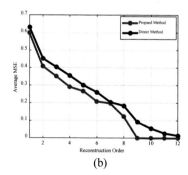

(a)   (b)

Fig. 5. Reconstruction error of binary images using two methods with Tchebichef moments of image as blocks of sizes **a** $[4 \times 4]$ and **b** $[8 \times 8]$

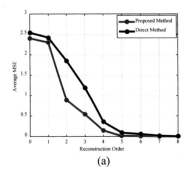
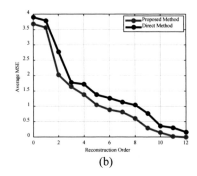

(a)   (b)

Fig. 6. Reconstruction error of gray-scale images using two methods with Tchebichef moments of image as blocks of sizes **a** [4 × 4] and **b** [8 × 8]

6 Conclusion

In this paper, we have suggested a fast and stable method for calculating discrete orthogonal moments of Tchebichef based on Clenshaw's recurrence formula and the block image representation lapped block-based image representation by Tchebichef's moments (LBBRM). The significant reduction of the image space during partitioning makes it possible to represent the minute details of the image with only low orders of Tchebichef's discrete orthogonal moments, which ensures the digital stability during the processing of the image. The ease of calculating the moments within each block constituting the overall image induces a significant improvement in the calculation time and the error becomes local.

References

1. Hu, M.K.: Visual pattern recognition by moment invariants. IRE Trans. Inform. Theory, **IT-8**, 179–187 (1962)
2. Abu-Mostafa, Y.S., Psaltis, D.: Recognitive aspects of moment invariants. IEEE Trans. Pattern Anal. Mach. Intell. **6**, 698–706 (1984)
3. M.R. Teague, "Image analysis via the general theory of moments", J. Opt. Soc. Amer., vol. 70, pp. 920–930, 1980
4. Khotanzad, A., Hong, Y.H.: Invariant image recognition by Zernike moments. IEEE Trans. Pattern Anal. Mach. Intell. **12**, 489–497 (1990)
5. Teh, C.H., Chin, R.T.: On image analysis by the method of moments. IEEE Trans. Pattern Anal. Mach. Intell. **10**(4), 496–513 (1988)
6. Hosny, K.M.: Image representation using accurate orthogonal Gegenbauer moments. Pattern Recogn. Lett. **32**, 795–804 (2011)
7. Zhang, H., Shu, H.Z., Haigron, P., Li, B.S., Luo, L.M.: Construction of a complete set of orthogonal Fourier-Mellin moment invariants for pattern recognition applications. Image Vis. Comput. **28**, 38–44 (2010)
8. Mukundan, R., Ong, S.H., Lee, P.A.: Image analysis by Tchebichef moments. IEEE Trans. Image Process. **10**(9), 1357–1364 (2000)

9. Yap, P.T., Paramesran, R., Ong, S.H.: Image analysis by Krawtchouk moments. IEEE Trans. Image Process. **12**(11), 1367–1377 (2003)
10. Zhu, H.Q., Shu, H.Z., Liang, J., Luo, L.M., Coatrieux, J.L.: Image analysis by discrete orthogonal Racah moments. Sig. Process. **87**(4), 687–708 (2007)
11. Hmimid, A., Sayyouri, M., Qjidaa, H.: Image classification using a new set of separable two-dimensional discrete orthogonal invariant moments. J. Electron Imaging. **23**(1), 013026, 18, 2014
12. Sayyouri, M., Hmimid, A., Qjidaa, H.: Improving the performance of image classification by Hahn moment invariants. J. Opt. Soc. Am. A **30**, 2381–2394 (2013)
13. Karmouni, H., Jahid, T., El affar, I., Sayyouri, M., Hmimid, A., Qjidaa, H., Rezzouk, A.: Image Analysis Using Separable Krawtchouk-Tchebichef's moments. In: International Conference On Advanced Technologies for Signal & Image Processing (Atsip'2017), Fez, Morocco, 22–24 May 2017
14. Karmouni, H., Jahid, T., Lakhili, Z., Hmimid, A., Sayyouri, M., Qjidaa, H., Rezzouk, A.: Image reconstruction by Krawtchouk moments via digital filter. In: International Conference on Intelligent Systems and Computer Vision, ISCV'2017, Fez, Morocco, 17–20 April 2017
15. Sayyouri, M., Hmimid, A., Karmouni, H., Qjidaa, H., Rezzouk, A.: Image classification using separable invariant moments of Krawtchouk-Tchebichef. In: 12th International Conference of Computer Systems and Applications (AICCSA), Marrakech, Morocco, 17–20 Nov 2015
16. Liao, S.X., Pawlak, M.: On image analysis by moments. IEEE Trans. Pattern Anal. Mach. Intell. **18**(3), 254–266 (1996)
17. Zhu, H.: Image representation using separable two-dimensional continuous and discrete orthogonal moments. Pattern Recogn. **45**(4), 1540–1558 (2012)
18. Hmimid, A., Sayyouri, M., Qjidaa, H.: Fast computation of separable two-dimensional discrete invariant moments for image classification. Pattern Recogn. **48**(2), 509–521 (2015)
19. Tsougenis, E.D., Papakostas, G.A., Koulouriotis, D.E.: Image Watermarking via Separable Moments. Multimedia Tools Appl. 1–28 (2014)
20. Wang, G., Wang, S.: Recursive computation of Tchebichef moments and its inverse transform. Elsevier Pattern recognition **39**, 47–56 (2006)
21. Jahid, T., Karmouni, H., Hmimid, A., Sayyouri, M., Qjidaa, H.: Image moments and reconstruction by Krawtchouk via Clenshaw's reccurence formula. In: 3rd International Conference on Electrical and Information Technologies (ICEIT), Rabat, Morocco, 15–18 Nov 2017
22. Karmouni, H., Hmimid, A., Jahid, T.: Fast and stable computation of the Charlier moments and their inverses using digital filters and image block representation. Circ. Syst. Signal Process (2018). https://doi.org/10.1007/s00034-018-0755-2
23. Jahid, T., Hmimid, A., Karmouni, H.: Multimed Tools Appl. (2017). https://doi.org/10.1007/s11042-017-5371-9
24. Aburdene, M.F., Zheng, J., Kozick, R.J.: Computation of discrete cosine transform using Clenshaw's recurrence formula. IEEE Signal Process. Lett. **2**(8), 155–156 (1995)
25. Kozick, R.J., Aburdene, M.F.: Methods for designing efficient parallel-recursive filter structures for computing discrete transforms. Telecommun. Syst. **13**(1), 69–80 (2000)
26. El Fadili, H., Zenkouar, K., Qjidaa, H.: Lapped block image analysis via the method of Legendre moments. EURASIP J. Appl. Sig. Process. **2003**(9), 902–913 (2003)
27. MPEG-7 DATA SET: http://www.dabi.temple.edu/ ~ shape/MPEG7/ dataset.html Jan 2014

The Effect of Transmit Power on MANET Routing Protocols Using AODV, DSDV, DSR and OLSR in NS3

Abdellah Nabou[1(✉)], My Driss Laanaoui[2], and Mohammed Ouzzif[1]

[1] RITM Laboratory, CED, Engineering Sciences, EST, ENSEM,
Hassan II University of Casablanca, Casablanca, Morocco
a.nabou@ensem.ac.ma, ouzzif@gmail.com
[2] Department of Computer Faculty of Sciences and Technology,
Cadi Ayyad University of Marrakesh, Marrakesh, Morocco
d.laanaoui@uca.ma

Abstract. Since last decades mobile ad hoc networks (MANETs) become very interesting subject of research. MANET is defined as the network without infrastructure that connects mobile devices named nodes like computers, smartphones, tablets or any other device by using wireless channel to communicate with each other, without aid of any additional equipment or admin intervention. Manet uses specific protocols intended for wireless ad hoc environment. These protocols experience constraints in their operation on several levels such as mobility, energy consumption, security, etc. In this paper we evaluate four MANET routing protocols are performances compared to the transmission power used by each node in the network to send data. We have chosen all the standard protocols available in the NS3 simulator AODV (Ad hoc On Demand Distance Vector Routing), DSDV (Destination Sequenced Distance Vector Routing), OLSR (Optimized Link State Routing) and DSR (Dynamic source routing). Also, we used five important metrics to analyze the performance for these protocols as Throughput, Packet Delivery Ratio, End-to-End delay, Jitter delay and Packet Lost.

Keywords: MANET · AODV · DSDV · DSR · OLSR · Transmission power · Performance

1 Introduction

MANET becomes very popular to use, thanks to its simplicity and ease of deployment, when there are lots of constraints to install wired network either for duration of the installation or for restrictively of wired infrastructure or for other reasons, MANET is can be a solution in these conditions. For example, MANET can be used in military networks; in emergency networks in temporary exhibition networks or corresponding to a particular event like conference room [1].

A dynamic topology, limited bandwidth, energy consumption, security and self-configuration are the biggest constraints when we want to use MANET [2]. There are many Wireless Ad hoc routing protocols divided into three categories reactive routing

© Springer Nature Switzerland AG 2019
M. Ezziyyani (Ed.): AI2SD 2018, AISC 915, pp. 274–286, 2019.
https://doi.org/10.1007/978-3-030-11928-7_24

protocols or (On Demand), proactive routing protocols or (Table Driven) and Hybrid routing protocols. Figure 1 presents some protocols are best known in literature. One of drawbacks in MANET is energy consumption, each node operates on limited battery energy or other consumable sources. For this reason many research activities are devoted in this area to reduce the energy consumption in the network in order to stronger the network life. The energy consumption must control during transmission and reception mode. One technique used to conserve energy in MANET is by changing the transmission power of a node. The adjustment of transmission power through the dynamic transmission power control protocol is an effective technique to reduce the power consumption of a network [3]. In this paper we focused to analyze performance of MANET routing protocols by considering transmit power as a factor for our study by using the recent Simulator Network NS3 [4].

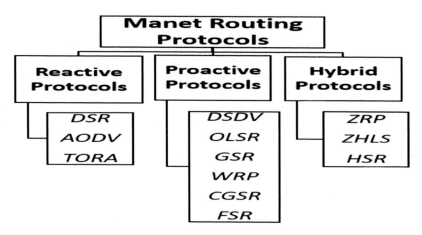

Fig. 1. MANET routing protocols

Rest of paper is organized as follows Sect. 2 define the routing protocols used in this study Sect. 3 gives an idea regarding energy consumption in MANET followed by related work in Sect. 4. Section 5 presents the simulation environment and metrics. The results and analysis are discussed in Sect. 6 finally, it concludes with conclusions and future work.

2   MANET Routing Protocols

The characteristics of the MANET network requires the use of specific protocols to ensure communication between nodes are mobile and have limited resources in terms of energy or bandwidth. MANET routing protocols are divided in three categories reactive, Proactive and Hybrid (combination of reactive and proactive) protocols, each type use different procedures for route discovery and route maintenance [5]. For our experiment we are using four routing protocols available in NS3 simulator [4], AODV (Ad hoc On Demand Distance Vector Routing) and DSR (Dynamic source routing) function as reactive routing protocols, on the other hand, DSDV (Destination Sequenced Distance Vector Routing) and OLSR (Optimized Link State Routing) function as proactive routing protocols.

2.1 Reactive Routing Protocols

In reactive routing protocols or On Demand a node start route discovery process, only when it wants to send packets to its destination [6]. This process of route discovery is completed once a route is determined or all possible permutations have been examined. After the completion of the first phase of discovery process, Once a route has been established, it is maintained by a route maintenance process until either the communication has stopped or the destination becomes inaccessible from the network or until the route is no longer desired [6]. The maintenance phase is performed only for active routes that have current use. In our evaluation we will mention two important reactive routing protocols AODV and DSR.

AODV (Ad hoc On Demand Distance Vector Routing). The Ad hoc On-Demand Distance Vector (AODV) algorithm enables dynamic, self-starting, multi-hop routing between participating mobile nodes wishing to establish and maintain an ad hoc network [7]. AODV use Route Requests (RREQs) for discovery a route to the destination, this process is finished just when a node source is reaching the destination node either by destination itself or by any node has the destination entry, by using another control message called Route Replies (RREPs). In case when there are errors in the path to establish route, another message is used Route Errors (RERRs). In order to avoid loop by given two routes to a destination, AODV use a destination sequence number for each route entry. The destination sequence number is created by the destination to be included along with any route information it sends to requesting nodes [7]. A requesting node is required to select the one that have a higher sequence number [7].

DSR (Dynamic source routing). The Dynamic Source Routing protocol (DSR) is a simple routing protocol designed specifically for use in multi-hop wireless ad hoc networks of mobile nodes [8]. DSR use two mechanisms, the first is "Route Discovery" allowed to discover a destination route and "Route Maintenance" allowed to maintain the route, Both of these mechanisms work together to allow nodes to discover and maintain routes to arbitrary destinations in the ad hoc network [8]. An advantage for optimization used in DSR the ability to reverse a source route to obtain a route back to the origin of the original route.

2.2 Proactive Routing Protocols

In Proactive or Table-Driven Routing Protocols, each node maintain the routes to all destinations of the network in hasty manner [6]. The proactive routing protocols use control messages to ensure the maintenance and update of routes if there is a change in the network topology. These messages are sending periodically, they incur additional overhead costs due to maintaining up-to-date information [9]. Destination Sequenced Distance Vector (DSDV) protocol, and Optimized Link State Routing (OLSR) are the most important example of proactive routing protocols.

DSDV (Destination Sequenced Distance Vector). DSDV use the above distance vector algorithm depends on the classical Distributed Bellman Ford (DBF) algorithm [10]. The DSDV protocol requires each node in the network to advertise its neighbors about it routing table is entries. The advertisement must be sent periodically in order to ensure that all new or mobile nodes can usually locate every other mobile node of the collection. To avoid the problem of traditional DBF algorithm regarding routing loops, DSDV adds a sequence number to each routing table entry. For that each node can quickly distinguish stale routes from the new ones by selecting the higher sequence number. The data broadcast by each node in the network will contain its new sequence number and the following information for each new route [10]: The destinations address, the number of hops required to reach the destination and the sequence number of the information received regarding that destination as originally stamped by the destination.

OLSR (Optimized link state routing protocol). The Optimized Link State Routing Protocol (OLSR) operates as a proactive protocol that mean it shares topology information with other nodes of the network in regular way [11]. OLSR uses specific concepts named multipoint relays (MPRs). MPRs are selected nodes that responsible for forwarding routing messages during the flooding process. One advance of using MPRs is reducing the message overhead forwarded in classical flooding mechanism by minimizing redundant retransmissions in the same region. Each OLSR node uses an algorithm to select its MPRs node, MPR selection algorithm allowed to each node to select its MPR set from among its 1-hop symmetric neighbors in order to reach all symmetric strict 2-hop nodes [11]. There are four type of OLSR message: HELLO_message to accommodate for links sensing, neighborhood detection and MPR selection signaling, TC_Message (Topology Control) generates and forward only by MPRs nodes to discover the topology of the network, MID_Message use in case of multiple OLSR interface nodes and HNA-message can be considered as a "generalized version" of the TC-message [11].

3 Energy Consumption in MANET

During the period of communication, each node in MANET exists in four modes as given in Equation "(1)". Each mode at a different consumption of energy for example "(2)" shows that node in active mode consumes most power as compared to sleep mode. On account of limited battery resources in MANET, it is better to put used node in sleep mode to save it powers Energy [12].

$$E_{pt} = E_{sleep} + E_{active} + E_{Idle} + E_{overhear} \qquad (1)$$

$$E_{active} = E_{transmit} + E_{recev} \qquad (2)$$

$$E_{sleep} \approx 0 \qquad (3)$$

where:

- E_{pt} = Packet Transmission Energy.
- E_{sleep} = Energy in Sleep Mode.
- E_{active} = Energy in Active Mode.
- E_{Idle} = Energy in Idle Mode.
- $E_{overhear}$ = Energy in Overhear Mode.
- $E_{transmit}$ = Energy in Transmission Mode.
- $E_{reception}$ = Energy in Reception Mode.

In following subsection we describe the amount of energy consumption in various models [13].

3.1   Power Consumption in Transmission Mode

In MANET each node sends data to another node in the network on the transmission mode consumes energy named transmission energy, it related with packet size (in bits) of data, "(4)" give the formula of energy transmission [12].

$$E_{transmit} = (330 \times P_{size})/2 \times 10^6 \tag{4}$$

$$P_{transmit} = E_{transmit}/T_{transmit} \tag{5}$$

where:

- P_{size} = Packet Size.
- $P_{transmit}$ = Transmission Power.
- $T_{transmit}$ = Time of Transmission.

From "(5)" it observes that transmit power depends on transmission energy and time of transmission.

3.2   Power Consumption in Reception Mode

In reception mode each node in network which receipts the data required energy named reception energy, also like transmission mode in reception mode the reception energy is depending on packet length of data, the formula of the reception energy is given as [12]:

$$E_{recev} = (230 \times P_{size})/2 \times 10^6 \tag{6}$$

$$P_{recev} = E_{recev}/T_{recev} \tag{7}$$

where E_{recev} is the reception energy P_{size} is the packet size of received data, P_{recev} is the reception power and T_{recev} is the Time taken to receive packet.

3.3   Power Consumption in Idle Mode

In the mode idle each node just listen to the wireless channel continuously without any communication either sending mode or reception mode it consumes unnecessary of energy. This energy is same as the amount of energy consumed in the reception mode [12]. Moreover, the power consumed in idle mode is same as the reception power the formulated of power in idle mode is:

$$P_{\text{Idle}} = P_{\text{recev}} \tag{8}$$

where P_{Idle} is the power consumed in Idle mode and P_{recev} is the reception power.

3.4   Power Consumption in Overhearing Mode

In this mode, a node listens to hear packets that is not destined for it. This listen consumes unnecessary energy like idle mode. The power consumption is the same as reception power in reception mode [12]. The formulated of power in idle mode is:

$$P_{\text{Overhear}} = P_{\text{recev}} \tag{9}$$

where P_{Overhear} is the power consumed in Overhearing mode and P_{recev} is the power consumed in reception mode.

In our study on focus of power in the transmission mode that evaluate the effect of transmit power on MANET routing protocols. The next section presents previous works that have related with our study.

4   Related Work

[14] The authors evaluate the performance of reactive routing protocols AODV and DSR by varying parameters number of sources, and transmission power they observed that Packet delivery fraction is more in AODV routing protocol than DSR routing protocol at high mobility condition and it increases in decrease in mobility. In addition, PDF of AODV and DSR increases with increases in transmission at high mobility [15] study three reactive routing protocols AODV, DSR and TORA by using two type of wireless LAN standard 802.11a and 802.11g, the authors use two scenarios of transmission power in order to calculate the transmission range corresponding to these values of transmission power. All results demonstrate that TORA protocol is more performance than AODV and DSR routing protocol. In [16] the authors analyze effect of transmit power in MANET routing protocols using three protocols AODV, DSDV and OLSR in NS3 simulator the results of this analysis shows an important rise of performance for all protocols when transmit power increases. However AODV protocol degrades in the last. OLSR routing protocol has shown better performance in terms of all the metrics calculated [17]. Test the performance of AODV routing protocol by varying packets Size and transmission power, the throughput gives high values when transmission power of nodes is in great value [18] authors analyze optimization of three MANET routing Protocols compared to the transmission range that varied by

changing transmission power, also the authors use two propagation model, two ray propagation model and free space model, the graphs of results demonstrate that DSR performs well if throughput is considered otherwise OLSR outperforms in terms of delay and average Jitter. In [19] the authors use transmission power value to calculate highest performance of three ad hoc routing protocol AODV, DSR and OLSR in Qualnet simulator; they mention that DSR has better performance for high transmission range. In addition, if the value of the transmission range is evaluated properly the performances of the network can be improved [20]. Analyze the impact of transmission power of three routing protocols AODV, DSDV and DSR, they choice two rays ground as propagation model then they calculate the transmission power needed compared to the transmission range or distance, the results of this work shown that the change in the transmission range/power has a significant impact on the performance of the routing protocol. DSR routing protocol is better in performance as compared as AODV and DSDV, however, all these protocols are the same performance after transmission range exceeds 300 m.

All these works studied just the performance of one; two or three routing protocols related to transmission power, most of it are reactive routing protocols. In this paper we will develop the work of [16] by adding DSR routing protocol and using five important metrics for analysis also we are choosing the recent version of NS3 (2.26) [4] as Network Simulator. The next section presents environment of simulation and the metrics of analysis.

5   Simulation Environment and Performance Metrics

5.1   Simulation Environment

To evaluate protocols are performances we use Network Simulator (NS3.25) as simulator environment. Ns-3 is a discrete-event network simulator for Internet systems, targeted primarily for research and educational use. Ns-3 is free software, licensed under the GNU GPLv2 license, and is publicly available for research, development, and use [4]. Table 1 present all parameters used in our simulation.

5.2   Simulation Environment

In our work, we choose metrics, which have a relationship with packets size and delay; we discussed about the following metrics:

Throughput. Define as the total of receiver bites from the source node to the destination node in a specified time is expressed in kilobits per second (Kbps) [21]. For the best performance, the throughput must be higher values.

$$Throughput = (\Sigma\ successfully\ receiver\ bits\ /\ Time\ of\ simulation \times 1024) \qquad (10)$$

Packet delivery ratio (PDR). Define as the total of receiver bites from the source node to the destination node in a specified time is expressed in kilobits per second (Kbps) [22]. For the best performance, the throughput must be higher values.

Table 1. Simulation parameters for MANET

N°	Parameter	Value
1	PC simulator	Dell Intel Xeon® CPU ES-2407 0 @ 2.20 GHz 7GiB
2	Number of nodes	50
3	Simulation time	200
4	Wi-Fi mode	Ad hoc
5	Wi-Fi rate	2 MB
6	Mobility model	Random waypoint mobility model
7	N. of source/sink	10
8	Sent data rate	2.048 Kbps
9	Packet size	64 Bytes
10	Protocols used	DSDV, OLSR, AODV and DSR
11	Connection type	UDP
12	Transmit power	1.5, 3, 4.5, 6, 7.5, 9 dBm
13	Propagation model	Friis propagation loss model
14	Pause time	0
15	Node speed	20 m/s
16	Network size	1000 × 1000 m

$$PDR = (\Sigma \, successfully \, receiver \, Packets / \Sigma \, Packets \, send \, by \, the \, sources) \times 100 \quad (11)$$

End to End Delay (EED). The average time taken by a data packet to arrive in the destination. It also includes the delay caused by route discovery process and the queue in data packet transmission. Only the data packets that successfully delivered to destinations that counted. It is expressing in miles second (ms). The lower value of end-to-end delay means the better performance of the protocol [22].

$$End \, to \, End \, Delay_i = |EndTime_i - StarTime_i| \quad (12)$$

where $EndTime_i$ is the time that packet i was sent by the source, is received successfully by the destination, $StartTime_i$ is the time of starting to send packet i by the source. We will use this formula for calculating the EED of all packets and then obtain the average EED.

Jitter Delay. Jitter is the delay variation between each received data packets. The variation in the packet arrival time should be minimum to have better performance in Mobile Ad hoc Network.

$$Jitter \, Delay_i = |(D_{i+1} - D_i) - (S_{i+1} - S_i)| \quad (13)$$

S_i is the time when packet i was sent from the source, D_i is the time is being received by the destination. We will use this formula for calculating the Jitter delay of all packets and then obtain the average of Jitter [23].

Packet Lost. The total number of lost packets during the simulation. The lower value of the packet lost means the better performance of the protocol.

$$Packet\ Lost = \left(\sum Packets\ send\ by\ sources - \sum Packets\ successfully\ received \right)$$

$$(14)$$

6   Results and Analysis

In this section, we present the simulation results for different transmission powers of reactive and proactive routing protocols. In order to make the analysis of the effect of variation in transmission power, we have chosen fixed the mobility of nodes (Node Speed and Pause Time) at (20 m/s and 0). The analysis is based on the comparison of different metrics stated in the last section. Different scenarios of transmission power are simulated many times and in many PC simulator, the same results were obtained.

Figure 2 indicates Throughput versus Transmit power for AODV, DSDV, DSR, and OLSR routing protocols. We observe that the Throughput of these protocols is increasing when Transmit power increases, For AODV routing protocol is more performance than all other protocols when Transmit power is very low for example 1.5 dBm. However, the Throughput of AODV, OLSR and DSR gives approximate results when Transmit power equal 3 dBm. DSDV protocol is less performance than other protocol. With further increase in transmission power from 4.5 to 9 dBm, there is an increase in throughput for all routing protocols with a preference of DSR and OLSR protocols. The performance of MANET routing protocols are more performance with higher value of Transmission Power.

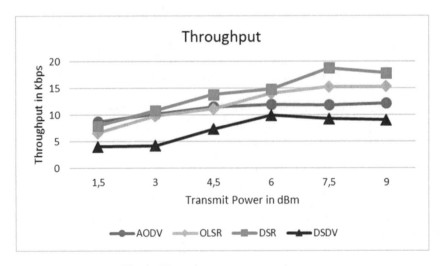

Fig. 2.   Throughput versus transmit power

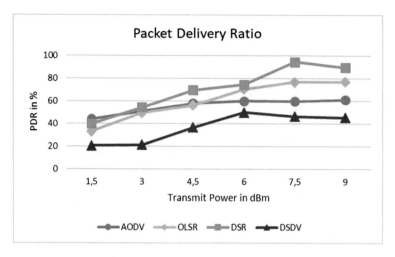

Fig. 3. PDR versus transmit power

Figure 3 presents the results of Packet Delivery Ratio versus Transmit power, these results are symmetric with Throughput metrics. When Transmit power increases, the PDR increases too. AODV protocol was more performance when Transmit power is very low, further to 3 dBm DSR and OLSR are starting to increase. However DSDV protocol is less in PDR than other protocols, for this metric DSR and OLSR are performance for higher transmit power, on the other hand, AODV protocol is the best for low transmit power.

Figure 4 indicates Average End-to-End delay versus Transmit Power, DSDV and OLSR routing protocols have fewer values of EED delay compared to DSR and AODV routing protocols, thanks to proactive routing protocols OLSR and DSDV keep the routes in routing table of each node, that is why DSDV and OLSR are more rapid in this metric, DSR protocol had high EED delay when transmit power was low for example in 1.5 and 3 dBm. All MANET routing protocols take a long time in EED delay when there are lower Transmit Power, with an exception of OLSR protocol, it keeps almost the same delay in different Transmit Power.

Figure 5 presents the results of Jitter delay versus Transmit Power, the jitter delay is better for proactive protocols than reactive protocols. For this reason, OLSR and DSDV are performance in Jitter term than DSR and AODV, by analyzing Jitter delay with previous results of Throughput, PDR and EED we observe that OLSR is more per-formance in this metric of performance due to fewer time taking in Jitter Delay.

Figure 6 shows Packet Lost versus Transmit Power, by analyzing these results, we note that all MANET routing protocols lose lots of routing packets in lower Transmit Power. Each node sends packets with 1.5 dBm of Transmit Power, these Packets are losing before reaching the destination, in addition when Transmit Power increases, the packet loss decreases, DSR and OLSR are the most performance compared to AODV and DSR protocols in Packet Lost metric.

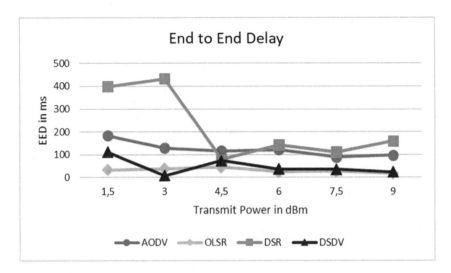

Fig. 4. EED versus transmit power

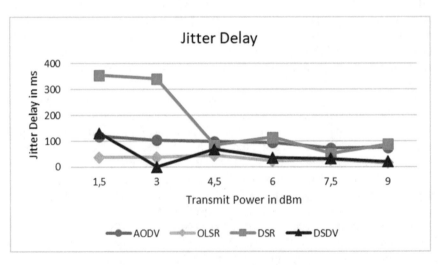

Fig. 5. Jitter Delay versus transmit power

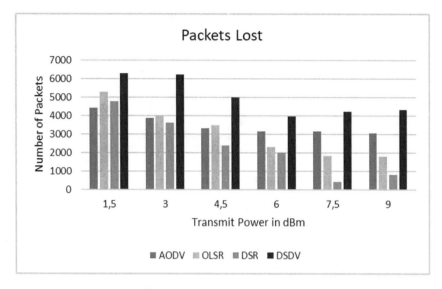

Fig. 6. PL versus transmit power

7 Conclusion

In this paper, we evaluated four MANET routing protocols AODV and DSR as reactive routing protocols, OLSR and DSDV as proactive routing protocols by choosing an essential criterion in MANET is Transmit Power. MANET is characterized by limited battery resources, Transmit power is the power used for sending data, our analysis shows that lower Transmit Power used by source node give poor results for all routing protocol with little preference of AODV. In the other hand when transmit power increases the performance of all protocols increases too, DSR and OLSR are the best in this situation of higher transmit power. However, performance of the routing protocols rest on various technical aspects like mobility models, packet size, transmission range, number of source/sink connections, speed and pause time, Wi-Fi rate, propagation models, etc. Further, our current research is focusing to improve OLSR routing protocol thanks to its rapidity and performance.

References

1. Frodigh, M., Johansson, P., Larsson, P.: Wireless ad hoc networking—the art of networking without a network (2000)
2. Goyal, P., Parmar, V.: MANET: vulnerabilities, challenges, attacks, application. IJCEM Int. J. Comput. Eng. Manag. **11** (2011)
3. Misra, S., Woungang, I., Misra, S.C.: Guide to Wireless Ad Hoc Networks. Springer (2009)
4. NS3 Homepage: https://www.nsnam.org
5. Patel, A., Patel, S., Verma, A.: A review of performance evaluation of AODV protocol in Manet with and without black hole attack. Int. J. Emerg. Technol. Adv. Eng. **2** (2012)

6. Raut, S.H., Ambulgekar H.P.: Proactive and reactive routing protocols in multihop mobile ad hoc network. Int. J. Adv. Res. Comput. Sci. Softw. Eng. **3** (2013)
7. Perkins, C., Belding-Royer, E., Das, S.: Ad Hoc On-Demand Distance Vector (AODV) Routing (2003)
8. Johnson, D., Hu, Y., Maltz, D.: The Dynamic Source Routing Protocol (DSR) for Mobile Ad Hoc Networks for IPv4. Network Working Group (2007)
9. Hemagowri, J., Baranikumari, C., Brindha, B.: A study on proactive routing protocol in ad-hoc network. Int. J. Mod. Eng. Res. (IJMER) 01–04
10. Perkins, C.E., Bhagwat, P.: Highly dynamic destination sequenced distance vector routing (DSDV) for mobile computers. ACM SIGCOMM Comput. Commun. Rev. **24**, 234–244 (1994)
11. Clausen, T., Jacquet, P.: Optimized Link State Routing Protocol (OLSR) (2003). https://tools.ietf.org/html/draft-ietf-manet-olsr-11
12. Rout, S., Turuk, A.K., Sahoo, B.: Review of transmission power control techniques in MANET. Int. J. Comput. Appl. (2013)
13. Tantubay, N., Gautam, D., Dhariwal, M.: A review of power conservation in wireless mobile adhoc network MANET. Int. J. Comput. Sci. **8**, 379–383 (2011)
14. Panda, B.K., Swain, J., Mishra, D.P., Sahu, B.: Analysis of Effect of Mobility and Transmission Power on AODV and DSR in Mobile Adhoc Network. IEEE, 978-1-4799-3156-9/14 (2014)
15. Nawaz, H., Mansoor Ali, H.: Analysis of routing protocol metrics in MANET. J. Indep. Stud. Res. Comput. **12** (2014)
16. Lakshman Naik, L., Khan, R.U., Mishra, R.B.: Analysis of transmit power effects in ad-hoc network protocols using network simulator-3. Int. Res. J. Eng. Technol. (IRJET) **03** (2016)
17. Agarwal, K., Sejwar, V.: Effect on throughput due to changes in transmission power of nodes in MANETs. Int. J. Future Gener. Commun. Netw. **8**, 207–212 (2015)
18. Fatima, M., Tiwari, A.: Node transmission power value optimization in MANET. Int. J. Innov. Res. Comput. Commun. Eng. **5** (2017)
19. Tiwari, A., Fatima, M., Manoria, M.: Survey of Impact of Transmission Range on MANET Routing Protocol (2017)
20. Lalitha, V., Rajesh, R.S.: The impact of transmission power on the performance of MANET routing protocols. IOSR J. Eng. (IOSRJEN) **3**, 34–41 (2013)
21. Rajeshkumar, V. sivakumar, P.: Comparative study of AODV, DSDV and DSR routing protocols in MANET using network simulator-2. Int. J. Adv. Res. Comput. Commun. Eng. **2** (2013)
22. Lakshman Naik. L., Khan, R.U., Mishra, R.B.: Analysis of node density and pause time effects in MANET routing protocols using NS-3. I. J. Comput. Netw. Inf. Secur. (2016)
23. Reena, Pandit, R., Richariya, V.: Performance evaluation of routing protocols for Manet using NS2. Int. J. Comput. Appl. (0975–8887) **66** (2013)

Transition Model from Articulatory Domain to Acoustic Domain of Phoneme Using SVM for Regression: Towards a Silent Spoken Communication

Aouatif Bencheikh[✉] and Abdeljabbar Cherkaoui

Laboratory of Innovative Technologies, National School of Applied Sciences,
Tangier, Morocco
{Bencheikh.aouatif,Cherkaoui.lti}@gmail.com

Abstract. This work is part of our project entitled: "Reconstitution speech by ultrasound imaging and video of the vocal apparatus: towards a silent spoken communication". Our objective is producing a normally articulate speech and not vocalized, from the vocal apparatus activity during a silent articulation. Our objective is to conceive a system which is based on tongue and lips images in silent articulation. So, it becomes necessary to conduct the recognition based on smaller speech units (typically phonemes). Several studies have been developed in the speech recognition, but our work treats more recent issue that is based on image analysis in order to produce speech. In this study, we propose a model of transition from a database of images corresponding to the forms of tongue and lips (Articulatory domain), to another database of frequencies (Acoustic domain). Our method is based on a regression analysis to predict the acoustic destination for each articulatory phoneme.

Keywords: Reconstitution speech · Silent spoken communication · Tongue and lips images forms · Phonemes · Silent articulation · Speech recognition · Image analysis · Model of transition · Regression analysis

1 Introduction

Among the principal components of our subject is speech and phoneme. Actually, speech is a continuous flux composed of a sequence of words, themselves made up of a sequence of phonemes and articulatory noises. Phoneme is the smallest discrete or distinctive unit of the spoken chain. It is the smallest unit of sound can produce a change in meaning by commutation. In literature many studies have been developed in the speech recognition, but our work treats more recent issue that is based on tongue and lips images forms in order to produce speech. In this paper, our objective is to constitute a model of transition from a first database (composed of images of tongue and lips corresponding to phonemes of French language) to a second database (composed of characteristics of these phonemes in a frequency domain). Firstly we extract

© Springer Nature Switzerland AG 2019
M. Ezziyani (Ed.): AI2SD 2018, AISC 915, pp. 287–296, 2019.
https://doi.org/10.1007/978-3-030-11928-7_25

features from the first database using HOG and SIFT. Then, we use acoustic features. Finally, we used two different regression methods based on support vector machine (SVM) to predict the acoustic destination for each image. Figure 1 represents an overview of our approach.

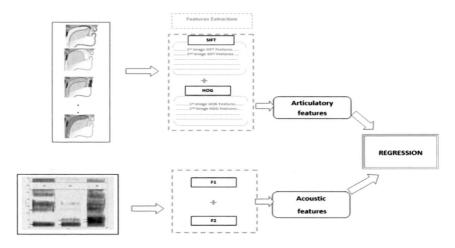

Fig. 1. Overview of the proposed approach

2 Related Works

In [1] authors presents a system built around an audio-visual dictionary which associates visual to acoustic observations for each phonetic class. Thus, they extract visual features from ultrasound images of tongue and from video images of the lips using PCA-based image coding technique. Later, they combine a phone recognition step with corpus-based synthesis.

In another work [2], researchers expose a new addition on "silent speech interface" that converts tongue and lip motions, captured by ultrasound and video imaging, into audible speech. Actually, they investigate the use of statistical mapping techniques, based on the joint modelling of visual and spectral features, using respectively Gaussian Mixture Models (GMM) and Hidden Markov Models (HMM). They predict voiced/unvoiced parameters from visual articulatory data using an artificial neural network (ANN). Also, they record continuous speech database consisting of one-hour of high-speed ultrasound and video sequences to evaluate the proposed mapping techniques.

In [3], authors present a video-only speech recognition system for a "silent speech interface" application, using ultrasound and optical images of the voice organ. Thus, they label phonetically a one-hour audio-visual speech corpus using an automatic speech alignment procedure and robust visual feature extraction techniques. HMM-based stochastic models were estimated separately on the visual and acoustic corpus.

Then, they compare the performance of the visual speech recognition system to a traditional acoustic-based recognizer.

This paper focuses on an experimental evaluation of phoneme recognition using features extracted from images and features related to acoustic domain. Thus, we employ SIFT and HOG descriptor to extract features from tongue and lips images. Then, we use two features from acoustic experiments. We investigate and evaluate the performance of different regression methods on images data set. The results of the evaluation are presented in the form of correlation coefficient and mean squared Error. Finally, the results of different regression methods are discussed.

3 Features Extraction Using Tongue and Lips Images

In our study, we use two methods to extract features from images: Histogram of Oriented Gradients (HOG) [4] and Scale Invariant Feature Transforms (SIFT) [5]. HOG and SIFT belong to a set of methods which aim to detect and describe local features in images.

3.1 Histogram of Oriented Gradients Features

The Histogram of Oriented Gradient (HOG) feature descriptor is popular for object detection [4]. Histogram of oriented gradients (HOG) is a feature descriptor used to detect objects in computer vision and image processing. The HOG descriptor technique counts occurrences of gradient orientation in localized portions of an image—detection window, or region of interest (ROI).

Implementation of the HOG descriptor algorithm is as follows:

1. Divide the image into small connected regions called cells, and for each cell compute a histogram of gradient directions or edge orientations for the pixels within the cell.
2. Discretise each cell into angular bins according to the gradient orientation.
3. Each cell's pixel contributes weighted gradient to its corresponding angular bin.
4. Groups of adjacent cells are considered as spatial regions called blocks. The grouping of cells into a block is the basis for grouping and normalization of histograms.
5. Normalized group of histograms represents the block histogram. The set of these block histograms represents the descriptor.

3.2 Scale Invariant Feature Transforms Features

For any object there are many features, interesting points on the object, which can be extracted to provide a "feature" description of the object. This description can then be used when attempting to locate the object in an image containing many other objects. There are many considerations when extracting these features and how to record them. SIFT [5] image features provide a set of features of an object that are not affected by many of the complications experienced in other methods, such as object scaling and rotation. While allowing for an object to be recognized in a larger image SIFT image features also allow for objects in multiple images of the same location, taken from different positions within the environment, to be recognized. SIFT features are also very resilient to the effects of "noise" in the image.

The SIFT approach, for image feature generation, takes an image and transforms it into a "large collection of local feature vectors". Each of these feature vectors is invariant to any scaling, rotation or translation of the image.

4   Features Extraction from Acoustic Domain

4.1   Acoustic Domain Description (Formants)

A formant, as defined by James Jeans, [6] is a harmonic of a note that is augmented by a resonance. Speech researcher Fant [7] defined formants as "the spectral peaks of the sound spectrum $|P(f)|$". In acoustics generally, a very similar definition is widely used: the Acoustical Society of America defines a formant as: "a range of frequencies [of a complex sound] in which there is an absolute or relative maximum in the sound spectrum" [8, 9]. In speech science and phonetics, however, a formant is also some-times used to mean acoustic resonance [10] of the human vocal tract. Thus, in phonetics, formant can mean either a resonance or the spectral maximum that the resonance produces. Formants are often measured as amplitude peaks in the frequency spectrum of the sound, using a spectrogram in Fig. 2 or a spectrum analyzer and, in the case of the voice, this gives an estimate of the vocal tract resonances. In vowels spoken with a high fundamental frequency, as in a female or child voice, however, the frequency of the resonance may lie between the widely spaced harmonics and hence no corresponding peak is visible.

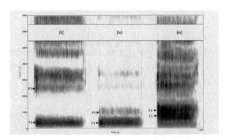

Fig. 2.   Spectrogram of Frensh vowels [i, u, ɑ] showing the formants F1 and F2

4.2   Acoustic Features

Formants are distinctive frequency components of the acoustic signal produced by speech or singing. The information that humans require to distinguish between speech sounds can be represented purely quantitatively by specifying peaks in the amplitude/frequency spectrum. The formant with the lowest frequency is called F1, the second F2, and the third F3. Most often the two first formants, F1 and F2, are enough to disambiguate the vowel.

The first two formants are important in determining the quality of vowels, and are frequently said to correspond to the open/close and front/back dimensions (which have traditionally, though not entirely accurately, been associated with the shape and position of the tongue). Thus the first formant F1 has a higher frequency for an open vowel (such as [a]) and a lower frequency for a close vowel (such as [i] or [u]); and the second formant F2 has a higher frequency for a front vowel (such as [i]) and a lower frequency for a back vowel (such as [u]) [11, 12] as can be seen in Fig. 3.

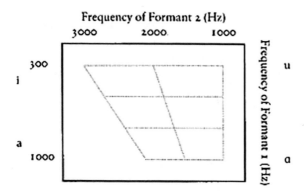

Fig. 3. Schematic diagram of formant plot

5   Regression Methods

To evaluate the proposed approach we use regression methods. Actually, regression analysis is a form of predictive modelling technique which investigates the relationship between a dependent (target) and independent variable (s) (predictor). We use two different regression methods based on Support Vector Machine (SVM) for regression.

5.1   SVM for Regression

Support Vector Machine (SVM)
SVM is a supervised machine learning algorithm used in classification and regression problems [13]. This algorithm performs classification tasks by constructing the hyper planes that separate different class labels in a multidimensional space. SVM is designed for binary classification problems. In the case of multi-class classification, the solution is to transform the single multiclass problem into diverse binary classification problems. Actually, SVM uses a set of mathematical functions that are defined as the kernel. The function of kernel is to take data as input and transform it into the required form. Different SVM algorithms use different types of kernel functions. These functions can be of different types, such as linear, non-linear, polynomial, RBF and sigmoid.

The kernel functions return the inner product between two points in a suitable feature space. Thus, by defining a notion of similarity, we get little computational cost even in very high dimensional spaces.

The SVM for regression (SVR) [6] uses the same principles as the SVM for classification, with few differences only when the output is a real number. Actually, SVM can also be used as a regression method, maintaining the main idea that characterises the algorithm: minimise error, detect the hyperplane which maximises the margin.

SVM for regression methods

To construct an optimal hyperplane, SVM employs an iterative training algorithm, which is used to minimize an error function. Thus, the task is to find a functional form that can correctly predict new cases that the SVM has not been presented with before. This can be achieved by training the SVM model on a sample set (training set). According to the form of the error function, SVM for regression models can be classified into two distinct groups: regression SVM type 1 (also known as epsilon-SVM regression) and regression SVM type 2 (also known as nu-SVM regression).

Regression SVM Type1: epsilon-SVM.

For this type of SVM the error function is:

$$\frac{1}{2} w^T w + C \sum_{i=1}^{N} \xi_i + C \sum_{i=1}^{N} \xi_i^* \tag{1}$$

Which we minimize subject to:

$$
\begin{aligned}
& w^T \phi(x_i) + b - y_i \leq \varepsilon + \xi_i^* \\
& y_i - w^T \phi(x_i) - b_i \leq \varepsilon + \xi_i \\
& \xi_i, \xi_i^* \geq 0, i = 1, \ldots, N
\end{aligned}
\tag{2}
$$

Regression SVM Type 2: Nu-SVM.

For this SVM model, the error function is given by:

$$\frac{1}{2} w^T w - C \left(v\varepsilon + \frac{1}{N} \sum_{i=1}^{N} (\xi_i + \xi_i^*) \right) \tag{3}$$

Which we minimize subject to:

$$
\begin{aligned}
& \left(w^T \phi(x_i) + b \right) - y_i \leq \varepsilon + \xi_i \\
& y_i - \left(w^T \phi(x_i) + b_i \right) \leq \varepsilon + \xi_i^* \\
& \xi_i, \xi_i^* \geq 0, i = 1, \ldots, N, \varepsilon \geq 0
\end{aligned}
\tag{4}
$$

Actually, there are number of kernels that can be used in SVM models. These include linear, polynomial, radial basis function (RBF) and sigmoid:

Kernel Functions.

$$K(\mathbf{X_i}, \mathbf{X_j}) = \begin{cases} \mathbf{X_i} \cdot \mathbf{X_j} & \text{Linear} \\ (\gamma \mathbf{X_i} \cdot \mathbf{X_j} + C)^d & \text{Polynomial} \\ \exp\left(-\gamma |\mathbf{X_i} - \mathbf{X_j}|^2\right) & \text{RBF} \\ \tanh(\gamma \mathbf{X_i} \cdot \mathbf{X_j} + C) & \text{Sigmoid} \end{cases} \tag{5}$$

where:

$$K(\mathbf{X_i}, \mathbf{X_j}) = \phi(\mathbf{X_i}) \cdot \phi(\mathbf{X_j}) \tag{6}$$

That is, the kernel function, represents a dot product of input data points mapped into the higher dimensional feature space by transformation ϕ. *Gamma* is an adjustable parameter of certain kernel functions. The RBF is by far the most popular choice of kernel types used in Support Vector Machines. This is mainly because of their localized and finite responses across the entire range of the real X-axis.

Performance measure
Correlation Coefficient.

The quantity r, called the linear correlation coefficient, measures the strength and the direction of a linear relationship between two variables. The linear correlation coefficient is sometimes referred to as the Pearson product moment correlation coefficient in honor of its developer Karl Pearson.

The mathematical formula for computing r is:

$$r = \frac{n - \sum xy - (\sum x)(\sum y)}{\left(\sqrt{n(\sum x^2) - (\sum y^2)}\right)\left(\sqrt{n(\sum x^2) - (\sum y^2)}\right)} \tag{7}$$

where n is the number of pairs of data.

- The value of r is such that $-1 < r < +1$. The + and − signs are used for positive linear correlations and negative linear correlations, respectively.
- Positive correlation: If x and y have a strong positive linear correlation, r is close to +1. An r value of exactly +1 indicates a perfect positive fit. Positive values indicate a relationship between x and y variables such that as values for x increases, values for y also increase.
- Negative correlation: If x and y have a strong negative linear correlation, r is close to −1. An r value of exactly −1 indicates a perfect negative fit. Negative values indicate a relationship between x and y such that as values for x increase, values for y decrease.
- No correlation: If there is no linear correlation or a weak linear correlation, r is close to 0. A value near zero means that there is a random, nonlinear relationship between the two variables. Note that r is a dimensionless quantity; that is, it does not depend on the units employed.

- A perfect correlation of ±1 occurs only when the data points all lie exactly on a straight line. If r = +1, the slope of this line is positive. If r = −1, the slope of this line is negative.
- A correlation greater than 0.8 is generally described as strong, whereas a correlation less than 0.5 is generally described as weak. These values can vary based upon the "type" of data being examined. A study utilizing scientific data may require a stronger correlation than a study using social science data.

Mean squared Error.

In statistics, the mean squared error (MSE) measures the average of the squares of the errors. MSE is a risk function, corresponding to the expected value of the squared error loss or quadratic loss [14].

If $\hat{Y}$ is a vector of n predictions, and Y is the vector of observed values of the variable being predicted, then the within-sample MSE of the predictor is computed as

$$MSE = \frac{1}{n} \sum_{i=1}^{n} \left(\widehat{Y_i} - Y_i \right)^2 \tag{8}$$

The MSE is always non-negative, and values closer to zero are better.

6 Setting and Results

We conduct experiments using data set containing (here number of images do you have). We extracted the groups of feature sets from images in the data set, and used features in each set to train many regressors. Then, we compare the features performance by comparing the regressors performances.

6.1 Settings

We employ the database that we propose, which is composed of 119 images representing different phonemes. We use the popular tool MATLAB for our approach features extraction, evaluation and analysis.

6.2 Results

We use settings cited in the previous Subsection A. The utilisation of SIFT descriptor results and HOG results are summarised in Table 1.

Among combinations (Features and regression methods) used in Table 1, (SIFT + nu-SVR) combination obtains the best accuracy rates: So, we notice that using SIFT gives performed results compared to HOG.

Therefore, we remark that MSE is closer to 0 and SCC is closer to 1 in the combination (SIFT + nu-SVR). Actually, considering calculation time for both SIFT and HOG features can be negligible.

Our reached results show that the proposed approach as attempt to assess phoneme recognition is interesting. These results provide evidence that both features extracted

Table 1. Regression results using SVR and the proposed features

	s	t	c	p	F1		F2	
					MSE	SCC	MSE	SCC
Test SVR-HOG	NU-SVR	0	10	0.01	14.1658	0.030827	19.1435	0.006997
		0	10	1	21.081	0.065582	22.2304	0.00603567
		0	100	0.1	18.0194	0.0029360	21.7751	0.0024361
		0	100	1	24.8865	0.0199017	14.831	0.0309928
		1	100	1	17.9056	0.0487527	16.6339	0.00290196
		1	10	1	15.1890	0.03678	18.1237	0.005908
	EPSILON-SVR	0	10	0.01	19.078	0.6548	20.91745	0.00534
		0	10	1	17.1567	0.2476	19.7591	0.09876
		0	1000	1	6.8935	0.1239	16.1831	0.061872
		0	1000	3	9.8354	0.7654	24.3739	0.0036096
Test SVR-SIFT	NU-SVR	0	10	0.01	6.72409	0.622342	8.88821	0.607228
		0	10	1	11.4758	0.487474	8.04091	0.75496
		0	100	0.1	**1.88551**	**0.87041**	**3.27063**	**0.779734**
		0	100	1	**2.6826**	**0.90033**	**3.25283**	**0.812224**
		1	100	1	15.6333	0.335372	16	0.314327
		1	10	1	20.2	0.075079	15.3333	0.35082
	EPSILON-SVR	0	10	0.01	11.8665	0.602137	10.951	0.658765
		0	10	1	10.632	0.449117	9.764	0.7987
		1	1000	1	**2.50566**	**0.904631**	**15.4**	**0.468784**
		1	1000	3	**2.08489**	**0.856153**	**14.65**	**0.310511**

Where

s—Regression type; t = 0—Linear SVR; t = 1—Polynomial SVR; c—Cost; p—epsilon

from images and features related to acoustic domain can affect the transition from articulatory domain to acoustic domain of phoneme.

7 Conclusion

In this paper we have presented an approach to model the transition from articulatory domain based on tongue and lips forms images to acoustic domain. The reached results represent a good attempt concerning this transition. In future works, we will add other acoustic features for speech recognition prediction.

References

1. Hueber, T., Benaroya, E., Chollet, G., Denby, B., Dreyfus, G., et al.: Development of a silent speech interface driven by ultrasound and optical images of the tongue and lips. Speech Commun. **52**(4), 288 (2010)

2. Hueber, T., Benaroya, E., Denby B., Chollet, G.: Statistical mapping between articulatory and acoustic data for an ultrasound-based silent speech interface. In: INTERSPEECH 2011, 12th Annual Conference of the International Speech Communication Association, Florence, Italy, 27–31 Aug 2011
3. Hueber, T., Chollet, G., Denby, B., Dreyfus G., Stone, M.: Continuous-speech phone recognition from ultrasound and optical images of the tongue and lips. In: INTERSPEECH 2007, 8th Annual Conference of the International Speech Communication Association, Antwerp, Belgium, 27–31 Aug (2007)
4. Dalal, N., Triggs, B.: Histograms of oriented gradients for human detection. In: IEEE Computer Society Conference on Computer Vision and Pattern Recognition, San Diego, CA, USA (2005)
5. Lowe David, G.: Object recognition from local scale-invariant features. In: Proceedings of 7th International Conference on Computer Vision (ICCV'99) (Corfu, Greece), pp. 1150–1157 (1999)
6. Jeans, J.H.: Science & Music, reprinted by Dover, 1968
7. Fant, G.: Acoustic Theory of Speech Production. Mouton & Co., The Hague, Netherlands (1970)
8. Acoustical Society of America: ANSI S1.1-1994 (R2004) American National Standard Acoustical Terminology, (12.41). Acoustical Society of America, Melville, NY (1994)
9. Titze, I.R., Baken, R.J., Bozeman, K.W., Granqvist, S., Henrich, N., Herbst, C.T., Howard, D.M., Hunter, E.J., Kaelin, D., Kent, R.D., Löfqvist, A., McCoy, S., Miller, D.G., Noé, H., Scherer, R.C., Smith, J.R., Story, B.H., Švec, J.G., Ternströmand, S., Wolfe, J.: Toward a consensus on symbolic notation of harmonics, resonances, and formants in vocalization. J. Acoust. Soc. Am. **137**, 3005–3007 (2015)
10. Titze, I.R.: Principles of Voice Productio. Prentice Hall. ISBN 978-0-13-717893-3 (1994)
11. Ladefoged, P.: A Course in Phonetics, 5th ed., p. 188. Thomson Wadsworth, Boston, MA. ISBN 1-4130-2079-8 (2006)
12. Ladefoged, P.: Vowels and Consonants: An Introduction to the Sounds of Language, p. 40. Blackwell, Maldern, MA. ISBN 0-631-21412-7 (2001)
13. Cortes, C., Vapnik, V.: Support-vector networks. Mach. Learn. **20**(3), 273–297 (1995)
14. Lehmann, B., Casella, E.L.: George:Theory of Point Estimation. 2nd ed., Springer, New York. ISBN 0-387-98502-6. MR 1639875 (1998)

Code Verification Based on TPM Solutions for Internet of Things Platforms

Toufik Ghrib[1,2,3]([⊠]), Mohamed Benmohammed[4],
Abdelkader Hadj Seyd[2], Mohamed Redouane Kafi[6],
and Abdelkader Guzzi[5]

[1] Department of Informatics,
University of Mohamed Khider Biskra, Biskra, Algeria
gharib.toufik@univ-ouargla.dz
[2] Departement of Production of Hydrocarbons, Faculty of Hydrocarbons,
Renewable Energies, Earth Sciences and the Universe,
University of Kasdi Merbah Ouargla, Ouargla, Algeria
[3] Laboratory of Mathematics and Applied Sciences,
University of Ghardaia, Ghardaia, Algeria
[4] Department of Software Technologies and Information Systems Faculty
of New Technologies of Information and Communication
University Constantine 2, Constantine, Algeria
[5] Faculty of New Technologies of Information and Communication,
University of Kasdi Merbah Ouargla, Ouargla, Algeria
[6] Laboratoire de Génie Electrique, Department of Electronics
and Telecommunication, University Kasdi Merbah Ouargla, Ouargla, Algeria

Abstract. Today's Internet of Things (IoT) is achieving more and more importance, since networks of physical objects embedded with electronic components, software and sensors are gaining popularity. The connectivity of such objects becomes crucial for the services and functionalities provided by the Internet of Things, which can be used for a great range of purposes: a network of cars sharing traffic information, a network of medical services, etc. more applications require the use of embedded code. This code usually exchanged in a pre-compiled form (byte code), can be naturally the product of the compilation of a source program written in a given language (smart cards,), but can also be of a unknown source (network games, hackers,). It is therefore appropriate, before running it, to make sure it is free of errors and that its execution on the host platform will not affect the proper functioning, both in terms of the calculation time and the level of the memory resources used. We are interested here in different techniques and methods to specify and to verify the veracity of the code exchanged between the different machines, In this case, we have to focus in two different sources of action: Device authentication: to ensure that any device can be replaced by a fake one and Software state attestation: to ensure that the current software state matches the system state. The way to address this issue is through trusted element-based TPM solutions.

Keywords: Internet of things · Security · Embedded systems · Verification · TPM

© Springer Nature Switzerland AG 2019
M. Ezziyyani (Ed.): AI2SD 2018, AISC 915, pp. 297–301, 2019.
https://doi.org/10.1007/978-3-030-11928-7_26

1 Introduction and Motivation

Internet of Things (IoT) is a network that inter- connects ordinary physical objects with the identifiable addresses so that provides intelligent services.

Ordinary objects are instrumented. It means that ordinary objects can be individually addressed by means of being embedded with chip, RFID, bar code and so autonomic terminals are interconnected. It means that the instrumented physical objects are connected as autonomic network Pervasive services are intelligent.

Compliance with coding rules, such as the MISRA rules, and mastering the complexity of your code by measuring industry-recognized metrics are some of the best practices in place for improving the quality of your code quality and reliability of the code [1].

In this case study, is in progress at security solutions for embedded systems and the Internet of Things application codes, the major objective of this work is to develop a model designed for the Internet of Things Platforms with TPM (Trusted Platform Module) to understand and improve a source code written in embedded language. In particular, it automates the analysis of control flows and dependencies, and detects problems in the use of data and the interaction of tasks.

Systems designed for these applications must therefore follow this complexity by integrating more and more features heterogeneous and complex. So you have to agree particular attention to the development of methods of design; Due to the heterogeneity of the targets, tools and multidisciplinary specification methods and especially verification and validation tools. It is also necessary to accentuate the automation of high design phase's level.

2 Methods and Tools

The first processors of security, developed following this principle, mainly focused on the applications of security of networks., that is why a consortium is mounted to develop a standard for crypto-processors for these targets. The Trusted Computing Group (TCG) brings together industrialists of the IT sector in order to define open standards that meet the needs of the applications of Security [2].

Among these different works, the TCG proposes architecture of crypto-coprocessor called Trusted Platform Module (TPM) a block diagram of this architecture (see Fig. 1).

TPM (Trusted Platform Module): is integrated security module, which protects sensitive data, authentication of individual platforms, generation of protection keys and random numbers, digital signature and encryption and platform approval [3].

Trusted modules can be used in computing devices other than PCs, such as mobile phones or network equipment [4]. The TPM specification was written to be platform independent, with the idea that additional specifications would be written to govern implementation on specific platforms.

The security policy is the same as that applied by the byte code verification step in a Java verifier byte code. The main difference by a byte code checker is that the code that is checked is the same code that is executed, It is to be noted that the different actors can very well be victims or attackers to a same system. The attacks implemented can

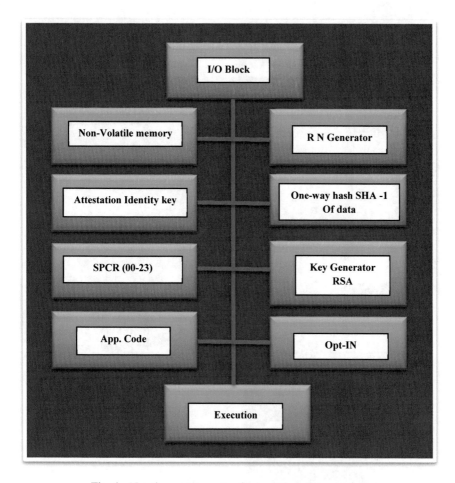

Fig. 1. Notation components of a trusted platform module

aim, for example, to destroy the system, the diverted from its normal functioning, the take in hand, make it unusable (denial of service) or extort of sensitive information. To achieve these objectives, the attacker uses both software techniques and material.

We tried to make a countermeasure to cope to type confusion attacks that are produced through the use of vulnerability present in the transaction mechanism offered by the platform, We used environment ECL to develop our new verification module and introduced it into the verification tool offered, a very important task. This is due to the sensitivity of the data that can be contained and the constraints related to the hardware devices (limited resources and constraints of power) which may be an obstacle to the implementation of protection mechanisms (Fig. 2).

The safety of operation focuses on the ability of a system to perform a function in the event of failure and, in a complementary way, is studying the IOT scenery of failures that lead to the inability to fulfill this function. A model for the safety of operation therefore represents both include functional and dysfunctional of a system.

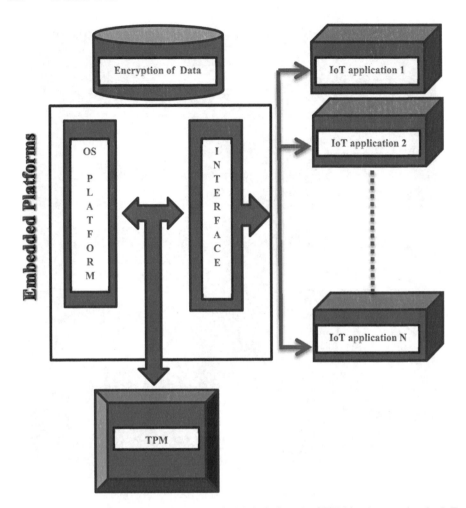

Fig. 2. Development device architecture (embedded platforms) of TPM implementation for IoT application

3   Conclusions

This work will eventually have a chain to code verification in the IoT platform; will serve as a basis for other problems such as property management (traceability and semantics) or modeling of platform.

Trusted Platform Module tries to solve one of the top problems in today's computing, It builds a complex and interesting architecture, using innovative hardware components.

The verification code does not ensure the total security of the IoT platform, but it reduces the risk to be attacked by facing as many types of attacks as possible.

The method of verification of the Code is, today, not supported by tools in the case Dynamic. Nevertheless; we have written the verification forms in order to be able to automate their appeal. An implementation in an industrial tool as the TPMs.

References

1. Roques, P.: Mbse with the arcadia method and the capella tool. In: 8th European Congress on Embedded Real Time Software and Systems (ERTS 2016) (2016)
2. Trusted Computing Group: Mobile Working Group. http://www.trustedcomputinroup.org developers/mobile
3. Trusted Computing Group: Guidance for Securing IoT Using TCG Technology, Version 1.0. TCG. http://opsy.st/TCGIoTSecurityGuidance
4. Bernard, R.: Analyses de sûreté de fonctionnement multi-systèmes. Modélisation et simulation. Université Sciences et Technologies - Bordeaux I, Français (2009)
5. Young, M.: The Technical Writer's Handbook. University Science, Mill Valley, CA (1989)

On the Security Communication
and Migration in Mobile Agent Systems

Sanae Hanaoui[⊠], Yousra Berguig, and Jalal Laassiri

Informatics Systems and Optimization Laboratory, Faculty of Science,
Ibn Tofail University, Kenitra, Morocco
{sanae.hanaoui, LAASSIRI}@uit.ac.ma, yousra.
berguig@gmail.com

Abstract. Mobile agent a new technology that satisfies the requirements of intelligence in distributed systems; also, it's a paradigm that accepts networking and distribution as a basic concept. But this it's still lacking when it comes to security which is a very important concept in the growth and development of this technology. In this paper we investigate the security of the distributed mobile agent system. We will present its benefits and we propose a new approach to improve the security of mobile agent communication while its migration, to grant the security agent, data, code and its environment.

Keywords: Mobile agents · Network security protocol · Security
mechanisms · Communication · Cryptography

1 Introduction

Nowadays we all hear the terms smart computers, smart phones, smart systems …, the term smart always turns toward intelligence, therefore the last three decades has been directed toward building computer systems that can act and think effectively on our behalf, and operates independently without human intervention, and interact with other computer systems to cooperate and reach agreements. Therefore, multi-agent systems come to existence which guarantees these needs, and they are becoming very popular and used in several domains. The idea of a multi-agent system is very simple. An agent is a computer system that is capable of independent action on behalf of its user or owner [1]. A multi-agent system is one that consists of a number of agents, which interact with one another, typically by exchanging messages through some computer network infrastructure [1]. The security of the mobile agent system is the most important issue for this technology which still unresolved. The use of multi-agent systems for security monitoring, control and management is increasing due to growing complexity of distributed systems. Therefore, it is essential to consider security issues of multi-agent systems [2]. In mobile agents several security issues arise so many scholars have discussed these issues [3, 4] which includes access control policies, authentication and authorization also intrusion detection etc. Because of the mobility of mobile agent, the security problems become more complicated and a bottleneck for development and maintenance of mobile agent technology especially in security

© Springer Nature Switzerland AG 2019
M. Ezziyyani (Ed.): AI2SD 2018, AISC 915, pp. 302–313, 2019.
https://doi.org/10.1007/978-3-030-11928-7_27

sensitive applications [3] such as electronic commerce [3–5], information retrieval and dissemination [5], personal assistance [6] (see Fig. 1).

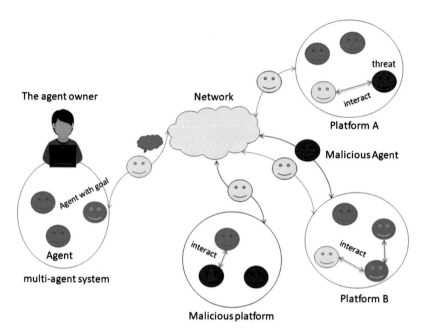

Fig. 1. Schema of multi agent system

The paper is organized as follows: Sect. 2 investigates the security problematic in the mobile agent systems and exposes various communication threats on mobile agents also explores some security requirements to protect it. Section 3 discusses and elaborates the background of research. While Sect. 4 introduces our approach by proposing a model to integrate it in our future solution and discusses the results of our current model. Finally, Sect. 5 concludes the paper.

2 Mobile Agents Security Overview

Threats to mobile agent security are classified into: agent-to-agent threats, agent-to-agent platform threats, agent platform-to-agent threats, and others-to-agent platform threats.

2.1 Communication Attacks on Mobile Agents While Its Migration

The mobile agent faces more severe security risks in case of its strong mobility all its code, data and state are exposed to the mobile agent platform in which it migrates for execution of operation or retrieval information [3].

The following are possible attacks by malicious platforms [7]:

(a) *Leak out or modify mobile agent's code*

Malicious platform can read and remember the instructions that are going to be executed by the arrived mobile agent to infer the rest of the program. By this process the platform knows the strategy and purpose of mobile agents [8]. Sometimes the malicious platform knows a complete picture of mobile agent's behavior and it might find out the physical address and then accesses its code memory to modify its code. It can even change code temporarily, execute it and finally resuming original code before the mobile agent leaves [3].

(b) *Leak out or modify mobile agent's data*

The malicious platform might get to know the original location of the data bit holed by the agent and then modify the data in accordance with the semantics of data [9] which might cause the leak of privacy or loss of money that lead to severe consequences even if the data is not sensitive.

(c) *Leak out or modify mobile agent's execution flow*

The malicious platform can predict what will be set of instructions to be executed next and deduce the state of that mobile agent by knowing the mobile agents physical location of program counter, mobile agent's code and data, consequently it can change the execution flow according to its will to achieve its goal [1]. It can even modify mobile agent's execution to deliberately execute agent's code in the wrong way.

(d) *Denial of Service (DoS)*

This attack is one of the most dangerous attacks that might causes mobile agent to miss some good chances if it can finish its execution on that platform in time and travel to some other platform. It causes not to execute the mobile agent migration and put it in waiting list carrying delays [10].

(e) *Masquerading*

Here malicious platform pretends as if it is the platform on which mobile agent has to migrate and finally becomes home platform where mobile agent returns. By this mechanism, it can get secrets of mobile agents by masquerading and even hurts the reputation of the original platform [2].

(f) *Leak out or Modify the interaction between a mobile agent and other parties*

Here the malicious platform eavesdrops on the interaction between a mobile agent and other parties (agent or platforms). This leads to extraction of secret information about mobile agent and third party. It can even alternate the contents of interaction and expose itself as part of interaction and direct the interaction to another unexpected third party. In this way, it might perform attacks to both mobile agent and third party.

2.2   Security Requirements to Protect the Mobile Agents

The protection of mobile agent-based systems in a distributed environment needs to guarantee the following five key security properties system, mobile agents traverse network freely to access [11]: Confidentiality, Integrity, Accountability, Availability, and Non-repudiation. In order to prevent the above threats we have to consider these security requirements which are the following [3, 4]:

- Authentication and Authorization: by requiring digital signatures in addition to password access to secure the source and integrity of mobile agents.
- Privacy and Confidentiality: by assuring confidentiality of exchanges and interactions in a mobile agent system in order to secure the communication of a mobile agent with its environment.
- Non-Repudiation: by logging important communication exchanges to prevent later denials.
- Accountability: by recording not only unique identification and authentication but also an audit log of security relevant events, which means all security related activities must be recorded for auditing and tracing purposes. In addition, audit logs must be protected from unauthorized access and modifications.
- Availability: Agent platform should be able to detect and recover from software and hardware failures. It should have the ability to deal with and avoid Dos attacks as well.
- Anonymity: the mother platform should keep agent's identity secret from other agents and maintains anonymity so as to determine agent's identity when necessary and legal.
- Fairness or trust: the necessity to ensure fair agent platform interaction where the agent should be able to assess the trustworthiness of information received from another agent or from an agent platform.

2.3   Security Mechanisms for Mobile Agent Protection

Mobile agent attack counter measures are categorized into detection mechanisms and prevention mechanisms which are classified according to whether they aim to detect or prevent violations against a mobile agent.

Where detection mechanisms make it possible to find actual identity of remote host and tries to partially or fully repairmen of tampered results. This includes solutions to detect unauthorized modifications of code, state or execution flow of a mobile agent [12]. While prevention mechanisms try to make it impossible or very difficult to access or modify code, state or execution flow of a mobile agent [13] (see Fig. 2).

3   Related Works

During the past years many attempts have been made either to improve the security issues for the MAS or to solve security issues using the MAS.

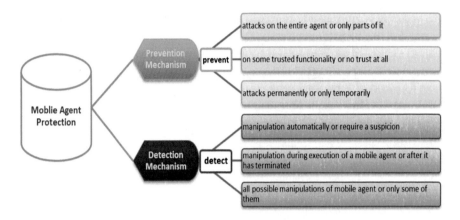

Fig. 2. Security mechanisms in MAS model

3.1 Models that Incorporates Security Considerations

Some Research have focused on proposing models to solve security issues of MAS, in this section we are going to focus on solutions based on models.

(a) *Securing the mobile agent during the communication*

Zrari et al. [5] have proposed a model for security properties in order to protect stationary agents during their communications with visitor mobile agents in the design phase of the mobile agent based system development process to secure stationary agents during their communications with visitor mobile agents by introducing new security concepts in the design stage. With the same objective Hedin and Moradian [6] presented a model for securing multi-agent systems, which is developed, based on the concepts and models regarding agent's role and communications.

These researches focused on proposing models that improve some of the security issues.

(b) *Security solutions based on architecture for mobile agent*

Some proposed solution based on architecture for making better security solutions in the mobile agent context.

Pinzón, Paz, Tapia, Bajo, and Corchado [7] tried to improve the FUSION@ multi-agent architecture by proposing a secure new perspective to address the DoS attacks problem in service oriented architectures. The model is not intended to replace the existing security solutions, but to be established as an additional layer to existing security measures, providing advanced knowledge that can support the decision-making process in those cases where the security and availability of the service information are at risk.

(c) *Securing the migration of the mobile agent*

The most unresolved issues for the mobile agents is the alteration while its migration therefore some research worked on solving some of the issues on the migration of the agent.

Karzan and Erdogan [9] they proposed a layered security architecture which can be applied to mobile agent systems in general, and specifically for agents which migrates via topic based publish/subscribe paradigm. The approach they proposed identifies if the incoming mobile agent is malicious (indeed untrusted) or not before it starts execution on the host via the use of a specific information which is appended to the mobile agent by the sending entity before the agent is transmitted onto the transmission channel. And for Hsu and Lin [14] proposed a secure, robust, and efficient hierarchical key management scheme for MANETs so the mobile agents can manage rights to access its own resources for the visited mobile nodes. As compared with Huang et al.'s scheme, their proposed scheme can provide better security assurance, while requiring smaller key-size, lower computational complexities, and constant key management costs which is independent on the number of the confidential files and the visited nodes. The proposed scheme consists three phases as those of Huang et al.'s scheme.

(d) *Security solutions for integrity protection*

Securing communication contents, data or code is becoming more important, in this section we will present some works proposed solution for empowering the integrity of the mobile agents.

Zwierko and Kotulski [10] they presented a new concept for providing mobile agents with integrity protection, based on a zero-knowledge proof system. The proposed solution fulfills the forward integrity definition: none of data and corresponding values can be changed without a future detection by the manager. a promising solution to the problem of providing agent with effective countermeasures against attacks on the integrity but still lacking in preventing any attacks that are aimed at destroying the agent's data, code or both. While Esfandi and Rahimabadi [15] they illustrated a novel distributed protocol for multi agent environments to improve the communication security in packet-switched networks. To enrich the overall system security, the approach makes use of distribution and double encryption and some other traditional methods such as digital signature. But for Vitabile, Conti, Militello, and Sorbello [12] they extended JADE-S based framework for developing secure Multi-Agent Systems. The framework functionalities are extended by self-contained FPGA biometric sensors providing secure and fast user authentication service, Each agent owner, by means of biometric authentication, acquires his/her own X.509v3 digital certificate [13]. In addition, a mechanism based on the agent reputation is used to grant the integrity of the agent.

In the same context our proposed approach comes to improve and to empower the security issues of the MAS by combining different security requirements to focus on solving many communication problems in mobile agent system.

4 Proposed Model for Secure Mobile Agent

There is no 100% secure system and it is not possible to stop or predict all the possible attacks for distributed systems. However, if we considered during development the security issues and threats it will certainly multi-agent system is going to be more secure. Therefore, we decided to consider a model which can help our system to be more secure by adapting both detection and prevention mechanism into our model and based on the security requirement we proposed the following solution which is improving the security agent communication while its migration as a result we grant security at agent and the system level (see Fig. 3).

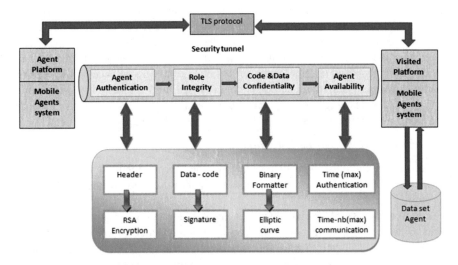

Fig. 3. Proposed model for secure mobile agent

4.1   Description of the Model

In this model we decided to adopt both prevention and detection mechanism to minimize the security threats on the agent and its environment. Following are the security requirements that are incorporated in our communication tunnel for the secure migration process.

To establish a cryptographically secure communication channel for our mobile agent we opted for the TLS protocol because its designed to provide three essential services to all applications running above it: encryption, authentication, and data integrity. before performing an agent migration, each platform must authenticate each other. A successful authentication indicates that each host is who it claims to be [11]. Authentication is performed via public-key cryptography. During the authentication process, each platform keeps a private known-host file containing public keys of all other platforms with which agent migration is allowed, and its own public and private key file.

Authentication process
Authentication refers to a process in which the platform ensures that the other platform in the communication is in fact who it is declared to be. Before the secure transfer of a mobile agent between the two platforms, they must authenticate each other. Therefore in our approach we opted to communicate a public key with the visited platform via the secure communication protocol TLS [8] (see Fig. 4), before transferring our mobile

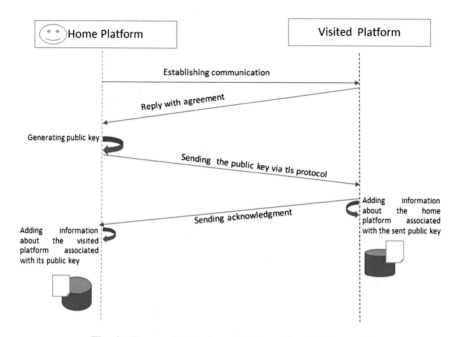

Fig. 4. Communicating the public key using TLS protocol

agent to the visited platform. And in order to make our agent identification and authentication more secure an encrypted formatted header using RSA algorithm (see Fig. 5) that consists of the owner id, code for the agent's permissions and agent id also a signature of data or code is sent with agent to assure that the right agent does the right things (see Fig. 6).

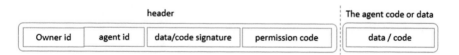

Fig. 5. Proposed AgentHeader

Role Integrity

Is to ensure that the agent was not tampered while the transit from the agent platform to the receiving platform. Therefor to grant the integrity of our mobile agent our proposed solution is based on using a signature to our code. in which the visited platform compares two hash codes. If the hash code does not match, it informs the agent platform. Then, another agent migration is attempted (see Fig. 7).

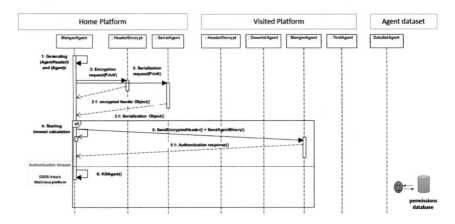

Fig. 6. Authentication scenario

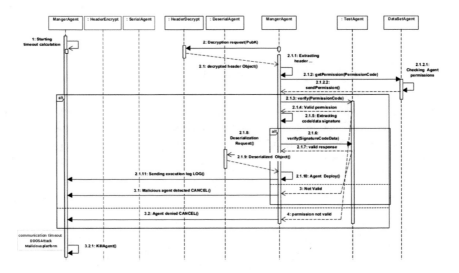

Fig. 7. Communication scenario

Agent Confidentiality

Is to grant the confidentiality of the agent while its migration to the visited platform, in our proposed approach we decided to use the binary serialization and to encrypt the mobile agent at the agent platform and to decrypt it at the receiver platform, using the Elliptic curve encryption. So that our mobile agent would not be accessible in an understandable form by any adversary (see Fig. 7).

Agent Availability

To avoid denial of service attack (DDOS) and subsequently ensure the availability of our agent, we proposed time max authentication (authentication timeout) which is the maximum time allowed to establish the authentication with the visited platform (see Fig. 6), and number max of communication it defines the maximum number of communication time attributed to our agent. This property can guarantee that the visited platform does not exploit the agent more than allowed. And for communication time max (communication timeout) this property defines the maximum time allowed to the agent to communicate with the visited platform. Thus, to guarantee the availability of our agent by eliminating the denial of service (see Fig. 7).

In our proposed approach we proposed a dataset agent which contains all sets of agent permissions in order to grant the certainty of our agent, in this way the visited platform will verify the agent permission before its execution in this way it will assure that agent will do only what it is supposed to do.

4.2   Test and Validation

In this part we will present the execution time of our solution composed of several security mechanisms to guarantee the security of our agent during his communication with an external platform. We are limiting our simulation on containers located in the same physical platform. We intend to develop this solution to a distributed one.

(a) *Analysis*

The practical tests of the implementation are carried out in a Machine which contains two containers that will represent the destination machines. The technical characteristics of the machine are: Intel Core i3 processor has 2.3 GHz with 4 GB of RAM. For the creation, management, mobility and execution of Agents we adopt JADE Snapshot from version During the Trip of the agent from the native platform to the hosting platform, it performs many operations to ensure the necessary security aspects needed. From the results it is observed that for communicating the public key between the agent platform and the visited platform it took 140 ms using TLS protocol and for encrypting the header which will contain information that verify the agents using RSA have taken almost 173 ms, while for using schnorr signature to insure the integrity of our data have taken 700 ms, and for the ECC elliptic curve have taken 1200 ms to encrypt our agent which guarantee the confidentiality.

The Total period includes many processes represented by sub-durations Illustrated in the figure (see Fig. 8). According to the graph (see Fig. 8), if we take in consideration checking the agent availability, which is defined in 3000 ms also the migration time of the agent which is 10 ms, given the use of a distributed platform in a single machine. We might conclude the total execution time has a value of 5223 ms.

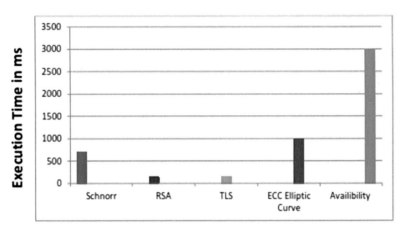

For one Agent

Fig. 8. Execution time in ms for each adopted mechanism

5 Conclusion

In this paper we have discussed the security problem in mobile agent system, we focused on the security of communication and we exposed various communication threats on mobile agents. We explored some security requirements also we presented some related work. After this we proposed our solution to secure the mobile agent during its migration, which is based on a set of cryptography techniques such as the elliptic curve, the cryptosystem RSA and the signature to guarantee the authentication the confidentiality and the integrity as well as a time-based technique to ensure availability, all those mechanisms present our secure tunnel that will protect the agent during his migration.

References

1. Madsen, M.W.: An introduction to multi-agent statistics. CEUR Workshop Proc. **1208**, 16–20 (2014)
2. Zrari, C., Hachicha, H., Ghedira, K.: Agent's security during communication in mobile agents system. Proc. Comput. Sci. **60**(1), 17–26 (2015)
3. Dadhich, P., Dutta, D.K., Govil, D.M.C.: Security issues in mobile agents. Int. J. Comput. Appl. **11**(4), 1–7 (2010)
4. Kaur, M., Saxena, S.: A review of security techniques for mobile agents 807–812 (2017)
5. Alami-Kamouri, S., Orhanou, G., Elhajji, S.: Overview of mobile agents and security. In: Proceedings of—2016 International Conference on Engineering MIS, ICEMIS 2016, 2016
6. Gupta, J.K., Egorov, M., Kochenderfer, M.: Cooperative multi-agent control using deep reinforcement learning. Adapt. Learn. Agents (2017)

7. Alfalayleh, M., Brankovic, L.: An overview of security issues and techniques in mobile agents. In: Communications and Multimedia Security: 8th IFIP TC-6 TC-11 Conference on Communications and Multimedia Security, 15–18 Sept 2004, pp. 59–78. Windermere, The Lake District, United Kingdom, 2005

8. Hedin, Y., Moradian, E.: Security in multi-agent systems. Proc. Comput. Sci. **60**(1), 1604–1612 (2015)

9. C.M.-F.: For S. M. Code and undefined 1997, Detecting attacks on mobile agents pdfs. semanticscholar.org

10. Lau, F., Rubin, S.H.S.S.H., Smith, M.H., Trajkovic, L.: Distributed denial of service attacks. Syst. Man Cybern. **3**, 2275–2280 (2000)

11. Wilhelm, U.G.: A technical approach to privacy based on mobile agents protected by tamper-resistant hardware (1999)

12. Ogunnusi, O.S., Ogunlola, O.O.: Solutions to mobile agent security issues in open multi-agent systems. Int. Res. J. Eng. Technol. **2**(5), 601–609 (2015)

13. Amro, B.: Mobile Agent Systems, Recent Security Threats and Counter Measures

14. Dagade, V., Kulkarni, C., Dhotre, S.R.: Mobile agent security based on code obfuscation and locator mechanism. Int. J. Comput. Appl. 975–8887

15. Chess, D.M.: Security Issues in Mobile Code Systems, pp. 1–14. Springer, Berlin (1998)

16. Pinzón, C.I., De Paz, J.F., Tapia, D.I., Bajo, J., Corchado, J.M.: Improving the security level of the FUSION@ multi-agent architecture. Expert Syst. Appl. **39**(8), 7536–7545 (2012)

17. Karzan, A.A.: Erdogan, N.: Securing mobile agent systems in which the agents migrate via publish/subscribe paradigm. Lect. Notes Softw. Eng. **2**(1) 2014

18. Hsu, C.L., Lin, Y.L.: Improved migration for mobile computing in distributed networks. Comput. Stand. Interfaces **36**(3), 577–584 (2014)

19. Zwierko A., Kotulski, Z.: Security of mobile agents: a new concept of the integrity protection. Arxiv Prepr. cs/0506103 (2005)

20. Esfandi, A., Rahimabadi, A.M.: Mobile agent security in multi agent environments using a multi agent-multi key approach In: Proceedings of—2009 2nd IEEE International Conference on Computer Science and Information Technology ICCSIT 2009, pp. 438–442 (2009)

21. Vitabile, S., Conti, V., Militello, C., Sorbello, F.: An extended JADE-S based framework for developing secure multi-agent systems. Comput. Stand. Interfaces **31**(5), 913–930 (2009)

22. Chau, J.: Digital certificates—is their importance underestimated? Comput. Fraud Secur. **2005**(12), 14–16 (2005)

23. Wang, Y.H., Wu, I.C.: Achieving high and consistent rendering performance of java AWT/Swing on multiple platforms. Softw. Pract. Exp. **39**(7), 701–736 (2009)

24. Warnier, M., Oey, M., Timmer, R., Brazier, F., Overeinder, B.: Enforcing integrity of agent migration paths by distribution of trust. Int. J. Intell. Inf. Database Syst. **3**(4), 382 (2009)

A Temporal Data Warehouse Conceptual Modelling and Its Transformation into Temporal Object Relational Model

Soumiya Ain El Hayat[(✉)] and Mohamed Bahaj

Faculty of Science and Technologies, Hassan 1st University, Settat, Morocco
{soumya.ainelhayat,mohamedbahaj}@gmail.com

Abstract. The Conventional data warehouses (DWs) are information repositories specialized in supporting decision making. Since the decisional process requires an analyzing of historical data, DWs systems have been increasingly feeling the need to collect temporal data for accountability and traceability reasons. On the other hand, the temporal object relational Model has been successfully used to handle and maintain past, present and future information. In this paper, we propose a Novel conceptual design for temporal data warehouse (TDW) including bitemporal data. Our solution provides a transformation method into temporal star and snowflake schemas, which incorporate features of object relational data warehouse and integrate Bitemporal data, to meet the requirement of integrating heterogeneous types of data to support decision making with an efficient manner. We have focused on the creation of a conceptual model for designing a temporal object-relational data warehouse based on UML technology and EER (Enhanced entity-relationship) model. The proposed method comprises a Meta Model using UML mechanism to express the varying time data in data warehousing applications that allow easily realizing and transforming the conceptual model into a logical design schema.

Keywords: Data warehouse · Object relational model · UML · Snowflake schema · Star schema · Temporal data warehouse · Bitemporal data · EER model

1 Introduction

A Data warehouse is a multidimensional database that is used to store and provide access to large volumes of historical data, based on indicators for supporting the strategic decisions of organizations. Data in data warehouse has features of being a collection of subject-oriented, integrated, non-volatile and time-varying data. The two last characteristics allow changes to the data values without overwriting the existing values. Furthermore, data in a DWs must be stored in a way thus is secure, reliable, easy to retrieve and to manage [1]. It is mainly used only for using querying and consequently, it is important that querying technique performance is as high as possible. The structure of DWs is based on a multidimensional view of data usually represented as a start or a snowflake schema, consisting of fact and dimension tables [2].

© Springer Nature Switzerland AG 2019
M. Ezziyyani (Ed.): AI2SD 2018, AISC 915, pp. 314–323, 2019.
https://doi.org/10.1007/978-3-030-11928-7_28

In the recent decades, another active research, temporal database, deals with recording the history of the objects or the database activity. The need to retain and audit the change made to a data and the ability to plan based on past or future assumptions are important uses case for temporal data [3]. Even today, a large number of database applications based on time in nature, to make a better description and clearly some tasks of database systems. The literature on temporal database offers three dimensions of time for temporal data support: transaction time, valid time and bitemporal data which support the both. Bitemporal data model our changing knowledge of the changing world, hence associate data values with facts and also specify when the facts are valid [4].

The Knowledge acquired from these two research area, Management varying time data and data warehouse, led to the emergence of temporal data warehouse (TDW). A TDW is considered as a repository of historical information associated with time, and originating from multiple and heterogeneous sources, for the purpose to analyze, plan, react to changing business conditions and identify the relevant trends fast as possible.

In this paper, we attempt to propose a new conceptual model for TDW including Bitemporal data. Our aim goal is to provide a general strategy for transformation process from Conceptual model to logical model which is represented by the temporal snowflake object relational schema (SW-TORDW) and the temporal star object relational(S-TORDW). This model based on data warehouse schema design using temporal object relational concepts and based on nested approach. Each dimension in S-TORDW and SW-TORDW contains a varying time attributes. In addition, we create a meta-Model that defines a new modeling of TDW including bitemporal data aspects which is accomplished by using UML specification, stereotype, constraint and tagged values. In the other hand, we introduce the temporal extension of EER diagram for preserving the characteristics of logical schema and providing a more abstract conceptual schema.

2 Related Works

Significant researchers address the problem of the storage and retrieval of historical data in DWs. A research work in [5] proposed a general design for abject relational Slowly changing dimension (SCD) data type 1–4, illustrated with an example that allows comparing the performance, in order to improve response time for queries with a data warehouse design for changing dimension tables.

Gosain and saroha introduced an approach for bitemporal versions of the schema in TDW design modelling that allows for retroactive and proactive schema modification [6]. Malinowski and Zimanyi proposed the translation method of spatial hierarchies from the conceptual to physical schema represented in the MultiDimER oracle 10 g Spatial [2]. In the other work, they presented the transformation of temporal MultiDim Model based on temporal databases aspects into ER and the object-relational models [7]. The research [8] provided a semi-automatic methodology for deriving the model from the standard documentation of the object-relational database and presented the results of transformation method from conceptual model into logical and physical model. Saxena and Agarwal focused on comparison of dimensional modeling and ER modeling in the data warehouse, they proposed the conceptual design approaches by combining star schema and E-R model specifications [9].

Grani, helmer proposed a starnest schema which is based on the nested approach for supporting time [10]. Also, they presented a novel design with star and snowflake schema to provide the temporal starnest schema [11].

A new data Model is discussed in [12] that incorporate the star schema with the object-relational concepts and multidimensional characteristics to integrate complex data in a data warehouse. Garani and atay introduced two different approaches: Object-relational temporal data warehouse and starnest temporal data warehouse, for dealing with temporal data in data warehouse, and they presented a comparison between these two models [1].

In Summary, we conclude that some previous works made a number of assumptions which contain limited and simple mechanisms compared to our work, especially at conceptual and representation level in time-varying data management field. We noticed that articles about the transformation from UML into temporal data warehouse are not frequent.

Our research work presented in this study is focused completely on the conceptual model based on UML notation and its transformation into TEER and logical modelling. The TEER representation of the TDW meta-Model allows a better understanding of temporal data warehouse semantics.

We provide our solution by combine several results from the existing methods and applying our enhancement using meta-model approach. This study presents the translation of UML class diagrams into TEER model that facilitate the mapping method into S-TORDW and SW-TORDW models based on bitemporal data and nested approach to express the hierarchies, in order to give a complete description of the different analysis dimension of data.

3   Process of Modeling and Transforming UML into Logical Model

In this section, we outline the important phase for modeling the conceptual and logical design schema. The process starts by defining a meta-model for temporal data warehouse, which is based on UML diagram class specification integrating bitemporal data features. In the Next, we propose EER representation of Temporal Meta-model which allows a better description of the entities, their attributes and their relationships. Through this model, we precede to the last step, we will develop S-TORDW and SW-TORDW as a logical design uses the star and snowflake structure according to the specifications provided by Object relational Models such as Structured Type, References and nested table (NT) to manipulate the complex data.

3.1   Creation of Meta-Model for TDW

UML mechanism has a very rich notation offers many aspects of software and applications development. It allow to experts to define and provide a new kind of modelling elements which are related by relationships. This is enriched by stereotype, constraints and tagged values concepts to define a several graphical diagram in term of the views of systems. In data warehousing field, UML can help system designer to build a DW model and make records of data over time (Fig. 1).

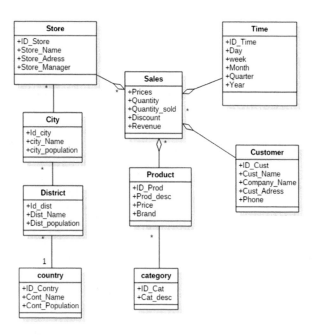

Fig. 1. Presents the class diagram modeling data of store department as an example used along this paper

We need in this work to develop a meta-model which task is to record the changes of data in past, present or in the future. Although a class diagram is a general purpose language for system modeling, the temporal data warehouse has not been addressed. For this reason, it is necessary to propose a novel model for TDW modeling operation.

A meta-Model is involved in system engineering to understand the data semantic meaning because it describes the elements, the relationships, constraints and attributes (Fig. 2).

Where:

TC   Temporal Class (Class contains temporal attributes)

SC   Simple Class (Class without temporal attribute)

TA   Temporal Attribute.

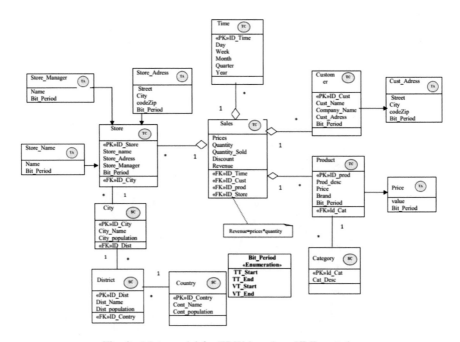

Fig. 2. Meta-model for TDW based on UML notation

3.2   Identification and Definition of TEER Model

We choose the enhanced entity-relationship (EER model) since it is well known and widely used conceptual data model for database design. In this work, the proposed EER model is implemented by transforming the previous meta-Model and its specification into object Relational model. Therefore, this migration requires additional attributes and concepts for supporting time varying data to make a better description of temporal data. The aim goal of the EER model enriched with object relational features and bitemporal data is to simplify the comprehension of the essential information stored in temporal data warehouse, and facilitate the implementation of the logical model. The TEER modeling plays a pivot role between the conceptual schemes expressed by UML and implementation of temporal data warehouse schema.

Consider the TEER model example as shown in Fig. 3. In This example, we produce a TEER model of sales, product and category class described in the previous conceptual model.

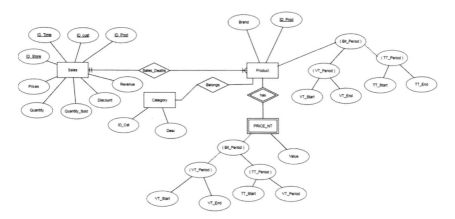

Fig. 3. The TEER model of sales, product and category tables

3.3   S-TORDW and SW-TORDW Model

The SW-TORDB Model and S-TORDBW uses the snowflake and star schema for representation of DW structure including the specifications provided by the Object relational model to handle the complex data and objects. It consists of the fact table connected to several Dimension contain varying time data which are called temporal dimensions. To provide a history of the data and store their changes, the Bitemporal period should be kept at the attribute level. Attributes can be temporal or non temporal. SW-TORDW and S-TORDW are based on Nested Approach to express hierarchy levels by the clustering of data in nested tables.

In Fig. 4, the schema of S-TORDW is represented in star schema at the logical design. In the S-TORDW a dimension's hierarchy is expressed as a structured type and Nested Table.

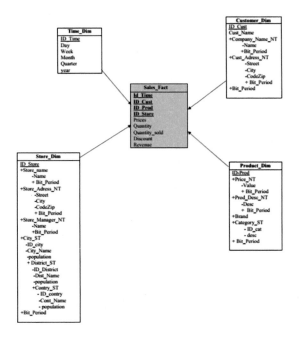

Fig. 4. Temporal star OR DW (S-TORDW) model

Figure 5 presents the SW-TORDW model which uses a snowflake schema. Each dimension table has a hierarchical attribute which is referred by a REFERENCE feature to express the foreign key attribute.

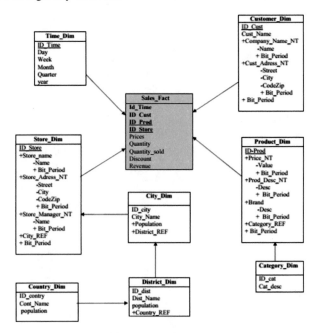

Fig. 5. Temporal snowflake OR DW (SW-TORDW) model

3.4 TORDB Queries Implementation

We can translate the S-TORDW and SW-TORDW models into temporal relational queries (for the sake of simplicity, we will create TORDB queries only for Product Dimension) using Oracle 12 C (Figs. 6 and 7).

```
CREATE TYPE BIT_PERIOD AS OBJECT(
TT_START DATE,
TT_END DATE,
VT_START DATE,
VT_END DATE
)/

    Create price_Type as object (
Value Number,
Bit-NT Bit_Period
)/
    Create price is table of price_Type;
Create Type category_T as Object(
    Id_cat Number,
    Cat_Desc varchar(20))/
    Create table category of category_T;
    Create Product_Type as Object (
ID_prod,
Price_NT price,
Prod_desc varchar(20),
Brand varchar(20),
Category  REF category_Type
)/
    Create table Product_Dim of product_Type
Constraint
Prod_Key Primary Key (Id_Prod), Nested table
Price_NT
Store AS Price_Tab.
```

Fig. 6. TORDB queries for product dimension in SW-TORDW based on snowflake schema

CREATE TYPE BIT_PERIOD AS OBJECT(
TT_START DATE,
TT_END DATE,
VT_START DATE,
VT_END DATE
)/

    Create price_Type as object (
Value Number,
Bit-NT Bit_Period
)/
    Create price is table of price_Type;

    Create Type category_T as Object(
Id_cat Number,
Cat_Desc varchar(20))/

    Create Product_Type as Object (
ID_prod,
Price_NT price,
Prod_desc varchar(20),
Brand varchar(20),
Category category_Type,
)/
    Create table Product_Dim of product_Type Constraint
Prod_Key Primary Key (Id_Prod), Nested table Price_NT
Store AS Price_Tab.

Fig. 7. TORDB queries for product dimension in S-TORDW based on star schema

4 Conclusion

In this paper, we have presented a novel approach for conceptual modeling of TDW. This study simplifies comprehension of the transformation process of UML class diagram into TDW using ORDB and Bitemporal data.

From UML class diagram we have extract data behaviour, relationships between class and constraint rules in order to provide our meta-Model in which contains varying time attributes. The advantage of meta_Model proposed its ability to promote the visualization of different navigational paths between objects. The obtained meta-Model was transformed into an enhanced entity-relationship and then into S-TORDW and SW-TORDW.

This solution is considered a complete study at representation level that show how can the collection semantics stated in the conceptual model into TDW.

Future Work includes comparison results between two temporal data warehouse models(S-TORDW, SW-TORDB), based on object relational concepts for efficient evaluation of complex Temporal queries. Also, we will present the results description based on several criteria to define the better approach which can be able to support temporal data warehouse.

References

1. Garani, G., Atay, C.E.: Comparison of different temporal data warehouses approaches. The Online J. Sci. Technol. **7**(2) (2017)
2. Malinowski, E., Zimanyi, E.: Logical representation of a conceptual model for spatial data warehouses. GeoInformatica **11**(4), 431–457 (2007)
3. Kaufmann, M., Fischer, P.M., May, N., Kossmann, D.: Benchmarking bitemporal database systems: ready for the future or stuck in the past? In: Proceedings of the: EDBT, pp. 738–749 (2014)
4. Ain El Hayat, S. Bahaj, M.: Converting UML class diagrams into temporal object relational databases. IJECE J. **7**(5) (2017)
5. Loyola, R., Sepulveda, A., Hernandez, M.: Optimization slowly changing dimensions of a data warehouse using object-relational. In: Conference: 24th International Conference of the Chilean Computer Science Society (SCCC) (2015)
6. Gosain, A., Saroha, K.: Bitemporal versioning of schema in temporal data warehouses. Data Eng. Intell. Comput. **542**, 357–367 (2017)
7. Malinowski, E., Zimanyi, E.: A conceptual model for temporal data warehouses and its transformation to the ER and the object-relational models. Data Knowl. Eng. **64**(1), 101–133 (2008)
8. Yu-Chih Liu, J., Ya Lai, S.: Constructing an object-relational data warehouse using semi-automated methods. J. Inf. Manag. 205–225 (2008)
9. Saxena, G., Agarwa, B.B.: Data warehouse desining: dimensional modelling and E-R modelling. Int. J. Eng. Invent. **3**, 28–34 (2014)
10. Garani, G., Helmer, S.: Integrating star and snowflake schemas in data warehouses. Int. J. Data Warehous. Min. **8**(4), 22–40 (2012)
11. Garani, G., Adam, G., Ventzas, D.: Temporal data warehouse logical modeling. Conf. Int. J. Data Min. Mod. Manag. **8**(2) (2016)
12. Lin, W.Y., Wu, C.A., Wu, C.C.: An object-relational datawarehouse modeling for complex data. In: Conference: 9th International Conference in Information Sciences (JCI) (2006)

Adherent Raindrop Detection Based on Morphological Operations

Elhassouni Fouad[(⊠)] and Ezzine Abdelhak

Laboratory of Information and Communication Technologies,
National School of Applied Sciences, Tangier, Morocco
elhassouni.fouad@gmail.com

Abstract. The presence of raindrops in an image can highly impact the performance of applications used in Advanced Driver Assistance Systems (ADAS). Therefore, the detection of raindrops remains a necessity, especially in rainy conditions to improve the ADAS performance. In this paper, we present a new approach to detect adherent raindrops in a single image based on the raindrops characteristics and using a combination of image processing techniques.

Keywords: Adherent raindrops · Morphological operations · ADAS · Ellipse fitting

1 Introduction

Recently, the Advanced Driver Assistance Systems (ADAS) have been gaining an interesting importance in traffic safety. These systems used different algorithms like obstacle detection, tracking, object recognition, etc. However, the results of these algorithms are limited and less effective in bad weather conditions (like rain, fog, snow, etc.), hence it is necessary to have a preprocessing step for detecting these obstacles, either to alert the driver to be more vigilant or to restore the image.

In this article, we discuss particularly raindrops detection on windshield to verify if the weather is rainy or clear. Previous work on this matter can be mainly presented in three categories; the first one considers the drop as a model, while the second classifies it with a statistical learning method, and the last one proposes to detect it based on certain features like gradient, color or texture.

For instance, Cord and Aubert [1] proposed an approach based on image processing techniques combined with pattern recognition systems to detect focused rain. But, its results are still limited to the case of a non-moving vehicle. As for Ito and Ito et al. [2], they used the Maximally Stable Eternal Regions (MSER) and quantitative metrics to detect adherent raindrop. However, their method needs a significant execution time. Moreover, Harsha et al. [3] developed an algorithm based on the principle intensity of raindrops in a scene and morphological operations. Unfortunately, the algorithm is still limited due to the high rates of false detections. Cord and Gimonet [4] detected raindrops based on photometric properties. Their method relies on low and high image processing techniques (watershed algorithm, background subtraction). But, it's limited on the case of a non-moving vehicle. And in [5] the authors proposed a method to

© Springer Nature Switzerland AG 2019
M. Ezziyyani (Ed.): AI2SD 2018, AISC 915, pp. 324–331, 2019.
https://doi.org/10.1007/978-3-030-11928-7_29

detect raindrops with various shapes, by examining the blur between the raindrop and surrounding areas, but they failed to reduce the number of false detections.

Furthermore, Wu et al. [6] proposed detecting rain by generating a raindrop saliency map based on color, texture and shape characteristics of raindrops. Despite of providing good results when applied in moderate rain scenarios, the approach is not performing well in heavy rain scenarios. In the other hand, Kurihata et al. [7, 8], have proposed a detection method based on a statistical learning method; the principal component analysis (PCA), that generates raindrop templates as known Eigen-drop. Their results are promising on clear background, but showed a lack of robustness on a complex image's background. In their paper [9], Machot and al. developed a method based on pattern recognition by a support vector machine and a cellular neural networks for the classification. Hence, the method is still limited in detecting small raindrops, and requires a large size of templates.

In [10, 11], Roser et al. presented a new geometric-photometric model for adherent raindrops. This model is used to generate a virtual raindrop which they compare with the image features to check the drop's presence. Even if the method is very robust, it requires a high computational time.

In this work we present an approach to detect adherent raindrop in a single image considering its edge and shape. We combine different algorithms such as image segmentation, pattern recognition and ellipse fitting. We focus on method based on image features because it provides an analogy between robustness and complexity of method compared to the other categories.

The rest of this paper is organized as following: Sect. 2 contains the new method's description. Results and experiments are discussed in Sect. 3. Finally, we conclude in Sect. 4.

2 Raindrop Detection Algorithm

2.1 Visual Raindrop Characteristics

Rain can be seen in different forms, such as rain streaks, focused and unfocused raindrop [12]. In the literature, a raindrop is defined by several characteristics, as its physical form, and the visual effects produced in an image.

The characteristics of a static raindrop and rain streaks has been studied by Garg and Nayar [13]. While Halimeh and Roser [10] has provided a new model for raindrop, which is based on the drop's photometric and geometric properties (spherical forms). Moreover [12] tried to characterize a raindrop on windshield by different visual effects like: its circular form, the blurring region, and its texture.

Our method investigates how to detect focused raindrop in a scene. By analyzing the raindrop appearances in different scenes, and according to the works described in [1] and [14], we conclude that raindrop can be characterized by:

- A significant change of the gradient around the boundary.
- The area of the raindrop should be between 10 and 160 pixels.
- The shape of raindrop is similar to an eclipse.

Based on this properties, we propose an algorithm deploying three main steps; first we select a ROI (Region Of Interest) by applying an image segmentation based on morphological operations. Then, we apply a pattern recognition on ROI to eliminate false detections. Finally, we remove regions that do not fulfill the third property using an ellipse fitting. Figure 1 shows the process of our work.

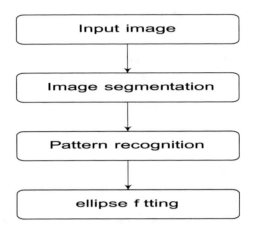

Fig. 1. Flowchart for proposed method

2.2   Image Segmentation

First of all, we apply an image segmentation based on morphological operations to detect raindrop candidates. Then we start our segmentation by searching for the frame edges. To extract them, we use a canny filter, which proves to be a powerful filter due to its insensitivity to noise. As illustrated in Table 1, the used canny filter [15] has a 5 × 5 window size, and a threshold value between 100 and 150, because the gradient change is important between the drop regions and its surrounding area. Figure 2b represents the image given by the canny filter.

Table 1. Parameters of segmentation

Steps	Properties
Canny filter	Windows size: 5 × 5
	Threshold value is between 100 and 150
Morphological gradient	Structural element: disk of size 20 pixels

Next, we apply a morphological gradient using a disk as a structural element with a diameter of 20 pixels. The morphological gradient is a powerful tool to detect regions with high intensity variations in an image [16]. It can be obtained from morphological processes (dilatation, erosion) as described by [16] in Eq. 1.

$$g(f) = \delta_B(f) - \in_B (f) \tag{1}$$

Having f as the image, B as the structural element, $\delta_B(f)$ represents the dilated image by B, and $\in_B(f)$ represents the eroded image by B. Figure 2c shows the results of applying the morphological gradient.

The image given after applying morphological gradient contains some dark pixels, which mislead the detection of exact region of raindrops. To resolve this problem, we apply a region filling. The term region filling consists on filling the dark pixels in the region. Therefore, the region of dark pixels in the binary image is removed or replaced. The results obtained by region filling is represented in Fig. 2d.

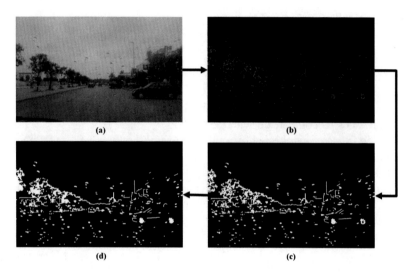

Fig. 2. **a** Original image. **b** The canny image. **c** The image given by applying morphological gradient. **d** The raindrop candidates after applying region filling

2.3 Pattern Recognition

For each connected component detected during the image segmentation, we apply some tests to eliminate false raindrop detections, based on the following raindrop characteristic:

- The number of pixels of each candidates' raindrops edges must be between 10 and 160 pixels.

2.4 Ellipse Fitting

To extract final candidate raindrops, we apply an ellipse fitting to select only elliptical regions from the image given by the second step, which fulfills the last raindrop characteristic.

We begin by generating an ellipse from the previous step's detected edges. This ellipse is described by the Eq. 2, where f_0 is a constant for the scale.

$$Ax^2 + 2Bxy + Cy^2 + 2f_0(Dx + Ey) + f_0^2 F = 0 \qquad (2)$$

To fit the regions, we search their ellipse parameters by applying least square approach [17]. Then we evaluate the results by calculating the rates between the edges area and the fitted ellipse area. We consider a raindrop if the rate is higher than threshold value as described in Eq. 3:

$$R = Q/E \geq th \qquad (3)$$

where Q is the edges area, E is the ellipse fitted area, and th is the threshold value to select an ellipse.

3   Results and Discussion

This section shows the results of our method using a video frame with adherent raindrops, besides its comparison with the method of [2].

The video frames are collected by a phone camera (Samsung galaxy S5) in a rainy day, installed under the car's inner rear mirror and located 10 cm away from the windshield. Moreover, we took three different video frames with a frequency of 29 frames per second, under various weather conditions (moderate rain; light rain), different road types (highway; urban road), and with different sizes (720×1280; 1080×1920). The algorithm is written in C++ using OPENCV library, and simulated on computer having an Intel(R) Core™ i5-2520M CPU@2.50 GHz processor, and 4Go of RAM.

Figure 4 shows some examples of raindrop detection by the proposed method and the Mser one under different situations. In order to evaluate the performance of the proposed method, we compare the accuracy of each method, by measuring the rate of missed and false detections as described in Eq. 4:

$$RMD = \frac{TN}{P}; \quad RFD = \frac{FP}{ND} \qquad (4)$$

where RMD is the rate of missed detection, RFD is the rate of false detection, TN is the true negative, FP is the false positive, P is the number of raindrops in a frame, and ND is the number of detections in a frame.

We summaries in Fig. 3 the results obtained by each method. In (a) and (b), the red curve represents the rates given by our method. while the blue one represents the rates obtained by Mser method. As we can see in Figs. 3 and 4, [2] has an important false detection rates, while our method exhibits a better performance in this field. However,

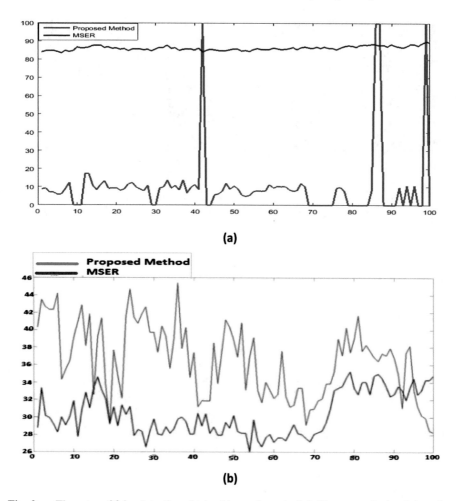

Fig. 3. **a** The rates of false detection obtained by each method. **b** The rates of missed detection obtained by each method

Further analysis showed that the missed detections rates of the proposed method is higher than Mser algorithm. But, we can have better results if we eliminate the regions of trees or give a solution to detect raindrops in these regions. For this, more data collection and analysis are required to determine how exactly the regions of trees affects the raindrop detection algorithm.

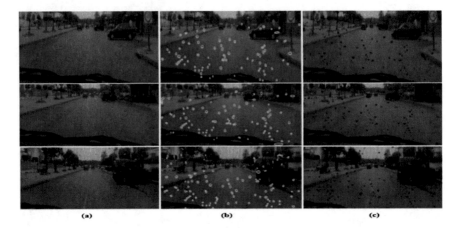

Fig. 4. Results of the raindrops detection using MSER and proposed method. **a** represents original images. **b** Represents the images produced by our method. **c** Represents the images produced by MSER

4   Conclusion

In this paper, we propose an approach to detect adherent raindrop in order to notify the driver of the rainy weather. The approach is based on Morphological operations and pattern recognition. The results demonstrated that our method succeed to reduce the number of false detections compared to the conventional method. But, our approach still limited on detecting raindrops in trees. Furthermore, we aim to reduce the rate of missed detections in the image and reduce more the algorithm's time of execution, all to remove raindrops from the scene and provide better frames to the ADAS.

References

1. Cord, A., Aubert, D.: Towards rain detection through use of in-vehicle multipurpose cameras. IEEE Intell. Veh. Symp. Proc. 399–404 (2011)
2. Ito, K., Noro, K., Aoki, T.: An adherent raindrop detection method using MSER. Proc. APSIPA Annu. Summit Conf. **2015**, 105–109 (2015)
3. Harsha, K., Reddy, V., Basha, M.S., Srinivasulu, J.: A simple approach for efficient detection and estimation of drops during the rainfall. Int. J. Innov. Sci. Eng. Technol. **2**, 203–207 (2015)
4. Cord, A., Gimonet, N.: Detecting unfocused raindrops. IEEE Robot. Autom. Mag. 49–56 (2014)
5. Ishizuka, J., Onoguchi, K.: Detection of raindrop with various shapes on a windshield. In: Proceedings of 5th International Conference on Pattern Recognition. Application Methods, pp. 475–483 (2016)
6. Wu, Q., Zhang, W., Kumar, B.V.K.V.: Raindrop detection and removal using salient visual features. Icip **2012**, 941–944 (2012)

7. Kurihata, H., Takahashi, T., Ide, I., Mekada, Y., Murase, H., Tamatsu, Y., Miyahara, T.: Rainy weather recognition from in-vehicle camera images for driver assistance. IEEE Intell. Veh. Symp. Proc. 205–210 (2005)

8. Kurihata, H., Takahashi, T., Ide, I., Mekada, Y., Hiroshi Murase, Y.T.† and T.M.†: Detection of raindrops on a windshield from an in-vehicle video camera. Int. J. Innov. Comput. Inf. Control. **3**, 1583–1591 (2007)

9. Al Machot, F., Ali, M., Haj Mosa, A., Schwarzlmüller, C., Gutmann, M., Kyamakya, K.: Real-time raindrop detection based on cellular neural networks for ADAS. J. Real-Time Image Process. 1–13 (2016)

10. Halimeh, J.C., Roser, M.: Raindrop detection on car windshields using geometric-photometric environment construction and intensity-based correlation. IEEE Intell. Veh. Symp. Proc. 610–615 (2009)

11. Roser, M., Geiger, A.: Video-based raindrop detection for improved image registration. 2009 IEEE 12th Int. Conf. Comput. Vis. Work. ICCV Work. 570–577 (2009)

12. Wahab, M.H.A., Su, C.H., Zakaria, N., Salam, R.A.: Review on raindrop detection and removal in weather degraded images. 2013 5th Int. Conf. Comput. Sci. Inf. Technol. CSIT 2013 - Proc. 82–88 (2013)

13. Garg, K., Nayar, S.K.: When does a camera see rain? Tenth IEEE Int. Conf. Comput. Vis. **2**, 1067–1074 (2005)

14. Fouad, E., Abdelhak, E., Salma, A.: Modelisation of raindrops based on declivity principle. Proc. - Comput. Graph. Imaging Vis. New Tech. Trends, CGiV 2016. 2, 6–9 (2016)

15. Canny, J.: A computational approach to edge detection. IEEE Trans. Pattern Anal. Mach. Intell. PAMI-8, 679–698 (1986)

16. Rivest, J.-F., Soille, P., Beucher, S.: Morphological gradients. (1992). http://proceedings.spiedigitallibrary.org/proceeding.aspx?doi=10.1117/12.58373

17. Fitzgibbon, A.W., Fisher, R.B., Pilu, M.: Direct least squares fitting of ellipses. IEEE Trans. Pattern Anal. Mach. Intell. **21**, 1–15 (1996)

Collaborative Filtering Recommender System

Yassine Afoudi[✉], Mohamed Lazaar, and Mohamed Al Achhab

New Trends Technology, Abdelmalek Essaadi University, Tetuan, Morocco
{yassine.afoudi,lazaarmd,alachhab}@gmail.com

Abstract. Recently, with the presence of a lot of information and the emergence of many programs, sites and companies that provide items to customers like Amazon for products or Netflix for movies …, it was necessary to exploit this data to achieve a quantum leap in the world of technology and specially do not leave the customer confused in the item to be chosen among other huge options, so many of sciences that are interested in the field of Big data and using the large information to meet the needs of users intervened to improve the area of recommendation such as data science, machine learning…. however there is one solution to give suggestions for customers is recommender systems. Recommender systems is a useful information filtering tool for guiding users in a personalized way of discovering products or services they might be interested in from a large space of possible options. It predicts interests of users and makes recommendation according to the interest model of users. On one hand, there is a traditional recommender systems recommend items based on different criteria of users or items like item price, user profile …on another hand we have recommender systems using deep learning techniques even if not been well explored yet. In this article, we first introduce different kinds of the most famous category of recommender systems and focus on one type to do movies recommendations and then make a quantitative comparison.

Keywords: Collaborative filtering · Information filtering · Movies
recommendation · Recommender system

1 Introduction

In the last decade, we have seen a very significant increase in all kind of information; especially information shared via smart phones the most well-known device in our generation. As a result, the amount of information available does not allow the average user to know all of his options. In this context, recommendation systems use several techniques to help the user to find the desired product. Hence, nowadays, recommendation systems play an important role.

1.1 Recommender Systems

In recent decades, with the emergence of various products and services provided by many companies to meet the needs of the customer, this customer is in the circle of confusion about the product to be chosen from the huge number of choices. Recommendation systems are designed to help customers by offering product or service

© Springer Nature Switzerland AG 2019
M. Ezziyyani (Ed.): AI2SD 2018, AISC 915, pp. 332–345, 2019.
https://doi.org/10.1007/978-3-030-11928-7_30

recommendations. These products and services are likely to be preferred by them. These recommendations are taken based on user preferences, item features, user-item past interactions and some other additional information such as temporal and spatial data needs, and purchase history…. Nowadays, the recommendation systems have been used to buy online, watch movies, listen to songs, find hotels, and even give jobs proposition…, a recommender systems is designed to give and recommend items I to the users U according to their preferences or rating, because often the customer provides an assessment of the items he has taken. Usually the work done by the recommendation systems are making predicting ratings or providing a ranked list of items for each user. Recommendation models are mainly categorized into three kinds of techniques collaborative filtering, content-based recommender system and hybrid recommender system. However, these models have their own limitations in dealing with data sparsity that mean cells of the dataset are either not filled with data or are zeros, and cold-start problems.

1.2 Techniques of Recommender Systems

Collaborative Filtering

Collaborative filtering (CF) follows a simple observation that users tend to buy items preferred by users with similar tastes for example if user u_1 likes products p_1, p_2, p_3 and user u_2 likes products p_2, p_3, p_7 then they have similar interests and user u_1 should like product p_7 and user u_2 should like p_1. This technique is based entirely on the past behavior and not on the context, that's why it's much known and useful in the field of recommendation. For example, a list of X users (u_1, u_2, …, u_x) and a list of Y items (i_1, i_2,…, i_Y) are given. A list of items, i_{ui}, has been rated by user u_j. The ratings can either be explicit indications on a 1–5 scale, or implicit indications. Implicit indications are generally implicit feedback, such as purchases or click-through, from users. A good overview of Collaborative Filtering is presented in Fig. 1.

CF techniques can be either memory-based or model-based.

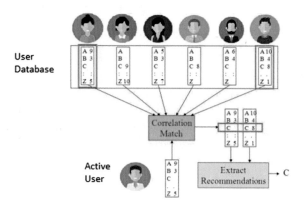

Fig. 1. Collaborative Filtering

Content-based Recommender System

Even that Collaborative Filtering is much known and useful but this model have limitations, and among them we have the most known problem is sparsity problem in another why those users who provide no ratings, in that case our model is unable to generate reasonable recommendations.

To deal with sparsity problem, researchers propose Content-based Recommender Systems is based on the observation between auxiliary information such as text, images and videos, and users such as their profiles. Suppose someone likes science fiction, romantic and action movies, and doesn't like fantasy movies. Overtime the algorithm can accumulate this and figure out that the user has positive rating on genres like science fiction, romance and action, and lower rating for fantasy. The algorithm might also find out that there were some actors that user likes or dislikes. In this way even with small notes, the user's preference can still be deduced.

The main difference between Content Based Filtering and Collaborative Filtering is that Collaborative Filtering works on preferences of users with similar preferences for some items to recommend new items whereas Content Based Filtering is based on the observation between auxiliary information and not at all concerned with preferences of the other users. The main difference is illustrated in Fig. 2.

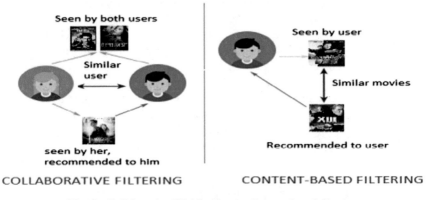

Fig. 2. Collaborative Filtering versus Content-based filtering

Hybrid Recommender System

The hybrid recommendation system refers to the recommendation system that uses two or more types of recommendation strategies to gain better performance with fewer of the drawbacks of any individual one. Most commonly, collaborative filtering is combined with some other technique.

2   Collaborative Filtering for Recommender Systems

In this article, we are interested in the technique of collaborative filtering to make a small comparison on existing methods. Collaborative recommendation is probably the most familiar, most widely implemented and most mature of the technologies. Collaborative recommender systems aggregate ratings or recommendations of objects, recognize commonalities between users on the basis of their ratings, and generate new recommendations based on inter-user comparisons.

This technique can be either Memory-Based Collaborative Filtering, comparing users against each other directly using correlation or other measures, or Model-Based Collaborative filtering, in which a model is derived from the historical rating data and used to make predictions.

2.1   Memory-Based Collaborative Filtering

In memory-based systems, recommendations or predictions are based on similarity values. Also to calculate similarity or weight between users or items we use rating data.

There are several advantages of memory-based CF. First of all, since we only need to calculate similarity, it is easy to implement. Second, memory-based CF systems are scalable to large size data. Third, most of memory-based systems are online learning models. Thus, new arrival data can be handled easily. At last, the recommendations results can be understood and can provide feedback to explain why recommend these items. However, several limitations are also existed in memory-based CF techniques. For example, since the similarity values are based on common items, when data are sparse and common rated items are very few, the recommendation results are unreliable and not accurate.

Neighbor-based CF is one of the most representative memory-based CF models, neighbor-based CF involves in two steps: similarity calculation and prediction. In the similarity calculation step, the similarity values can be measured between users or items. Users are similar if their vectors are close according to some distance measure such as Jaccard or cosine distance.

For Jaccard distance as show in Eq. 2, only considers the number of common ratings between two users. The basic idea is that users are more similar if they have more common ratings. The drawback is that it does not consider the absolute ratings. For example, user U1 rates 5 and 4 on item I1 and item I2, user U2 rates 1 and 2, user U3 rates 4 and 5. Obviously, user U 1 and user U3 are more similar.

As we say Vector Cosine-based Similarity is another similarity metric used to measure the difference between documents. Documents are represented as a vector of word frequency. In neighbor-based CF, Vector Cosine-based Similarity is adopted to compute the similarity across users or items. As shown in Eq. 1, Vector Cosine-based Similarity between item i and item j can be derived.

$$\mathrm{W}i,j = \cos(\vec{i},\vec{j}) = \frac{\vec{i}.\vec{j}}{\left\|\vec{i}\right\| \times \left\|\vec{j}\right\|} \tag{1}$$

$$\sin(u, v)^{\text{Jaccard}} = \frac{|Iu| \cap |Iv|}{|Iu| \cup |Iv|} \tag{2}$$

In neighbor-based CF, to generate recommendations or predictions for user U, we use similarity to generate a set of users that are close to user U. Then, the prediction of user U can be calculated by using ratings from the set of users.

Memory-Based Collaborative Filtering approaches can be divided into two main sections user-item filtering and item-item filtering.

User-Item Collaborative Filtering

The user-Item CF is quite like item-item CF. Instead of computing the similarity between two items, we focus on the similarity between two users. We use Jaccard-based method of computing similarity between two customers u, v.

This technique takes a particular user, find users that are similar to that user based on similarity of ratings, and recommend items that those similar users liked, as seen in Fig. 3, the similarity values between users are measured by observing all the items that are rated by both users.

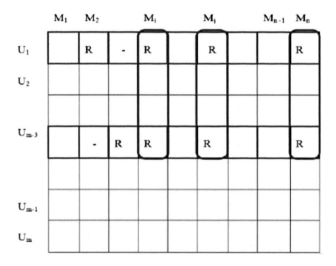

Fig. 3. Principe of user-item collaborative filtering

Item-Item Collaborative filtering

Computing the similarity between items is the fundamental step of our recommendation system, since we want to recommend similar items to users based on what they have bought before. The basic idea of similarity computation between two items i and j is to firstly isolate the users who have rated both of these items and then to apply a similarity computation technique to determine the similarity.

It's takes an item, find users who liked that item, and find other items that those users or similar users also liked, as seen in Fig. 4, the similarity values between items are measured by observing all the users who are rated both items.

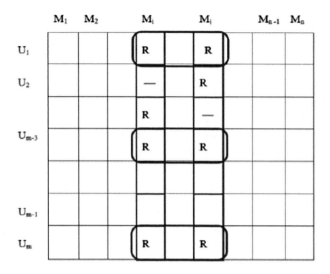

Fig. 4. Principe of item-item collaborative filtering

The user-based CF has some limitations. One is its difficulty in measuring the similarities between users, and the other is the scalability issue. As the number of users and products increases, the computation time of algorithms grows exponentially. The item-based CF was proposed to overcome the scalability problem as it calculates item similarities in an offline basis. It assumes that a user will be more likely to purchase items that are similar or related to the items that he or she has already purchased. Another one is the ratings, which are some discrete values, cannot provide us much information about relationship between users and items.

2.2   Model-Based Collaborative Filtering

Model-based CF is based on machine learning or data mining models, finds rating using training data. After the training process, model-based CF becomes capable of making intelligent and personalized prediction, also doing better recommendations for users. Model-based CF algorithms are developed to counter the shortcomings of memory-based CF models.

The most successful model-based CF techniques is Matrix Factorization. Matrix factorization techniques get the matrix containing all available ratings in the datasets and find a feature set for each user and item (for as the movies are our items) as the result of the factorization process. Then, the rating of each user assigns to each item can get estimated by the scalar product of the two feature vectors of those user and item. As shown in Fig. 5 we have 3 users and 4 movies for each movie we have the rating giving by user but the problem that many users doesn't give rating to items, that's why we use matrix factorization for find two vectors of user and item, like that if we want to estimate or predict the rating that may be giving to a movie by a user we can do just the scalar product of those two feature vectors. In this way, items which are favored by similar users will share similar latent features.

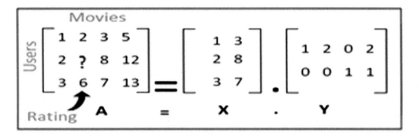

Fig. 5. Example of matrix factorization technique

As shown in Eq. 3, Matrix Factorization approximates the rating matrix R with two matrices: U and I, which are latent factors of users and items, respectively. Each row of matrix U and each column of matrix I are the latent factors of a user or item respectively. By multiplying latent factors of a user to latent factors of an item, we get an estimation of the corresponding rating.

$$R \approx U \times I \tag{3}$$

3   Dataset

We use in this purpose the MovieLens dataset. It has been collected by the GroupLens Research Project at the University of Minnesota. The dataset consists of movies released on or before July 2017, we extract only ratings data for training and testing contains 100,000 ratings from 700 users on 9000 movies. The sparseness of the collected dataset is hence more than 95.5%.

4   Implementation

4.1   Experimental Steps

First of all, we will split the whole dataset into the training set and the test set. We will build two recommendation system using two techniques of collaborative filtering which filters information of a user based on a collection of user ratings in the training set, after that predict and give recommendations on what items that user will buy in the future. We will test and evaluate our predictions by searching whether the items that we recommend to a user according to the training set, are in the item list the user have bought in the test set.

To implementing what we are defining above we choose Item similarity model for Memory-Based Collaborative Filtering and Singular-value decomposition SVD for Model-Based Collaborative filtering.

For Item similarity model we firstly build a co-occurrence matrix item by item, that mean we take all available unique movies and we create a matrix with all possible combination between movies, and for values of this matrix is that how many users have seen movie A and movie B for example, after that we normalize this matrix by using Jaccard similarity as shown in Eq. 4. After that we calculate a weighted average of the scores in co-occurrence matrix as shown in Fig. 6.

$$\frac{\text{Number of users common for movies } i \text{ and } j}{\text{Number of user for either movies } i \text{ or } j} \qquad (4)$$

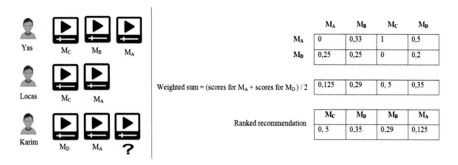

Fig. 6. Example of recommendation using item similarity

For the second method of collaborative Filtering is Singular-value decomposition, SVD is the well-known matrix factorization method. Collaborative Filtering can be formulated by approximating a matrix X by using singular value decomposition. In 2006, Netflix, a global provider of streaming movies and TV series, announced an open competition to predict user ratings for films, based on previous ratings without any information about the users or the films, SVD matrix factorization models are using by the winning team at this competition, the general equation can be expressed as Eq. 5, SVD result gives three matrices as output: U, S and V^T (T means transpose), matrix U represents user vectors and Matrix V^T represents item vectors. In simple terms, U represents users as two dimensional points in the latent vector space, and V^T represents items as two dimensional points in the same space. Elements on the diagonal in S are known as singular values of X. For making prediction of ratings using this method we simply taking the dot product of U, S and VT as shown in Eq. 6. We apply for our study this technique on the train matrix that contains rows represents users and columns represents movies and as values all available ratings.

$$X = U \times S \times V^T \qquad (5)$$

$$\hat{X} = U \cdot S \cdot V^T \qquad (6)$$

4.2 Experimental Platform

All our experiments were implemented using Python and compiled using Jupyter notebook. We ran all our experiments on a Windows7 based PC with Intel core i5 processor having a speed of 2.5 GHz and 4 GB of RAM.

4.3 Experiment Results

After building our models, we have tested the item-similarity and singular value decomposition on user 1, Table 1 show us result of the experiment.

Table 1. Result experiment of the two collaborative filtering models on user 1

	Recommended movies	
	Using item similarity	Using SVD
Movie1	Eraser (1996)	Star Trek VI: The Undiscovered Country (1991)
Movie2	Star Maps (1997)	Air Bud (1997)
Movie3	Hate (Haine, La) (1995)	First Kid (1996)
Movie4	Free Willy 3: The Rescue (1997)	Local Hero (1983)
Movie5	Fall (1997)	Once Upon a Time... When We Were Colored (1995)

5 Evaluation and Quantitative Comparison

5.1 Evaluation

In recommender systems, the most important result for the final user is to receive an ordered list of recommendations, from best to worst. In fact, in some cases the user doesn't care much about the exact ordering of the list, a set of few good recommendations is fine. Taking this fact into evaluation of recommender systems, there are many evaluation techniques to evaluate accuracy of predicted ratings such as Root Mean Squared Error (RMSE) and Precision-Recall method, for this study we used the second technique to evaluate our result.

Precision and recall are the most popular metrics for evaluating information retrieval systems. In 1968, Cleverdon proposed them as the key metrics, and they have held ever since. For the evaluation of recommender systems, they have been used by Billsus and Pazzani (1998), Basu et al. (1998), and Sarwar et al. (2000a, b).

The item set must be separated into two classes—relevant or not relevant. That is, if the rating scale is not already binary, we need to transform it into a binary scale. For example, the MovieLens dataset has a rating scale of 1–5 and is commonly transformed into a binary scale by converting every rating of 4 or 5 to "relevant" and all ratings of 1–3 to "not relevant." For precision and recall, we also need to separate the item set into the set that was returned to the user (selected/recommended), and the set that was not. We assume that the user will consider all items that are retrieved.

In another way Precision and Recall are two measurements for statistics, which are used to evaluate the quality of statistic result. Precision is used to calculate the ratio of related items with selected items. Recall is used to calculate the ratio of related items with all related items in selected items.

For this method, data is first divided in a training set and a test set. The algorithm runs on the training set, giving a list of recommended items. The concept of 'hit set' is considered, 'hit set' containing only the recommended (top-N) items that are also in the test set. Recall and precision are then determined as Eqs. 7 and 8.

$$Recall = \frac{Size\ of\ hit\ set}{Size\ of\ test\ set} \tag{7}$$

$$Precision = \frac{Size\ of\ hit\ set}{N} \tag{8}$$

The precision is the proportion of recommendations that are good recommendations, and recall is the proportion of good recommendations that appear in top recommendations.

Generally we should comprehensively consider precision and recall, then we introduce F-Measure, which is defined in Eq. 9.

$$F - Measure = \frac{2 \times Precision \times Recall}{Precision + Recall} \tag{9}$$

5.2   Quantitative Comparison Between the Models

After building and testing the models we want to evaluate which model gives us much better recommendation for our database of movies, that's why we use precision-recall curves and Fig. 7 show us a plot precision recall curve, by reading and observing the results we can't assume which model give us better recommendation, that's why we made a comparison of results calculated by Equations above. The result is in Table 2.

As we can see in Table 2, Figs. 7 and 8, the precision, Recall and F-Measure by Item similarity are all higher than that of SVD. We conclude that the item similarity provides much better performance in recommendation of our database over the Singular-value decomposition SVD, even that SVD have a very important role to predict the ratings in the case of sparsity but can be very slow and computationally expensive.

6   Conclusion and Future Work

In this work we decided to give an overview about the recommendation systems and the role of evolution of science to give best recommendations and better predictions. We also talked about kinds of techniques involved in recommender systems.

Collaborative Filtering, Content-based Recommender System and Hybrid recommender System, for this study we are focused on Collaborative Filtering that can be

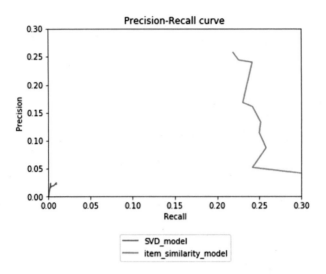

Fig. 7. Precision-Recall curve of our models

Table 2. Comparison of item similarity model and SVD model

Users id	Item similarity model			SVD model		
	P	R	F	P	R	F
User 416	0.4	0.153	22.13	0.1	0.038	5.50
User 575	0.2	0.016	2.96	0.2	0.016	2.96
User 518	0.4	0.028	5.23	0.2	0.014	2.59
User 15	0.6	0.017	3.30	0.1	0.002	0.39
User 547	0.7	0.014	2.74	0.1	0.0021	0.41
User 94	0.4	0.111	17.37	0.1	0.0277	4.33

divided into Memory-Based Collaborative Filtering and Model-Based Collaborative filtering, also we tested item similarity model for Memory-Based and Singular-value decomposition the most known Matrix Factorization method on MovieLens dataset. The result of our study indicates that Memory-Based collaborative filtering does improve the performance over the Model-Based Collaborative filtering in movies recommendation.

By necessity, as masses of information become ubiquitously available, collaborative filtering will not give us better recommendation. In the process, with the development of machine learning, large-scale network and high performance computing is promoting new development in this field we will continue in another study to explore others techniques used in recommended systems and we will consider the following aspects in future work.

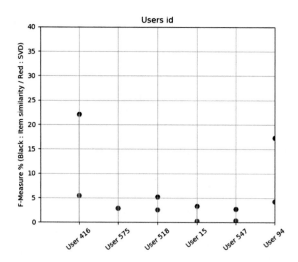

Fig. 8. Comparison of Item similarity model and SVD model in histogram format

- Use content-based recommendation techniques
- Use Term Frequency- Inverse Document Frequency technique for making recommendation.
- Use features instead of rating for making recommendation.
- Use more techniques to evaluate our models
- Introduce machine learning.

Acknowledgements. We would like to express our sincere thanks to members of new technology trends our research laboratory. Their advices and comments are gratefully acknowledged.

References

Koren, Y., Bell, R., Volinsky, C.: Matrix factorization techniques for recommender systems. Computer (2009)

Zhang, S., Yao, L., Sun, A.: Deep learning based recommender system: a survey and new perspectives. ACM J. Comput. Cult. Herit. **1**, 1, Article 35 (2017)

Hegde, A., Shetty, S.K.: Collaborative filtering recommender system. Int. J. Emerg. Trends Sci. Technol. (2015)

Ben Schafer, J., Frankowski, D., Herlocker, J., Sen, S.: Collaborative Filtering Recommender Systems

Wang, N., Yeung, D.-Y.: Collaborative Deep Learning for Recommender Systems (2015)

Saga, R., Hayashi, Y., Tsuji, H.: Hotel recommender system based on user's preference transition. In: IEEE International Conference on Systems (2008)

Yao, G., Cai, L.: User-Based and Item-Based Collaborative Filtering Recommendation Algorithms Design

Adomavicius, G., Tuzhilin, A.: Toward the next generation of recommender systems: a survey of the State-of-the-Art and possible extensions. IEEE Trans. Knowl. Data Eng. **17**(6), 734–749 (2005)

Balabanovíc, M., Shoham, Y.: Fab: content-based, collaborative recommendation. Commun. ACM **40**(3), 66–72 (1997)

Basu, C., Hirsh, H., Cohen, W.W.: Recommendation as classification: using social and content-based information in recommendation. In: Proceedings of the Fifteenth National Conference on Artificial Intelligence, pp. 714–720. AAAI Press, Madison, Wisconsin (1998)

Breese, J.S., Heckerman, D., Kadie, C.: Empirical analysis of predictive algorithms for collaborative filtering. In Proceeding of the Fourteenth Conference on Uncertainty in Artificial Intelligence (UAI). Morgan Kaufmann, Madison, Wisconsin (1998)

Canny, J.: Collaborative filtering with privacy via factor analysis. In: Proceedings of the 25th Annual International ACM SIGIR Conference on Research and Development in Information Retrieval. ACM Press, Tampere, Finland (2002)

Claypool, M., Gokhale, A., Miranda, T., Murnikov, P., Netes, D., Sartin, M.: Combining content-based and collaborative filters in an online newspaper. In: Proceedings of the ACM SIGIR '99 Workshop on Recommender Systems: Algorithms and Evaluation. Berkeley, California (1999)

En-Naimani, Z., Lazaar, M., Ettaouil, M.: Architecture optimization model for the probabilistic self-organizing maps and speech compression. Int. J. Comput. Intell. Appl. (2016)

Cosley, D., Lam, S.K., Albert, I., Konstan, J.A., Riedl, J.: Is seeing believing?: How recommender system interfaces affect users' opinions. In: Proceedings of the SIGCHI Conference on Human Factors in Computing Systems. ACM Press, Ft. Lauderdale, Florida, USA (2003)

Ettaouil, M., Lazaar, M., Elmoutaouakil, K., Haddouch, K.: A new algorithm for optimization of the kohonen network architectures using the continuous hopfield networks. WSEAS Trans. Comput. (2013)

Dahlen, B.J., Konstan, J.A., Herlocker, J., Riedl, J.: Jump-starting Movielens: User Benefits of Starting a Collaborative Filtering System with "Dead Data". TR 98-017, University of Minnesota

Delgado, J., Ishii, N.: Memory-based weighted majority prediction for recommender systems. In 1999 SIGIR Workshop on Recommender Systems, pp. 1–5. University of California, Berkeley (1999)

Harper, F., Li, X., Chen, Y., Konstan, J.: An economic model of user rating in an online recommender system. In: Proceedings of the 10th International Conference on User Modeling. Edinburgh, UK (2005)

Konstan, J.A., Miller, B., Maltz, D., Herlocker, J., Gordon, L., Riedl, J.: GroupLens: applying collaborative filtering to usenet news. Commun. ACM **40**(3), 77–87

Linden, G., Smith, B., York, J.: Amazon.Com Recommendations: item-to-item collaborative filtering. IEEE Internet Comput. **7**(1) (2003)

Oard, D.W., Kim, J.: Implicit feedback for recommender systems. In: Proceedings of the AAAI Workshop on Recommender Systems. Madison, Wisconsin (1998)

Popescul, A., Ungar, L.H., Pennock, D.M., Lawrence, S.: Probabilistic Models for Unified Collaborative and Content-Based Recommendation in Sparse-Data Environments, pp. 437–444 (2001)

Hofmann, T.: Latent semantic models for collaborative filtering. ACM Trans. Inf. Syst. **22**(1), 89–115 (2004a)

Das, A., Datar, M., Garg, A., Rajaram, S.: Google news personalization: scalable online collaborative filtering. In: Proceedings of the 16th International Conference on World Wide Web (WWW) (2007)

Liu, J., Dolan, P., Pederson, E.: Personalized news recommendation based on click behavior. In: Proceedings of the 14th International Conference on Intelligent User Interface (IUI) (2010)

Hu, Y., Koren, Y., Volinsky, C.: Collaborative filtering for implicit feedback datasets. In: Proceedings of 8th International Conference on Data Mining (2008)

Parra, D., Karatzoglou, A., Amatriain, X., Yavuz, I.: Implicit feedback recommendation via implicit-to-explicit ordinal logistic regression mapping. In: Workshop on Context-Aware Recommender Systems in 5th ACM Conference on Recommender Systems (2011)

Poriya, A., Patel, N., Bhagat, T., Sharma, R.: Non-personalized recommender systems and user-based collaborative recommender systems. Int. J. Appl. Inf. Syst. 6(9), 22–27 (2014)

Herlocker, J., Konstan, J.A., Terveen, L.G., Reidl, J.: Evaluating collaborative filtering recommender systems. ACM Trans. Inf. Syst., 5–53 (2004)

Herlocker, J.L., Konstan, J.A., Riedl, J.: Explaining collaborative filtering recommendations. In: Proceedings of the 2000 ACM Conference on Computer Supported Cooperative Work, pp. 241–250. ACM Press, Philadelphia, Pennsylvania (2000)

Hofmann, T.: Latent semantic models for collaborative filtering. ACM Trans. Inf. Syst. (TOIS) 22(1), 89–115 (2004b)

Karypis, G.: Evaluation of item-based Top-N recommendation algorithms. In: 10th Conference of Information and Knowledge Management (CIKM), pp. 247–254 (2001)

Lam, S.K. Riedl, J.: Shilling recommender systems for fun and profit. In: Proceedings of the 13th International Conference on World Wide Web, pp. 393–402. ACM Press, New York, NY, USA (2004)

Lin, W.: Association rule mining for collaborative recommender systems. Master's Thesis, Worcester Polytechnic Institute, May 2000

McLaughlin, M., Herlocker, J.: A collaborative filtering algorithm and evaluation metric that accurately model the user experience. In: Proceedings of the SIGIR Conference on Research and Development in Information Retrieval, pp. 329–336 (2004)

Miller, B.N., Konstan, J.A., Riedl, J.: Pocketlens: toward a personal recommender system. ACM Trans. Inf. Syst. 22(3), 437–476 (2004)

O'Connor, M., Cosley, D., Konstan, J.A., Riedl, J.: PolyLens: a recommender system for groups of users. In: Proceedings of ECSCW 2001, pp. 199–218. Bonn, Germany (2001)

Adomavicius, G., Tuzhilin, A.: Toward the next generation of recommender systems: a survey of the state-of-the-art and possible extensions. IEEE Trans. Knowl. Data Eng. 17(6), 734–749 (2005)

Agichtein, E., Brill, E., Dumais, S., Ragno, R.: Learning user interaction models for predicting web search result preferences. In: ACM SIGIR '06, pp. 3–10. ACM, New York (2006)

Ali, K., van Stam, W.: TiVo: Making Show Recommendations Using a Distributed Collaborative Filtering Architecture. In: ACM KDD '04, pp. 394–401. ACM, New York (2004)

Ansari, A., Essegaier, S., Kohli, R.: Internet recommendation systems. J. Mark. Res. 37(3), 363–375 (2000)

Avery, C., Zeckhauser, R.: Recommender systems for evaluating computer messages. Commun. ACM 40(3), 88–89, ACM ID: 245127 (1997)

Balabanović, M., Shoham, Y.: Fab: content-based, collaborative recommendation. Commun. ACM 40(3), 66–72 (1997)

Billsus, D., Pazzani, M.J.: Learning collaborative information filters. In: AAAI 2008 Workshop on Recommender Systems (1998)

Brand, M.: Fast online SVD revisions for lightweight recommender systems. In: SIAM International Conference on Data Mining, pp. 37–46. SIAM (2003)

Burke, R.: Evaluating the dynamic properties of recommendation algorithms. In: ACM RecSys '10, pp. 225–228. ACM, New York (2010)

Introducing a Traceability Based Recommendation Approach Using Chatbot for E-Learning Platforms

Kamal Souali[1]([✉]) [iD], Othmane Rahmaoui[1], and Mohammed Ouzzif[2]

[1] RITM ESTC Laboratory, Hassan II University, ENSEM, Casablanca, Morocco
{kml.souali,othmane.rahmaoui}@gmail.com
[2] RITM ESTC Laboratory, Hassan II University, EST, Casablanca, Morocco
ouzzif@gmail.com

Abstract. For many years, the use of recommender systems has increased and reached a new level recently. These systems are widely used in different areas, as they tend to offer and provide customers with the most suitable products or items that can satisfy their needs to the best. Especially in e-Learning environments, the purpose of such systems is to help students improve their learning by suggesting relevant resources and increase their knowledge through a selection of tips, hints, and tutorials. The process of recommendation considers the user's profile which is a set of preferences and interests and is based on various techniques, often combined to provide improved results. However, due to the huge amount of data, the selection process becomes more and more difficult to handle and the same items get proposed repeatedly. Traceability, on the other hand, can either mean the history or the composition of something. It is a collection of actors, actions, objects and most importantly, time. In this paper, we introduce the use and the benefits of traceability and discuss how it can enhance recommendations. We also propose a traceability based approach for recommendations in e-Learning platforms, by means of a chatbot.

Keywords: Recommendation · Recommender systems · Traceability · Trace · E-Learning · Chatbot

1 Introduction

Recently, teaching through the internet, without the traditional classroom limitations, has become a trend. E-Learning is an online interactive way meant for educational purposes and used for sharing information, following courses and communicating with other teachers and students. This form of communication can be established either through forums, through a messaging system or online, during a live classroom. Due to the huge number of available resources in an e-Learning environment, which are continuously improved and changed, there is always a need to provide guidance and offer the most interesting and relevant materials to learners and students. A Recommendation is a suggestion or a proposal that can fulfill best the needs of a user, given by someone who has more experience on a specific field or subject. It is generally considered as good or suitable for a certain job or purpose.

© Springer Nature Switzerland AG 2019
M. Ezziyyani (Ed.): AI2SD 2018, AISC 915, pp. 346–357, 2019.
https://doi.org/10.1007/978-3-030-11928-7_31

As stated in [1], a recommender system primarily helps students who lack adequate personal experience or competent to evaluate and to make better choices from the potentially overwhelming number of alternative items. This system is able to assist the learners and students to discover suitable resources that match their profiles and thus provide them with personalized contextual contents at the right time and in the right way [2].

Sawant et al. [3], explained that recommender systems are considered as information filtering systems that select carefully vital information fragments (items), and predict which item would be a subject of interest or satisfaction to the active user. To suggest these top n items, the process of recommendation always considers the user's preferences and interests, as well as his ratings of current items [4].

These systems tend to use a variety of techniques such as filtering techniques (collaborative, content-based, knowledge-based). They even apply various data mining methodologies to recommend efficiently for all active users, based on their ratings given for previous items and on similar users as well [5]. But for more improved recommendations, they may combine other techniques like graphs and ontologies to form a hybrid recommender system.

In fact, as described by Anuvareepong et al. [6], hybrid recommender systems are more reliable in many fields. They overcome the issues of traditional systems, and the combination of algorithms focusing on user-centric and real-time relevance feedback, provide strong and accurate recommendations. Whether they are based on ratings, on preferences or on implicit feedback, recommender systems are taking part of our life and are being used widely by many people so far. Nowadays, they are no longer personal recommender systems, rather they are group recommender systems which list out recommendations for a group of users [4].

The rest of this paper is organized as follows: In Sect. 2, we give definitions of traceability and its benefits. Section 3 presents the main filtering techniques used in recommender systems. A discussion about the traceability roles in the process of recommendation will be the object of Sect. 4. Section 5 contains recent related works in e-Learning. We will present our traceability based recommendation (TR) approach in Sect. 6 and in Sect. 7, we will give a brief conclusion.

2 Traceability

In general, the definition and the use of "traceability" follows certain standards and laws like the European General Food Law (EGFL) [7], the Global Standard (GS1) [8] and the International Organization for Standardization (ISO) [9] (ISO 9001:2000, ISO 22005:2007). There are many definitions on the internet for traceability, and each one of them has a different meaning and describes a specific object. Even though it is limited to a set of criteria and rules, it always reflects the context in which it is being used.

Traceability is a two ways process: one from upstream to downstream called "tracking" and the other, is from downstream to upstream, known as "tracing". Bruno Schiffers explained in a training manual [10] the following:

- Tracking answers the questions of "Where?" and "When?" and takes interest in the product's logistics.
- Tracing focuses on the product's contents and answers the questions of "What?", "With what?", "How?", "By whom?" and "Why?".

Traceability is a well-coordinated and a well-documented movement of a product or an artefact from one state to another. As previously mentioned in [11], we defined "traceability" as the ability to keep a detailed history of all activities and changes that an object can undergo throughout its entire life cycle, considering the different relationships that may appear. This object can be a resource, a material, a product, a model or even a class or an artefact in a software development platform.

Traceability can be used in many ways and has several benefits. In software development, for instance, it is represented as links or associations between pair of artefacts: between a source and a target. It is used not only to provide insights and demonstrate that a rigorous development process has been followed [12], but also to certify a safety-critical product and to show that all requirements were implemented [13]. Additionally, it is a way to support the maintainability, changeability and sustainability of these artefacts within a software system [14].

In the industry, whether the activity concerns food, fish, or other kinds of consumable products, traceability represents the relations between a material and its composition or transformations, through all the production's stages. It is then used to keep a complete record of these processes, including customer requirements, test measurements, and metrics, and ensure the final product's quality and safety. The same thing is applied in heavy industries, where the safety and security of humans is questioned.

In e-commerce, these links represent the relations between users and items (e.g. orders, purchases, ratings), while in e-Learning, they represent the relations between students and resources (e.g. ranks, lessons, scores), including their browsing's history.

Traceability Systems are considered as important tools in a production environment. They are used to ensure data reliability, as well as to help companies or institutions improve their processes, their productivity and efficiency and hence, reduce their costs (time, privacy, budget, … etc.).

3   Filtering Techniques

Recommender Systems have been praised for many years due to their ability to predict and suggest relevant items that meet users' interests and expectations and hence, solve the problem of information overload. To achieve this goal, these systems use several filtering techniques that exploit users' profiles, browsing activities and history, demographic data, rating matrixes and other textual information.

Among the techniques that are used in a recommendation, collaborative filtering and content-based filtering are the most dominants. The first is based mainly on ratings while the second is based on textual characteristics. Nevertheless, other combined techniques known as hybrid, are becoming more and more popular, due to their ability to overcome techniques' limitations and to their improved ability to generate quick and relevant suggestions.

3.1 Collaborative Filtering

According to [15], Collaborative Filtering is an efficient and well organized method for recommendation systems and its core scheme is to calculate the relation among the products and users based on preferences. In fact, authors in [16], explained that this filtering is mainly based on the ratings which are collected from users to identify others with similar interests and to predict which items the active user may be interested in.

The recommendation process using this filtering is based on a user-item matrix. Once created from the behaviour history data of the user (ratings), the degree of similarity between any two users or between any two items is calculated from this matrix. Therefore, user participation is a vital key to the success of CF based recommendation.

Collaborative Filtering has various methods such as memory-based and model-based. In the model-based approach, a model is built based on previous ratings then it learns and improves recommendations using machine learning techniques. We will only consider the memory-based approach in this study, since it is based on behaviour history data such as users' browsing and interacting activities.

Kawasaki and Hasuike [17] said that there are two types of collaborative filtering: user-based and item-based. User-based Collaborative Filtering finds users with similar preferences to the target user, then recommends items that similar users are purchasing but the target user does not purchase. Item-based Collaborative Filtering recommends items that are similar to the items that the target user prefers. Simply put, the first method attempts to estimate or predict the products based on the interests and the behaviour of other users related to the customer, while the second method tends to estimate or predict the products by computing similarity amongst the products [15].

Even though it uses several techniques, the Collaborative Filtering has yet to be improved, as it still suffers from a so-called sparse issue. At first, the number of total items available for recommendation is always much larger than the number of items previously seen or rated. Secondly, the time-consuming task of rating items, in case it was performed, can only be done once obtaining experience on them. Finally, newly added items could never be recommended because of insufficient ratings.

3.2 Content-Based Filtering

Content-based filtering approaches always operate based on textual representation. It utilizes a series of discrete characteristics of an item to recommend additional items with similar properties [18].

This filtering uses a machine learning algorithm to induce a profile of the user's preferences from training examples based on a content's description feature. It compares the profile of a user with the items that are analysed. Each item consists of descriptors or words that are related to the item. The same goes for the user's profile; its descriptors are added depending on the items previously seen by the user [19].

The process of recommendation is executed through two phases. In the first phase, the preferred items' descriptions are analysed to extract the preferences that can be utilized to describe these items and which will be stored in a user profile. The second phase consists of comparing each items' attributes with the user profile so that only related items which have a high degree of similarity with it would be recommended to the active user [20].

Several techniques and measurements are used to compute recommendations. However, the content-based filtering does not consider multimedia data types and does not take into account duplicated keywords or new users during the recommendation.

3.3   Knowledge-Based Filtering

Knowledge is data which was acquired through experience or education. Recommender systems that usually use this kind of filtering, build suggestions based mainly on knowledge about the user's need for an item and therefore, can reason about the relationship between a need and a possible item [4].

Although this type of filtering successfully overcome the problem of cold start, it still needs a quick and a strong knowledge acquisition process. It is only applied when facing difficulties using collaborative or content-based filtering.

3.4   Hybrid Filtering

Hybrid filtering approaches attempt to combine different techniques to eventually eliminate their drawbacks. In recent researches, both collaborative and content-based filtering are combined.

For instance, by proposing a novel movie recommender system, Pal et al. [21] have modified the content based algorithm that takes into consideration the tags and genres specified in the dataset, and instead of using Naive Bayes for text matching, they have used a simple comparator which compares and matches the tags and genres of two movies. Following their results, the algorithm reduced the sparsity of the user rating matrix.

Herath and Jayaratne [22] combined both collaborative (group clustering) and content-based filtering (media and content analysis), and proposed a system which provides effective recommendations of courses and assignments to students, in an e-Learning environment. Within the same context, a book recommender system was presented in [23]. The authors combined features of content-based filtering, collaborative filtering and association rule mining into a single algorithm that is executed through six steps and can produce efficient and effective recommendations.

Authors in [24] have also proposed a hybrid model that incrementally update similarity table of items and improve the relevance of the recommendation results by combining incremental update item-based collaborative filtering and content-based algorithm. As in [25], the authors presented a mixed approach based on complex attributes of goods. By combining the subjective scoring of users and objective scoring of commodities, the algorithm reflects user preferences, gets a hybrid rating and then computes data. The proposed model can solve the problem of extremely sparse user data through the scene classification, takes users' objective grading into account, overcomes the internet ghost-writers malicious rating and reflects user preferences.

Even though the hybrid approach is well known for providing relevant suggestions, there was no interest, in recent researches, in using and including traceability as a way of filtering technique for recommendations.

4   Gaps in Recommender Systems

Having said that recommender systems use hybrid filtering approaches to build efficient suggestions, they still suffer from some issues. According to a review made by Patel et al. [20], there are five issues with Recommender Systems. We will try in this section, to provide ideas and guidance on how to overcome these gaps using traceability.

4.1   Changing User Preferences

Recommender systems are mainly based on the user's interest and profile. The user's attraction and preferences are subject to changes after some time.

As shown in Fig. 1, traceability can be used to trace and record these changes. P_n is the resource while t_n represents is the time of change. When a preference or an interest is modified, depending on its status if it was added (P_4) or removed (P_3), we may as well adapt the suggestions and remove the items that do no longer belong to the new profile. There are always links between a preference and a resource and the user can also perform recalls to restore his previous preferences.

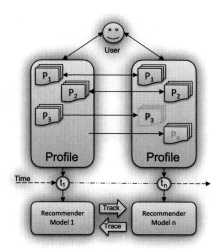

Fig. 1.   Traceability versus user preferences

4.2   Sparsity

The time-consuming task of rating items, can only be done once obtaining experience on them. If the user has rated just small number of items, then it is hard to conclude his taste and he could be related to false neighbourhood. Also, newly added items could never be recommended because of insufficient ratings.

Once an item is added, the recommendation process is launched to calculate a first similarity degree. As shown in Fig. 2, while this similarity remains low or incorrect, the item (R_n) will be kept in the selection until it gets the correct rating. If this item doesn't receive a feedback from the user to whom it was suggested (R_3) within a period of time (t_n) or gets a negative feedback (R_2, R_4), then it is automatically discarded. Traceability in this case is applied to track possible similarities.

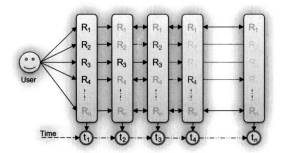

Fig. 2. Traceability versus sparsity

4.3 Scalability

The number of total items available for recommendation is always much larger than the number of items previously seen or rated and with the growth of numbers of users and items, the system needs more resources for processing information and giving recommendations.

Figure 3 represents how traceability can improve the time needed to generate a recommendation, where R_n are the previously seen items and R'_n are the items to be recommended. While computing similarities between a user and an item, we can introduce a measure or an attribute and assign it to every item in the database.

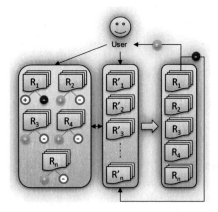

Fig. 3. Traceability versus scalability

Negative values are assigned to already viewed items which do not attract sufficiently the user. Thus, when adding new items and calling for recommendations, only
items with positive values are processed.

4.4 Synonymy

Synonymy is the likelihood of very nearer items to have dissimilar names or entries.
Most recommender systems find it hard to make distinction between nearer related
items.

By fixing this issue manually the first time, whether by correcting its name or
adjusting its position in the similarity matrix, the system will remember this change as a
form of traceability; thus, the synonymy issue of the same item will be bypassed during
next recommendations.

4.5 Privacy

The system must acquire the most amount of information possible about the user,
including demographic data and data about the location of a particular user. Such idea
to include demographic attributes was explained and presented as an ethical-based
recommender system [26].

Traceability can be used to track the user's positions and time events (Fig. 4). For
each position and time Pt_n, there are specific foods or items that can be subject of
recommendation, based on inputs such as the weather or the season. Based on that, we
can for sure render the user's profile much richer by adding new confirmed preferences
about his tastes and needs. Hence, recommendations will be improved based on new
acquired preferences every time.

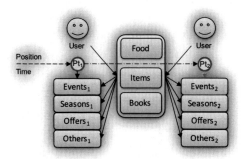

Fig. 4. Traceability versus privacy

5 Related Works

According to a recent literature review, there was a limited number of studies that dealt
with e-Learning recommendation with a user-item centric focus, using any form of
traceability.

For instance, authors in [22] proposed a personalized web content recommendation system for e-learners, which is based on navigation behaviors and access logs, to follow e-learners' activities. By analyzing usage and navigation records, the system is able to monitor e-learners' performance and deliver suitable contents.

Atallah et al. [27] focused more on the instant messaging features of MOODLE. They presented a recommender model that prevents messages containing taboo words from reaching instructors, issues a notification to monitors for security purposes, and suggests recommended materials to the students based on their sent questions. Thus, the system can reduce the number of unwanted messages and deliver fast responses to students.

6 Proposed Approach

The main concern of a student is to find courses or any kind of resource that can best improve his abilities and enrich his knowledge about a specific subject. Since the number of available resources is very large and contains a variety of elements (lessons, courses, explanations, hints, tips, … etc.), the recommendation can be challenging. On the other hand, the tutor or the instructor cannot stay available all the time and may need a considerable amount of time, to judge and decide which course or resource needs to be assigned or recommended, considering the number of active sessions.

When applying traceability in an e-Learning environment, the choice of tracking and tracing a student or a resource depends on the platform's strategy. If the focus is on the student, we may learn more about his records, his performances, and his activities. On the contrary, if it is meant for resources, then we may catch learning and rating indicators to decide whether to keep the resource or to discard it.

Figure 5 represents our Traceability-Recommendation approach which consists of three main components: Chatbot which is the communication interface between a student and the recommendation process, the TR-Model which applies a customized unique representation on the extracted data and provides the key decision indicators,

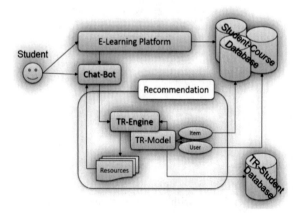

Fig. 5. The TR-recommendation approach

and the TR-Engine which considers the input of the traceability model and computes the recommendation.

The recommendation process begins once the student starts the chatbot and asks for help or instructions. While engaged in a conversation, the chatbot analyses the request to select relevant keys and asks for more inputs in case the recommendation is item-oriented. Based on the user's inputs, the TR-Engine collects data from the original database, proceeds with a cleaning phase to discard records with missing values and applies the predefined TR-Model, which converts all extracted information into a unique historical representation, upon which the recommendation is based. Once this representation is finished, it is stored in a separated database and may be accessed and updated in case of new requests or changes.

As previously mentioned in [9], the purpose of the TR-Model is to consolidate data and represent it in a customized and standard way. Figure 6 shows the implementation example of the model, which adapts the extracted artifacts into a set of three main elements {item, stages, activities}.

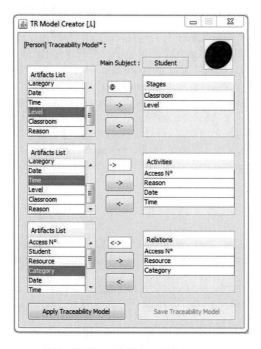

Fig. 6. Traceability model creator

The "Main Subject" is the main traceable item; it can be either a user or a resource. The "Stages" represent the positions or movement points. The "Activities" reflect the different variations or transformations that occurred to the resources or the different operations that were conducted by the user. The "Relations" represent the links between the main traceable item and the remaining artifacts. Additionally, two measures were added: TR-Frequency which represents the number of times a resource is viewed or used and TR-Weight, which is the duration of time that was spent on a resource. In the end, the TR-Model will provide key-decision factors including details about ratings, time and appreciations to the TR-Engine. Thus, based on these keys, the role of the TR-Engine is to suggest the suitable resources using recommendation techniques.

7 Conclusion

Although recommender systems are becoming more and more complex, they are considered as very useful tools that deal with the information overload in a way that can help users gain time, by suggesting a Top-N list of items that can best satisfy their needs and expectations.

In this paper, we have introduced traceability which is an ability to trace and track an item's movement from one position to another, by keeping a complete record over all activities, changes, and relations that this item undergoes, including attributes and metrics, and attempted to present the benefits of using it within recommender systems. We have also proposed an accessible e-Learning approach that combines both Traceability and Recommendation for students through Chatbots, which consists first, in creating and applying a traceability model then, providing the results as inputs and indicators for the traceability recommendation engine and finally, suggesting the resulted resources as a form of recommendation.

Future research direction will be mainly centered on conducting more tests on a real e-Learning platform such as Moodle, and studying the feasibility and performance of this approach, with an increased focus on the Traceability Model. We will then check its ability to adapt and to be used in other environments. We are hoping that, through this study, we can refine this model and render it as generic as possible, for more applications.

References

1. Alharbi, H., Sandhu, K.: Toward a model for E-Learning recommender system adoption: a pilot study. In: International Conference on New Trends in Computing Sciences (ICTCS) (2017)
2. Maravanyika, M., Dlodlo, N., Jere, N.: An adaptive recommender system based framework for personalised teaching and learning on e-learning platforms. In: IST-Africa Week Conference (IST-Africa) (2017)
3. Dilip Sawant, S., Vijay Sonawane, K., Jagani, T., Chaudhari, A.N.: Representation of recommender system in IoT using cyber physical techniques. In: International Conference on Electronics, Communication and Aerospace Technology (ICECA) (2017)
4. Dwivedi, S., Roshni, V.S.: Recommender system for big data in education. In: 5th National Conference on E-Learning & E-Learning Technologies (ELELTECH) (2017)
5. Anitha, L., Kavitha Devi, M.K., Anjali Devi, P.: A review on recommender system. Int. J. Comput. Appl. 82(3), 0975–8887 (2013)
6. Anuvareepong, S., Phooim, S., Charoenprasoplarp, N., Vimonratana, S.: Course recommender system for student enrollment using augmented reality. In: 6th IIAI International Congress on Advanced Applied Informatics (IIAI-AAI) (2017)

7. European General Food Law (EGFL). https://ec.europa.eu/food/safety/general_food_law_en
8. Global Standard/Global Language of Business (GS1). https://www.gs1.org/
9. International Organization for Standardization (ISO). https://www.iso.org/obp/ui#home
10. Schiffers, B.: Goals and components of a traceability system. In: Training Manual: Traceability, COLEACP, 6–35(118) pages, October 2011
11. Souali, K., Rahmaoui, O., Ouzzif, M.: An overview of traceability: towards a general multi-domain model. Adv. Sci. Technol. Eng. Syst. J. 2(3), 356–361 (2017)
12. Rempel, P., Mäder, P.: Continuous assessment of software traceability. In: IEEE/ACM 38th IEEE International Conference on Software Engineering Companion (ICSE) (2016)
13. De Lucia, A., Marcus, A., Oliveto, R., Poshyvanyk, D.: Information retrieval methods for automated traceability recovery. In: Software and Systems Traceability, pp. 71–98 (2012)
14. Gayer, S., Herrmann, A., Keuler, T., Riebisch, M., Antonino, P.O.: Lightweight traceability for the agile architect. Computer 49(5), 64–71 (2016)
15. Khan, B.M., Mansha, A., Khan, F.H., Bashir, S.: Collaborative filtering based online recommendation systems: a survey. In: International Conference on Information and Communication Technologies (ICICT), December 2017
16. Xu, L., Jiang, C., Chen, Y., Ren, Y., Ray Liu, K.J.: User participation in collaborative filtering-based recommendation systems: a game theoretic approach. IEEE Trans. Cybern. (2018)
17. Kawasaki, M., Hasuike, T.: A recommendation system by collaborative filtering including information and characteristics on users and items. In: IEEE Symposium Series on Computational Intelligence (SSCI) (2017)
18. Li, Y., Wang, H., Liu, H., Chen, B.: A study on content-based video recommendation. In: IEEE International Conference on Image Processing (ICIP) (2017)
19. Jena, K.C., Mishra, S., Sahoo, S.: Principles, techniques and evaluation of recommendation systems. In: International Conference on Inventive Systems and Control (ICISC) (2017)
20. Patel, B., Desai, P., Panchal, U.: Methods of recommender system: a review. In: International Conference on Innovations in Information, Embedded and Communication Systems (ICIIECS) (2017)
21. Pal, A., Parhi, P., Aggarwal, M.: An improved content based collaborative filtering algorithm for movie recommendations. In: 10th International Conference on Contemporary Computing (IC3) (2017)
22. Herath, D., Jayaratne, L.: A personalized web content recommendation system for E-learners in E-Learning environment. In: National Information Technology Conference (NITC) (2017)
23. Mathew, P., Kuriakose, B., Hegde, V.: Book recommendation system through content based and collaborative filtering method. In: International Conference on Data Mining and Advanced Computing (SAPIENCE) (2016)
24. Wang, H., Zhang, P., Lu, T.: Hybrid recommendation model based on incremental collaborative filtering and content based algorithms. In: IEEE 21st International Conference on Computer Supported Cooperative Work in Design (CSCWD) (2017)
25. Zhou, L., Tang, H., Dong, T.: A hybrid collaborative filtering recommendation model-based on complex attribute of goods. In: International Conference on Security, Pattern Analysis and Cybernetics (SPAC) (2017)
26. Souali, K., El Afia, A., Faizi, R.: An automatic ethical-based recommender system for e-commerce. In: International Conference on Multimedia Computing and Systems (ICMCS) (2011)
27. Atallah, R.R., Barhoom, T.S., Elejla, O.E.: Recommender model for messaging system at MOODLE. In: Palestinian International Conference on Information and Communication Technology (PICICT) (2017)

Optimization of Makespan in Job Shop Scheduling Problem by Hybrid Chicken Swarm Algorithm

Soukaina Cherif Bourki Semlali[✉], Mohammed Essaid Riffi, and Fayçal Chebihi

LAMAPI Laboratory, Department of Mathematics, Faculty of Sciences,
University of Chouaib Doukkali, El Jadida, Morocco
Soukaina.cherif.b.s@ucd.ac.ma

Abstract. This paper presents an adaptation of a new metaheuristic called Chicken swarm optimization with simulated annealing (CSOSA) to solve the job shop scheduling problem (JSSP). The objective is to optimize the makespan by involving chicken swarm algorithm which take into consideration the behavior and the hierarchical order of chicken swarm while seeking for food. The performance of the proposed algorithm is enhanced with an hybridization of CSO with simulated annealing (SA). Furthermore, we propose to integrate the pair-exchange method which is used on each machine to improve the solution quality. The empirical results are obtained by applying the new algorithm on some instances of OR-Library. The computational results demonstrate the effectiveness of the CSOSA comparing to other existing metaheuristics from literature in term of quality of solution and run time for the various benchmark.

Keywords: Chicken swarm optimization · OR-library · Combinatorial optimization · Simulated annealing · 2-opt neighborhood · Makespan.

1 Introduction

The job shop scheduling problem is known to be the most difficult problems in the planning of manufacturing processes [1]. The job-shop scheduling problem (JSSP) was formulated by Muth and Thompson in 1963 [2] in order to allocate a shared resources to different activities over time, which is called also scheduling.

In literature, several exact, heuristic and metaheuristics algorithms have been proposed to solve the job shop scheduling problem. The objective of the job-shop scheduling problem is to find the solution or the schedule to minimize the time required to complete a group of jobs called makespan. The proposed algorithms include branch and bound (B&B) [3], Tabu search (TS) [4,5], simulated annealing (SA) [6], genetic algorithms (GA) [7–9], neural networks (NN) [10], Particle swarm optimization (PSO) [11,12], Bee colony optimization (BCO) [13], ant colony optimization (ACO) [14] and firefly algorithm (FA) [15]. Furthermore,

© Springer Nature Switzerland AG 2019
M. Ezziyyani (Ed.): AI2SD 2018, AISC 915, pp. 358–369, 2019.
https://doi.org/10.1007/978-3-030-11928-7_32

hybrid optimization strategy has been developed for JSSP such as a parallel GRASP with path-relinking [16] and a new hybrid genetic algorithm [17].

The remainder of this paper is organized as follows: in Sect. 2, we represent a brief review from literature and the mathematical formulation of the job shop scheduling problem. In Sect. 3, we describe the proposed CSO algorithm with simulated annealing (CSOSA). In Sect. 4, we discuss the empirical results obtained while applying the new proposed algorithm on some instances of OR-Library. Finally, in the conclusion we give some prospect for further works.

2   Job Shop Scheduling Problem

The job-shop scheduling problem (JSSP) can be formulated by assigning a set of n jobs consists of a set of operations to a set of m machines. The aim purpose is to find a schedule with minimum makespan C_{max}, then a solution can be depicted as a vector $n \times m$ of a sequence of operation, which optimizes the completion time of all jobs.

$$C_{max} = max_{t_{ij}}(t_{ij} + p_{ij}) \tag{1}$$

$$minC_{nm+1} \tag{2}$$

Where

$$C_{kl} \leq C_{ji} - d_{kl}; \quad j = 1, \cdot, n; \quad i = 1, \ldots, m; \quad kl \in P_{ji} \tag{3}$$

$$\sum_{ji \in O(t)} r_{ji} \leq 1; \quad i \in M; \quad t \geq 0 \tag{4}$$

$$C_{ji} \geq 0; \quad j = 1, \ldots, n; \quad i = 1, \ldots, m \tag{5}$$

- The constraint (2) minimizes the finish time of operation o_{nm+1} (the makespan).
- The constraint (3) represents the fact that between operations the precedence relations should be respected.
- The constraint (4) describes that each machine can process one operation at a each time.
- The constraint (5) guarantees that the finish times to be positive.

let's consider the following example with $m = 3$ machines and $n = 3$ jobs, where:
$J = \{J1, J2, J3\}$ and $M = \{1, 2, 3\}$
   $J1 = \{(1; 3), (2; 3), (3; 3)\}$
   $J2 = \{(1; 2), (3; 3), (2; 4)\}$
   $J3 = \{(2; 3), (1; 2), (3; 1)\}$

The representation of the information matrix will be as below:

$$\begin{pmatrix} o1 & o2 & o3 & o4 & o5 & o6 & o7 & o8 & o9 \\ jo1 & jo2 & jo3 & jo4 & jo5 & jo6 & jo7 & jo8 & jo9 \\ 1 & 2 & 3 & 1 & 2 & 3 & 1 & 2 & 3 \\ 1 & 2 & 3 & 1 & 3 & 2 & 2 & 1 & 3 \\ 3 & 3 & 3 & 2 & 3 & 4 & 3 & 2 & 1 \end{pmatrix}$$

Then

$$\begin{pmatrix} 1\,2\,3\,4\,5\,6\,7\,8\,9 \\ 1\,1\,1\,2\,2\,2\,3\,3\,3 \\ 1\,2\,3\,1\,2\,3\,1\,2\,3 \\ 1\,2\,3\,1\,3\,2\,2\,1\,3 \\ 3\,3\,3\,2\,3\,4\,3\,2\,1 \end{pmatrix}$$

The first line contains the operations, the second line contains the jobs, the third line indicates the sequence number, the forth line refers to the machine number and the last line contains the processing time of each operation.

The aim purpose is to find the sequence of operations with the minimum makespan. The valid solution as indicated by the Gant chart in Fig. 1 as the minimum makespan is Cmax = 12.

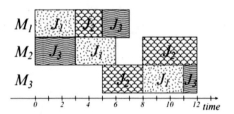

Fig. 1. Gantt chart representation

3 Chicken Swarm Algorithm with Simulated Annealing to Solve Job Shop Scheduling Problem

In this paper, we used the original version of chicken swarm algorithm which was introduced by Meng et al. [18]. This algorithm is based on the behavior of a chicken swarm while searching for food.

The chicken swarm is divided into several groups contains several individuals, which are the leader of the group or the rooster, many hens and their chicks. In order to establish the hierarchical order in the swarm, the fitness value is used. In this paper, the fitness value is equivalent to the sequence of operations. Consequently, a chicken can search food in a set of solutions S defined as the search space. The number of roosters, hens and chicks are depicted by RN, HN and CN, then

$$CN = PS - (NR + NH) \tag{6}$$

In this paper, we used the position update equation from [19], then the equation of the rooster can be represented as:

$$x_{i,j}^{t+1} = x_{i,j}^{t} * (1 + Randn(0, \sigma^2)) \tag{7}$$

$$\sigma^2 = \begin{cases} 1, \ if \ f_i \leq f_k, \\ \exp\left(\left(\frac{f_k - f_i}{|f_i| - \varepsilon}\right)\right), \\ otherwise \quad k \in [1, N], \quad k \neq i \end{cases} \tag{8}$$

where

- $Randn(0, \sigma^2)$ refers to a Gaussian distribution
- σ^2 represents a standard deviation
- The rooster index k which is randomly selected.
- f is the fitness value of the corresponding individual.

Moreover, the position update equation of the hen can be formulated as below:

$$x_{i,j}^{t+1} = x_{i,j}^{t} + S1 * Rand * (x_{r1,j}^{t} - x_{i,j}^{t}) + S2 * Rand * (x_{r2,j}^{t} - x_{i,j}^{t}) \tag{9}$$

and

$$S1 = \exp\left(\left(\frac{f_i - f_{r1}}{|f_i| + \varepsilon}\right)\right) \ and \ S2 = \exp((f_{r2} - f_i))$$

where $Rand \in [0, 1]$, r_1 is the index of the rooster and r_2 is the index of a random chicken from the swarm (where r1 $\neq$ r2).

Otherwise, the position update equation of the chick is expressed by [19] as follows:

$$x_{i,j}^{t+1} = W * x_{i,j}^{t} + FL * (x_{m,j}^{t} - x_{i,j}^{t})) + C * (x_{r,j}^{t} - x_{i,j}^{t})) \tag{10}$$

Where W represents a self-learning factor for chicks, $FL \in [0, 2]$ is a randomly selected parameter for the relationship between the chicks and its mother where $m \in [1, N]$. Besides, C is a learning-factor from the rooster.

In our new adaptation, we proceed the redefinition of operators quoted in Eqs. 7, 9 and 10. In this adaptation, the subtraction $\ominus$ operator represents the crossover operator, the multiplication $\otimes$ refers to the chosen crossover. Finally, the addition $\oplus$ operator indicates that the randomly chosen crossover is applied to the movement.

We integrate the uniform crossover (UX) [20] in the position update equation of hens and chicks for the movement towards the leaders of groups and the sequential constructive crossover (SCX) [21] to simulate the movement towards the neighbors. The difference between the chosen crossover ensures the competition between group in the swarm.As well, we incorporate the pair-exchange method used on each machine by exchanging jobs pairwise to realize the auto-improvement in the position equation of the leaders and the chicks. Furthermore, the pair-exchange method will be used as a simple method for generating neighborhood solutions.

In this paper, we propose an adaptation of Chicken swarm algorithm mixed with Simulated Annealing (CSOSA) to solve the job shop scheduling problem (JSSP) by employing certain probability to avoid becoming trapped into the local optima, the new strategy allows to explore a large search space, which guarantees the basic concept of the main algorithm CSO. In this study, the simulated annealing (SA) is hybrid with the chicken swarm algorithm to ensure the redistribution of the swarm. Accordingly, we realize a great balance between the effectiveness of initialization, mutation crossover and a strategy to improve the performance of our new algorithm.

The simulated annealing algorithm (SA) was introduced by Kirkpatrick et al. [22], SA is based on the physical annealing process introduced by Metropolis et al., which starts with a high temperature in the beginning of the process in order to attempt a cooling phase and then the solid regains its form which improve the quality of solution. The search process can be controlled by the cooling schedule. Each phase is characterized by state. Otherwise a solid passes with a sequence of successive states, if the energy produced by this change of state decreases. Then the new solution is accepted if the objective function value is improved, the new solution is accepted with the probability defined by the following Eq. (11) of the fitness value f:

$$p = e^{(-\Delta E/C_b T)} \tag{11}$$

Where

ΔE is the energy difference produced by this change of state. In the new adaptation, we consider that:

$\Delta = f(S') - f(S)$

C_b is Boltzmann constant produced by this change of state and where B is a parameter called decreasing rate.

T is the temperature of the solid which refers to the number G, after G iterations a redistribution of the swarm is made. On the other hand the redistribution will be the same in applying the hybridization of CSO and SA.

The new CSOSA in pseudo-code is represented as below:

4   Experimental Results and Discussion

The new CSOSA was coded in python and run on a DELL in visual studio 2017, the CSOSA was simulated with Intel(R) Core(TM) i7-6500 U CPU 2.5 GHZ (4 CPUs) 2.6 GHz and 16.00 GB of RAM and Microsoft Windows 10 Professional (64-bit) operating system. The performance of CSOSA was tested on different instances of OR-Library 20 runs in 100 iterations.

Algorithm 1: Hybrid optimization algorithm CSOSA
1. Initialize the size of population PS
2. Generate PS chickens using GRASP
3. Initialize parameters: PS, G=T_k, FL, C and w.
4. Evaluate the fitness values at t=0 for each chicken
5. Establish a hierarchical order by ranking the swarm
6. Create groups in the swarm
7. Assign chicks to mother-hens.
8. Update the position by Eqs. 7, 9 and 10
9. For S_{best} of the swarm SA is used
10. Generate a new solution S' in the neighborhood of S by pair-exchange method (SA) Compute fitness fo S'
11. $\Delta = f(S') - f(S)$ and $p = exp(-\Delta/T_k)$
12. If $p > random[0,1]$, the new solution S' is accepted and $T_k = BT_{k-1}$
13. Return to step 10 if G is reached until the termination temperature T_{end}
14. Return optimization results

The parameter values used in the new adaptation CSOSA are indicated in Table 1. We execute different tests to choose the values which allow that CSOSA converge towards the good results.

Table 1. The parameters for the CSOSA algorithm

Parameters of CSOSA	Values
PS: Population size	500
RN: Number of roosters (%)	14
HN: Number of hens (%)	20
CN: Number of chicks (%)	66
G: Number of iterations to update the algorithm	8
W: Self-learning factor	0.5
FL: Learning factor from the mother hens	0.4
C: Learning factor from the rooster	0.65
B: Decreasing rate	0.97
T_{end}: Termination temperature	0.1

Moreover, Table 2 summarizes the obtained results when applying CSOSA. The first column represents different instances in OR-Library, the second column indicates the best Known solution (BKS), the third column describes the average of the best found solution or the makespan reported by the algorithm δ_{avg}, the fourth column represents the average of time T_{avg}, the last column indicates the

Table 2. Numerical results by CSOSA applied to some instances of OR-library

n × m	Instance	BKS	δ_{avg}	$T_{avg}(s)$	Err (%)
10 × 10	Abz5	1234	1234	13	00
10 × 10	Abz6	943	943	15	00
20 × 15	Abz7	656	672	1572	1.8
20 × 15	Abz8	646	698	3120	6.4
20 × 15	Abz9	662	740	2105	6.4
11 × 5	Car1	7038	7038	01	00
13 × 4	Car2	7166	7166	01	00
12 × 5	Car3	7312	7312	162	00
14 × 4	Car4	8003	8003	02	00
10 × 6	Car5	7702	7702	28	00
8 × 9	Car6	8313	8313	30	00
7× 7	Car7	6558	6558	02	00
8 × 8	Car8	8264	8264	05	00
10 × 10	Orb1	1059	1062	1204	0.3
10 × 10	Orb2	888	889	219	0.1
10 × 10	Orb3	1005	1034	149	1.03
10 × 10	Orb4	1005	1009	259	0.04
10 × 10	Orb5	887	890	221	0.2
10 × 10	Orb6	1010	1011	96	0.1
10 × 10	Orb7	397	400	91	0.3
10 × 10	Orb8	899	899	141	00
10 × 10	Orb9	934	934	852	00
10 × 10	Orb10	944	944	209	00
6 × 6	Ft06	55	55	01	00
10 × 10	Ft10	930	930	549	00
20 × 5	Ft20	1165	1181	633	0.6
10 × 5	LA01	666	666	01	00
10 × 5	LA02	655	655	04	00
10 × 5	LA03	597	597	09	00
10 × 5	LA04	590	590	17	00
10 × 5	LA05	593	593	01	00
15 × 5	LA06	926	926	05	00
15 × 5	LA07	890	890	01	00
15 × 5	LA08	863	863	03	00
15 × 5	LA09	951	951	05	00

(*continued*)

Table 2. (*continued*)

n × m	Instance	BKS	δ_{avg}	$T_{avg}(s)$	Err (%)
15 × 5	LA10	958	958	01	00
20 × 5	LA11	1222	1222	06	00
20 × 5	LA12	1039	1039	07	00
20 × 5	LA13	1150	1150	05	00
20 × 5	LA14	1292	1292	02	00
20 × 5	LA15	1207	1207	07	00
10 × 10	LA16	945	945	09	00
10 × 10	LA17	784	787	168	0.06
10 × 10	LA18	848	848	45	00
10 × 10	LA19	842	842	52	00
10 × 10	LA20	902	905	02	0.3
15 × 10	LA21	1046	1049	2285	0.03
15 × 10	LA22	927	927	982	00
15 × 10	LA23	1032	1032	14	00
15 × 10	LA24	935	941	663	0.13
20 × 10	LA26	1218	1218	704	00
20 × 10	LA30	1355	1355	176	00
30 × 10	LA31	1784	1784	27	00
30 ×10	LA32	1850	1850	26	00
30 ×10	LA33	1719	1719	28	00
30 × 10	LA34	1721	1721	108	00
30× 10	LA35	1888	1888	29	00

results obtained from Eq. 12 use to perform the quality of the solution. The proposed CSOSA allows to find the best-known solution about 73.6% from all tested instances.

The mathematical formulation of the percentage of error ERR (12) is represented as below:

$$Err = \frac{(\delta_{avg} - BKS)}{BKS} \times 100 \tag{12}$$

where BKS is the best known value and δ_{avg} the average of the best found solution.

The new algorithm CSOSA allows to obtain good results in term of the global optimum compared to other algorithms from literature, CSOSA seems to be promising to solve jssp in a reasonable time compared to the D-PSO algorithm [23] in term of relative percent in makespan ($Err\%$) as represented in Table 3 and Fig. 2. Furthermore, comparison with the Cat Swarm algorithm (CSO) [24] shows that our algorithm allows to obtain better results in term of average time as represented in Fig. 3.

Table 3. Relative percent in makespan % by CSOSA and D-PSO

Instance	BKS	CSOSA (*Err%*)	D-PSO (*Err%*)
Abz5	1234	0	0.32
Abz6	943	0	0.21
Abz7	656	1.8	4.88
Abz8	646	6.4	9.6
Abz9	626	6.4	7.7
Orb2	888	0.1	0.11
Orb3	1005	1.03	2.19
Orb4	1005	0.04	0.1
Orb8	899	0	0
Orb9	934	0	0
Orb10	944	0	0
Ft06	55	0	0
Ft10	930	0	0.86
Ft20	1165	0.6	0
LA01	666	0	0
LA02	655	0	0
LA03	597	0	0
LA04	590	0	0
LA05	593	0	0
LA06	926	0	0
LA07	890	0	0
LA08	863	0	0
LA09	951	0	0
LA10	958	0	0
LA11	1222	0	0
LA12	1039	0	0
LA13	1150	0	0
LA14	1292	0	0
LA15	1207	0	0
LA16	945	0.06	0
LA17	784	0	0
LA18	848	0	0
LA19	842	0	0
LA20	902	0.3	0.89
LA21	1046	0.03	0.1
LA22	927	0	0

(*continued*)

Table 3. (*continued*)

Instance	BKS	CSOSA (*Err%*)	D-PSO (*Err%*)
LA23	1032	0	0
LA24	935	0.13	0.43
LA26	1218	0	0
LA30	1355	0	0
LA31	1784	0	0
LA32	1850	0	0
LA33	1719	0	0
LA34	1721	0	0
LA35	1888	0	0

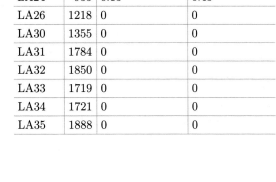

Fig. 2. Average time (s) by CSOSA and CSO algorithm

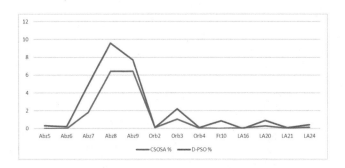

Fig. 3. *Err%* by CSOSA and D-PSO algorithm

5 Conclusion

In this work, we proposed a new Chicken Swarm algorithm by integrating the Simulated Annealing search and the 2-opt mechanism to solve the job shop scheduling problem (CSOSA). The results of the proposed adaptation show that the CSOSA algorithm is promising, comparison with other results in the literature such as Cat Swarm algorithm (CSO) and D-PSO indicates that CSOSA is effective to solve the job-shop scheduling problem and yields a better solution. In further research, we suggest to apply CSOSA to solve other NP-hard combinatorial optimization problems such as vehicle routing problem (VRP).

References

1. Jain, A.S., Meeran, S.: Deterministic job-shop scheduling: past, present and future. Eur. J. Oper. Res. **113**(2), 390–434 (1999)
2. Adams, J., Balas, E., Zawack, D.: The shifting bottleneck procedure for job shop scheduling. Manag. Sci. **34**(3), 391–401 (1988)
3. Brucker, P., Jurisch, B., Sievers, B.: A branch and bound algorithm for the job-shop scheduling problem. Discr. Appl. Math. **49**(1–3), 107–127 (1994)
4. Zhang, C.Y., Li, P., Rao, Y., Guan, Z.: A very fast ts/sa algorithm for the job shop scheduling problem. Comput. Oper. Res. **35**(1), 282–294 (2008)
5. Peng, B., Lü, Z., Cheng, T.: A tabu search/path relinking algorithm to solve the job shop scheduling problem. Comput. Oper. Res. **53**, 154–164 (2015)
6. Kolonko, M.: Some new results on simulated annealing applied to the job shop scheduling problem. Eur. J. Oper. Res. **113**(1), 123–136 (1999)
7. Cheng, R., Gen, M., Tsujimura, Y.: A tutorial survey of job-shop scheduling problems using genetic algorithms-I. Representation. Comput. Ind. Eng. **30**(4), 983–997 (1996)
8. Wang, Y., et al.: A new hybrid genetic algorithm for job shop scheduling problem. Comput. Oper. Res. **39**(10), 2291–2299 (2012)
9. Asadzadeh, L.: A local search genetic algorithm for the job shop scheduling problem with intelligent agents. Comput. Ind. Eng. **85**, 376–383 (2015)
10. Foo, S.Y., Takefuji, Y., Szu, H.: Scaling properties of neural networks for job-shop scheduling. Neurocomputing **8**(1), 79–91 (1995)
11. Sha, D., Hsu, C.-Y.: A hybrid particle swarm optimization for job shop scheduling problem. Comput. Ind. Eng. **51**(4), 791–808 (2006)
12. Xia, W.-J., Wu, Z.-M.: A hybrid particle swarm optimization approach for the job-shop scheduling problem. Int. J. Adv. Manufact. Technol. **29**(3–4), 360–366 (2006)
13. Sundar, S., Suganthan, P.N., Jin, C.T., Xiang, C.T., Soon, C.C.: A hybrid artificial bee colony algorithm for the job-shop scheduling problem with no-wait constraint. Soft Comput. **21**(5), 1193–1202 (2017)
14. Nazif, H., et al.: Solving job shop scheduling problem using an ant colony algorithm. J. Asian Sci. Res. **5**(5), 261–268 (2015)
15. Khadwilard, A., Chansombat, S., Thepphakorn, T., Thapatsuwan, P., Chainate, W., Pongcharoen, P.: Application of firefly algorithm and its parameter setting for job shop scheduling. J. Ind. Technol. **8**(1) (2012)
16. Aiex, R.M., Binato, S., Resende, M.G.: Parallel grasp with path-relinking for job shop scheduling. Parallel Comput. **29**(4), 393–430 (2003)

17. Gonçalves, J.F., de Magalhães Mendes, J.J., Resende, M.G.: A hybrid genetic algorithm for the job shop scheduling problem. Eur. J. Oper. Res. **167**(1), 77–95 (2005)
18. Meng, X., Liu, Y., Gao, X., Zhang, H.: A new bio-inspired algorithm: chicken swarm optimization. In: International Conference in Swarm Intelligence, pp. 86–94. Springer (2014)
19. Wu, D., Kong, F., Gao, W., Shen, Y., Ji, Z.: Improved chicken swarm optimization. In: 2015 IEEE International Conference on Cyber Technology in Automation, Control, and Intelligent Systems (CYBER), pp. 681–686. IEEE (2015)
20. Tate, D.M., Smith, A.E.: A genetic approach to the quadratic assignment problem. Comput. Oper. Res. **22**(1), 73–83 (1995)
21. Ahmed, Z.: A simple genetic algorithm using sequential constructive crossover for the quadratic assignment problem (2014)
22. Kirkpatrick, S., Gelatt, C.D., Vecchi, M.P.: Optimization by simulated annealing. Science **220**(4598), 671–680 (1983)
23. Rameshkumar, K., Rajendran, C.: A novel discrete PSO algorithm for solving job shop scheduling problem to minimize makespan. In: IOP Conference Series: Materials Science and Engineering, vol. 310, p. 012143. IOP Publishing (2018)
24. Bouzidi, A., Riffi, M.E.: Cat swarm optimization to solve job shop scheduling problem. In: 2014 Third IEEE International Colloquium in Information Science and Technology (CIST), pp. 202–205. IEEE (2014)

Arabic Stop Consonant Acoustic Characterization

Mohamed Farchi[1], Karim Tahiry[1($\boxtimes$)], Badia Mounir[2], Ilham Mounir[2],
and Ahmed Mouhsen[1]

[1] Faculty of Sciences & Technics, University Hassan First, Settat, Morocco
{simo.farchi,karim.tahiry}@gmail.com,
ahmed.mouhsen@uhp.ac.ma
[2] Graduate School of Technology, University Cadi Ayyad, Safi, Morocco
{mounirbadia2014,ilhamounir}@gmail.com

Abstract. The present study investigates Arabic stop consonants. Our goal is to give sufficient acoustic cues for detecting and characterizing such consonants. In general, speech is made with sequences of consonants (fricatives, nasals and stops), vowels and glides. The first task is then to separate stop consonants from other phonemes. From an acoustic point of view, stop consonants are characterized by abrupt changes in speech signal. To detect such changes, we exploit landmarks method. The second purpose of this work is to give a relevant characterization of stop consonants by using normalized closure and release durations and computing the spectral moments.

Keywords: Arabic stop consonants · Landmarks · Spectral moments · Closure duration · Release duration

1 Introduction

The simplest method for the production of a number of distinctive speech sounds is to vary the degree of closure that constricts the air flow passing through the articulatory system. These different types of constructions are responsible for the consonants classification (fricatives, stops, nasals).

Several works were interested in acoustic study of consonants in different languages, with different methods and tools. In our study, we focus on stops consonants in Arabic language. Which are produced by forming a closure in the vocal tract, building up pressure in the mouth behind this closure, and releasing the closure. Or the closure is formed by a particular articulator: the lips, the tongue blade, or the tongue body [1]. Therefore, we can say that the production of the stop consonants is done in two phases: the phase of the complete closure of the vocal tract and the accumulation of the pressure of the air behind this closure.

Many studies have been realized on temporal information with different purposes. In order to characterize stop consonants, some researchers have been interested to voice onset time (VOT), [2, 3]. They concluded that VOT is an important cue to place of articulation. Moreover, Lisker [2] and Abramson [4] have established that VOT is an important cue for distinguishing word-initial voiceless and voiced stops in many

© Springer Nature Switzerland AG 2019
M. Ezziyyani (Ed.): AI2SD 2018, AISC 915, pp. 370–382, 2019.
https://doi.org/10.1007/978-3-030-11928-7_33

languages. Furthermore, Kiefte [5] has suggested that Dynamic properties of stop bursts are important only when they include VOT information. Indeed, he noticed that dynamic spectral properties within isolated bursts appear to contain no phonetic information up to 20 ms. In addition, Chodroff and Wilson [6] have showed that burst spectrum influences category typicality for voiceless stops even when voice onset time is unambiguous. Blumstein and Stevens [7] have reported that the 10–20 ms of the speech signal immediately following oral release contained the most of the phonetically relevant acoustic information.

Other Research have exploited some frequency factors for stop consonants characterization, Suchato and Punyabukkana [8], have showed that there are four key sets of factors: 'normalized burst amplitude', 'burst shape', 'formant frequency' and 'formant transition' that describe the acoustic properties significant to the place classification. Liberman et al. [9] found that the first formant F1 onset and transition influence the perception of stop voicing. Some researchers reported that formant transitions can be a very important cue in place perception [10, 11, 12].

Another aspect that has been considered in the study of stop consonants is its characterization by the spectral moments. Jayan et al. [13] have investigated the addition of spectral moments and Mahalanobis distance on energy bands variation for burst onset detection. Zue [14] has indicated that the spectral means differentiate voiceless and voiced stops. Some researchers have studied stop consonants in terms of place and manner of articulations, Atiwong Suchato has reported that stop consonant can be classified according to three places of articulation: labial, alveolar and velar [15].

Thereafter, many studies have been realized on localization of acoustic events, the behavior of speech signal leads to abrupt acoustic changes. It is believed that acoustic cues for speech perception are most obvious around those points with rapid acoustic variation. These points act as landmarks in human speech perception [16]. These landmarks offer several possibilities. They allow detecting the beginning or abrupt acoustic changes, such as close and releasing consonants [17]. They also indicate the maximal point of acoustic energy for sonorant [18] and the voiced or unvoiced parts of speech. Furthermore, combined with perception models (MFCC, PLP …) or stochastic models (GMM, HMM, SM, SVM), they were used in the construction of speech recognition systems for stop consonants.

Most of the studies carried out on plosive consonants have been made on the languages like English, Frensh, German, Chinese, etc. Few works have been dedicated to the Arabic language. The principal motivation of this work is, first, to contribute to the experimental literature on stop consonant in Arabic language in different context. Second, all studies have agreed that the energy distribution of plosive consonants differs between closure and release phases. So, in addition to the durations of these phases, we thought about using the spectral moments to highlight this difference. This tool has been little used in the description of the energetic distribution of the plosive consonants. The aim of this work is to identify the Arabic stop consonant and to determine the two production phases (closure and release) according to factors such as spectral moments, normalized release and closure durations.

This paper is organized as follows. The first section outlines the methods and tools employed and the experiments carried out. The second section comprises presentation and discussion of the results. In the last section, there is a summary of the findings and presentation of conclusions.

2   Methods

2.1   General Processing

For our experiments, we constructed a corpus of Arabic language containing stop consonants (/b/, /d/, /t/, /k/ and /q/) used with vowels /u/, /a/ and /i/. Five Moroccan speakers (three males and two females) were asked to pronounce four times the sequences CVCVCV (C is an Arabic stop consonant and V a vowel within /a/, /i/ or /u/). We then compute the energy band parameters (Landmarks) in order to isolate each stop consonant (Fig. 1).

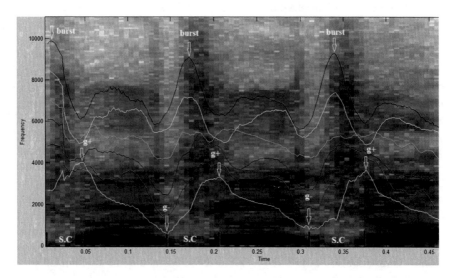

Fig. 1. Stop consonants (S.C) localized between g+ and g− landmarks (white represent energy in first band, purple in second band, blue in third band, green in forth band, yellow in fifth band and red in sex band)

2.2   Landmarks

Figure (2) shows a flowchart of the landmarks detection algorithm (g and b). The input of the algorithm is a speech signal that goes through a general processing step, the output is a series of acoustic cues specified by time and type. In general processing, a spectrogram is calculated and divided into six frequency bands. An energy waveform is constructed in each of these six bands, the energy derivative is calculated, and peaks in the derivative are detected and localized over time. These peaks represent the times of abrupt spectral change in the six bands. Localized peaks undergo a direct processing to determine both types of acoustic cues. The g-landmark pinpoints a time when vocal folds start vibrating (g+) and when the vibration ends (g−). The landmark (b) indicates the beginning of the explosion (b+) during the production of a stop consonant and the end of the aspiration (b−).

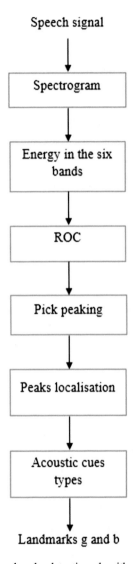

Fig. 2. Landmarks detection algorithm (g and b)

The speech sampled at 22,050 Hz is divided into time segments of 11.6 ms with an overlap of 9.6 ms. Each segment is Hanning windowed and followed by zero-padding. 512-point fast Fourier transform (FFT) is then computed. The magnitude spectrum for each frame is smoothed by a 20-point moving average taken along the time index n.

From the smoothed spectrum X(n, k), peaks in six different frequency bands (Band 1: 0–400 Hz; Band 2: 800–1500 Hz; Band 3:1200–2000 Hz; Band 4: 2000–3500 Hz; Band 5: 3500–5000 Hz and Band 6: 5000–8000 Hz) are selected as:

$$Eb(n) = 10 \log 10(\max X \, |(n,k)|2) \tag{1}$$

where the band index b ranges from 1 to 6: Band 1 reveals the presence or absence of glottal vibration, Bands 2–5 for detecting sonorant, stop, fricatives and affricate consonants, Band 6 is one of bands used for silence detection for stops. The frequency index k ranges from the DFT indices representing the lower and upper boundaries for each band.

Landmark detection involves measurement of rate of variation of a set of parameters extracted from the speech signal on a short-time basis, and locating regions with a significant variation characterizing the landmark. A rate of change measure based on first difference operation with a fixed time step is generally used to get the rate of variation of parameters. For band energy parameter Eb(n), ROC measure is defined as:

$$rEb(n) = Eb(n) - Eb(n - K) \tag{2}$$

where K is the time step. This measure indicates the difference in parameter value of the current frame, from a frame preceding it by K frames. An abrupt transition is indicated by a well-defined peak in the ROC track, while the track has a very low value during steady-state segments.

The detection of voicing offsets (g−) and voicing onsets (g+) are performed using the peak energy variation in the frequency band from 0 to 400 Hz. The peak energy is computed as:

$$Eg(n) = 10 \log 10 \, (\max|X(n,k)|) \tag{3}$$

where $k1 \leq k \leq k2$, k1 and k2 being the DFT indices corresponding to 0 and 400 Hz respectively. A rate of rise measure of Eg(n) is computed with a time step of 50 ms (K = 50) as:

$$rEg(n) = Eg(n) - Eg(n - K) \tag{4}$$

The crossing points rEg (n) below and above threshold values of −9 dB and +9 dB respectively are taken as the voicing offset and voicing onset points. An intervocalic burst onset is located at the most prominent peak in the ROC, between the g− and g+ points.

2.3   Computation of the Normalized Closure and Release Durations

The first step to compute the normalized closure and release durations of stop consonant consists on extracting stop consonants contained in each CVCVCV sequence. For this purpose, we used landmark method [19], which provides segments that can be fully specified by a feature bundle. In our process, we operate two types of landmarks (Fig. 1). The first one is g-landmark that pinpoints a time when vocal folds start vibrating (g+) and when the vibration ends (g−). These times correspond to the crossing points ROC in the first band above and below threshold values of 9 dB (g+) and −9 dB (g−) respectively. The second one is b-landmark which corresponds to the existence of turbulence noise during obstruent regions. It pin-points the time of the beginning of stop consonant release (burst). This burst is located at the most prominent peak in the ROC of bands 2–6, between the (g−) and (g+) points. The stop consonant is then localized in the region between (g−) and (g+) which contain the burst.

The closure and release normalized durations of each stop consonant (Fig. 2) were computed as:

$$dclosure = (Tburst - Tonset)/dc \tag{5}$$

$$drelease = (Tend\text{-}Tburst)/dc \tag{6}$$

where Tburst is the time where the consonant onset burst is located (b +), Tonset is the time corresponding to the consonant onset (g−), Tend is the time when the consonant takes end (g+) and dc is the overall consonant duration (Fig. 3).

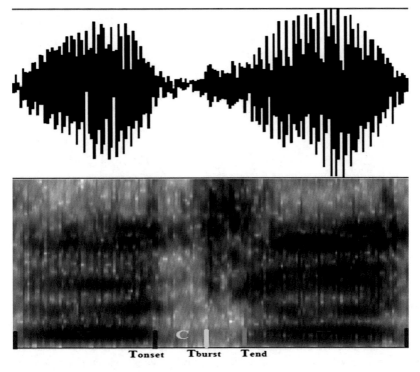

Fig. 3. Stop consonant in VCV context (V: vowel, C: closure and R: release) plotted with waveform and wideband spectrogram

2.4   Spectral Moments

Spectral moments are characteristics that describe the distribution of spectral energy in the frequency range. There are four different spectral moments: the center of gravity, standard deviation, skewness and kurtosis. The center of gravity (CoG) or spectral mean represents the average of the frequencies across the entire spectrum. The standard deviation describes the extent to which the frequencies of the spectrum deviate from the CoG. The skewness presents the asymmetry in the shape of the spectrum between the frequencies above and below the CoG and the kurtosis of the spectrum describes the extent to which the spectrum differs from the Gaussian distribution of the spectrum.

After general processing, for each frame, the probability density function for the spectrum can be estimated by normalization over all frequency components [20]:

$$\frac{P(f_k)}{\sum_{k=0}^{\frac{N}{2}-1} P(f_k)} \tag{7}$$

where $P(fk)$ is the power spectrum $fk = 2\ fNq\ k/N$, $k = 0, 1,\ldots, (N/2) - 1$), and N is the window length. fNq indicates the Nyquist frequency. The coefficients of the normalized power spectrum were computed as:

$$\text{Mean, } \mu = \sum_{k=0}^{\frac{N}{2}-1} P(f_k)f_k \tag{8}$$

$$\text{Standard deviation, } \sigma = \sqrt{\sum_{k=0}^{\frac{N}{2}-1} (f_k - \mu)^2\, P(f_k)} \tag{9}$$

$$\text{Skewness,} = \sum_{k=0}^{\frac{N}{2}-1} \left(\frac{f_k - \mu}{\sigma}\right)^3 P(f_k) \tag{10}$$

$$\text{Kurtosis,} = -3 + \sum_{k=0}^{\frac{N}{2}-1} \left(\frac{f_k - \mu}{\sigma}\right)^4 P(f_k) \tag{11}$$

3   Results and Discussions

3.1   The Closure and Release Normalized Durations

In this section, we were interested to investigate the acoustic temporal cues for each stop consonant. We have measured the consonant overall, closure and release durations. We have also computed the consonant closure and release normalized durations.

The analysis of the overall and release duration of stop consonants (Figs. 4 and 5b) shows that the voiced consonants /b/ and /d/ present a small duration in comparison with the voiceless consonants /t/, /k/ and /q/. For consonant closure durations (Fig. 5a), the voiceless /q/ and /k/ have a longer duration than /b/, /d/ and /t/. These behaviors can be explained by the position and shape of the oral constriction as well as the articulators involved in forming the constriction. Indeed, during the production of the voiceless velar stops /q/ and /k/, the principal used articulator is the tongue body which is rather massive and cannot move away from the palate too rapidly. Hence, their closure and release phases have longer durations. Otherwise, during the production of the stop consonants /b/, /d/ and /t/, the principal used articulators are the lips and the blade of the tongue which move rapidly to form the constriction. So the closure and release phases take small durations. The high intensity of the consonant /t/ through the constriction contributes to the appearance of a long burst. Consequently, the release phase of the consonant /t/ takes longer than /b/ and /d/.

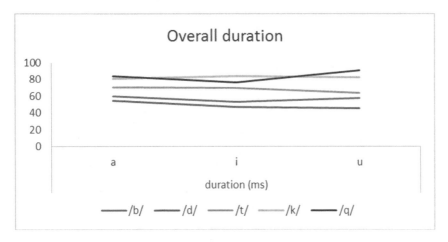

Fig. 4. Stop consonant overall durations used with vowels /a/, /i/and /u/

The investigation of the closure and release normalized durations (Fig. 6) shows that, for all consonants, the closure duration pre-sent more than 50% of the overall consonant duration. This result indicates that the closure phase takes longer than the release one. We can also noticed that, at variance of the voiceless consonants /t/, /k/ and /q/, the voiced stop consonants /b/ and /d/ have the same closure and release percentages with all the following vowels /a/, /i/ and /u/. Moreover, we can see that the release or closure normalized durations help to distinguish between the voiced and the voiceless consonants.

Regarding the results obtained in the acoustic temporal cues section, we can see that the release or closure normalized durations help to distinguish between the voiced (/b/ and /d/) and the voiceless consonants (/t/, /k/ and /q/). Moreover, for all stop consonants, the closure phase is longer than the release one. At the difference of the voiceless consonants /t/, /k/ and /q/, the voiced stop consonants /b/ and /d/ have the same closure and release percentages with all the following vowels /a/, /i/ and /u/.

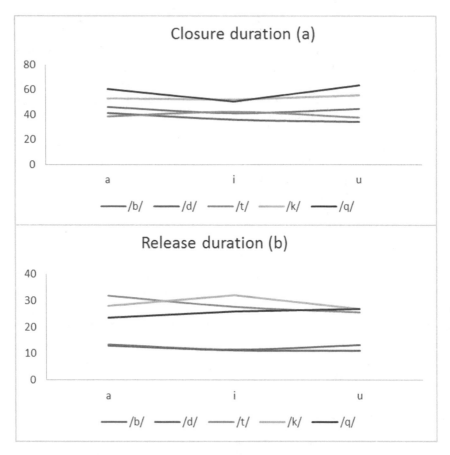

Fig. 5. Stop consonant closure (**a**) and release (**b**) durations used with vowels /a/, /i/and /u/

3.2 Spectral Moments

The objective of this section is to examine the spectral moments namely the center of gravity (CoG), standard deviation (STD), the skewness (Sk) and the kurtosis (K) of Arabic stop consonants (/b/, /d/, /t/, /k/ and /q/) accompanied by Arabic vowels (/a/, /i/ and /u/). The results obtained are summarized in (Figs. 7, 8, 9, 10 and 11). We can see that the behavior of these spectral moments depends on the vowel following the stop consonant. When the Arabic stop consonant is followed by the vowel /i/, its spectral mean is of the order of 2000 Hz. If the consonant is followed by the vowel /a/, its spectral mean is of the order of 1400 Hz. On the other hand, accompanied by the vowel /u/, the spectral mean of the consonant is of the order of 1000 Hz. This behavior is due to the values of the formants of each vowel (/a/ is characterized by $F1 > 600$ Hz and $F2 > 1000$ Hz, /u/ is known by $F1 > 300$ Hz and $F2 < 1000$ Hz and /i/ By $F1 < 300$ Hz and $F2 > 2000$ Hz) [21].

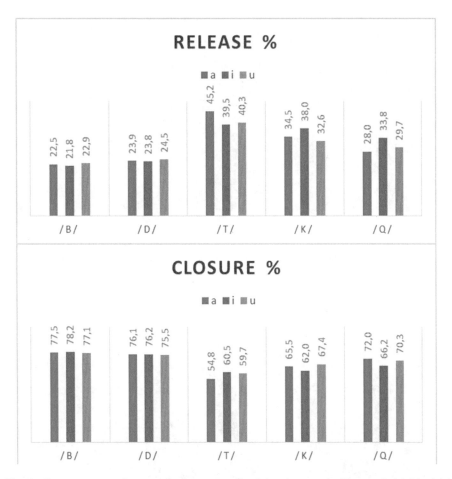

Fig. 6. Stop consonant closure and release normalized durations used with vowels /a/, /i/and /u/

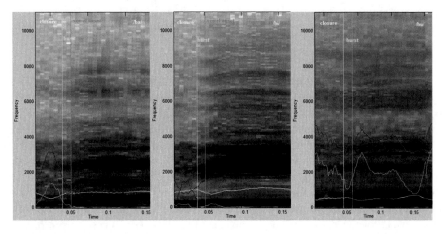

Fig. 7. The spectral moments of the stop consonant /b/with the vowels /a/, /i/and /u/ (red: spectral mean, white: standard deviation, blue: skewness coefficient, green: kurtosis coefficient)

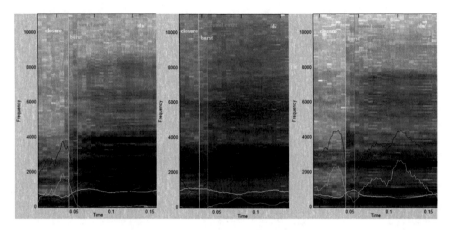

Fig. 8. The spectral moments of the stop consonant /d/ with the vowels /a/, /i/ and /u/ (red: spectral mean, white: standard deviation, blue: skewness coefficient, green: kurtosis coefficient)

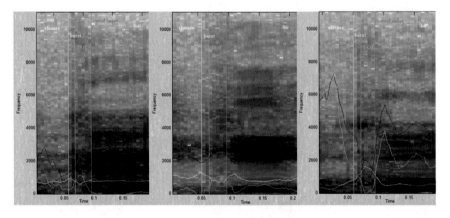

Fig. 9. The spectral moments of the stop consonant /k/ with the vowels /a/, /i/ and /u/ (red: spectral mean, white: standard deviation, blue: skewness coefficient, green: kurtosis coefficient)

We can also notice that this spectral mean increases remarkably during VOT (VOT is the time interval from the release time until the start of the glottal vibration) that characterizes the consonants (/k/ and /t/). This increase is due to the migration of energy to the high frequencies during the phase of release [22].

We can also observe that the skewness (Sk) and kurtosis (K) coefficients are always positive indicating that the maximum energy is localized to lower frequencies and that energy distribution is more pointed than the normal distribution. These positive values of skewness and kurtosis are important when the consonant occlusive Arabic is followed by the vowel /u/. This behavior is due to the fact that during the release phase, the energy is localized to the high frequencies whereas the maximum energy of the vowel /u/ is localized to the low frequencies; this passage of energy from high frequencies to low frequencies leads to remarkable changes in skewness and kurtosis.

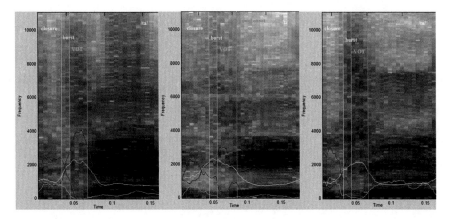

Fig. 10. The spectral moments of the stop consonant /t/ with the vowels /a/, /i/ and /u/ (red: spectral mean, white: standard deviation, blue: skewness coefficient, green: kurtosis coefficient)

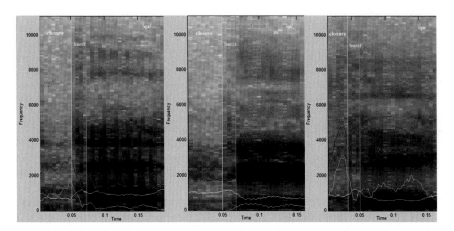

Fig. 11. The spectral moments of the stop consonant /q/ with the vowels /a/, /i/ and /u/ (red: spectral mean, white: standard deviation, blue: skewness coefficient, green: kurtosis coefficient)

4   Conclusion

In this paper, we present an approach to study Arabic stop consonants in terms of detection and characterization. This approach is based on landmarks method for stop consonants extraction in order to compute the normalized closure, release durations and spectral moments of each stop consonant.

The results show that the release or closure normalized durations help to distinguish between the voiced (/b/ and /d/) and the voiceless consonants (/t/, /k/ and /q/). Moreover, for all stop consonants, the closure phase is longer than the release one. Furthermore, the behavior of spectral moments depends on the vowel following the stop consonant. Likewise, the spectral mean during VOT leads to classify the Arabic voiceless stop consonants (/t/ and /k/) from the Arabic stop consonants (/b/, /d/ and /q/).

References

1. Stevens, K.N.: Models for the production and acoustics of stop consonants. Speech Commun. **13**, 367–375 (1993)
2. Lisker, L., Abramson, A.S.: A cross language study of voicing in initial stops: acoustical measurements. Word **20**(3), 384–422 (1964)
3. Oden, G.C., Massaro, D.W.: Integration of featural information in speech perception. Psych. Rev. **85**(3), 172–191 (1978)
4. Lisker, L., Abramson, A.S.: The voicing dimension: some experiments in comparative phonetics. In: Proceedings of the 6th ICPhS, pp. 563–567. Prague, Czech Republic (1970)
5. Kiefte, M.: Temporal information in gated stop consonants. Speech Commun. **40**, 315–333 (2003)
6. Chodroff, E., Wilson, C.: Burst spectrum as a cue for the stop voicing contrast in American English. J. Acoust. Soc. Am. **136**(5), 2762–2772 (2014)
7. Blumstein, S.E., Stevens, K.N.: Perceptual invariance and onset spectra for stop consonants in different vowel environments. J. Acoust. Soc. Amer. **67**, 648–662 (1980)
8. Suchato, A., Punyabukkana, P.: Factors in classification of stop consonant place of articulation. In: Proceedings of the Interspeech, pp. 2969–2972 (2005)
9. Liberman, A.M., Delattre, P.C., Cooper, F.S.: Some cues for the distinction between voiced and voiceless stops in initial position. Lang. Speech **1**(3), 153–167 (1958)
10. Cooper, F.S., Delattre, P.C., Liberman, A.M., Borst, J.M., Gerstman, L.J.: Some experiments on the perception of synthetic speech sounds. J. Acoust. Soc. Amer. **24**, 597–606 (1952)
11. Liberman, A.M., Delattre, P.C., Cooper, F.S., Gerstman, L.J.: The role of consonant–vowel transitions in the perception of the stop and nasal consonants. Psychol. Monogr. **68**(8), 1–13 (1954)
12. Sussman, H.M., Fruchter, D., Hilbert, J., Sirosh, J.: Linear correlates in the speech signal: the orderly output constraint. Behav. Brain Sci. **21**, 241–299 (1998)
13. Jayan, A.R., Rajath Bhat, P.S., Pandey, P.C.: Detection of burst onset landmarks in speech using rate of change of spectral moments. In: National Conference on Communications— NCC (2011)
14. Zue, V.W.: Acoustic characteristics of stop consonants: a controlled study. Sc. D. thesis. MIT, Cambridge, MA (1976)
15. Suchato, A.: Classification of stop place of articulation. Ph.D. Thesis, MIT (2004)
16. Stevens, K.N., Manuel, S.Y., Shattuck, S., Liu, S.: Implementation of a model for lexical access based on features. In: Proceedings of the ICSLP, vol. 1, pp. 499–502. Banff, Alberta (1992)
17. Liu, S.A.: Landmark detection for distinctive feature-based speech recognition. J. Acoust. Soc. Am. **100**(5), 3417–3430 (1996)
18. Schutte, K., Glass, J.: Robust detection of sonorant landmarks. In: Proceedings of the Interspeech, pp. 1005–1008 (2005)
19. Liu, S.A.: Landmark detection for distinctive feature based speech recognition. J. Acoust. Soc. Am. **100**, 3417–3430 (1996)
20. Feng, Y., Grace, J.H., Steve, A.X., Max, L.: Detecting anticipatory effects in speech articulation by means of spectral coefficient analyses. Speech Commun. **53**, 842–854 (2011)
21. Tahiry, K., Mounir, B., Mounir, I., Farchi, A.: Energy bands and spectral cues for Arabic vowels recognition. Int. J. Speech Technol. **19**(4), 707–716 (2016). (Springer)
22. Tahiry, K., Mounir, B., Mounir, I., Elmazouzi, L., Farchi, A.: Arabic stop consonants characterization and classification using the normalized energy in frequency bands. Int. J. Speech Technol. **20**(4), 869–880 (2017). (Springer)

Combined Mixed Finite Element, Nonconforming Finite Volume Methods for Flow and Transport -Nitrate- in Porous Media

Omar El Moutea[✉] and Hassan El Amri

Laboratoire de Mathématiques et Applications. ENS-Casablanca, Hassan II University of Casablanca, Casablanca, Morocco
mouteaomar@gmail.com

Abstract. In this paper, we have applied a numerical method, to Simulate a coupled partial differential equation, applied in groundwater flow. For our study, we want to predict the development of nitrate in our reservoir, for 30 years.

Keywords: Flow and transport in porous media · Mixed finite element · Nonconforming finite volume methods

1 Introduction

In this paper, we have applied a new numerical method for solving a coupled partial differential system (1)–(2), this system modeling the flow and transport contaminants, in heterogeneous porous media.

We use Mixed finite element method, to obtain a precise approximation of the flow, the elliptic equation, and a nonconforming finite volume method to the concentration, the diffusion-convection equation. For our study area, we want to study with this model the development of nitrate pollution in the 2D aquifer for the next 30 years, for more information about this model (see, e.g., [1, 2]).

2 Model of Problem

For a reason of simplicity, let's neglect gravity effects. Consider the single-phase flow of an incompressible fluid, in a two-dimensional horizontal reservoir with a dissolved solute in a porous media.

By adding the boundary conditions for the two equations, and the initial condition for transport Eq. (2), we have:

© Springer Nature Switzerland AG 2019
M. Ezziyyani (Ed.): AI2SD 2018, AISC 915, pp. 383–392, 2019.
https://doi.org/10.1007/978-3-030-11928-7_34

The Pressure equation, defined by:

$$\begin{cases} \vec{q} = -\frac{K(x)}{\mu}\nabla p & in \quad \Omega \\ div\vec{q} = 0 & in \quad \Omega \\ \vec{q}.\vec{n}_{|\Gamma_1^1} = q_0, \vec{q} \cdot \vec{n}_{|\Gamma_2^2} = q_0, p_{\Gamma_3} = p^0 & in\,]0, T[\end{cases} \quad (1)$$

where $\Gamma = \Gamma_1 \cap \Gamma_2 \cap \Gamma_3$ is the boundary of Ω, μ is the viscosity of the mixture. p, $\vec{q}$ are the pressure respectively Darcy velocity of the fluid mixture, K is the porosity and Φ the permeability of the medium,

The Concentration equation, defined by:

$$\begin{cases} \Phi(x)\frac{\partial c}{\partial t} - div(D(x,\vec{q})\nabla c) + divc \cdot \vec{q} = f(x,t)\,in\,Q \\ c|\Gamma = 0 & in\,]0, T[\\ c(x,0) = c_0(x) & on\,\Omega \end{cases} \quad (2)$$

where, c is the concentration of the contaminant solute, and f is the external rate of flow.

3   Numerical Methods

Let's say the following notations and assumptions,

(1) Ω is a bounded open polygonal subset of R^2, and $Q = \Omega \times]0,T[$.
(2) $\Phi \in L^\infty(\Omega), 0 \le \Phi(x) \le 1$ a.e in Ω, $f \in L^2(Q)$ and $f(x,t) \ge 0$ a.e in Q.
(3) μ is a lipschitz continuous function such that, $0 < \mu_- \le \mu(x) \le \mu^+$.
(4) $c \in C^2(\Omega), c_0 \in L^\infty(\Omega), 0 \le c_0(x) \le 1$ a.e in Ω and $c \in [0, 1]$.
(5) D and K are bounded, uniformly positive definite symmetric tensors (that is to say.
   $\forall \zeta \ne 0, d_-|\zeta|^2 \le D\zeta \cdot \zeta \le d^+|\zeta|^2 < \infty$ a.e in Ω).
(6) $\vec{q} \in (L^\infty(\Omega))^2$ a.e in $]0,T[$, $q_0 \ge 0$.

Note that, these assumptions are very important to prove the existence, uniqueness classic and discrete solutions.

3.1   Mixed Finite Element Method (MFEM)

The hybrid mixed finite element method, is a robust technique performs well in every case. The popularity of this method has increased considerably as consequence of hard work made in recent years, in developing efficient algorithms (see, e.g., [3]). For the accurate approximation of the pressure-velocity equation $(\vec{q}_h^n, p_h^n)$, at time $t = t_n$, (For suitability in notation, in this subsection we will denote, $(\vec{q}_h^n, p_h^n) = (\vec{q}_h, p_h)$ and $\mu(c) = \mu(c(x, t_n))$ and using this method, (see, e.g., [3, 4]). Accurate simulation requires an accurate approximation of the velocity $\vec{q}$, because the transport term is governed by the fluid velocity in (2), a sequential approach is adopted.

Before you start, we introduce some finite element spaces $RT_0(T)$, X_0^h and P_0^h (see, e.g., [3, 4]). The lowest Raviart-Thomas space $R_{0,T}$ is defined in [1].

We defined a Lagrangian multiplier λ_h (see [3]). The solution of the following mixed hybrid finite element scheme, is finds $(\vec{q}_h, p_h, \lambda_h) \in X_0^h \times P_0^h \times L_h^{P_0}$ such that:

$$
\begin{cases}
\int_T \mu K^{-1} \vec{q}_h \cdot s_h - p_h \, divs_h \, dT + \sum_{T' \in T} \int_{T'} \lambda_h s_h \cdot ndT' = 0 & \forall s_h \in R_{0,T} \\
\int_T v_h div \, \vec{q}_h dT = 0 & \forall v_h \in P_0^h \\
\sum_{T \in T_K} \sum_{T' \in T} \int_{T'} w_h q_h \cdot ndT' + \sum_{T' \in \Gamma_1} \int_{T'} q_0 w_h dT' & \forall w_h \in L_h^0
\end{cases}
\tag{3}
$$

To solve the linear system of very large equations, can be write in a very big matrix, (see, e.g., [3, 4]) and decrease the solution of the system (3), the solution of this linear system obtained by involving only the Lagrangian multipliers vector λ_h, it is a symmetric positive definite and sparse matrix.

3.2 The Discrete Problem for Transport Equation

In this section, we will define a semi-implicit scheme: explicit approximation of the convection term and implicit approximation of the diffusion-dispersion term. For discretization the convection term using a Godunov scheme and we use Nonconforming Finite Volume method for the diffusion term, these methods of the finite volumes require the construction Dual mesh, (see, e.g., [1]).

Note that, the unstructured meshes allow treat geometrically complex geological structures, this is real because the coefficients in (1), (2) can be discontinuous, depended on the lithology of the reservoir and the physical situation like. To start our study, we can see some very useful notation and definitions in [5, 8]. The first step in this part is defining the discrete solution to the concentration equation. Then, the aim of the second parts is to prove the existence and uniqueness these solutions.

Domain Discretization's: Some Definitions and Notations

Before represent the numerical discretization of the transport equation, let T be a partition of time, the size time step is $\Delta t_n = t_{n+1} - t_n$. The next figures, resume the space discretization we can see more notations and definitions in [5].

Let P be a primary meshes of the polygonal Ω (not necessarily convex) domain, such that $\Omega = \bigcup_{L \in P} L$. We define the vertex $x_K, \forall K \in P$, it's necessaire to obtain the corresponding dual cell $K^* \in D$, the Dual mesh $D = \bigcup_{K^* \in D} K^*$ is a partition of our domain Ω. obtained by connecting x_K with the medium of the edge (see Figs. 1 and 2).

Formulation of the Discrete Problem

Let us now concentrate on investigating the transport Eq. (2) in general mesh, by nonconforming finite volume, this scheme obtained should be a linear system involving discrete unknowns the quantities (c_P^n, c_{P*}^n). These unknowns (noted by c_P^n, c_{P*}^n just for simplify where $c_M^n = c(x_1^M, x_2^M, t_n)$, $M = P, P*; \forall(P, P*) \in P \times D$ see [5].

3.3 Nonconforming Finite Volume Method and Computation of Fluxes

We integrate the two sides of the Eq. (2) in $K \times \Delta t^n$. Applying the Ostrogradski's theorem to the integral in the left-hand side of this equation leads to computing the flux

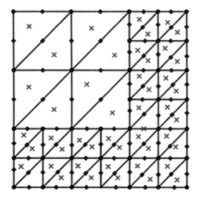

Fig. 1. Example of a primary unstructured mesh edgepoints and cellpoint

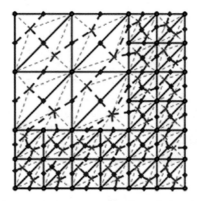

Fig. 2. Dual mesh (blue discontinuous lines) Diamond cell (red discontinuous lines)

across the boundary of K. The diffusion tensor of the cell K noted by D^K, $n^K_{[x_{K*},x_{L*}]}$ is the unit normal vector to $[x_{K*},x_{L*}]$ exterior to K, see Fig. 3.

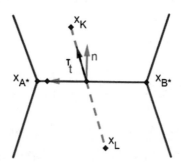

Fig. 3. Two molecules for a DDFV computation of the flux

The convective numerical flux is approached as:

$$\int_{[x_{K*},x_{L*}]} div\, c\,\overrightarrow{.q}\, ds = \left(c_L^n - c_K^n\right)\left(-q_{K,L} \cdot n_{K,L}\right)^+ \tag{4}$$

where $\overline{K} \cap \overline{L} = [x_{K*}, x_{L*}]$, in a similar way approach the term in a dual mesh. We are only interested in the diffusion term, for the other terms remained the same, see [5].

Because the orthogonality is not satisfied see [5], using the decomposition of the tensor $D^K n_{[x_{K*},x_{L*}]}^K$, in the following identity holds:

$$D^K n_{[x_{K*},x_{L*}]}^K = a^h(D^K)\tau_{[x_K,x_L]}^K - b_h(D^K)\tau_{[x_{K*},x_{L*}]}^K \tag{5}$$

where $a^h(D^K)$ and $b^h(D^K)$ is defined as:

$$\begin{cases} a^h(D^K) = \frac{1}{\cos\theta_h^{K,\mathrm{I}}} \left(n_{[x_{K*},x_{L*}]}^K\right)^t D^K n_{[x_{K*},x_{L*}]}^K \\ b_h(D^K) = \frac{1}{\cos\theta_h^{K,\mathrm{I}}} \left(n_{[x_{K*},x_I]}^{K*}\right)^t D^K n_{[x_{K*},x_{L*}]}^K \end{cases} \tag{6}$$

Proposition (Consistency property) Let (P, E) is a regular mesh system, under the assumptions, there exists a strictly positive number C, mesh independent such that:

$$\mathrm{Err} = Ch^2. \tag{7}$$

The relation (7), is a consistency property, and so naturally allows to approximate the flux F_{L*K*}, where $F_{L*K*} = \overline{F_{L*K*}} + \mathrm{Err}$ by $\overline{F_{L*K*}}$.

$\overline{F_{L*K*}}$ present the diffusive numerical flux of F_{L*K*}, defined by:

$$\overline{F_{L*K*}} = \Delta t_n \left(b_h(D^K)\left(c_{K*}^{n+1} - c_{L*}^{n+1}\right) + a^h(D^K)\frac{h_{K*I}}{h_{KI}}\left(c_K^{n+1} - c_I^{n+1}\right) \right). \tag{8}$$

To eliminate c_I^{n+1} in (8), we set the projection of $D^L n_{[x_{K*},x_{L*}]}^L$,

$$D^L n_{[x_{K*},x_{L*}]}^L = a^h(D^L)\tau_{[x_{K*},x_{L*}]}^L - b_h(D^L)\tau_{[x_K,x_L]}^L \tag{9}$$

where $\widehat{a}^h(D^L)$ and $\widehat{b}^h(D^L)$ is real numbers defined as:

$$\begin{cases} \widehat{a}^h(D^L) = \frac{1}{\cos\theta_h^{L,\mathrm{I}}} \left(n_{[x_{K*},x_{L*}]}^L\right)^t D^L n_{[x_{K*},x_{L*}]}^L \\ \widehat{b}^h(D^L) = \frac{1}{\cos\theta_h^{L,\mathrm{I}}} \left(n_{[x_{K*},x_I]}^L\right)^t D^L n_{[x_{K*},x_{L*}]}^L \end{cases} \tag{10}$$

By using the consistency of flux, we have the following first semi-implicit scheme, based on DDFV scheme, We can see the consistency and stability of this scheme in [5, 6].

The scheme defined by for all $K \in P$ we have:

$$c_K^{n+1}(1 + \frac{D_{KK}^1}{|K|\Phi_K}) - \sum_{\substack{L \in P \\ \overline{L} \cap \overline{K}}} (\frac{D_{LK}^1}{|K|\Phi_K} c_L^{n+1} - \frac{D_{L*K}^2}{|K|\Phi_K}(c_{L*}^{n+1} - c_{K*}^{n+1})$$

$$= c_K^n(1 - \frac{\Delta t_n}{|K|\Phi_K})(-q_{K,L} \cdot n_{K,L}^+) + \frac{\Delta t_n}{|K|\Phi_K} \sum_{\substack{L \in P \\ \overline{L} \cap \overline{K}}} c_L^n(-q_{K,L} \cdot n_{K,L})^+ + (\frac{\Delta t_n}{\Phi_K})f_K^n$$

$$(11)$$

where $\overline{L} \cap \overline{K} = [x_{K*}, x_{L*}]$ and

$$\begin{cases} D_{LK}^1 = \Delta t_n \frac{a^h(D^K)a^h(D^L)h_{K*L*}}{a^h(D^K)h_{IL} + a^h(D^L)h_{KI}}, \\ D_{LK}^2 = \Delta t_n \frac{b_h(D^K)a^h(D^L)h_{KI} + a^h(D^K)b_h(D^L)h_{IL}}{a^h(D^K)h_{IL} + a^h(D^L)h_{KI}}. \end{cases}$$

$$(12)$$

Necessity of Defining a Dual Grid

To solve a system, it is necessary that: the number of unknown equals equations number, which is not satisfied we can sees that discrete unknowns $(c_P)_{P \in P}$ and $(c_{P*})_{P* \in D}$ is superior than the number of equations in (11). To solve the problem, corresponding to the equilibrium number of unknowns and equations. To do this, we define a Dual mesh, as described in [5] see Fig. 2. To apply our technique, we must introduce a new notion the notion of pseudo-cutting associated with Dual mesh. Under the same assumptions and thanks to consistency property see (7), the scheme is a consistence.

We start, with integrating the two sides of Eq. (2), in a dual cell D, represented [5], applying the Ostrogradski's theorem, using the following identity holds:

$$D^K n_{[x_I, x_L]}^{K*} = c_h(D^K)\tau_{[x_I, x_L]}^{K*} - d_h(D^K)\tau_{[x_{K*}, x_{L*}]}^{K*},$$

$$(13)$$

where $c_h(D^K)$ and $d_h(D^K)$ is a real number are given by the relations:

$$\begin{cases} c_h(D^K) = b_h(D^K) \\ d_h(D^K) = \frac{1}{\cos \theta_h^{p,1}} (\tau_{[x_{K*}, x_I]}^{K*})^t K^P \tau_{[x_{K*}, x_{L*}]}^{K*} > 0 \end{cases}$$

$$(14)$$

Similarly, let us focus on the computation of the flux across edge $[x_I, x_L]$, for this purpose, we set:

$$D^L n_{[x_I, x_L]}^{K*} = -c_h(D^L)\tau_{[x_I, x_L]}^{K*} - d_h(D^L)\tau_{[x_{K*}, x_{L*}]}^{K*}$$

$$(15)$$

Finally, we summarize the flux approximation across the pseudo-edge $[x_K, x_L], \forall K*, L* \in D^2$, and $\overline{L*} \cap \overline{K*} = [x_K, x_L]$, in the following way, we have the second semi-implicit finite volume scheme,

$$c_{K*}^{n+1}(1 + \frac{D_{K*K*}^2}{|K*|\Phi_{K*}}) - \sum_{\substack{L* \in P \\ L* \cap K*}} \frac{D_{L*K*}^2}{|K*|\Phi_{K*}} c_{L*}^{n+1} + \frac{D_{LK*}^1}{|K*|\Phi_{K*}}(c_L^{n+1} - c_K^{n+1})$$

$$= c_{K*}^n(1 - \frac{\Delta t_n}{|K*|\Phi_{K*}} (-q_{K,L}.n_{K,L})^+) + \frac{\Delta t_n}{|K*|\Phi_{K*}} \sum_{\substack{L* \in P \\ L* \cap K*}} c_{L*}^n(-q_{K,L} \cdot n_{K,L})^+$$

$$+ \frac{\Delta t_n}{|K*|\Phi_{K*}} f_{K*}^n$$

(16)

where $\overline{L*} \cap \overline{K*} = [x_K, x_L]$ and

$$\begin{cases} D_{LK*}^1 = -D_{KL*}^1 \\ D_{L*K*}^2 = D_{L*K*}^2 \end{cases}$$

(17)

In this part, we sum up the Eqs. (11) and (16), we define a semi implicit non-conforming FV scheme to transport equations as:
Find $C^{n+1} = (c_K^{n+1}, c_{K*}^{n+1})$ such that:

$$A^n C^{n+1} = F^n$$

(18)

The components of the matrix A^n, and vertex F^n is defined in previous section.

4   Existence and Uniqueness for a Solution of the Discrete Problem

Existence and uniqueness for a solution of the discrete problem is proved, in another article submitted. for convergence this scheme is proved see [6].

5   Numerical Results

In this section, we present some numerical results in 2D, based on the combined mixed finite element and nonconforming finite volume methods presented in this paper. The modeled hydrogeological domain is of a rectangular shape of 300 m long, and 150 m high, devised a four-part see Fig. 4. The choice of the conceptual model has been conditioned not only by the search for a high degree of precision but also by the quantity and quality of the data available. The evolution of the pollutant concentration

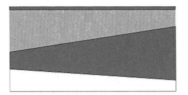

Fig. 4. Permeability distribution

defined by this model is followed for a period of 30 years. The boundary conditions are
the two types, Dirichlet and Neumann defined as follows:

$$
\begin{cases}
P = 15 & \text{on} &]30, 110] \times \{300\} \\
P = 10 & \text{on} &]110, 145] \times \{300\} \\
P = 5 & \text{on} &]70, 145] \times \{0\} \\
P = 3 & \text{on} &]0, 70] \times \{0\} \\
P = 0 & \text{on} &]145, 150] \times \{0\}.\{0\} \times]0, 300] \\
P = p^0 - P & \text{on} & \{150\} \times \{150\} \\
\vec{q} \cdot \vec{n} = 0 & \text{on} &]0, 30] \times \{300\}.\{150\} \times]0, 300]
\end{cases}
$$

For our simulations, we take real coefficients see [7], and we put them according to
this model. The hydraulic conductivity distribution resulting from this model revealed
three zones of permeability, between 2.9 and $2.9 10^{-4}$ m/s see [2]. An area with very
low permeability with values less than $2.9 10^{-4}$ m/s, generally located first part at the
top and third part see previous Fig. 4, a zone with good permeability with values
greater than $2.9 10^{-2}$ m/s. This area is located mainly to the second part. The rest of the
domain corresponds to intermediate permeability is 2.9 m/s. The values of the storage
coefficient resulting from this calibration vary between $5 10^{-4}$ and $2 10^{-1}$, these variations are due mainly to lateral facies changes in the aquifer. The effective porosity is
estimated at 3% see [2]. The calibration of the hydro dispersive model made it possible
to determine longitudinal dispersivity values α_L varying between 98 and 103 m over
the entire domain, the anisotropy ratio (α_T/α_L) being chosen equal to 0.1 [9]. We
simplify these coefficients for better results or we will have very complicated and
difficult calculations [2, 3]. The permeability distribution, and pressure contours are
presented in the next Figs. 4 and 5.

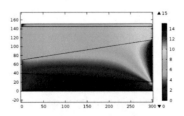

Fig. 5. Pressure

The initial values of the concentration are null on the whole domain except the high part equal to one at instant zero. We show the concentration contours at three times step at t = 0, 10, 15, 20 years in the next Figs. 6, 7, 8 and 9.

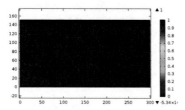

Fig. 6. Concentration at T = 0 years

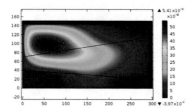

Fig. 7. Concentration at T = 10 years

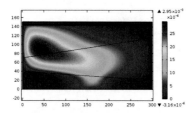

Fig. 8. Concentration at T = 15 years

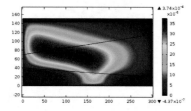

Fig. 9. Concentration at T = 30 years

References

1. Sachse, A., Nixdorf, E., Jang, E., Rink, K., Fischer, T., Xi, B., Beyer, C., Bauer, S., Walther, M., Sun, Y., Song, Y.: Reactive nitrate transport model. In: Open GeoSys Tutorial. SpringerBriefs in Earth System Sciences. Springer, Cham
2. El Bouqdaoui, K., Aachib, M., Blaghen, M., Kholtei, S.: Modélisation de la pollution par les nitrates de la nappe de Berrechid, au Maroc
3. Amaziane, B., El Ossmani, M.: Convergence analysis of an approximation to miscible fluid flows in porous media by combining mixed finite element and finite volume methods. Numer. Methods Partial Differ. Equ. **24**, 799–832 (2008)
4. Chou, S.H., Kwak, D.Y., Kim, K.Y.: A general framework for constructing and analyzing mixed finite volume methods on quadrilateral grids: the overlapping covolume case. SIAM J. Numer. Anal. **39**(4), 1170–1196 (2001)
5. Njifenjou, A., Moukouop-Nguena, I.: Traitement des anisotropies de permèabilitè en simulation d'ècoulement en milieu poreux par les volumes finis. In: Tchuente, M. (ed.) Proceedings of an International Conference on "Systèmes Informatiques pour la Gestion de l'Environnement", pp. 245–259. Douala, Cameroon (2001)
6. Eymard, R., Gallouet, T., Herbin, R.: A new finite volume scheme for anisotropic diffusion problems on general grids: convergence analysis. C.R. Math. Acad. Sci. Paris **344**(6), 40340 (2007)
7. Bourgeat, A., Kern, M. (eds.): Simulation of Transport around a Nuclear Waste Disposal Site: The Couplex Test Cases, Computational Geosciences, vol. 8. Kluwer Academic, Dordrecht (2004)
8. Njifenjou, A., Mbehou, M., Moukouop Nguena, I.: Analysis on General Meshes of a DDFV Type Method for Subsurface Flow Problems
9. NF-PRO: Understanding physical and numerical modelling of the key processes in the near field, and their coupling, for different host rocks and repository strategies, contract FI6W-CT-2003-02389 (2004)

Artificial Neural Network Optimized by Genetic Algorithm for Intrusion Detection System

Mehdi Moukhafi[1]([✉]), Khalid El Yassini[1], Seddik Bri[2], and Kenza Oufaska[3]

[1] Department of Mathematics and Computer Sciences,
Faculty of Sciences, Informatics and Applications Laboratory,
Moulay Ismail University, Meknes, Morocco
{mehdi.moukhafi,khalid.elyassini}@gmail.com
[2] Department of Electrical Engineering, Materials and Instrumentations (MIN),
ESTM, Moulay Ismail University, Meknes, Morocco
briseddik@gmail.com
[3] Faculty of Computer Science and Logistics,
International University of Rabat, Rabat, Morocco
kenza.oufaska@uir.ac.ma

Abstract. Due to the convergence of new communication technologies to compatible platforms, the number of intrusions into computer systems is growing the attacks carried out by malicious users to exploit the vulnerabilities of these systems are more and more frequent; In this context, intrusion detection systems (IDS) have emerged as a group of methods that combats the unauthorized use of a network's resources. Recent advances in information technology, especially in machine learning, have produced a wide variety of methods, which can be integrated into an IDS. This paper presents a technique of intrusion detection based on pre-treatment of data set and classification intrusions with a Self Organizing Map (SOM) Artificial Neural Network method optimized with Genetic algorithm (GA) to develop a model for intrusion detection system. The simulation results show a significant improvement in detection rate. The performance of the proposed method of intrusion detection was evaluated on all UNSW-nb15 and KDD99 data sets.

Keywords: Anomaly intrusion detection system (IDS) · Machine learning based intrusion detection · Self organizing map (SOM) · Neural network, genetic algorithm

1 Introduction

The connectivity of data and objects is the critical component of new production technologies such as sensor networks, connectivity of software, equipment's, massive data processing etc.... In this context, the cybersecurity become essential elements that allow to create the intelligence in a manufacturing system capable of greater adaptability in production and a more efficient allocation of resources. these are essential for

© Springer Nature Switzerland AG 2019
M. Ezziyani (Ed.): AI2SD 2018, AISC 915, pp. 393–404, 2019.
https://doi.org/10.1007/978-3-030-11928-7_35

the monitoring of the state of large installations of agriculture, photovoltaics, wind farm etc. … and any interruption or pane, due to an attack, can cause loss of performance as well as damage, sometimes irreversible. The number of intrusions into computer systems is constantly growing, the attacks carried out by malicious users to exploit the vulnerabilities of these systems are more and more frequent; These intrusions, increasingly complex, are easy to implement, especially with the easy access to security test tools which are accessible to professionals as well as hackers. As the complexity of the attacks keeps increasing, new and more robust detection mechanisms need to be developed.

Intrusion detection systems (IDS), presented for the first time by Anderson in 1980 [1], and later formalized by Denning [2], aim to identify and respond to malicious activity that compromises network and computer security [1]. There are two types of IDSs: Network Intrusion Detection Systems (NIDSs) detect attacks by observing various network activities, while Host-based Intrusion Detection Systems (HIDSs) detect intrusions in an individual host.

Actual IDS's based on heuristic rules, such as Snort, are signature based system. The problem with this method is that cannot detect novel attacks whose signature is not available and hence generates a high rate of alerts. the major drawback of approaches based signature is that detect only known attacks, and the system need to be constantly database updating. To overcome the mentioned problem above, many techniques have been developed [3], Especially using Artificial Intelligence (AI) technologies.

Indeed, the new searches approaches the problem of detection of intrusion from a different perspective, instead of trying to detect the intrusion by comparing its signature with a database, it seeks to establish a model of behavior of each type Intrusion, in other words, To detect the attacks (and these variations) it is necessary to study the behavior of this last one, the behavior of the legitimate traffic in order to establish a model capable of classifying the traffic circulating within the network in two categories: normal and abnormal.

This paper presents intrusion detection system model based on neural network, using self-organizing map (SOM) optimized with Genetic Algorithm (GA). SOM classifier is employed to classify a network traffic into normal and abnormal connections.

The paper is organized as follows: Related works are discussed in Sects. 1, 2 gives an overview of methods used in this work and a description of the proposed method, Sect. 3 describes the system model, Sect. 4, evaluates the proposed system and at last, Sect. 5 presents the conclusion of this work.

2 Related Work

Anomaly detection has been an important subject in intrusion detection research. Various anomaly detection approaches based on Artificial Intelligence technologies are utilized in IDSs due to their flexibility and learning capability. These intelligent systems construct a general model of existing patterns which will be able to detect new attacks. Additionally, the IDS's performances are considerably improved at the network level. The machine learning algorithm obtains a good detection performance in terms of classifying the flow of a network into normal or abnormal behaviors. Feng et al. [4] introduced an approach combining SVM with self-organized ant colony network.

Kuang et al. [5] propose a solution based on a combination of the Support Vector Machine (SVM) model with kernel Principal Component Analysis (KPCA) and genetic algorithm. KPCA was used to reduce the dimensions of feature vectors, where GA was employed to optimize the SVM parameters.

Wathiq et al. [6] propose a solution based on hybrid SVM and Extreme Learning Machine (ELM) model learned with data set built by a modified K-means. The modified K-means is used to build new small training datasets representing the entire original training dataset.

Intrusion detection technique used by Saied et al. [7] to detect Distributed Denial of Service (DDOS) attacks known and unknown in real time, based on Artificial Neural Network (ANN). The model classifies legitimate traffic and attacks traffic using learning by back propagation coupled with a sigmoid activation function, the authors has selected three ANN topological structures, one for the most used protocols (TCP, UDP, ICMP) in DDOS attacks, each one with three layers (input, hidden and output). The number of nodes in each topological structure is different, the ICMP topological structure consists of three inputs and four hidden nodes, the topology structure TCP consists of five inputs and four hidden nodes and the topological structure of UDP consists of four inputs and three hidden nodes that treat the calculation process with respect to input and output nodes. The output layer consists output node for the attacks and an output node for legitimate traffic.

Bhuyan et al. [8] introduced a procedure based on a mutual and general information, an entropy function selection technique for selecting a non-redundant subset of features, based on a clustering and trees to generate a set of reference points and a function of aberrant score, to classify incoming network traffic to identify anomalies.

Nadiammai and Hemalatha [9] were establish a DOS attack detection with a hybrid mechanism which is based on two steps, the first is the analysis of the traffic flow with a SNORT intrusion detection system (based signature), for preliminary detection of the incoming flow and detecting known attacks, the second step is the recovery of the classified flows as legitimate and applies a classification based supervised learning (SVM) with the use of the kernel function Radial Basis Function (RBF).

The present study proposes propose an intrusion detection method based on the combination of two algorithms Genetic Algorithm (GA) and self-organizing map (SOM), the method is evaluated on the data set KDD 1999, to show that the system performance intrusion detection is significantly promoted by our method.

3   Proposed Work

In this section, we first describe self-organizing map algorithm, Genetic algorithm and discuss our proposed method for IDS.

3.1   Self-Organizing Map

Artificial Neural Network (ANN) is defined as an information processing system that has characteristics resembling biological nervous systems [10]. The ANN provides a new technology to help solve problems that require thinking of experts and computer based routine.

Il this paper the ANN method which applied is SOM method, that to be classify the network traffic into normal and attacks traffics.

Self-Organizing Map (SOM) originally proposed by Kohonen [11], its main characteristic of is its ability to recognize patterns in complex sets via an unsupervised methodology is a fully connected single-layer linear network, where the output generally is organized in a two-dimensional arrangement of nodes, see Fig. 1. The fundamental of the SOM is the soft competition between the nodes in the output layer; not only one node (the winner) but also its neighbors are updated.

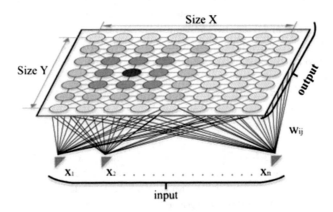

Fig. 1. Classical example of self-organizing map

In this method, a measure is used to determine the distribution of an input space over an output space (generally of a lower dimension). This measure is defined by a group of neurons distributed over a line, rectangular, or hexagonal plane, thus preserving the properties of the patterns in the input space.

The SOM system is adaptively to classify samples into classes determined by selecting the winning neurons are competitive and the weights are modified. Figure 1 shows a very small Kohonen's network, the input space is represented by a vector of inputs, while the output space is given by the values of the diagram of nodes that are activated with different colors depending on the input. All neurons in the output layer are well connected to adjacent neurons by a neighborhood relation depicting the structure of the map.

The Self-Organizing Map algorithm can be broken up into 6 steps:

1. Each node's weights are initialized. The weight vector of the neuron j is defined as $w_j = (\omega_{j1}, \ldots \omega_{jn})$, where the weights ω_{ji} is related to the input x_i.
2. A vector x is chosen at random from the data set of training and presented to the network.
3. Every node in the network is examined to calculate which ones' weights are most like the input vector. The winning node is commonly known as the Best Matching Unit (BMU) by:

$$\text{DistFromInput}^2 = \sum_{i=0}^{i=n} (I^i - W^i) \tag{1}$$

where I is the current input vector, W the node's weight vector And n is the number of weights.

4. Determine the radius of the neighborhood of the BMU. This value starts large. Typically, it is set to be the radius of the network, diminishing each iteration by:

$$\sigma(t) = \sigma_0 e^{(-t/\lambda)} \tag{2}$$

where σ_0 is the radius of the map, t is the current iteration and λ is the time costant.

5. Adjust weights of nodes within in the BMU t neighbourhood towards the chosen datapoint by:

$$W(t+1) = W(t) + \theta(t)L(t)(I(t) - W(t)) \tag{3}$$

where (t) is the weight vector of the neuron x, L(t) is the learning rate, and θ (t) is a neighboring function.

6. Repeat steps 2–5 for N iteration.

3.2 Genetic Algorithm

Genetic Algorithm (GA), refers to a model introduced and investigated by Holland [12], It is a general adaptive optimization search methodology based on a direct analogy to Darwinian's principle of evolution of fittest to optimize a population of candidate solutions towards a predefined fitness [13].

The algorithm by natural selection can be formulated in many ways, but the following encapsulates its essential elements:

- Successive generations can differ from previous ones.
  Children inherit characteristics of their parents. But combining and mutating these characteristics introduces variation from generation to generation.
- Less fit individuals are selectively eliminated ('survival of the fittest').
  The procedure for a genetic algorithm is:

1. Create an initial random population of individuals.
2. Evaluation—Each individual x of the population is then evaluated and we calculate a 'fitness' for that individual.
3. Repeat:

   • Selection—Select Best individuals from a population, based on their fitness (the better fitness, the bigger chance to be selected).
   • Crossover—create new individuals by combining aspects of our selected parent.
   • Mutation—The algorithm creates mutation children by randomly changing the genes of individual parents. Mutation typically works by making very small changes at random to an individual genome.
   • Replace the worst chromosomes of the population by the best new chromosomes.
   • Evaluate the fitness of de new Chromosomes.

4. Test—If the end condition is satisfied, stop, and return the best solution in current population.

3.3   Benchmark KDD-99

• **KDD-99**

Cyber Systems and Technology Group of MIT Lincoln Laboratory [14] simulated LAN US Air Force LAN with multiple attacks and captured nine weeks TCPdump data. This database was first used for competitions kdd99, but since it has become the database test to the IDS's based on a behavioral approach. KDD Cup 1999 provided both the training dataset, it is called KDd99_10p. Each connection record consists of approximately 100 bytes. This was converted into about 49 * 105 connection vectors each one contains 41 fields.

This database is collected by simulating attacks on different platforms such as Windows, Unix… Four gigabytes of raw data compressed TCP dump is transformed into five million connections files. The attacks are divided into four main categories: Denial of Service Attack (DOS), Probing, User to Root Attack (U2R), Remote to Local Attack (R2L) (Table 1).

Table 1. List of attacks present in KDD99 Dataset

Attack groups	Attacks
Probe	Ipsweep, mscan, nmap, portsweep, satan
DOS	apache2, back, land, mailbomb, Neptune, processtable, pod, udpstorm, smurf, teardrop
U2R	buffer_overflow, httptuneel, loadmodule, perl, rootkit, xterm, ps, sqlattack
R2L	ftp_write, imap, guess_passwd, named, multihop, phf, sendmail, snmpgetattack, snmpguess, spy, warezclient, worm, warezmaster, zsnoop, xlock

Connection Examples:

0,tcp,smtp,

SF,946,494,0,0,0,0,0,1,0,0,0,0,0,0,0,0,0,0,1,1,0.00,0.00,0.00,0.00,1.00,0.00,0.00,

64,243,0.94,0.05,0.02,0.02,0.00,0.00,0.00,0.00,normal.

25,tcp,telnet,

SF,269,2333,0,0,0,0,0,1,0,1,0,2,2,1,0,0,0,0,1,1,0.00,0.00,0.00,0.00,1.00,0.00,0.00,

69,2,0.03,0.06,0.01,0.00,0.00,0.00,0.00,0.00,smurf.

- **UNSW-NB15**

A recent network intrusion detection data set, UNSW-NB15, proposed in [15], as a modernized dataset which reflects the contemporary network traffic characteristics and new low-footprint attack scenarios. UNSW-NB15 is a collection of the raw network traffics which is created by the Cyber Range Lab of the Australian Centre for Cyber Security (ACCS), it was developed by using IXIA tool to extract a hybrid of modern normal and modern attack behaviors. 100 GB of the raw traffic was transformed into 2,540,044 connections, each connection is represented by 49 features. This dataset was divided into 175,341 and 82,332 records for training and testing. This data set involves nine different moderns attack types (compared to 4 attack types in KDD'99 dataset) wide varieties of real normal activities [16]:

- The Fuzzers attack is an unauthorized attempt to discover security loopholes in the victim system by feeding it with a massive inputting of random data.
- The Analysis attack is an unauthorized attempt to penetrate the web applications via ports (e.g. port scans), emails (e.g. spam) and web scripts (e.g. HTML files).
- The Backdoor attack is an unauthorized access from a remote machine. The DoS attack is an unauthorized attempt to disrupt the normal functioning of a victim host or a network.
- The Exploit attack is a sequence of instructions that takes advantage of a glitch, bug or vulnerability on the victim system.
- The Generic attack is an attempt to cause a collision on the victim system without respecting the configuration of the block-cipher.
- The Reconnaissance attack is an unauthorized attempt to gather information about a victim system to evade its security controls.
- The Shell-code attack is an unauthorized attempt to penetrate a slight piece of code starting from a shell to control the com-promised machine.
- The Worms attack is an attack in which the attacker replicates itself to spread on other computers.

3.4 Proposed Approach

The Genetic Algorithm begins with n individuals chosen randomly. Each individual is an M-dimensional vector which represents a candidate's solution. The Self-Organizing map (for this ability to recognize patterns in complex sets) to *build* a wide range candidates solution to evaluate its performance until the optimal solution (combination of features). The GA algorithm guide the selection of potential subsets that lead to better prediction accuracy. The algorithm uses the best individuals to contribute to the generation of the next generation. Thus, on average, each successive population of candidate particles is better than its predecessor. Figure 2 describes the proposed solution.

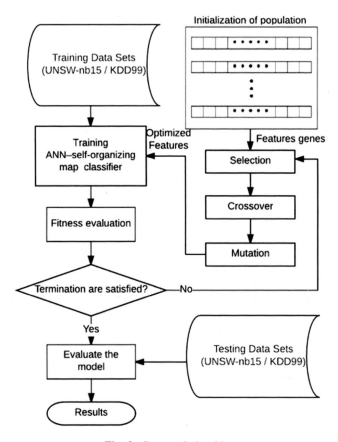

Fig. 2. Proposed algorithm

At each iteration the classifier is trained with an individual and evaluated by his fitness, the evaluation function used is the maximization of the accuracy. each individual is given a probability of being selected that is directly proportionate to its fitness score. After this step, the algorithm selects half of the individuals evaluated for applying a crossover to produce offspring with them.

After selection and crossover, the algorithm applies a mutation to the reproduced population by randomly changing 1% of genes of each individual in order to ensure that the individuals are different from the previous population.

The technique 10-folds crossover validation is used. The k-folds crossover validation is typically used to reduce the error resulting from random sampling in comparing accuracies of a number of predictive models. The study divided training data into 10-folds where 1 was to test and 9 folds were for training. This process continues until the performance is satisfactory SOM. After that, we evaluate our optimized model on the entire KDD99 data set.

4 Experiment Setup and Performance Evaluation

In this section, we summarize our experimental results to detect intrusions using the Self-Organizing map optimized with GA over the UNSW-nb15 and KDD'99 datasets. All experiments were conducted on a calculation station 24 CPU Intel Core 2.13 GHz, 48 GB RAM, running under Linux CentOS 7. The implementation was coded using the Java language.

For a binary classifier, confusion matrix shows the results of the real class compared to the predicted result. In these experiments, normal connections are positive events while abnormal represent negative events. To evaluate our approach, we have used four performance indicators from intrusion detection research [17]: True Positive (TP) is the number of real normal logon events that were correctly classified as normal. false positive (FP) is the number of abnormal connections of events that have been incorrectly classified as normal connections. False negative (FN) is the number of normal connections of events that have been incorrectly classified as abnormal connections. True negative (TN) is the number of abnormal connections of events that were correctly classified as abnormal.

The performance of the proposed method of intrusion detection was evaluated on all UNSW-nb15 and KDD99 data sets, UNSW-nb15_Training-Set data set and 10% of the KDD99 were used for training the GA-SOM model. The performance of the proposed method of intrusion detection was evaluated on all KDD99 and UNSW-nb15 data sets. Tables 2 and 3 illustrate the confusion matrix for KDD99 and UNSW-nb15 respectively. this system achieves a top performance of up to 94.35% in accuracy with a detection rate of 99.69% for KDD99 and 82.91% in accuracy with 89.43% in detection rate for UNSW-nb15.

Table 2. KDD99 confusion matrix

	Normal	Intrusion
Normal	TN = 732,335 73.69%	FN = 261,446 26.31%
Intrusion	FP = 1321 0.03%	TP = 3,824,449 99.97%

Table 3. UNSW-nb15 confusion matrix

	Normal	Intrusion
Normal	TN = 32,665 88.28%	FN = 4335 11.72%
Intrusion	FP = 4792 10.57%	TP = 40,540 89.43%

Figure 3 shows the detection rate classified by attack in KDD99, the proposed algorithm has detected 99.89% of DOS attacks whom are the most used by hackers. For Probe attacks a rate of 84.38% is correctly classified, 67.31% for R2L attacks and 84.90% for U2R, the low rate of detection of R2L and U2R attacks can be explained by the insufficient number of data learning about these, unlike the DOS attacks and Probe's which are quite numerous and diversified to build a more accurate detection model.

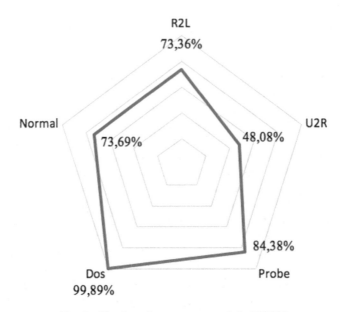

Fig. 3. The detection rate per attack in KDD99

Figure 4 shows the detection rate classified by attack in KDD99, the proposed algorithm has detected 78.1% of Reconnaissance attacks. For Generic attacks a rate of 89.1% is correctly classified, 79.1% for Exploits attacks and 65.9% for Worms.

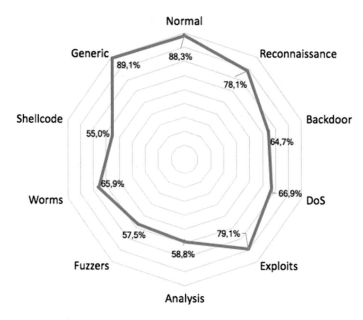

Fig. 4. The detection rate per attack in UNSW-nb15

5   Conclusion and Futures Works

This paper deals the Self-Organizing Maps optimized with a genetic algorithm to detect four types of attack (DOS, probe, U2R and R2L) in KDD99 data set, and nine types of attack (Reconnaissance, Backdoor, DoS, Exploits, Analysis, Fuzzers, Worms, Shellcode, Generic) in UNSW-nb15. We adopted 10 cross validation applied for classification. The GA is applied on the data set to reduce dimensionality and remove redundant and irrelevant features. The proposed approach is evaluated using KDD99 data set. For future work, we will apply clustering to improve the quality of the learning data and thus increase the performance of the prediction model. We will also exploit the characteristics of multi-agent system to speed up data analysis and facilitate model retraining on new attacks to increase the efficiency of the system.

References

1. James, P.: Anderson: Computer Security Threat Monitoring and Surveillance. Technical Report, Fort Washington, PA, USA (1980)
2. Denning, D.E.: An intrusion-detection model. IEEE Trans Softw. Eng. **SE–13**(2), 222–232 (1987)
3. Forrest, S., Hofmeyr, S.A., Somayaji, A., Longstaff, T.A.: A sense of self for Unix processes. In: Proceedings 1996 IEEE Symposium on Security and Privacy. pp. 120–128. IEEE Comput. Soc. Press, Oakland, CA, USA (1996)

4. Feng, W., Zhang, Q., Hu, G., Huang, J.X.: Mining network data for intrusion detection through combining SVMs with ant colony networks. Future Gener. Comput. Syst. **37**, 127–140 (2014)

5. Kuang, F., Xu, W., Zhang, S.: A novel hybrid KPCA and SVM with GA model for intrusion detection. Appl. Soft Comput. J. **18**(C), 178–184 (2014)

6. Al-Yaseen, W.L., Othman, Z.A., Nazri, M.Z.A.: Multi-level hybrid support vector machine and extreme learning machine based on modified K-means for intrusion detection system. Expert Syst. Appl. **67**, 296–303 (2017)

7. Saied, A., Overill, R.E., Radzik, T.: Detection of known and unknown DDoS attacks using Artificial Neural Networks. Neurocomputing **172**, 385–393 (2016)

8. Bhuyan, M.H., Bhattacharyya, D.K., Kalita, J.K.: An effective unsupervised network anomaly detection method. In: Proceedings of the International Conference on Advances in Computing, Communications and Informatics—ICACCI '12. pp. 533–539. ACM Press, New York, USA (2012)

9. Nadiammai, G.V., Hemalatha, M.: Effective approach toward intrusion detection System using data mining techniques. Egypt. Inform. J. **15**(1), 37–50 (2014)

10. Koprinkova-Hristova, P.: Artificial Neural Networks Methods and Applications in Bio-/Neuroinformatics. (2014)

11. Kohonen, T., Kaski, S., Lagus, K., Salojarvi, J., Honkela, J., Paatero, V., Saarela, A.: Self organization of a massive document collection. IEEE Trans. Neural Networks **11**(3), 574–585 (2000)

12. Holland, J.H.: Adaptation in natural and artificial systems. First edn (1992)

13. Sendra, S., Parra, L., Lloret, J., Khan, S.: Systems and algorithms for wireless sensor networks based on animal and natural behavior. Int. J. Distrib. Sens. Netw. **11**(3), 625972 (2015)

14. Tavallaee, M., Bagheri, E., Lu, W., Ghorbani, A.A.: A detailed analysis of the KDD CUP 99 data set. In: IEEE Symposium on Computational Intelligence for Security and Defense Applications, CISDA 2009. pp. 1–6. IEEE, Ottawa, ON, Canada (2009)

15. Moustafa, N., Slay, J.: UNSW-NB15: a comprehensive data set for network intrusion detection systems (UNSW-NB15 network data set). In: 2015 Military Communications and Information Systems Conference (MilCIS). pp. 1–6, Canberra, ACT, Australia (2015)

16. Moustafa, N., Slay, J.: The evaluation of Network Anomaly Detection Systems: Statistical analysis of the UNSW-NB15 data set and the comparison with the KDD99 data set. Inf. Secur. J. **25**(3), 18–31 (2016)

17. Hassan, M.M.M.: Current studies on intrusion detection system, genetic algorithm and fuzzy logic. Int. J. Distrib. Parallel Syst. **4**(1), 35–47 (2013)

Single-Valued Neutrosophic Techniques for Analysis of WIFI Connection

Said Broumi[1]($\boxtimes$), Prem Kumar Singh[2], Mohamed Talea[1],
Assia Bakali[3], Florentin Smarandache[4], and V. Venkateswara Rao[5]

[1] Laboratory of Information Processing, Faculty of Science Ben M'Sik,
University Hassan II, Sidi Othman, B.P 7955, Casablanca, Morocco
broumisaid78@gmail.com, taleamohamed@yahoo.fr
[2] Amity Institute of Information Technology, Amity University,
Sector 125, Noida, Uttar Pradesh, India
premsingh.csjm@gmail.com
[3] Ecole Royale Navale, Boulevard Sour Jdid, B.P 16303, Casablanca, Morocco
assiabakali@yahoo.fr
[4] Department of Mathematics, University of New Mexico,
705 Gurley Avenue, Gallup, NM 87301, USA
fsmarandache@gmail.com
[5] Mathematics Division, Department of S&H, Chirala Engineering College,
Chirala 523157, India
vunnamvenky@gmail.com

Abstract. Wireless ad hoc network (WANET) is self-configured networking. It does not rely on pre-existing routers or access points. Mobile ad hoc network (MANET) is an application of WANET where mobile devices are connected wirelessly without any infrastructure. Such networks are either considered as truly connected, not connected and may disconnected due to noise in network or some other uncertainty in connectivity. In this case, characterizing the truth, indeterminacy and falsity information communicated in the mobile network is difficult while utilizing the traditional mathematical set theories. To resolve this issue, in current paper authors' focus on estimating information processing in MANET via mathematics algebra of Single-Valued Neutrosophic Set (SVNS). In addition, an example is given for better understanding of MANET in the neutrosophic environment.

Keywords: Neutrosophic sets · WANET · MANET · Network connection · Low-medium-high estimations

1 Introduction

Wireless ad hoc network (WANET) is a decentralized network which works without access points as compared to ordinary networks having an access point or router for their performance. WANET is further classified in MANET [1], VANET [2], smart phones ad hoc networks [3], army, air force, navy ad hoc networks [4–6], disaster rescue and hospital ad hoc networks [7, 8] etc.

© Springer Nature Switzerland AG 2019
M. Ezziyyani (Ed.): AI2SD 2018, AISC 915, pp. 405–412, 2019.
https://doi.org/10.1007/978-3-030-11928-7_36

A mobile ad hoc network (MANET) is wireless ad hoc network and it is incessantly self-configuring, infrastructure-less net of mobile devices. All node in a MANET can be dynamic or autonomously moves in different direction and alter the connectivity with distinct nodes regularly. Each of the node used to promote traffic unconnected to its own use, and therefore be a router. The most important challenge in building a MANET is equipping each device to constantly maintain the information required to properly route traffic [9].

There are many protocols which are related to this work one can refer to [10–12]. The growth of laptops and 802.11/Wi-Fi wireless networking has made MANETs a popular research topic since the mid-1990s. Similarly, the smart phone technology has made the MANET more popular since 2016 with high speed even for a common man. Even now a day's all members are using smart phone in that they use networks in travels from one place to another places. In that sometimes network connection signals are good or sometimes it's disconnected. This one explains clearly using fuzzy system but sometimes signals are appear while the data transformation contains uncertainty, which cannot be represented precisely using unipolar fuzzy environment. It used to become more complex when the given information contains acceptation, rejection and uncertain part based on information sent. In this case traditional fuzzy set cannot represent these information of MANET. Due to which, authors aimed at neutrosophic logic based MANET network information processing at given threshold.

Smarandache [13, 14] developed the mathematics of neutrosophic set (NS) as generalization of conventional fuzzy set (FS) [15] for handling the uncertainty in a better way. Single-valued neutrosophic set (SVNS for short) is proposed by Wang et al. [16] which is a discrete form of NS theory. So far, SVNSs have been applied extensively to different real-life challenges to measure the information based on three-way decision space [17–19] and its dynamic changes [20]. The single valued neutrosophic sets and their hybrid are applied on graph theory [21–28]. One of the suitable example is information communication through WIFI network is also based on three-way decision space. Many times the user unable to know the information is truly reached, not reached or uncertain. At moment, there is no mathematical model, which can precisely represent this scenario of information processing in WIFI network. To fulfil the objective, the current paper focuses on introducing the properties of single-valued neutrosophic set in MANET. The motivation is to find the confirmed, unconfirmed as well as uncertain information communicated in the MANET at user defined threshold. To accomplish this task, a mathematical model based on single-valued neutrosophic set and its logic is established in this paper. The article also described different situations of MANETs and its modelling at user defined threshold values. To analyze the sent, received, unreceived and uncertain information in the given WIFI connection. The obtained results are also compared with recently available approaches.

2 Single Valued Neutrosophic Sets

This section provides some basic notation about Single valued neutrosophic set as given below:

For a space X of objects, a SVNSs is of the form $A = \{x, \langle T(x), I(x), F(x)\rangle : x \in X\}$ where $T, I, F : X \to [0,1]$ denote the truth, indeterminacy and falsity membership degrees respectively and $0 \le T(x) + I(x) + F(x) \le 3$. An ordinary FS describe fuzziness only by membership T whereas IFS [29] describe uncertainty with membership T as well as non-membership F under a constraint $0 \le T + F \le 1$ with uncertainty factor $\pi = 1 - T - F$. SVNS on the other hand describe not only membership and non-membership grades but also discussed indeterminacy degree I independently, with a condition that $0 \le T + I + F \le 3$. Hence, the concept of SVNS is more general than the existing tools and has the capability of dealing with uncertainty based on their acceptation, rejection and uncertain part more precisely in three-way decision space $[0, 1]^3$.

Let us consider a universal set region R is given, one of the neutrosophic geometrical interpretation is shown using the Fig. 1. The diversity of SVNS and IFS is illustrated in the Figs. 1 and 2 to understand their graphical comparison. The space of SVNS is described geometrically and SVN region is shown in Fig. 1 while the space of IFS is presented in Fig. 2.

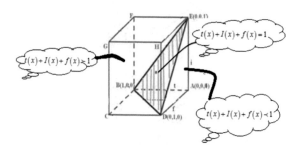

Fig. 1. An understanding of three distinct regions using neutrosophic cube

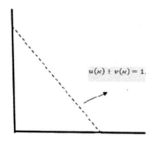

Fig. 2. Intuitionistic fuzzy space

In MANET, there are three types of regions. One region is where receiver received all the information without any disruption due to shadowing, path loss or multi-path propagation. The second region is where the receiver may receive data sometime but could not receive at other time i.e. there are some sort of fluctuations in receiving data due to above mentioned reasons like shadowing etc. The third region is no coverage area i.e. receiver did not receive any information. These three regions are independent to each other and can be precisely characterized via properties of neutrosophic set as shown in Fig. 1. The IFS does not allow representing the uncertainty independently when compared to neutrosophic set which can be observed from Fig. 2. Hence, the mathematical paradigm of SVNN to deal with information processing in WIFI connection as shown in Fig. 3. It can be observed that the first region exists inside the network; second region is indeterminate or uncertain whereas the third region exists outside of the network which is also popularly known as out-off coverage area as shown in the Fig. 3 in context of MANET.

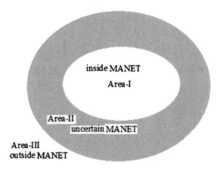

Fig. 3. Communication areas according to MANET

The proposed method in this paper establishes following three-distinct regions for information processing in MANET based on Fig. 3:

Area-I is inside of the MANET, which is the truth or acceptance membership region for the sent information.

Area-II is in between Area-I and Area-III of the MANET represents the information which are not reached and uncertain. It can be represented as indeterminacy region of a defined SVNS.

Area-III is outside of the MANET which is the non-membership region which is also well known as out-off coverage area. It can be represented by falsity membership-value for the defined SVNS.

3   Estimation for Information Transformation of MANET by Using CRC-16

Traditionally the information processing and its estimation based on Cyclic Redundancy Check (CRC). In which, the initial message was used to converted into series of bytes and register then final out puts check different parameters width, poly serial order register and receiver then only send the data from one node to another node. During the transformation of the data via MANET, there are three possibilities.

1. The sent data is confirmed that the receiver has received it. This information can be considered as truth membership.
2. The data is transmitted but no confirmation from the other end. This information can be considered as false membership.
3. At this situation, it is sure that the data cannot be reached. This information can be considered as indeterminacy membership.

The above three cases estimate the rate of the good connection (U), the non- good connection (V) and uncertain connection (I) of the information obtained in the MANET. It will be helpful in analyzing the intelligent of MANETs network by considering the information processing as one of the parameters. This information is represented by triplet (U, I, V) of real numbers from the neutrosophic set defined in three-way decision space $[0, 1]^3$.

It can be observed that the uncertain information in the MANET used to exist due to indeterminate or uncertain error exists in the obtained information. It means that the uncertainty connection contains the transformation of data is coming with wrong CRC. Everywhere the triplet (U, I, V) has been defined in the neutrosophic sets as defined above.

All the fields in the protocol are protected with the CRC-16 frame check sequence (FCS). For more details about CRC-16, the readers can see the ref. [10–12, 30, 31].

Initially when no information is obtained all values become (0, 0, 0) in Fig. 4. In case, $k \geq 0$, the current $(k+1)th$ estimation can be calculated based on previous estimations using the recurrence relation.

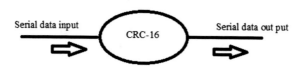

Serial data input   CRC-16   Serial data out put

Fig. 4. Model of working CRC-16

$$(U_{k+1}, I_{k+1}, V_{k+1}) = \left(\frac{U_k k + p}{k+1}, \frac{I_k k + q}{k+1}, \frac{V_k k + r}{k+1}\right)$$ where (U_k, I_k, V_k) is the previous estimation, and (p, q, r) is the estimation of the latest message, for $p, q, r \in [0, 1]$ and $0 \leq p + q + r \leq 3$. In this way, final estimation of information can be computed. To achieve this goal, the proposed method considers following threshold values for the U, I and V as follows:

$$U(p+, p-), I(q+, q-), V(r+, r-)$$

If $U \geq p+$, $I \leq q-$, $V \leq r-$, then the data is transformation received is confirmed.
If $U \leq p-$, $I \geq q+$, $V \leq r-$, then the data is transformation received is uncertain.
If $U \leq p-$, $I \leq q-$, $V \geq r+$, then the data is transformation not received is confirm.

In rest of the cases, the received data may be incorrect which may contain wrong CRC. It should be noted that the proposed method utilizes the properties of CRC only for checking the error. The following are the steps for the proposal:

Step 1. Initially when still no information has been obtained, all estimations are given initial values of (0, 0, 0).

Step 2. Characterize the truly confirmed information, uncertain information and rejected information as the previous estimation (U, I, V) about sent information.

Step 3. The current $(k+1)th$ estimation is calculated based on the previous estimations according to the recurrence relation.

$$(U_{k+1}, I_{k+1}, V_{k+1}) = \left(\frac{U_k k + p}{k+1}, \frac{I_k k + q}{k+1}, \frac{V_k k + r}{k+1} \right)$$

Step 4. Define the threshold value to find the reliability of given WIFI network as follows $U(p+, p-), I(q+, q-), V(r+, r-)$.

Step 6. If $U \geq p+, I \leq q-, V \leq r-$.

It shows that acceptance rate of sent information crossed the threshold of defined its truth, indeterminacy and falsity values. Hence, in this case the data transformation and received is confirmed.

Step 7. If $U \leq p-, I \geq q+, V \leq r-$.

It shows that truth membership-values about the sent information is less than the given threshold, the indeterminacy about them is maximum from the defined threshold, whereas the falsity values is less than the given threshold. It means the data transformation and received is indeterminate or uncertain.

Step 8. If $U \leq p-, I \leq q-, V \geq r+$.

It shows that the truth and indeterminacy values about the sent information is less than the given threshold whereas the falsity values is more than the defined threshold. In this case, the data transformation is confirmed as not received.

Step 9. The most interesting part about the proposed method is that it provides flexibility to refine or coarser the given information for analysis of defined WI-FI network.

Step 10. The obtained neutrosophic values provide an information that how much data can be sent, rejected or uncertain while choosing the given network as its reliability. This can be decided totally based on user required threshold values.

Above proposals shows that the neutrosophic set gives more general way to deal with indeterminacy in WIFI connection when compared to intuitionistic fuzzy sets [32]. In the same time, it uses the threshold value for precise measurement of path based on user requirement which concordant with [18]. However, the proposed method is unable to provide any analysis when the dynamic changes happens in the given MANET at the particular interval of time. It means the proposed method unable to process the information when the observed mobile network in different areas, or even we are traveling which will be our future research.

4   Conclusion

This paper aimed at precise mathematical representation of Wi-Fi connection and its quality based on neutrosophic logic. One of the proposition is also introduced based on previous (U_k, I_k, V_k), and latest message (p, q, r) estimation where $p, q, r \in [0, 1]$ and

$0 \leq p + q + r \leq 3$. Moreover, the neutrosophic logic based estimation is introduced based on defined threshold values on previous (U_k, I_k, V_k) and sent information (p, q, r). Hence, the introduced method in this paper helps more precisely towards quality analysis of MANET in term of information transformation characterized by its acceptance, rejection and uncertain part. In near future, we will focus on introducing a real life example to extract some useful information using the proposed method and its applications in various fields for providing an intelligent MANET.

References

1. Toh, C.K.: Ad hoc mobile wireless networks: protocols and systems. Pearson Education (2001)
2. Eze, E.C., Zhang, S., Liu, E.: Vehicular ad hoc networks (VANETs): current state, challenges, potentials and way forward. In: Automation and Computing (ICAC), 2014 20th International Conference on IEEE. pp. 176–181 (2014)
3. Alam, T., Aljohani, M.: Design and implementation of an Ad Hoc network among android smart devices. In: Green Computing and Internet of Things (ICGCIoT), 2015 International Conference on. pp. 1322–1327, IEEE (2015)
4. Fossa, C.E., Macdonald, T.G.: Internet working tactical manets. In: Military Communications Conference, 2010-Milcom IEEE. pp. 611–616 (2010)
5. Rosati, S., Kruželecki, K., Heitz, G., Floreano, D., Rimoldi, B.: Dynamic routing for flying ad hoc networks. IEEE Trans. Veh. Technol. **65**(3), 1690–1700 (2016)
6. Meagher, C., Olsen, R., Cirullo, C., Ferro, R.C., Stevens, N., Yu, J.: Directional ad hoc networking technology (DANTE) performance at sea. In: Military Communications Conference, 2011-Milcom IEEE, pp. 950–955 (2011)
7. Reina, D.G., Toral, S.L., Barrero, F., Bessis, N., Asimakopoulou E.: Evaluation of ad hoc networks in disaster scenarios. In: Intelligent Networking and Collaborative Systems (INCoS), IEEE Third International Conference on. pp. 759–764 (2011)
8. Bader, R., Pinto, M., Spenrath, F., Wollmann, P., Kargl, F.: Bignurse: A wireless ad hoc network for patient monitoring. In: Pervasive Health Conference and Workshops IEEE. pp. 1–4 (2006)
9. Djenouri, D., Kheladi, L., Badache, N.: A survey of security issues in mobile Ad hoc and sensor networks. IEEE Commun. Surv. Tutorials. **7**, 4 (2005)
10. IEEE Std. 802.11–1999, Part 11: Wireless LAN Medium Access Control (MAC) and Physical Layer (PHY) specifications, Reference number ISO/IEC 8802-11:1999(E), IEEE Std 802.11, 1999 edition (1999)
11. IEEE Std. 802.11a, Supplement to Part 11: Wireless LAN Medium Access Control (MAC) and Physical Layer (PHY) specifications: High-speed Physical Layer in the 5 GHZ Band, IEEE Std. 802.11a- (1999)
12. IEEE 802.11 g/D3.0, Draft Supplement to Part 11: Wireless LAN Medium Access Control (MAC) and Physical Layer (PHY) specifications: Further Higher-Speed Physical Layer Extension in the 2.4 GHz Band, July (2002)
13. Smarandache, F.: Neutrosophy. neutrosophic probability, set, and logic. In: ProQuest Information & Learning, Ann Arbor, Michigan, USA (1998)
14. Atanassov, K.: Intuitionistic Fuzzy Sets. Springer, Heidelberg (1999)
15. Zadeh, L.A.: Fuzzy sets. In: Fuzzy Sets, Fuzzy Logic, And Fuzzy Systems: Selected Papers by Lotfi A Zadeh. pp. 394–432 (1996)

16. Wang, H., Smarandache, F., Zhang, Y., Sunderraman, R.: Single valued Neutrosophic Sets. In: Multisspace and Multistructure 4. pp. 410–413 (2010)

17. Singh, P.K.: Three-way fuzzy concept lattice representation using neutrosophic set. Int. J. Mach. Learn. Cybernet. **8**(1), 69–79 (2017). https://doi.org/10.1007/s13042-016-0585-0

18. Singh, P.K.: Interval-valued neutrosophic graph representation of concept lattice and its (α, β, γ)-decomposition. Arab. J. Sci. Eng. 43(2), 723–740 (2018). https://doi.org/10.1007/s13369-017-2718-5, ISSN: 2193-567X

19. Singh, P.K.: Complex vague set based concept lattice. Chaos, Solitons Fractals **96**, 145–153 (2017). https://doi.org/10.1016/j.chaos.2017.01.019

20. Singh, P.K.: m-polar fuzzy graph representation of concept lattice. Eng. Appl. Artif. Intell. **67**, 52–62 (2018)

21. Broumi, S., Bakali, A., Talea, M., Smarandache, F., Kumar, P.K.: Shortest Path Problem on Single Valued Neutrosophic Graphs. In: 2017 International Symposium on Networks, Computers and Communications (ISNCC) (2017)

22. Broumi, S., Smarandache, F., Talea, M., Bakali, A.: Decision-making method based on the interval valued neutrosophic graph. In: Future Technologie. pp. 44–50, IEEE (2016)

23. Broumi, S., Talea, M., Smarandache, F., Bakali, A.: Single valued neutrosophic graphs: degree, order and size. In: IEEE International Conference on Fuzzy Systems (FUZZ), pp. 2444–2451 (2016)

24. Broumi, S., Dey, A., Bakali, A., Talea, M., Smarandache, F., Son, L.H., Koley, D.: Uniform Single Valued Neutrosophic Graphs". Neutrosophic Sets Syst. **17**, 42–49 (2017)

25. Broumi, S., Bakali, A., Talea, M., Smarandache, F.: A matlab toolbox for interval valued neutrosophic matrices for computer applications. Uluslararası Yönetim Bilişim Sistemleri ve Bilgisayar Bilimleri Dergisi **1**(1), 1–21 (2017)

26. Broumi, S., Bakali, A., Talea, M., Smarandache, F., Dey, A., Son, L.H.: Spanning tree problem with neutrosophic edge weights. Procedia Comput. Sci. **127**, 190–199 (2018)

27. Broumi, S., Bakali, A., Talea, M., Smarandache, F., Vladareanu, L.: Computation of shortest path problem in a network with SV-trapezoidal neutrosophic numbers. In: Proceedings of the 2016 International Conference on Advanced Mechatronic Systems. pp. 417–422, Melbourne, Australia (2016)

28. Broumi, S., Bakali, A., Talea, M., Smarandache, F., Vladareanu, L.: Applying dijkstra algorithm for solving neutrosophic shortest path problem. In: Proceedings of the 2016 International Conference on Advanced Mechatronic Systems, pp. 412–416. Melbourne, Australia, 30 Nov–3 Dec (2016)

29. Smarandache, F.: Neutrosophic logic-generalization of the intuitionistic fuzzy logic. arXiv preprint math/0303009 (2003)

30. Behrouz, F.: Data Communications and Networking. McGraw Hill, 5th edition (2013)

31. Myung, S., Yang, K., Kim, J.: Quasi-cyclic LDPC codes for fast encoding. IEEE Trans. Inform. Theor. 51(8), pp. 2894–2901 (2005)

32. Atanassov, K., Sotirov, S., Kodogiannis, V.: Intituionistic fuzzy estimations of the wifi connections. In: First International Conference on IFSs, GNs, KEs. pp. 76–79, London (2006)

Capturing Hadoop Storage Big Data Layer Meta-Concepts

Allae Erraissi$^{(\boxtimes)}$ and Abdessamad Belangour

Laboratory of Information Technology and Modeling LTIM, Faculty of Sciences
Ben M'sik, Hassan II University, Casablanca, Morocco
{erraissi.allae,belangour}@gmail.com

Abstract. Nowadays, producing streams of data is not helpful if you cannot store them somewhere. Applications, software, and objects generate huge masses of data, which need to be collected, stored, and made available for analysis. Moreover, these data are very valuable and need to be preserved. That is why Big Data has attracted global interest from all leaders of information technology and new ways of storing information have emerged and flourished. Accordingly, while proceeding our analysis on this subject, we note that in terms of Big Data architecture, the storage layer is very useful and is essential for the proper functioning of any Big Data system. In fact, there are two types of storage at this layer: Hadoop distributed file system (HDFS) and NoSQL databases. We relied on previous works in which we identified key storage concepts through comparative studies of main big data distributions. The storage layer is located directly above Data Sources and Data ingestion layers for which we already proposed a meta-model. Thus, in this paper, we applied techniques related to Model Driven Engineering 'MDE' to provide a universal Meta-modeling for the storage layer at the level of a Big Data system.

Keywords: Meta-model · Big data · Storage layer · Model driven engineering · NoSQL databases · HDFS

1 Introduction

Today, Big Data, which appears to be a vague term, is, in reality, a massive phenomenon that has quickly become an obsession for scientists, entrepreneurs, governments and the media. An indication of the growing concern about this phenomenon is that companies focus their efforts on deploying the most efficient and secure architecture to collect, store and process an abundance of increasingly heterogeneous data, in real time while integrating machine-learning technologies [1].

According to our earlier research studies of the distributions of leading Big Data solution providers [2–4], we found that each distribution of Hadoop has its own vision for a Big Data system. We also deduce that Programmers do not have the necessary meta-models to create standard applications that can be compatible with each provider because each provider has his own policy for a Big Data system. Indeed, this work comes after our first Meta-modeling of the two layers Data Sources and Ingestion [5]. In this paper, we propose a meta-model for the Storage layer. This meta-model together

© Springer Nature Switzerland AG 2019
M. Ezziyyani (Ed.): AI2SD 2018, AISC 915, pp. 413–421, 2019.
https://doi.org/10.1007/978-3-030-11928-7_37

with previous ones we proposed for the other layers, can be used as an independent cross-platform Domain Specific Language.

Correspondingly, we shall start in this article with the definition of Hadoop [6] and their main components. Then, we shall discuss the Hadoop distributed file system "HDFS" [7] and its architecture as well as the NoSQL databases [8]. Finally, we shall propose a meta-model for the Storage layer.

2   Hadoop

Hadoop, which is a framework written in Java, is an open-source Apache Foundation project. Originally, Doug Cutting developed it and gave him the name of his son's elephant toy. Hadoop is the most widely used framework for manipulating and making big data [9]. It allows the processing of massive data on a cluster ranging from one to several hundred machines. It is an open source project (Apache v2 license). The development of Apache Hadoop technology has changed the cost of data management completely. This is the first technology that has existed to virtually store, manage, and analyze unlimited amounts of data by assigning the right workload to the right system.

Technically, Hadoop consists of two key services: The storing of data using the Hadoop Distributed File System (HDFS) and the large-scale parallel processing of data using the technique called MapReduce [10].

3   Meta-Modeling of Hadoop Distributed File System

Hadoop distributed file system (HDFS) is a distributed file system that covers all nodes of a Hadoop cluster. It connects file systems on many local nodes in order to make it a large file system.

The Characteristics of a Hadoop Distributed File System:

- Distributed, scalability, fault-tolerant, broadband
- Access to data with MapReduce
- Files divided into blocks
- 3 replicas for each piece of default data
- Create, delete, and copy files without editing them
- Developed for streaming playback and no direct access
- Data localization: Data processing in the nearest physical location to reduce data transmission.

3.1   HDFS—Master /Slave Architecture

- **Master: NameNode**

Manages the file system's namespace and metadata. The FsImage stores the namespace of the entire file system, with mapping of blocks to files and properties of the file system [11]. This file is stored in the local file system of the NameNode. It contains the metadata on the disk (not an exact copy of what the RAM contains; but up to a certain point, a copy of control). The NameNode uses a transaction log file called EditLog to keep a record of each change in file system metadata and synchronizes with the RAM metadata after each writes. The NameNode has a knowledge of the DataNodes in which the blocks are stored. Thus, when a client requests Hadoop to recover a file, it is via the NameNode that the information is extracted. This NameNode will tell the client which DataNodes contain the blocks. All that remains for the customer is to recover the desired blocks [12]. In the event of a power failure on the NameNode, you must perform a recovery using FsImage and EditLog.

- **Slave: DataNode**

A cluster has multiple DataNodes. These DataNodes handle the storage attached to the nodes and periodically reports status for the NameNode. A DataNode contains the data blocks. They are under the command of the NameNode and are nicknamed the Workers. On that account, they are solicited by NameNodes during reading and writing operations. In reading, the DataNodes will transmit to the client the blocks corresponding to the file to be transmitted. In writing, the DataNodes will return the location of the newly created blocks [13].

This figure shows the Master/Slave architecture of the Hadoop distributed file system HDFS (Fig. 1):

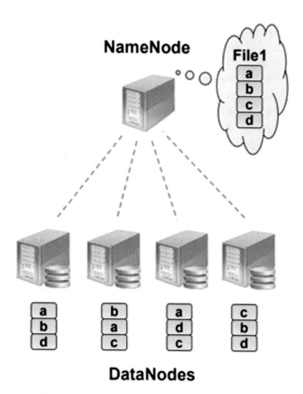

Fig. 1. Master/Slave architecture of HDFS [13]

3.2   HDFS—Blocks

The HDFS is developed to support very large files. Data in a Hadoop cluster is divided into smaller pieces, which are distributed throughout the cluster. These smaller pieces are called blocks. HDFS uses much larger block sizes than conventional operating systems. By default, the size is set to 64 MB. However, it is possible to increase to 128, 256, 512 MB or even 1 GB. Whereas on conventional operating systems, the size is usually 4 KB. Thus, Interest in providing larger sizes reduces the access time to a block. If the size of the file is smaller than the size of a block, the file will not occupy the total size of this block but just the size necessary for its storage. This figure shows the difference between HDFS blocks and classical operating systems blocks (Fig. 2).

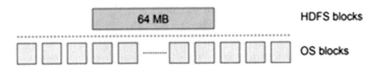

Fig. 2.   Difference between HDFS blocks and OS blocks [13]

3.3   HDFS—Replication

Replica placement is critical to HDFS in order to ensure reliability and performance. HDFS differs from most other distributed file systems by placing replicas. This characteristic requires adjustment and experience. The purpose of this placement policy is to increase data reliability and availability and to reduce network bandwidth usage. HDFS provides a block replication system with a configurable number of replications [12]. During the write phase, each block corresponding to the file is replicated on several nodes. As for the read phase, if a block is unavailable on a node, copies of this block will be available on other nodes.

Large instances of HDFS work on clusters that are spread across multiple arrays. Communication between two nodes in different racks must go through switches. In most cases, the bandwidth between machines in the same rack is larger than that of machines in a different rack. There is a simple but not an optimal policy, which consists of placing replicas in a unique rack. This, of course, avoids losing data if an array fails and allows the use of bandwidth from multiple racks in reading data. This policy evenly distributes replicas in the cluster, which makes load balancing easy if a component fails. However, this policy increases the cost of writing because a writing requires the transfer of blocks to several Rack. The figure below describes the replicas in HDFS (Fig. 3).

3.4   Meta-Model of Hadoop Distributed File System

The meta-model we proposed for the Hadoop distributed file system has seven meta-classes. These meta-classes define the HDFS Master/Slave architecture, the notion of blocks, which are small units of split data, and finally, the replication represented in this meta-model by the Racks to ensure reliability and the performance of Hadoop (Fig. 4).

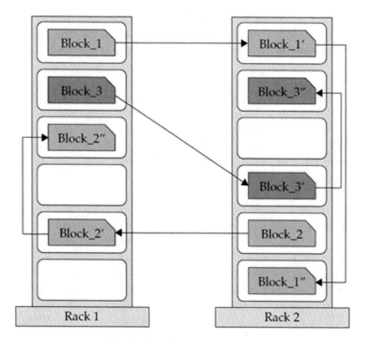

Fig. 3. Replicas in HDFS [12]

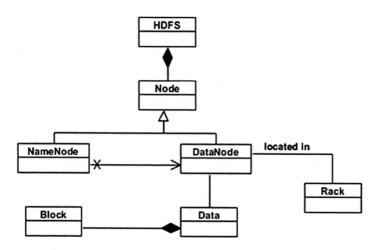

Fig. 4. Meta-model of HDFS

4 Meta-Modeling of NoSQL DataBases

NoSQL [8] stands for "Not Only SQL" and refers to a new class of database technologies, which was created to solve big data problems. In essence, NoSQL is a category of database management systems that cease its overall reliance on the classic relational database architecture. It appeared in order to counter the dominance of relational databases in the Internet domain [14, 15]. Indeed, relational databases reveal many complications. Firstly, one of its recurring problems is the loss of performance when dealing with a very large volume of data. Secondly, the proliferation of distributed architectures has brought to the surface the need for solutions that adapt natively to the mechanisms of data replication and load management. Eventually, unstructured and semi-structured data generate a variable number of fields and variable data content, which imposes a problem for the data model when designing the database. In this context, Pramod J.Sadalage and Martin Fowler [16] stressed the fact that the main reason for the emergence and adoption of NoSQL DBMS would be the development of data centers and the need to have a database paradigm adapted to this hardware infrastructure model.

Admittedly, existing NoSQL solutions can be grouped into four large families [17]:

Key/Value [18]: This model can be likened to a distributed hash map. It stores information in the form of a key/value pair where the value can be a string of characters, an integer or a serialized object. Hence, this lack of structure or typing has a significant impact on querying. In fact, all the intelligence, which was previously carried by the SQL requests, will have to be carried by the application that interrogates the database. Nevertheless, communication with the database will be limited to PUT, GET and DELETE operations. The best-known solutions are Redis [19], Riak [20], and Voldemort [21] created by LinkedIn. For example, a Redis database offers a very good performance by its simplicity. It can even be used to store user sessions or the cache of your site.

Column-oriented [22]: This model resembles relational databases because the data is saved in a row with columns. Nonetheless, it is distinguished from the relational database by the fact that the number of its columns can vary from one row to another [23]. Actually, in a relational table, the number of columns is fixed once the schema of the table is created. this number remains the same for all the records in this table. Conversely, with the Column-oriented model, the number of columns can vary from one record to another, and this, of course, results in avoiding the detection of columns with NULL values. As for the solutions, we mainly find HBase [24] (Open Source implementation of the Big Table model [25] published by Google) as well as Cassandra [26] (Apache project that respects the distributed architecture of Amazon Dynamo [27] and Google's Big Table model).

Document-oriented [28]: It is based on the key value paradigm. The value, in this case, is a JSON or XML document. The advantage of the document-oriented model is its ability to recover, via a single key, a hierarchically structured set of information. Obviously, the same operation in the relational world would involve several joins. The most popular implementations for this model are CouchDB from Apache [29], RavenDB [30] (intended for .NET/Windows platforms with the possibility of querying via LINQ) and MongoDB [31].

Graph-oriented [32]: This model of data representation is based on graph theory. It relies mainly on the notion of nodes, relationships, and properties attached to them. Indeed, this model facilitates the representation of the real world and makes it suitable for the processing of data from social networks. The main solution of this model is Neo4J [33] (Fig. 5).

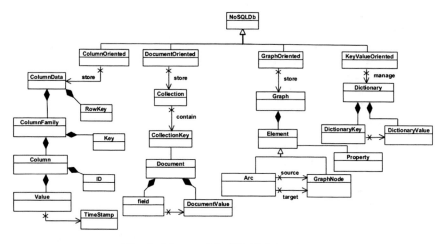

Fig. 5. Meta-model of NoSQL Databases

Our proposed meta-model includes the four types of NoSQL databases we have cited above. Firstly, we talked about The Key/Value databases. These are used to manage dictionaries that consist of a key/value pair. Then, We present Graph-oriented databases which can store graphs based on the notion of nodes, relationships, and properties attached to them. After that, We meta-modeled the Document-oriented databases with seven meta-classes that store collections containing documents. Finally, we have column-oriented databases that store data as rows with columns. However, this storage is distinguished by the fact that the number of columns can vary from one row to another.

5 Conclusion

We conclude that actually Hadoop is the main Big Data platform used for the storage and processing of huge amounts of data. This software framework and its various components are used by many companies for their Big Data projects. In this paper, we have dealt with the storage layer at the level of the Big Data architecture, which is very useful for the proper functioning of a Big Data system. We continued the application of techniques related to Model Driven Engineering (MDE) to propose a universal meta-modeling for this layer.

References

1. Richards, Ken: Machine Learning: For Beginners—Your Starter Guide For Data Management, Model Training, Neural Networks. CreateSpace Independent Publishing Platform, Machine Learning Algorithms (2018)
2. Erraissi, A., Belangour, A., Tragha, A.: A big data hadoop building blocks comparative study. Int. J. Comput. Trends Technol. Accessed 18 June 2017

3. Erraissi, A., Belangour, A., Tragha, A.: A comparative study of hadoop-based big data architectures. Int. J. Web Appl. IJWA. **9**(4) (2017)
4. Erraissi, A., Belangour, A., Tragha, A.: Digging into hadoop-based big data architectures. Int. J. Comput. Sci. Issues IJCSI. **14**(6), 52–59 (2017)
5. Erraissi, A., Belangour, A, Tragha, A.: Meta-Modeling of Data Sources and Ingestion Big Data Layers. SSRN Scholarly Paper. Rochester, Social Science Research Network, NY 26 May 2018. https://papers.ssrn.com/abstract=3185342
6. White, T.: Hadoop—The Definitive Guide 4e-. 4th ed. O'Reilly, Beijing (2015)
7. Alapati, S.R.: Expert Hadoop Administration: Managing, Tuning, and Securing Spark, YARN, and HDFS. Addison Wesley, Boston, MA (2016)
8. Raj, P., Deka, G.C.: A Deep Dive into NoSQL Databases: The Use Cases and Applications. S.l.: Academic Press (2018)
9. Dunning, T., Friedman, E.: Real-World Hadoop (2015)
10. Blokdyk, G.: MapReduce Complete Self-Assessment Guide. CreateSpace Independent Publishing Platform (2017)
11. N. Sawant, Shah, H.: Big data application architecture Q & A a problem-solution approach. Apress (2013)
12. Balasubramanian, S.: Big Data Hadoop The Premier Interview Guide (2017)
13. Borthakur, : HDFS architecture guide. Hadoop Apache Proj. http//hadoop apache …, pp. 1–13 (2008)
14. Banane, M., Belangour, A., El Houssine, L.: Storing RDF data into big data NoSQL databases. In: Mizera-Pietraszko J., Pichappan P., Mohamed L. (eds) Lecture Notes in Real-Time Intelligent Systems. RTIS 2017. Advances in Intelligent Systems and Computing. vol. 756. Springer, Cham
15. Banane, M., Belangour, A., Labriji, E.H.: RDF data management systems based on NoSQL Databases : a comparative study. Int. J. Comput. Trends Technol. (IJCTT). **V58**(2), 98–102 (2018)
16. Sadalage, P.: NoSQL Distilled: A Brief Guide to the Emerging World of Polyglot Persistence, 1st edn. Addison Wesley, Upper Saddle River, NJ (2009)
17. Nayak, A., Poriya, A., Poojary, D.: Type of NoSQL Databases and its Comparison with Relational Databases. Int. J. Appl. Inf. Syst. **5**(4), 16–19 (2013)
18. Seeger, M., Ultra-Large-Sites, S.: Key-value stores: a practical overview. … Sci. Media, pp. 1–21 (2009)
19. Carlson, J.L.: Redis in Action. Pap/Psc. Shelter Island. Manning Publications, NY (2013)
20. Meyer, M.: Riak Handbook (2011)
21. Akboka, B., Filipchuk, N., Zimanyi, E.:Advance database: Voldemort (2015)
22. Abadi, D.: The Design and Implementation of Modern Column-Oriented Database Systems. Found. Trends® Databases, **5**(3), 197–280 (2012)
23. VLDB 2009 Tutorial Column-Oriented Database Systems Column-Oriented Database Systems
24. George, L.: Hbase: The Definitive Guide: Random Access to Your Planet-size Data. 2nd Revised edition. O'Reilly Media, Inc, USA (2018)
25. Chang, F. et al.: Bigtable: A distributed storage system for structured data. 7th Symp. Oper. Syst. Des. Implement. (OSDI '06). pp. 205–218, Novemb. 6–8, Seattle, WA, USA (2006)
26. Carpenter, J., Eben Hewitt.: Cassandra—The Definitive Guide 2e. 2nd ed. Sebastopol, O'Reilly, CA (2015)
27. Amazon Web Services: Amazon DynamoDB Developer Guide API Version 2012-08-10 (2012)
28. Issa, A., Schiltz, F.: Document oriented Databases (2015)
29. Team, C.: CouchDB 2.0 Reference Manual. Samurai Media Limited (2015)

30. Syn-Hershko, I.: RavenDB in Action. Manning Publications (2016)
31. Bradshaw, Shannon, Chodorow, Kristina: Mongodb: The Definitive Guide: Powerful and Scalable Data Storage, 3rd edn. Place of publication not identified, O'Reilly Media Inc, USA (2018)
32. Robinson, I., Webber, J., Elfrem, E.: Graph Databases 2e. 2nd ed. O'Reilly, Beijing (2015)
33. Baton, J., Van Bruggen, R.: Learning Neo4j 3.x—Second Edition: Effective data modeling, performance tuning and data visualization techniques in Neo4j. 2nd Revised edition. Packt Publishing Limited (2017)

Audit and Control of Operations in the Insurance Sector Through the Application of the IT Reference System

Jamal Zahi and Merieme Samaoui[(⊠)]

Hassan 1st University, Settat, Morocco
mersamaoui@yahoo.fr

Abstract. The approach presented in this article is a contribution to understanding the issues and consequences in terms of governance and management of IT services considered as supporting the creation of value for the company. This work has the following objectives: to provide a global framework to help companies in the health insurance sector achieve their objectives, understand the need for a control framework based on the need of IT governance and learn the COBIT repository and its components which are control objectives and management directives.

Keywords: Systems governance · Health insurance · COBIT · ITIL · Audit of information systems · Risk management

1 Introduction

Information is a key resource for all businesses, and technology plays an important role from creation to destruction. Information Technologies are becoming more advanced and have become ubiquitous in business and social, public and commercial environments [1].

Companies and their leaders are striving to:

- Maintain a high quality of information to support decisions.
- Optimize the costs of IT services and technologies.
- Comply with laws, regulations, contractual agreements and policies.
- Achieve strategic goals and realize business benefits through the effective and innovative use of IT.

Corporate governance is a regulatory mechanism to ensure that the organization's strategy is effectively implemented in the field. It is increasingly seen as a mechanism to put in place a series of processes that will keep the business stable, empower all stakeholders and ensure that all stakeholders take ownership of the processes, in total transparency, with a clearly identified communication policy and clearly defined roles.

The governance of information systems is an integral part of corporate governance. It corresponds to the establishment of means by which stakeholders can ensure that their concerns are taken into account in the operation of the information system.

M. Ezziyyani (Ed.): AI2SD 2018, AISC 915, pp. 422–433, 2019.
https://doi.org/10.1007/978-3-030-11928-7_38

This document is organized in the following way, in the second section, the position of the problem is presented, in the third section the "COBIT" information systems audit reference framework is presented, its purpose as well as its principles and in the last section we give the results of a practical case of using the COBIT repository to audit the information system of a company in the insurance sector finally a conclusion.

2 Position of the Problem

Corporate governance is characterized by a set of decisions made throughout the life of the company and at all levels of responsibility in order to create lasting value:

- By ensuring the medium/long-term development of the company thanks to the relevance of the strategy developed and the optimization of the resources made available;
- By ensuring that the risks that may threaten it are quickly identified and controlled [2].

The IT Information Systems Directorate should be considered a "Business" Directorate and all stakeholders have an interest in working together, ensuring the implementation of a single strategy decided by management and broken down into all actors in the decision chain.

Good governance of the IT department therefore necessarily involves the control of the human factor by the CIO and his management team.

The audit of information systems aims to:

- Observe, examine and analyze facts, situations and information in relation to internal (company policy) or external (regulation) standards,
- Highlight discrepancies or dysfunctions,
- Investigate the causes and consequences in terms of risks and costs, thus enabling the auditor to present in a report short and medium term opinions and recommendations.

The ISACA (Information System Audit and Control Association) is an international professional association whose objective is to improve the governance of information systems through the improvement of computer audit methods and their approach based on the principle that companies get a return on an investment by taking risks.

As a result, the COBIT repository, developed by ISACA, contributes to the creation of IT value with respect to aspects of strategic alignment.

Based on the fact that health insurance aims to:

- Provide access to care for insured persons and their dependents,
- Ensure the payment of benefits and the treatment of diseases,
- Ensure the sustainability of its medical coverage system,
- Better match the required funds with the risks that insurance incurs in their activity.

It is therefore crucial to have an information system that can adapt and monitor upstream the changes in the business of the cover.

The objective of our research is to audit the information system of a health insurance company by applying the COBIT repository.

3   COBIT Repository

Before you begin to format your paper, first write and save the content as a separate text file. Keep your text and graphic files separate until after the text has been formatted and styled. Do not use hard tabs, and limit use of hard returns to only one return at the end of a paragraph. Do not add any kind of pagination anywhere in the paper. Do not number text heads-the template will do that for you.

Finally, complete content and organizational editing before formatting. Please take note of the following items when proofreading spelling and grammar.

3.1   Presentation and Evolution

COBIT (Control Objectives for Business Information and Related Technology), in French "Controlling the Objectives of Information Technologies" is a reference published by the ISACA IT Governance Institute in 1996, which was designed to ensure the coherence of the information system with the objectives and the overall strategy of the company (see Fig. 1).

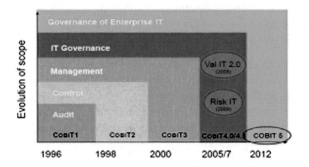

Fig. 1. Evolution of the COBIT repository

The COBIT offers a very powerful set of means to manage the levels of control to be exercised over the IT resources so that its last effectively support the achievement of the objectives of the company [3].

The COBIT reference system is intended for the three main actors of the company:

1. Management since it offers a means of decision support. It makes it possible to precisely estimate the level of risk that the company can bear to align IT resources in financial, organizational and technological terms.
2. Users to whom it provides security guarantees and controls of IT services. Indeed, the COBIT shows that trust in IT resources by the operational directorates is a factor for the alignment of resources.

3. Auditors to whom it proposes internationally recognized means of intervention. This standardization of the audit methodology makes analysis easier and more efficient, thus providing a less consistent result.

The COBIT repository is based on 5 Principles and 7 categories:
The 5 principles of the reference are:

Principle 1: Meeting the needs of stakeholders.
Principle 2: Cover the business from end to end.
Principle 3: Apply a single, integrated reference framework.
Principle 4: Provide a holistic approach to IT Governance and Management.
Principle 5: Separate Management Governance.

The 7 categories are:

- Principles, policies and terms of reference,
- Process,
- Organizational structures,
- Culture, ethics and attitudes,
- Information,
- Services, infrastructures and applications,
- People, know-how, skills.

The COBIT is a repository that breaks down any computer system into 34 processes divided into four functional areas [4]:
Planning and Organization (This field covers 6 processes);

1. Strategy and computer tactics

- Contribution to the objectives of the company,
- Planning, communication and management,
- Proper organization and technological infrastructure.

2. Acquisition and Implementation (This domain contains 11 processes);

- Implementation of the IT strategy,
- Identification, development or acquisition, implementation of solutions,
- Integration of solutions to management processes,
- Modification and maintenance of systems.

3. Distribution and Support (DS) (13 processes belong to this domain);

- Provision of necessary services,
- Operational safety,
- Implementation of support processes,
- Data processing by applications.

4. Monitoring, which contains 4 processes (4 processes in this area);

- Regular evaluation of all IT processes,
- Compliance with control requirements and quality of control,

- These 4 areas cover 34 processes (series of activities and grouped tasks) and 318 activities (tasks required to obtain a measurable result).

3.2   Maturity Model (See Fig. 2)

Legend used for ranking (see Fig. 3):

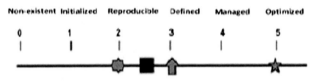

Fig. 2. .

0	Non-existent	Management processes are not applied at all
1	initialized	Processes are implemented on a case-by-case basis, and without methods
2	Reproducible	Processes follow the same pattern
3	Defined	Processes are documented and communicated
4	Managed	Processes are monitored and measured
5	Optimized	Best practices are tracked and automated

Fig. 3. .

Legend of symbols used (see Fig. 4):

⬡	Current state of the company
■	Current orientation of international standards
⬆	Best practice of the market
☆	Business Strategy

Fig. 4. .

3.3   Implementation Model of COBIT

To implement the COBIT repository, it is necessary to follow the following life cycle:

1. Initiate the program by defining the desired change and the need to act
2. Identify problems and opportunities: designate the project team, evaluate the existing one
3. Define the roadmap: Define the target goal and communicate the results
4. Plan the Program: Identify Stakeholder Roles
5. Execute the program: implement the improvement

6. Identify Benefits: Integrate the New Approach, Operate and Measure Benefits
7. Examine effectiveness: monitor and review processes.

3.4 COBIT and Other Standards

The COBIT is considered as a leader of the information systems department since it addresses the IS of the company and therefore it addresses all the directions of the company. It can be said that the other standard repositories are not competitors with COBIT, but they complement each other like ITIL and CMMI.

The two Information Technology Infrastructure Library (ITIL) and Capability Maturity Model Integration (CMMI) repositories are designed for internal or external development operations managers.

4 Case Application

4.1 Scope

Health insurance is a branch of social security, which aims to provide access to care, it allows many people to share the risks associated with the disease. The risks are generally divided into two groups:

- Big risks: this category includes serious illnesses that involve major expenses such as hospitalizations, surgical procedures and other specialized acts. the probability of occurrence of these events is low, on the other hand, the financial effort requested is more considerable for the families as well for the provident societies.
- The small risks: they concern the most benign cases which require less expense but on the contrary the frequency is higher. It's about ambulatory care.

Much of the health insurance is provided by the state or what may be called compulsory health insurance. It is one of the fundamental components of social security.

A public health insurance system can be managed by a state agency, delegated to private bodies or be mixed.

A mutual (or mutual) society is a non-profit partnership that organizes solidarity among its members, and whose funds come from membership fees. The operation of mutual is governed by the Mutuality Code.

4.2 Methodology

"In order to measure the maturity of the company in terms of governance, a synthetic questionnaire is proposed. This questionnaire must be used to start a process of analysis of governance. "The steering of our health insurance system has become progressively more complex to the point of being dual today, between the State on the one hand and the health insurance institution on the other," said a report in 2013. of the Health Innovation Circle with provocative title: "Is the Health Insurance still useful?" [5].

The imperatives to be examined are:

- Efficiency of the process: quality and relevance of information, consistent distribution,
- Efficiency in the use of resources: speed of delivery,
- Confidentiality of information: protection against disclosure,
- Integrity of information: the accuracy of information,
- Availability of information: accessibility on demand and protection (backup),
- Compliance with regulations: compliance with rules and laws,
- Reliability of the information: reliability of the information: the accuracy of the information transmitted by the management.

And the resources, being defined in:

- Data: information about the activity inserted or provided by the IT,
- Applications: automated information processing systems,
- Technologies
- Installations: equipment (servers, DB,…),
- Staff: engineers and technicians in charge of IT management.

Acknowledgment aims at listing information useful for the appreciation of these factors:

- The IT strategy can be defined as the process by which the IS professionals, confronted with a decision problem having for object the IS, will define and prioritize objectives for IT projects in coherence with the strategy of the organization, and consider action levers on the project portfolio based on quantitative evaluations that alone can support well-informed development choices (see Fig. 5).

IT Strategy			
Nature	Description	Qualif.	Return
- existence	the approach that allows a manager and his company to clarify the strategic plan of his IT	2	
- mastery	Ability to dominate strategic axes	2	
- speakers	The actors of the processes	2	
- procedure	The methods and means necessary to accomplish the tasks	1	
- change management	Allow driving changes effectively when driving IT projects	1	(*)

Fig. 5. .

(*) he cycle of change is shorter and shorter; the same is true of the technological life cycle. Today, over a quarter, we can witness major changes [6].

- The computer function is the set of tasks and/or applications giving results from the data, it is the management of IT processes in terms of management, development, operation (see Fig. 6).

Computer Function			
Nature	Description	Qualif.	Return
- internal – external (1)	internal : - software (Production + Accounting) - complementary applications (developed in-house) - Intranet external : - Company Website	4	
- type of organization	Entity attached to the management	3	
- internal functions	(1)		
- external functions	(1)		
- skills	Head of the IT entity /IT Framework	3	
- training	information systems engineer		
- workload	High : - Computer management - Operations - Development - Assistance and user training	2	
- documentation	• Accounting Software • Website	1	

Fig. 6. .

– The level of complexity allows for an assessment of the level of control over the risks associated with IT activities as it allows any company to pinpoint the capabilities and needs of its computer system in the most precise manner by the degree of automation and data availability (see Fig. 7).

Level of complexity			
Nature	Description	Qualif.	Returni
- level of automation	Computerization of all activities of the company without human intervention.	2	Objective of the implementation of complementary applications
- level of integration	The design and implementation of an information system covering all of the company's activities (for example the implementation of interfacing between the applications)	1	Separate applications
- availability level	Availability of information at any time	2	
- performance level	Measurable indicators of materials, systems, processes ...	1	
- characteristic syst. inf.		2	

Fig. 7. .

– Applications are the set of programs, software and packages used to perform a set of tasks (see Fig. 8).
– Interfaces are the set of devices allowing exchanges and interactions between several actors (software) (see Fig. 9).
– The treatments are the set of operations performed for the exploitation of the data (see Fig. 10).

Applications			
Nature	Description	Qualif.	Return
Production software	Management of activities (Accession and dependents, outpatient care, care, health provider, repository, users and their privileges ...)	2	
Accounting Software	Accounting management, payroll, in addition to disability pension (CAID)	4	
Receipt of requests TP	Receipt of requests for support	2	Internally developed
Release management	• Management of outpatient discharges and care • Convocation management	2	Internally developed
Payement of inactive contributions	Management of annual contributions of inactive members (retired, disabled, widowed ...)	2	Internally developed
Providers invoicing	Invoice management with care providers	2	Internally developed
Finance management	Follow-up of bank entries / exits	2	Internally developed
Management of UCITS	UCITS management	2	Internally developed
Management of payment orders	Management of payment orders (medical expenses, healthcare providers...)	2	Internally developed
Intranet	Consultation of medical expenses and care via the internal network (Online consultation)	3	Internally developed
Internet	Website (showcase of the company, consultation of the files)	4	Outsourced to a qualified provide

Fig. 8. .

Interfaces			
Nature	Description	Qualif.	Returni
	The technical means which allow the transmission of data of a system to another	1	Separate applications

Fig. 9. .

Treatments			
"Business" procedures	Procedures describing the process of processing "Business" activities (Membership, Ambulatory Care, Assumption of responsibility ...)	2	
Support Procedures	Procedures describing transversal functions (Accounting, treasury ...)	2	

Fig. 10. .

- Maintenance is the set of actions aimed at preventing (evolutionary maintenance) or correcting (corrective maintenance) the problems encountered in order to maintain its compliance with the specifications (see Fig. 11).
- Security helps to control the risks of access to data by unauthorized persons (internal or external) as well as the risks of data corruption or malicious acts (see Fig. 12).

Maintenance			
Nature	Description	Qualif.	*Return*
system maintenance	All technical and management actions to maintain or restore the system	2	Internally (IT team)
operating function		2	Internally (IT team)
software maintenance	- Accounting Software (Annual Maintenance Agreement) - other applications: internally	2	
user support		2	
newspaper analysis		3	

Fig. 11. .

Security			
access to the system	administrators	4	
access to software	Users according to their profiles - Membership: update, consultation - Refund files: reception, processing, consultation - Support: treatment, consultation -	4	
access to data	Users according to their profiles - Membership: update, consultation - Refund files: reception, processing, consultation - Support: treatment, consultation	3	
backups	According to the periodicity of each application	2	
Access management	According to the profile of each user	3	
password management	Depending on the profile of each user and the login session	4	
Internet protection	A proxy server is installed to bridge the gap between the production base and the back office of the online consultation	3	

Fig. 12. .

5 Conclusion

After the text edit has been completed, the paper is ready for the template. Duplicate the template file by using the Save As command, and use the naming convention prescribed by your conference for the name of your paper. In this newly created file, highlight all of the contents and import your prepared text file. You are now ready to style your paper; use the scroll down window on the left of the MS Word Formatting toolbar.

By studying the management of IT processes for this insurance company, we have been able to raise dysfunctions that the latter must take into consideration and put the necessary measures to address them.

In the strategy component, it must respect and follow the strategic priorities defined by the company and the regulations in force. And especially the change management of the components of the information system infrastructure that the company can undergo.

For the function and computer applications part, we can point out the existence of several applications developed internally or externally, which makes the availability and relevance of the information in question since all of these applications generate a lot of applications. Interventions and time to complete a task or respond to a request.

All applications are managed and maintained by the internal team of the company, and no maintenance contract is taken into account, it can be considered as a major malfunction, either on the availability of the team or on their ability to handle major incidents.

However, we can raise the average degree of security provided by the company and its team and especially the management of rights and privileges granted to users, and the existence of a proxy server to secure the production of external attacks.

As a result, and in order to manage the various risks that the company incurs, and to provide better services, it must adopt and invest on good measures and practices to ensure the proper management of its system, be they procedural, financial and human.

As a result, it became necessary to set up an ERP (Enterprise Resource Planning) integrated information system covering the areas of management and management of the company's activities (management, production, claims, control, finance and human resources).

With the help of this unified system, the various users can work in an identical intoxication and a single database. This model ensures data integrity and non-redundancy of information.

Lastly, the COBIT repository is a key piece in the application of the rules and principles of IT Governance. However, its scope alone cannot cover the entire IT governance process.

References

1. Information System Audit and Control Association: COBIT 5. ISACA p. 98 (2012)
2. The Academy of Accounting and Financial Sciences and Techniques: Corporate Governance: A Global Management Vision, N°14, p. 81 (2009)
3. Georgel, F.: IT Gouvernance. 2nd edn. DUNOD. p. 290 (2006)
4. Delvaux, J.-P.: COBIT, the reference system for the governance of the information system. ANDSI (2007)
5. The Health Innovation Circle, under the scientific direction of Jean de Kervasdoué. Is Health Insurance still useful? (2013)
6. Challande, J.-F., Lequeux, J.-L.: Big book DSI. Eyrolles, p. 354 (2009)
7. Bonneaud, A.: Gouvernance IT et Normalisation. AB Consulting
8. Morley, C., Bia-Figueiredo, M., Gillette, Y.: Business Processes and S.I. 3rd edition, DUNOD (2011)
9. Brunelle, D.: Governance. Theory and practices (2010)
10. Research Report Robert Joumard: The concept of governance. LTE 0910. p. 52 (2009)
11. Rafael, A.: Performance and Corporate Governance. editions of official journals (May 2013)

12. Guizouarn, J.-C., Marescaux, N.: Health insurance—Segmentation and competitiveness. Economica
13. The standards of the DSI, Cigref (2009)
14. Grojean, P., Morel, M., Nolin, S.-P., Plouin, G.: Performance of IT architectures., 2nd edition, Dunod

Performance and Complexity Comparisons of Polar Codes and Turbo Codes

Mensouri Mohammed[✉] and Aaroud Abdessadek

Faculty of Sciences, Department of Computer Science, El Jadida, Morocco
mensourimoh1@hotmail.com, a.aaroud@yahoo.fr

Abstract. Polar codes can be considered serious competitors to turbo codes in terms of performance and complexity. This paper provides a description of the Polar codes and the Turbo codes used by channel coding. Then, we undertake a comparison of Polar codes and Turbo codes based on several factors: BER performance, encoding complexity and decoding computational complexity. The performance of newly obtained codes is evaluated in term of bit error rate (BER) for a given value of Eb/No. It has been shown via computer simulations. They are employed as the error correction scheme over Additive White Gaussian Channels (AWGN) by employing Binary phase shift keying (BPSK) modulation scheme.

Keywords: Channel coding · Polar codes · Turbo codes · Coding · Decoding · Successive cancellation algorithm · Max-log-MAP algorithm

1 Introduction

Polar Codes are linear block codes. Their invention is recent and proposed in [1]. These are the only codes for which one can mathematically prove that they reach the Shannon limit for an infinite size code. In addition, they have low coding and decoding complexity using a particular algorithm called Successive Cancellation (SC). The construction of the code as well as the coding and the decoding are explained in the different parts of this section before locating the performances of the Polar Code with respect to the existing codes.

Polar Codes can be used in a variety of practical communication scenarios. Indeed, they are faced with the Holevo capacity in [2] and the ITU G.975.1 standard in [3] for optical communications. In [4], the authors consider Polar Codes for multiple access channels to two users. The application of Polar Codes for voice communications is discussed in [5]. The authors compare performance with systems using LDPC codes for AWGN and Rayleigh channels. In [6], the authors consider a symmetric and memory-free relay channel, they show that the Polar Codes are suitable for compression-transmission applications. Polar Codes can be implemented for quantum communication channels from [7]. Security applications may use Polar Codes. The authors in [8] showed that Polar Codes asymptotically reach the capacity region of a wiretap channel under certain conditions.

© Springer Nature Switzerland AG 2019
M. Ezziyyani (Ed.): AI2SD 2018, AISC 915, pp. 434–443, 2019.
https://doi.org/10.1007/978-3-030-11928-7_39

In 1993 a new class of concatenated codes called 'Turbo codes' was introduced [9]. These codes can achieve near-Shannon-limit error correction performance with reasonable decoding complexity. Turbo codes outperformed even the most powerful codes known at that date, but more importantly they were much simpler to decode. It was found that good Turbo codes can come within approximately 0.8 dB of the theoretical limit at a BER of 10^{-6}.

Turbo codes have advantages in terms of performance and implementation complexity of traditional solutions for error correction. Naturally, therefore, they have gradually been integrated into real systems. Today, they are found in many systems with requirements for enough variables of service quality. Some of the current applications of turbo codes Satellite links, Deep-space missions, 3G wireless phones, Digital Video Broadcast (DVB) systems, Wireless Metropolitan Area Networks (WMAN), Wi-Fi networks, Long Term Evolution (LTE) and LTE advanced [10–13].

Polar Codes theoretically reach the capacity of a channel for infinite code size. It is the only error-correcting code so far for which it is possible to mathematically prove this property [14]. It is therefore natural to wonder if they can replace the codes of literature. For that, it is necessary to compare the performances of different codes, as well as their computational complexity, for equivalent constraints like the size of the code or the rate of the code. The codes used in the latest generation standards are mainly Turbo codes and LDPC codes.

The paper is organized as follows. In Sect. 2, we provide the overview of Polar codes. In Sect. 3, we describe the encoding and the decoding method of Turbo codes. The main contribution of the paper is Sect. 4, where comparisons of Polar codes and Turbo codes based on several criteria are presented. Finally, we provide some conclusions in Sect. 5.

2 Polar Codes

2.1 Construction of Polar Codes

A Polar Code $PC(N, K)$ is a linear block code of size $N = 2^n$, with n is a natural integer, containing K bits of information. The generator matrix of the code is a submatrix of the nth power of Kronecker k, noted $F = k^{\otimes n}$:

$$k = \begin{pmatrix} 1 & 0 \\ 1 & 1 \end{pmatrix} \text{ and } F = \begin{pmatrix} k^{\otimes n-1} & 0_{n-1} \\ k^{\otimes n-1} & k^{\otimes n-1} \end{pmatrix} \tag{1}$$

The matrix F is composed of K lines. These K lines are chosen assuming a decoding Successive Cancellation (SC) which allows polarizing the error probability of the message bits. A Polar Code can be represented in matrix form from the matrix F and in the form of factor graph. The latter can be used for coding and decoding.

2.2   Process of Coding Polar Codes

Like any block code, the code words associated with Polar Codes are defined by a generative matrix G of dimension $(K \times N)$. This generating matrix G is obtained by removing $(N - K)$ rows of the matrix F. The equivalent encoding process then consists in multiplying a vector of size K by this matrix G. An alternative coding process consists of constructing a vector, denoted U, containing the K information bits and $N - K$ frozen bits set at 0. This vector is constructed in such a way that the information bits are located on the indices more reliable corresponding to K lines of $F^{\times n}$ previously selected. The corresponding code word X can then be calculated simply such that:

$$X = U \times F^{\times n} \tag{2}$$

A block code can be represented as a factor graph. In the case of the Polar Codes, we have seen that the construction of the generating matrix is recursive. It is then possible to show that the construction of the graph is also recursive. More generally, the factor graph of a Polar Code is presented in [14], of size $N = 2^n$ is composed of n stages of $\frac{N}{2}$ nodes of parity of degree 3 and $\frac{N}{2}$ nodes of variables of degree 3. The degree of a node represents its number of connections with other nodes. The factor graph can be used for coding and decoding.

2.3   Decoding of the Polar Codes by Successive Cancellation

The successive cancellation decoding algorithm can decode the Polar Codes. For the Polar Codes, a first algorithm has been proposed in [14] and is detailed in the following paragraph.

Once the message is transmitted through the communication channel, the noisy version, $Y = Y_0^{N-1} = [Y_0, Y_1, \ldots, Y_{N-1}]$, of the code word $X = X_0^{N-1} = [X_0, X_1, \ldots, X_{N-1}]$ is received. Arıkan showed in [1], as Polar codes reached the channel capacity under the assumption of a successive cancellation decoding. This decoding consists in estimating a bit u_i from the observation of the channel and the knowledge of the bits previously estimated. The value of the estimated bit is noted $\widehat{u}_i$. Each sample Y_i is converted into a format called Likelihood Ratio (LR). These LRs, denoted $L_{i,n}$. During the decoding the different values $L_{i,j} (0 \le j \le n)$ are updated as well as the values $S_{i,j}$. The latter, called partial sums represent the recoding of the bits $\widehat{u}_i$, as and when they are estimated. The particular sequencing of operations is explained below. First, it should be noted that the update of $L_{i,j}$ and partial sums $S_{i,j}$, can be calculated efficiently using the graphical representation of the Polar Codes.

To successively estimate each bit u_i, the decoder is based on the observation of the vector from the channel $\left(L \binom{N-1}{0}, n \right) = [L_{(0,n)} \ldots, L_{(N-1,n)}]$ and previously estimated bits $\widehat{u}_0^{i-1} = [\widehat{u}_0, \ldots, \widehat{u}_{i-1}]$. For this purpose, the decoder must calculate the values of LRs following:

$$L_{i,0} = \frac{Pr\left(Y_0^{N-1}, \widehat{u}_0^{i-1}|u_i = 0\right)}{Pr\left(Y_0^{N-1}, \widehat{u}_0^{i-1}|u_i = 1\right)} \tag{3}$$

During the decoding, when updating a stage $j > 0$, it is not the bits u_i that are used directly, but the partial sums, $S_{i,j}$ which are a combination of these estimated bits. When the decoding updates an LR of the stage $0, L_{i,0}$, then the decoder makes a decision as to the value of the bit u_i such that:

$$\widehat{u}_i = \begin{cases} 0 \; si \; L_{i,0} > 1 \\ 1 \; si \; non \end{cases} \tag{4}$$

The decoder knows the frozen bits. Therefore, if u_i is a frozen bit then $\widehat{u}_i = 0$ regardless of the value of $L_{i,0}$. The decoder successively estimates the bits $\widehat{u}_i$ from LRs, $L_{i,j}$ and partial sums $S_{i,j}$ which are calculated such as:

$$L_{i,j} = \begin{cases} F\left(L_{i,j+1}, L_{i+2^j,j+1}\right) & si \; B_{ij} = 0 \\ G\left(L_{i-2^j,j+1}, L_{i,j+1}, S_{i-2^j,j}\right) & si \; B_{ij} = 1 \end{cases} \tag{5}$$

$$S_{i,j} = \begin{cases} H_l\left(S_{i,j-1}, S_{i+2^{j-1},j-1}\right) & si \; B_{ij} = 0 \\ H_u\left(S_{i,j-1}\right) & si \; B_{ij} = 1 \end{cases} \tag{6}$$

With:

$$\begin{cases} F(a,b) = \frac{1+ab}{a+b} \\ G(a,b,S) = b \times a^{1-2S} \\ H_u(S) = S \\ H_l(S, St) = S \oplus St \\ B_{ij} = \frac{i}{2^j} \, mod \, 2, 0 \leq i < N \, and \, 0 \leq j < n \end{cases} \tag{7}$$

The partial sum $S_{i,j}$ corresponds to the propagation of hard decisions in the factor graph. The decoding algorithm can alternatively be represented by a complete binary tree. The branches symbolize the functions F, G, H_u and H_l. Nodes represent LRs and intermediate partial sums, computed during the decoding process. The functions F and G process the LRs from right to left and store the results in the nodes on the left. The H functions retrieve partial sums from the left node, process them and store them in the right node.

3 Turbo Codes

3.1 Turbo Code Encoding

The Turbo encoder is composed of two recursive systematic convolutional (RSC) encoders, as shown in Fig. 1. The input information d sequence is encoded twice by the two RSC encoders. The first encoder processes the information in its original order, while the second encoder processes the same sequence in a different order obtained by an interleaver π. As shown in the Fig. 1, the systematic bit sequence d is also transmitted to the decoder; sequence p_1 and p_2 are the output of each encoder. Sequence d is the systematic bit sequence and b is the interleaved systematic bit sequence. Note that only d is transmitted since b can be obtained by an identical interleaver on the decoder.

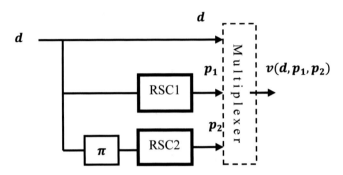

Fig. 1. Block diagram of the Turbo encoder

The input sequence d is passes through the convolutional encoder RSC1 and generates the coded bit p_1. The sequence d is then interleaved i.e. the data bit are loaded row-wise and read out column-wise. The bits are often readout in a pseudo random manner [15, 16]. The interleaved data sequence is passed to the second convolutional encoder RSC2 and coded bit p_2 is generated. After the step of coding, sequence information and two redundancy sequences (i.e.v) are transmitted on noise channel provided to receiver a sequence $r(d', p_1', p_2')$ of N bits, the relation between v and r to the Additive White Gaussian Noise channel (AWGN) is:

$$r = v + b \tag{8}$$

Or b is a randomized sequence representing the "noise" or "Error" additive.

3.2   Turbo Code Decoding

The scheme of the turbo decoding is composed of two SISO decoders, two of interleavers and a deinterleaver as illustrated in Fig. 2. d' is the sequence of information received corresponding to the transmitted information sequence d. p_1' and p_2' are the noisy information sequences respectively associated with the sequences p_1 and p_2 redundancy. The information exchanged between the elementary decoders is described as a conditional probability of the information bit transmitted on the observations at the input of decoder. In the case of the binary code, the extrinsic information bit di with $i \in (1...K)$ is formulated as P $(d_i = 1|v, p_1)$ or $P(d_i = 0|v, p_2)$. The quantities of this quantity are often considered as a logarithmic form such as logarithms Report Likelihood (LRV). The extrinsic information generated by a decoder are then considered as the a priori information input from the other decoder. The iterative decoding process of the turbo decoder can be divided into two steps:

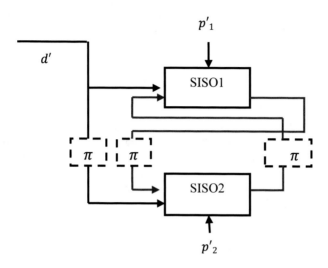

Fig. 2. Scheme of Parallel Turbo decoder

The first step: SISO2 decoder performs the decoding from three contributions: p'_2 redundancy sequence, the interleaved information sequence d' that matches the encoding process of the second RSC encoder, the interleaved extrinsic information output of the first decoder SISO1. Then the SISO2 decoder produces a weighted output that corresponds to the reliability of each decoded bit. From this information, the extrinsic information corresponding to the p_2 sequence is produced, interleaved and transmitted to the decoder SISO1.

The second step: SISO1 decoder uses the extrinsic information provided by the second SISO2 decoder to decode the information sequence based on its own observation sequences d' and p'_1. This decoder will then produce reliable information on each decoded bit sequence corresponding to the p_1. This information is subsequently used by the interlaced and SISO2 decoder during the next iteration.

These two steps of extrinsic information exchange between the two components decoders are defined as a decoding iteration. The process in which a decoder performs decoding on the received sequences and produces the extrinsic information for the other decoder is also defined as a half-iteration. During the iterations, transmission errors are corrected and the two decoders provide their information decoded sequences which are as near as possible to the transmitted information sequence. Conventionally, the turbo decoder makes a decision on the output of the first decoder SISO1 as the overall decision.

4 Comparisons of Polar Codes and Turbo Codes

In this section, we compare several aspects of coding and decoding Polar codes and turbo codes. We plot the bit error probability versus the signal-to-noise ratio Eb/N0 to compare the BER- FER performance of Polar codes and Turbo codes by using the simulation resultants.

4.1 BER-FER Performance Comparison of Polar Codes and Turb Codes

A comparison was made between a Turbo code from the Long Term Evolution (LTE) standard and a Polar Code. In terms of pure performance, the Polar Codes are below the Turbo codes with an original Successive Cancellation decoding (unsystematic). A loss of about 0.8 dB for a TER $= 2 \times 10^{-2}$ is observed in Fig. 3 between a Turbo code and a Polar Code. The turbo code is of size $N = 2^n = 1024$ and the rate $R = 1/2$ with $m = 3$ storage elements and performing iterations Imax $= 6$. The Polar Code is of size $N = 1024$, of rate $R = 1/2$ and unsystematic, as originally proposed.

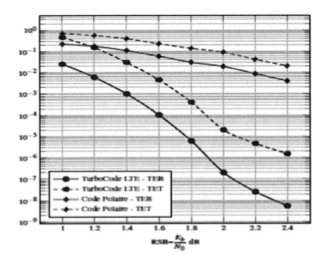

Fig. 3. Comparison of performances on a AWGN channel of a Turbo code and a Polar Code

The performances of a systematic Polar Code having a length 16 times greater, CP (16384,8192) are then compared to the performances of the previous Turbo code of Fig. 4. Systematic encoding and decoding do not alter the complexity of the algorithm but improve decoding performance. This is why a systematic Polar Code is retained. It appears that in this configuration of equivalent decoding complexity, the performance of the Polar Code is only about 0.2 dB of Turbo code performance for the BER $= 10^{-4}$.

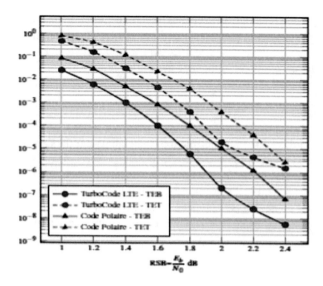

Fig. 4. Comparison of performances on a AWGN channel of a Turbo code and a Polar Code

4.2 Complexity Comparison of Polar Codes and Turb Codes

The complexities of the coding and decoding algorithms are summarized in Table 1. We can easily see that the coding of Turbo codes is very complex compared to the coding of Polar Codes. In addition, the complexity of the Turbo codes decoding algorithm is presented. The decoding algorithm used is the enhanced Max-Log-Map algorithm which is the same as the MAP but whose calculations are simplified (exponential, division and multiplication are replaced by additions, subtractions and maximum).

Table 1. Comparison of computational complexity of coding and decoding of Polar Codes and Turbo codes

	Coding		Decoding	
Code	Structure	Complexity	Algorithm	Complexity
Polar code	Recursive encoder	$o(Nn)$	Successive cancellation	$o(Nn)$
Turbo code	Convolutional encoder	$o(Nm)$	Max-Log-MAP	$o(I_{max}(4N2^m))$

On the other hand, the decoding complexity is much lower for a Polar Code, using a Successive Cancellation algorithm, systematic or not, for the following reasons:

- Decoding is not iterative.
- The Successive Cancellation algorithm is very simple to implement because it is recursive and regular.
- A relatively low memory fingerprint of $Qc + Qi + 1 = 2$. The variables Qc and Qi represent the number of bits on which a given is quantified.

According to the previous observations, the Polar Codes are particularly interesting in terms of their decoding complexity. Indeed, the SC decoding algorithm makes it possible to decode the Polar Codes with computational complexity 8 to 32 times lower compared to the decoding algorithms of the Turbo codes.

5 Conclusion

We have seen in this paper the construction, the coding and the decoding of the Polar Codes. The decoding algorithm used for Polar code is Successive Cancellation, which has been detailed because a lot of work derives from it. Then, we have presented an overview of turbo code. Finally, a comparison of the decoding performances with other current codes, for an equivalent computational complexity, shows that the Polar Codes have performances that make it possible to compete with the Turbo codes.

References

1. Arikan, E.: Channel polarization: A method for constructing capacity-achieving codes. IEEE Int. Symp. Inf. Theory, ISIT **2008**, 1173–1177 (2008)
2. GUHA, S., Wilde, M.: Polar coding to achieve the Holevo capacity of a pure-loss optical channe. In: Information Theory Proceedings (ISIT), 2012 IEEE International Symposium on, pp. 546–550 (2012)
3. Wu, Z., Lankl, B.: Polar codes for low-complexity forward error correction in optical access networks. In: ITG Symposium; Proceedings of Photonic Networks, 15, pp. 1–8 (2014)
4. Sasoglu, E., Telatar, E., Yeh, E.: Polar codes for the two-user binary-input multiple-access channel. In: Information Theory Workshop (ITW), 2010 IEEE, pp 1–5 (2010)
5. Zhang, C., Yuan, B., Parhi, K.: Low-Latency SC Decoder Architectures for Polar Codes (2011). arXiv:1111.0705
6. Lasco-Serrano, R., Thobaben, R., Andersson, M., Rathi, V., Skoglund, M.: Polar Codes for Cooperative Relaying. IEEE Trans. Commun., **60**, pp 3263–3273 (2012)
7. HIRCHE, C.: Polar codes in quantum information theory (2015)
8. Andersson, M., Rathi, V., Thobaben, R., Kliewer, J, Skoglund, M.: Nested Polar Codes for Wiretap and Relay Channels,. Commun. Lett. IEEE, 14, pp. 752–754 (2010)
9. Berrou, C., Glavieux, A., Thitimajshima, P.: Near Shannon limit error-correcting coding and decoding: Turbo Codes. In: Proceedings IEEE International Conference Communications ICC'93, pp. 1064–1070, Geneva, Switzerland, May (1993)
10. Evolved Universal Terrestrial Radio Access (EUTRA) and Evolved Universal Terrestrial Radio Access Network (EUTRAN), 3GPP TS 36.300
11. General UMTS Architecture, 3GPP TS 23.101 version7.0.0, June (2007)
12. Parkvall, S., Dahlman, E., Furuskar, A., Jading, Y., Olsson, M., Wanstedt S., Zangi, K.: LTE-advanced evolving LTE towards IMT—advanced. In: IEEE Vehicular Technology Conference, pp 1–5, Sep (2008)
13. Berrou, C., Amat, A.G., Mouhamedou, Y.O.C., Douillard, C., Saouter, Y.: Adding a Rate-1 Third Dimension to Turbo Codes. In: Proceedings IEEE Information Theory Workshop ITW '07, pp. 156–161, Sept 2–6 (2007)

14. Arikan, E.: Channel polarization: a method for constructing capacity-achieving codes for symmetric binary-input memoryless channels. IEEE Trans. Inf. Theory **55**, 3051–3073 (2009)
15. Mark Sum Chuen Ho, B.: Serial and Parallel Concatenated Turbo Codes. Doctoral Thesis. Unversity of South Australia, School of Electrical and information Engineering, Institute for Telecommunications Research (2002)
16. Berrou, C., Saouter, Y., Douillard, C., Kerouédan S., Jézéquel, M.: Designing good permutations for turbo codes: toward a single model. In: Proceedings IEEE International Conference Communications, pp. 341–345, Paris, France, Jun (2004)

A Survey on RDF Data Store Based on NoSQL Systems for the Semantic Web Applications

Mouad Banane[(✉)] and Abdessamad Belangour

Hassan 2 University, Casablanca, Morocco
{mouadbanane, belangour}@gmail.com

Abstract. Today the Resource Description Framework (RDF) that allows computers to understand and exploit Web data becomes very much in a progressive way, as well as the amount of web data that becomes very large. The storage and efficient management of this large RDF data is a real challenge in front of the classic RDF databases called triplestore. Recently, several researches focus on storing RDF data in triplestores based on NoSQL data management systems like HBase, Cassandra, Accumulo, and Couchbase. The majority of these researches are based on HBase. This NoSQL technology that is intended to handle this phenomenon of data explosion called Big Data, provided benefits like scalability and high availability compared to traditional triplestores. In this paper, we review existing works and systems that use NoSQL databases to store massive RDF data.

Keywords: Storing RDF data · RDF · Semantic web · NoSQL · Big data

1 Introduction

Making Web data understandable and exploitable by machines like human beings is the semantic Web's major goal, the technique is based on providing a common framework for data exchange. This framework, which is a W3C standard called RDF (Resource Description Framework), describes the Web resources. Using RDF, pro-grams and software agents can access and use Web data/resources. RDF is the Semantic Web data model that allows the representation and exchange of information. Thanks to RDF we can represent structured and unstructured data [1].

RDF data that is in the form of triplets we can simply store in a single relational database table, this table contains three columns for the subject, predicate, and object triplets.

Today with this explosion of data (Big Data) in different areas and especially on the Web with RDF data. Web giants have developed data management systems to manage this Big Data with NoSQL which is a new big data management approach that is not based on the traditional relational database management system architecture. These massive volumes of RDF data also require scalable data management systems, capable of effectively offering storage, indexing, and querying of RDF data. We find initiations that propose storing RDF data in databases. NoSQL data that is distributed and scalable databases.

© Springer Nature Switzerland AG 2019
M. Ezziyyani (Ed.): AI2SD 2018, AISC 915, pp. 444–451, 2020.
https://doi.org/10.1007/978-3-030-11928-7_40

The rest of this Survey is structured as follows. Section 2 reviews the RDF technology. The Big Data architecture and the NoSQL technology are presented in Sect. 3. Section 4 reviews existing works and systems that use NoSQL databases to store big RDF data. Finally, in Sect. 6, we conclude this study.

2 Resource Description Framework

2.1 RDF

The RDF system, which is a standard XML application, is a meta-language specialized in metadata to define arbitrarily complex relationships between documents or data. It allows representing the description of the content of a resource, to organize it, to control its access and to guarantee its availability. With this type of automatic data processing, that is to say, the automation of the information extraction task, it seems that the limits of use are hardly restrictive. Thus, thanks to the use of a different Uniform Resource Identifier (URI) for each specific concept, the power of RDF, and by extension of the Semantic Web, is to label each part of a resource in order to make it interoperable with all other resources that have received the same treatment, regardless of the computing platform on which these resources are based and regardless of their location on the networks. In other words, by categorizing the information, the RDF interprets the information to make it mutually intelligible.

2.2 RDF Data Storage

Generally RDF triplestores can be classified into three categories [2]:

- Native triplestores are blinds implemented from scratch, are based on the RDF data model for storage and efficient access to these RDF data. For example, AllegroGraph [3] 4Store [4], Sesame, Jena TDB.
- RDBMS-based triplestores: this category contains triplestores that are based on relational database management systems. They are created by adding a specific RDF layer to an existing database management system. For example: Virtuoso [5], Jena SDB.
- NoSQL Triplestores are RDF data storage solutions based on the new family of NoSQL databases, such as CumulusRDF [6], Jena-HBase [7], RYA [8].

3 Big Data and NoSQL

3.1 Big Data

Big Data is the accumulation of so much data that processing becomes difficult and highly technical. To manage this explosion of data we need a powerful and powerful ecosystem that is able to both store and process this large data, this ecosystem is Hadoop. Apache Hadoop is a distributed system that addresses these issues. On the one hand, it offers a distributed storage system via its Hadoop Distributed File System (HDFS) file system, which offers the possibility to store the data by duplicating it, so a Hadoop cluster does not need to be configured with a RAID system that becomes useless. On the other hand, Hadoop provides a data analysis system called MapReduce. The latter is working on the HDFS file system to perform processing on large volumes of data.

Today, Hadoop has become a complex ecosystem of components and tools, some of which are packaged into commercial distributions of the framework

The Hadoop framework includes a large number of open source components, all connected to a set of core modules designed to capture, process, manage and analyze large volumes of data. These core technologies are:

- Hadoop Distributed File System (HDFS). This file system supports a convention-al hierarchical directory, but distributes the files on a set of storage nodes on a Hadoop cluster.
- MapReduce. It is a programming model and an execution framework for parallel processing of applications in batch mode.
- YARN (Yet Another Resource Negociator). This module supports the scheduling of tasks (jobs) and allocates resources to the cluster to run the applications, and arbitrate when there is a resource conflict. It also monitors job execution.
- Hadoop Common. A set of library and tools on which the different components are based.

In a Hadoop cluster, these master pieces and other modules are placed above a system that takes into account computation and storage, in the form of nodes. These nodes are connected via a very high speed internal network to form a distributed and parallelized processing system. Alternative modules for managing and processing data, such as Spark that has the ability to run over YARN to either administer the cluster, manage the cache. Apache HBase is a columnar database management system based on Google's Big Table project that runs on top of HDFS. It also has development tools like Pig [9] and Hive that allow to build MapReduce applications. For configuration and administration tools, such as ZooKepper [10] and Ambari [11], that can be used for monitoring or administration. This Hadoop ecosystem also offers analytic environ-ments like Mahout [12] which provides templates analytics for machine learning, data mining and predictive analytics.

3.2 NoSQL

The NoSQL is a collection of four large database families that offer a different rep-resentation of the data, each having advantages and disadvantages depending on the context in which it is desired to use it. Among these are key-value databases. The key-value representation is the simplest and is very suitable for caches or quick access to information. This representation generally achieves much better performance in that reads and writes are reduced to a single disk access. There are three different imple-mentations: Riak [13], Redis [14] and Voldemort [15]. Then there are the columns oriented databases. The column-oriented representation is the one that is closest to the tables in a relational database. They allow to be much more scalable and flexible since we can have different columns for each line. There are two types of implementations: HBase [16] and Cassandra [17]. Then there are the document-oriented databases. The document-oriented representation is more suited to the world of the internet. This representation is very close to the key-value representation except that the value is represented as a document. Hierarchically organized data can be found in this document, such as what is found in an XML or JSON file. There are two types of implementations: CouchDB [18] and MongoDB [19]. Finally there are databases oriented graph. The graph-oriented representation is to overcome problems that cannot be solved with relational databases. The typical use case is on social networks where the graphical aspect makes sense, but also where complex relationships between actors need to be described. There are three different implementations: Neo4j [20], HypergraphDB [21] and FlockDB [22].

4 Storing RDF Triples into NoSQL Systems

The era of Big Data has arrived? We can say yes with this giant amount of data to create every day, data that comes everywhere social networks, sensors.etc. As a result, data management systems must be scalable to allow the storage, processing, and analysis of this big data. For this reason RDF stores are offered with RDF data storage techniques based on NoSQL data management systems, these databases which are designed for Big Data management (large data) offer and guarantee the distributivity and the scalability for efficient management of RDF triplets, the beginning with Jianling and al [23] who introduced a HBase-based RDF data store [16] for storage and indexing of RDF triplets and uses MapReduce for querying these data RDF. then Khadilkar and al propose scalable RDF triplestore called Jena-HBase [7] developed on the basis of HBase also, it uses Apache Jena for the querying of RDF triples. Another distributed triplestore based on the database Hbase is developed by Haque and Perkins [24] and takes as a query Hive [25]. Rainbow [26] provided by Gu and al, this triplestore that adopts a new distributed and hierarchical storage architecture based on HBase for scalable persistent storage and to accelerate query performance it combines a distributed memory storage. top uses HBase which is a column-oriented, non-relational and distributed open source database modeled on Google's BigTable [27] and written in Java. Developed as an Apache Hadoop [28] project from Apache Software Foundation, it runs on the Hadoop distributed file system. Apache HBase is ideal for accessing Big Data in real-time random read/write. The goal of the project is to host very large tables -billions of rows and millions of columns- on hardware clusters. In HBase the tables are stored in column orientation as explained above. Each table consists of a set of column families (logical groupings of columns) to be specified when it is created. Each family can then receive an arbitrary number of columns that can be added after the table is created, at any time. Unlike traditional RDBMSs, it is very easy to implement tables of millions of columns and billions of rows without having a significant impact on performance: it is simply necessary to increase the number of rows accordingly. Number of instances. The rows of the tables are partitioned into several regions. When creating a table, only one region is created, and then it is automatically subdivided when its size reaches a threshold. Each region is placed on a region server. The content of the region servers is indexed in a master server which routes the clients to the appropriate node. Data transfer between clients and region servers is done through a direct connection that does not include the master. Another approach proposes the storage of RDF data in another NOSQL database, CumulusRDF [6] which implemented on Apache Cassandra [17]. They studied the possibility of using an embedded key/value datastore. As the underlying storage component for a Linked Data server that provides functionality to process Linked Data via http searches. Based on Apache Cassandra, a distributed and open source key and value-based database management system, Cassandra is typically used to handle large amounts of data on many servers, this NoSQL database provides high availability. Without any point of failure. It provides robust support for clusters across multiple datacenters. Data is replicated to multiple nodes for fault tolerance, replication across multiple data-centers is supported, and failed nodes can be overwritten without any downtime. Cassandra regularly outperforms other NoSQL solutions for benchmarks and applications, mainly because of its fundamental architecture choices. note also that the CumulusRDF indexing scheme consists of only four indexes (SPO, PSO, OSP, CSPO). Punnoose and Crainiceanu have proposed Rya [8] which is a scalable RDF data management system that uses Accumulo [29], a column-oriented NoSQL data management system. With a new method of storage, indexing schemes and techniques for processing requests that are scalable across multiple nodes, you can also provide fast access to data through the classic SPARQL query tool. Rya [8] implemented on Accumulo Based on Google's BigTable, Apache Accumulo is a structured and highly elastic storage written in Java. Work at the top of the Hadoop distributed file system. Apache Accumulo supports the recovery and storage of structured and semi-structured data, including interval queries, and supports the use of Accumulo tables as inputs/sorts for MapReduce processing. This data management system provides a robust and scalable data storage and retrieval system. With some innovative features, such as cell-based access control and server-side programming mechanisms, Accumulo can be considered an efficient RDF data management systems. H2RDF [30] is a distributed RDFstore that is based on HBase and uses the MapReduce framework to process RDF data. SPIDER [31] is a scalable, parallel and distributed system for managing RDF data. In approach of Cuder et al. [32] they are based on Couchbase [33] which is a column-oriented NoSQL database. The RDF data is loaded into the system via the insertion of the RDF triples in a JSON document. The majority of this research is based on HBase [34]. For the Jena-HBase queries and Cuder's approach [32] uses Apache Jena, CumulusRDF, Rya and Rainbow used the Sesame tool. Hive-HBase requests RDF data with the HiveQL language of Hive. SPIDER converts SPARQL queries into MapReduce jobs. Schatzle et al. [35] proposed an RDF data query tool that uses Spark [36]. and finally we quote PigSPARQL [37] which is an A SPARQL Query Processing which transforms SPARQL queries into HiveQL language. In [38] they have reviewed the storage of large RDF data in NoSQL systems according to the different NoSQL models, and the work [39] presents a comparative study of RDF data storage systems into NoSQL databases.

5 Review of NoSQL-Based RDF Data Store

From these systems presented at the top we can conclude that the NoSQL technology that is intended to manage the phenomenon of Big Data is an effective solution for the management of large RDF data. Firstly the scalability and high availability of NoSQL systems are considered as the major point that makes the deference of these databases by contributing to traditional RDF triplestores like 4store, Virtuoso and other. Then if the RDF data is managed by a NoSQL system e.g. HBase, then we can apply queries on the different types of data stored in this database and among these types there are the RDF triples which is not the case for traditional RDF databases that are intended to handle only RDF data.

We noticed from this work that the proposed research works used different types of NoSQL: key-value-oriented databases, column-oriented, Document-oriented and graph-oriented. CumulusRDF uses Cassandra is a key/value-oriented systems, column-oriented systems like Jena-HBase, Hive-HBase, and Rainbow which are based on HBase and Rya implemented on Accumulo. Document-oriented we find Couchbase. This diversity of NoSQL models and NoSQL databases, proposes future research works such as: evaluation and comparison of these approaches based on a set of performance criteria and the possibility of migrating from a solution to other.

6 Conclusion

The limitations of traditional RDF triplestores such as distributivity, scalability and high availability are advantages of NoSQL data management systems. On the basis of these systems and to take advantage of these advantages several research works have been proposed which store the data. RDF data in NoSQL databases. This article reviewed these different approaches by describing their characteristics and the technologies used in these works. the approaches presented above, proposes the management of large RDF data through the use of a NoSQL database. This leads us to compare and evaluate these approaches based on standards such as LUBM [40]. In our future works, we propose an RDF data management system for storage will be based on NoSQL and for the querying we will use the MDA approach as [41–43].

References

1. Mnola, F., Miller, E., McBride, B.: RDF Primer. W3C Recommendation **10**(1–107), 6 (2004)
2. Sequeda, J.F., Miranker, D.P.: Ultrawrap: SPARQL Execution on Relational Data. 13
3. Aasman, J.: Allegro Graph: RDF Triple Database
4. Harris, S., Lamb, N., Shadbolt, N.: 4store: the design and implementation of a clustered RDF store. In: CEUR Workshop Proceedings, vol. 517, pp. 94–109 (2009)
5. Virtuoso Erling, O., Mikhailov, I.: RDF Support in the Virtuoso DBMS, pp. 7–24. Springer, Heidelberg (2009)

6. Ladwig, G., Harth, A.: CumulusRDF: Linked Data Management on Nested Key-Value Stores. 13 (2011)
7. Khadilkar, V., Kantarcioglu, M., Thuraisingham, B., Castagna, P.: Jena-HBase: A Distributed, Scalable and Efficient RDF Triple Store. 4
8. Punnoose, R., Crainiceanu, A., Rapp, D.: Rya: A Scalable RDF Triple Store for the Clouds (2012)
9. https://pig.apache.org/. Apache Pig. Accessed 05 June 2018
10. https://zookeeper.apache.org/. Apache ZooKepper. Accessed 07 July 2016
11. https://ambari.apache.org/. Apache Ambari. Accessed 21 June 2018
12. https://mahout.apache.org/. Apache Mahout
13. Klophaus, R., Rusty: Riak core. In: ACM SIGPLAN Commercial Users of Functional Programming (CUFP'10), p. 1 (2010)
14. Redis in Action. (n.d.). Retrieved 21 Jan 2018, from https://dl.acm.org/citation.cfm?id=2505464
15. http://www.project-voldemort.com/voldemort/. Accessed 28 June 2018
16. Apache HBase—Apache HBaseTM Home. https://hbase.apache.org/. Accessed 18 July 2018
17. Brown, M.: Learning Apache Cassandra : Build an Efficient, Scalable, Fault-Tolerant, and Highly-Available Data Layer into Your Application Using Cassandra (n.d.)
18. Anderson, J.C., Lehnardt, J., Slater, N.: CouchDB : The Definitive Guide. O'Reilly Media, Inc (2010)
19. Chodorow, K.: (n.d.). MongoDB : The Definitive Guide
20. Vukotic, A., Watt, N., Abedrabbo, T., Fox, D., Partner, J.: (n.d.). Neo4j in Action
21. Iordanov, B.: HyperGraphDB: A Generalized Graph Database, pp. 25–36. Springer, Heidelberg (2010)
22. Pointer, R., Kallen, N., Ceaser, E., Kalucki, J.: Introducing FlockDB
23. Sun, J., Jin, Q.: Scalable RDF store based on HBase and MapReduce, Aug 2010
24. Haque, A., Perkins, L.: Distributed RDF Triple Store Using HBase and Hive. 4
25. https://hive.apache.org/. Apache Hive. Accessed 18 July 2018
26. Gu, R., Hu, W., Huang, Y.: Rainbow: A Distributed and Hierarchical RDF Triple Store With Dynamic Scalability, Oct 2014
27. Chang, F., Dean, J., Ghemawat, S., Hsieh, W.C., Wallach, D.A., Burrows, M., Chandra, T., Fikes, A., Gruber, R.E.: Bigtable: a distributed storage system for structured data. ACM Trans. Comput. Syst. **26**, 1–26 (2008)
28. http://hadoop.apache.org/. Apache Hadoop. Accessed 11 June 2018
29. https://accumulo.apache.org/. Apache Accumulo. Accessed 27 June 2018
30. Papailiou, N., Konstantinou, I., Tsoumakos, D., Koziris, N.: H2RDF: Adaptive Query Processing on RDF Data in the Cloud (2012)
31. Choi, H., Son, J., Cho, Y., Sung, M.K., Chung, Y.D.: SPIDER: A System for Scalable, Parallel/Distributed Evaluation of Large-scale RDF Data (2009)
32. Cudré-Mauroux, P., Enchev, I., Fundatureanu, S., Groth, P., Haque, A., Harth, A., Keppmann, F.L., Miranker, D., Sequeda, J.F., Wylot, M.: NoSQL databases for RDF: an empirical evaluation. In: Alani, H., Kagal, L., Fokoue, A., Groth, P., Biemann, C., Parreira, J.X., Aroyo, L., Noy, N., Welty, C., and Janowicz, K. (eds.): The Semantic Web—ISWC 2013, pp. 310–325. Springer, Heidelberg (2013)
33. Brown, M.C.: Getting Started with Couchbase Server. Oreilly (2012)
34. https://mahout.apache.org/. Apache Mahout. Accessed 06 June 2018
35. Sch, A., Przyjaciel-zablocki, M., Skilevic, S., Lausen, G.: S2RDF : RDF Querying with SPARQL on Spark, pp. 804–815 (n.d.)
36. https://spark.apache.org/. Apache Spark. Accessed 09 June 2018

37. Sch, A., Przyjaciel-zablocki, M., Hornung, T., Lausen, G.: PigSPARQL : A SPARQL Query Processing Baseline for Big Data (n.d.)
38. Banane, M., Belangour, A., Houssine, L.E.: Storing RDF data into big data NoSQL databases. In: Lecture Notes in Real-Time Intelligent Systems, pp. 69–78. Springer, Cham (2017)
39. Banane, M., Belangour, A., Labriji, E.H.: RDF data management systems based on NoSQL databases: a comparative study. Int. J. Comput. Trends Technol. (IJCTT) **V58**(2), 98–102 (2018)
40. Guo, Y., Pan, Z., Heflin, J.: LUBM: A benchmark for OWL knowledge base systems. J. Web Sem. **3**(2–3), 158–182 (2005)
41. Erraissi, A., Belangour, A., Tragha, A.: A Big data Hadoop building blocks comparative study. Int. J. Comput. Trends Technol. Accessed 18 June 2017
42. Erraissi, A., Belangour, A., Tragha, A.: A comparative study of hadoop-based big data architectures. Int. J. Web Appl. IJWA **9**(4) (2017)
43. Erraissi, A., Belangour, A., Tragha, A.: Digging into hadoop based big data architectures. Int. J. Comput. Sci. Issues IJCSI **14**(6), 52–59 (2017)

Understanding Driving Behavior: Measurement, Modeling and Analysis

Zouhair Elamrani Abou Elassad$^{(\boxtimes)}$ and Hajar Mousannif

LISI Laboratory, Cadi Ayyad University, Marrakesh, Morocco
z.elamrani@uca.ma, mousannif@uca.ac.ma

Abstract. Human factors contribute in the manifestation of 95% of all accidents; recently there has been a research emphasis on driving behavior established as an outcome of individual actions as well as psychophysical values. This paper pursues the guidelines of systematic literature reviews to present an unbiased survey of the existing research on driving behavior in line with the psychophysical state as well as the behavioral operations of the driver and to develop unconventional taxonomies based upon the nature of the conducted study, measurement patterns and supervision motives underlying the detection and prediction models of driving behavior. A discussion on each classification is provided with a focus on the dominant mechanisms thought to be involved. The proposed overview gives insights into the scope of the problem and paves the way for grasping the major contributions and shortcomings in the state-of-the-art research.

Keywords: Driving behavior · Driving measures · Driving studies · Detection models · Prediction models

1 Introduction

The World Health Organization stated that 1.3 million people die each year and tens of millions are injured on the world's roads [1]. In Morocco, an average of 10 civilians are killed and another 33 are seriously wounded every day [2]. Many studies have been conducted to identify the causes of traffic road crashes. Based on the study of 2041 traffic accidents conducted by [3], it was inferred that human factors took part in the manifestation of 95% of all accidents. In [4], it was depicted that in three out of five crashes driver-related behavioral factors were the cause of motor vehicle accidents. Hence, it becomes crucial to study the driver behavior and attitudes that may lead to dangerous outcomes.

The psychophysical state aspects along with the behavioral actions of the driver are considered to be key components to enhance traffic efficiency and to mitigate hazards of accidents threatening not only the driver's safety, but also the safety of other road users. In this direction, it is substantial to be able to detect driver's state and behavior in order to assess the driving risk-level to avoid dangerous situations from happening. In contrast, anticipating such attitudes could prevent critical conditions even before they occur. The literature on detection and prediction of the driver behavior shows a variety

© Springer Nature Switzerland AG 2019
M. Ezziyyani (Ed.): AI2SD 2018, AISC 915, pp. 452–464, 2019.
https://doi.org/10.1007/978-3-030-11928-7_41

of approaches; although most research adopts the term "prediction", they only focus on the "detection" of an impaired conduct, rather than on its prediction [5].

Distinct study models have been carried out to monitor the behavioral features of the driver. Research based on the naturalistic driving studies along with field driving studies and driving simulator studies have been considered the major recognition sources of the objective driving data [6], whereas subjective self-reports have been always examined as more open to socially desirable responding than unobtrusive observations [7, 8]. Conversely, the present monitoring systems, and depending on how the observed data are collected, are classified into intrusive and non-intrusive, which influences the reliability and accuracy of the process [9].

In this paper, we review the field of driving behavior according to the psychophysical state and the behavioral operations of the driver. Generic study-type taxonomy is therefore proposed based on objective and subjective driver data thought to be involved. In addition, taxonomy of the data-source surveillance category, derived from the review of driving behavior is also presented. Moreover, until now, no overviews of the existing driving behavior detection and prediction models have been presented to remove confusion surrounding the terms. This survey aims to bridge the gap related to the absence of a valid taxonomic approach for accurately classifying driver behavior detection and prediction paradigms.

2 Background

Driving is overwhelmingly an underappreciated domain of self-sufficiency and major life activities, despite the fact that it is considered to be a substantial factor that facilitates most other adaptive domains, including employment, family care and responsibilities among others [10]. A multi-dimensional model has conceptualized driving into three hierarchically organized levels of qualifications and abilities where lower levels are being harnessed by higher levels so that larger goals are achieved [11], shortcomings in lower levels may have heavy effects on the higher hierarchy, whilst, deficits on higher levels may have little or no impact at all on the lower levels. The first and lowest level is the operational level; it involves primitive mental functions such as attention, concentration, reaction time and other basic neuro-psychological competencies. The second level known as the tactical level comprises behaviors and decisions implicated in maneuvers like lane change, turns and stops amongst others. The third level namely the strategic level is induced by the destination objectives and planning strategies such as the choice of the route, weather conditions and so on.

In [12], driving behavior models that emphasize the cognitive components have been studied such as the multi-dimensional hierarchical model and motivational models that give priority to non-fully tested situation-specific factors rather than stable and individual predictors. A review capturing drivers' tactical decisions in various traffic conditions have been displayed in [13]. The paper reviews the state-of-the-art on the areas of: acceleration, lane changing and gap acceptance. It was derived that most of the driving behavior models proposed in the literature were not estimated rigorously due to the limited amount of data, still, the advances in data collection technology and detailed trajectory data would make the estimation of improved models feasible. More research about tactical driving behavior was conducted by [14] who focused mainly on understanding intentional maneuvers. Another survey related to driving styles, i.e. subcategories of driving behavior satisfying the criteria of varying systematically between individual drivers or groups of drivers and also being habitual, was discussed by [15]; it has been chosen to exclude behavior patterns which are determined exclusively by the driving context such as traffic situation, road types, weather conditions, light conditions, etc.

Whilst a number of studies on driving behavior have been conducted using various types of data sources in order to detect or predict the psychophysical condition and the behavioral maneuvers of the driver [16, 17], there is still a lack of an underlying conceptual taxonomy to plainly shed light on the driver's attitudes. Here we make an attempt to capture most of the common elements in the reviewed literature in an effort to have a pertinent illustration for future work in this field and also to differentiate driving behavior detection from prediction, intrusive measurement from non-intrusive and distinguish between the different experimental studies.

3   Modeling Studies of Driving Behavior

3.1   Analysis of Objective Observations

Typically, objective driving assessments are obtained based on measurable facts independent from the driver thoughts. On this basis, the driver behavior is observable by any other entity supervising driving events, hence, all subjective biases have to be removed. Naturalistic driving studies as well as field driving studies and driving simulator studies are believed to be the major recognition sources of the objective driving data [6]. The three research methods are adopted to better outline perception of driving behavior and to contribute to the understanding of the actions resulting in crashes and rear-end collisions.

Naturalistic Driving Study
Naturalistic Driving Study (NDS) is a research method in which, typically, the subjects' own cars are equipped with devices that continuously monitor various aspects of their everyday driving behavior in an unobtrusive way and without the presence of a test supervisor [18].

Much research on driving behavior has been carried out based on Naturalistic Driving Studies. The National Highway Traffic Safety Administration (NHTSA) conducted an earnest study in which 100 vehicles automatically and continuously collect driving measures including vehicle's speed, acceleration, position, eye glance behavior and Time-to-Collision (TTC)—TTC represents the time after which a collision between the two vehicles will occur if the collision course and the speed difference are maintained - using advanced, unobtrusive instrumentation such as GPS, accelerometers, video cameras showing the inside and outside of the vehicle, radar sensors, lane trackers as well as on-board sensors [19, 20]. The trial was performed for over 13 months by 241 primary and secondary drivers. The data set is comprised of almost 43,000 h and approximately 2,000,000 vehicle miles resulting in a database that holds many drastic psychophysical states related to the driver, including severe drowsiness, impairment, judgment error, inattention. Moreover, the database contains analysis of behavioral driving events counting rear-ends events, lane changing, aggressive driving, and traffic violations.

The recently completed Second Strategic Highway Research Program Naturalistic Driving Study (SHRP 2 NDS) is the largest NDS of its kind, capturing more than 35 million miles of continuous naturalistic driving data and 2 petabytes (PB) of video, kinematic, and audio data from more than 3500 participants [21]. The objective of the SHRP 2 NDS is to reduce traffic injuries and fatalities by preventing collisions or reducing their severity by supporting detailed estimates of collision risk based on objective information on the role of driver behavior and performance in traffic collisions and on the interrelationship of the driver with vehicle, roadway, and environmental factors. Another NDS survey has been pursued in order to detect dangerous driving behavior of more than 100 participants [22]. The experiment using instrumented vehicles (IV) [23] in active mode, that is by monitoring the kinematics imposed on the vehicle by the driver and close by vehicles, as well as in passive mode where sensors observed the attitudes of the driver behind.

Analysis of right-turn driver behavior at signalized intersections with the SHRP 2 NDS was discussed in [24] and resulted in identifying five major influencing factors: vehicle type, traffic signal status, conflicting traffic, conflicting pedestrian and driver age group. SHRP 2 NDS was also conducted by [25] to study the driver lane-keeping performance under rainy weather condition by considering 196 trips in rain and additional 392 matching trips in clear weather conditions, representing 141 drivers. Driver anger has been monitored in [26] offering a special insight on the interplay between driving anger, driving behavior and other road.

Field Driving Study

Field Driving Studies (FDS) use instrumented vehicles in order to monitor the driver behavior; even with the use of surveillance gear, frequently instructors are present in the vehicle registering measures and coding driving performance. Field studies are frequently used to explore new areas of research and to provide preliminary input to surveys where the topic can be investigated in greater breadth [27].

A recognition algorithm of driving behavior using a smartphone examined twelve events which are brake, sudden brake, acceleration, sudden acceleration, turn left, sudden turn left, turn right, sudden turn right, lane change left, sudden lane change left, lane change right, and sudden lane change right, to provide real-time feedback while driving [28]. Another mobile based application with a server side storage and processing intended to link the negative driving and user motivation for a safer driving behavior was developed by [29]. Analysis of the driver confusion state was discussed in [30] using instrumented vehicle with multiple sensors. Recently, [31] proposed an interdisciplinary methodology using mobile sensing approach to observe bus drivers. In [32], a study was conducted to minimize distractions in high cognitive demanding situations and to promote stress-friendly driving behaviors.

Simulator Driving Study

Simulator Driving Studies (SDS) harness research tools to conduct fundamental research into the operation of the driver-vehicle-environment system in all types of weather, terrain, and traffic. They try to simulate driving in a safe environment, with the major advantage of having full experimental control over conditions. Another benefit of the simulator study is the ability to examine multiple design considerations through a factorial experiment design that assesses relative contributions and interactions among variables of interest [33].

A driver simulator study was conducted to observe dangerous driving situations using a physiological sensing system, Eye Alert Fatigue Warning System and a driver simulator to imitate different aspects of driving in various weather conditions [34]. The drowsiness state of the driver was studied based on driving a car simulator in drowsiness induced conditions in which participants were video-recorded and data on driving performance, eyelid and head movements, and physiological data were gathered [5]. Drowsiness-related lane departure maneuver was evaluated based on continuously collected data throughout each drive from the simulator and a dashboard-mounted eye-tracker [35]. Lane change right, lane change left and lane keeping were experimentally surveilled in the work of [36]. The study elaborates a novel prepro-cessing model for the advanced driver assistance system (ADAS).

3.2   Analysis of Subjective Observations

Subjective driving measurements are usually retrieved in accordance with personal opinions, interpretations and beliefs. In driving status inquiry, the judgement belongs to the driver's way of thinking; it comes from their perspective, and will express their particular experience. Subjective self-reports assorted as questionnaires and interviews, are useful when assessing internal, non-evaluative traits and states such as anxiety [37]. However, there have been some concerns with self-reported measurements; they may be subjects to errors of recall and reporting like social desirability bias [38].

The 100-naturalistic driving study phase 1 and phase 2 conducted by the NHTSA used questionnaires filled out by subjects before and after data collection (Telephone Screening Questionnaire, Sleep Hygiene Questionnaire, Medical Health Assessment ...) as several information will not be collected through hardware [19, 20]. The SHRP 2 NDS obtained non-DAS (Data Acquisition System) information through a variety of instruments, including questionnaires that were used to assess sleep, health, Attention Deficit Hyperactivity Disorder (ADHD), sensation seeking, risk and driving knowledge [21]. Also, pre-selection, pre and post-driving self-reports have been employed in the survey of [22]; pre-selection questionnaires were administered in random order to respondents to avoid distortion phenomena, as most people tend to provide the last answers hastily due to the annoyance. In [25], a Driver Demographics Questionnaire was adopted to merge geometric characteristics and driver demographics with one-minute segment data regarding non-freeway driving time in clear weather conditions.

A Demographic and Health Questionnaire was used in the survey on stress detection [31]. In [29], due to the small scale prototype testing, collected data were insufficient to gauge the effectiveness of integrating user motivation for safer driving. Instead, users were given a questionnaire to aid the measurement of user motivation and retention features. The drivers in [5] have been under examination for their sus-ceptibility to simulator sickness and circadian typology using the Motion Sickness Susceptibility Questionnaire, Short-form [39] and the Horne and Ostberg morning/evening questionnaire [40]. Also, drivers in [36] were given a questionnaire to aid training the driver intention detection module. In [41], the big five factors (openness to experience, conscientiousness, extraversion, agreeableness, and emotional stability), sensation seeking and driving anger have been measured to define the frequency of aggressive and risky driving. The Five Factor Model was assessed with the 50-item International Personality Item Pool [42], whereas the 35-item Driving Survey [43] was used to estimate the frequency of aggressive driving, risky and crash-related conditions. Sensation seeking and driving anger were measured based on the 40-item form of [44] and the 14-item short form of [45] respectively.

4   Intrusive and Non-intrusive Measurement Techniques

The existing monitoring systems for driving behavior, according to the source of the surveillance data, fall into two categories: intrusive and non-intrusive techniques, which influences the reliability and accuracy of the process [9]. Intrusive techniques use physiological data which are collected using ponderous attached devices to the driver with the aim of analyzing the driving process. The used instruments may distract the driver or perturb the driving behavior. This greatly restricts the application of these methods in engineering [46]. On the other hand, non-intrusive techniques are much more appealing to drivers for their naturalness [47]; they gather driving data without contact with the driver so the monitoring process will not interfere with the driver or by the use of self-reports [48].

Intrusive assessments, even though they require the user to wear potentially uncomfortable sensors, they may yield more accurate measures. In the study by [31], driver's stress state was monitored using The Vital Jacket (VJ), which is a wearable bio-monitoring platform in the form of a t-shirt that provides real time electrocardio-gram (ECG), 3 axis accelerometer and an event push-button. In [32] analysis of stress was assisted using of a Polar H7 band to record the Heart Rate Variability signal. Electrocardiography (EKG), pulse plethysmography (PPG), Electrodermal Activity (EDA) and Respiration were computed with the Biopac® MP150 system in order to evaluate the driver's drowsiness condition [5]. Stress was detected based on elec-troencephalography (EEG) in the study of [35].

5   Driving Behavior: Detection and Prediction Models

Identification of driving behavior is a decisive job which targets understanding the reasons for accidents and the precautions accounted for to prevent them from occurring. It is crucial to examine the driver's state and actions that relate to involvement in dangerous driving behavior. Hence, several studies have tackled the driving behavior Detection/Prediction paradigms to improve the safety and comfort of drivers, as well as other road users. Recognizing and anticipating the psychophysical state and the behavioral operations of the driver could enhance the driver's situation awareness and prevent critical conditions even before they happen.

The literature on detection and prediction of the driver's state and behavior shows a variety of approaches. Although most research adopts the term "prediction", they only focus on the "detection" of an impaired conduct, rather than on its prediction [5]. This finding have been shown in numerous studies, from which we mention a prototype of driver fatigue monitoring system that combines different visual cues and the contextual information to produce a consistent fatigue index [49]. In [28, 50] a detection algorithm using multi-sensory data on a smartphone was presented; it provided real-time feedback while driving. Enhanced measurements of the vehicle's state and the road surface condition were used to better detect the driver's intention of lane change as well as lane keeping [36]. The expression "prediction" is usually used even though the driving process is solely under "detection" because in machine learning, the term "prediction" is used to infer the label of an object not seen during the learning phase [5].

Other research delineated basically the adoption of a detection process, The work in [31] investigated daily sources of stress faced by bus drivers while driving in an ecological setting during their daily work and facilitated memory recall of the stressful situations. In [29], risky driving was detected to motivate the driver to act more cautiously. The twelve events studied in [28, 50] were detected using smartphone sensors such as GPS receiver and accelerometer sensor without the aid of any external hardware. As most of the previous studies on lane-keeping have made their investigation from the driver inattention perspective, [25] detected lane keeping performance under rainy weather conditions. Confusion has been supervised applying deep network architectures based on data collected from heterogeneous sensors and driving conditions in [30]. In [24], the turn right event was examined to study the influence of different factors on the driver behavior at signalized intersections. The driver's fatigue and anger conditions were detected based on a fatigue detection system in [46, 49], and on 10 min anger video segments in [26]. The 100 Car NDS Phase 1 and Phase 2 [19, 20] as well as [21] detected various attitudes including rear-end events, lane change events, inattention, drowsiness, distraction-related events, etc.

While some studies intended to detect the driving status, others planned at prediction it in the future. The driving danger-level system built in by [34] can accurately predict driving risks due to sharp turning, sudden acceleration/deceleration, continuous weaving and so on; it converts any coming data to a numerical danger-level using machine learning algorithms. The studies [41, 51] predicted risky driving too based on the detection of the driver's sensation seeking and anger conditions. In [22], Time-to-Collision was estimated, TTC was also monitored in [19, 20] along with the frequency of near-crashes and driver errors. In [32], single user with cross users scenarios were conducted to forecast the driver's perceived stress using machine learning techniques. The best results for drowsiness prediction analysis in [5] were obtained using data-set of behavioral features, driving time and participant information with a mean square error of 4.18 ± 1.17 min.

Table 1 summarizes the major studies described above, grouped by the driver's psychophysical state and behavioral operations, along with the proposed observation-based and measurement-type taxonomies discussed in this review, in addition to the classification of motives underlying the detection and prediction models.

Table 1. The selected taxonomies in this review grouped by driving behavior

Driving event/State	Paper	Subjective observation	Type of study			Type of measurement		Type of model	
			Objective observation			Non instrusive	Instrusive	Predictive	Detective
			Naturalistic driving study	Driving simulator study	Field driving study				
Various attitudes[a]	[19]	✓	✓			✓		✓	✓
	[20]	✓	✓			✓		✓	✓
	[21]	✓	✓			✓			✓
Stress	[32]				✓		✓	✓	
	[31]	✓			✓		✓		✓
Danger	[41]	✓				✓		✓	
	[34]			✓		✓		✓	
	[51]	✓				✓		✓	
	[22]	✓	✓			✓		✓	
	[29]	✓				✓			✓
Drowsiness	[5]	✓		✓	✓		✓	✓	✓
	[35]			✓			✓		✓
Confusion	[30]				✓	✓			✓
Brake	[50]				✓				✓
Sudden brake	[50]				✓				✓
Acceleration	[50]				✓				✓
Sudden acceleration	[50]				✓				✓
Turn left	[50]				✓				✓
Sudden turn left	[50]				✓				✓
Turn right	[50]				✓			✓	✓
	[24]		✓			✓			✓

(continued)

Table 1. (*continued*)

Driving event/State	Paper	Type of study					Type of measurement		Type of model	
		Subjective observation	Objective observation				Non instrusive	Instrusive	Predictive	Detective
			Naturalistic driving study	Driving simulator study	Field driving study					
Sudden turn right	[50]				✓					✓
Lane change left	[50]				✓					✓
	[36]	✓		✓			✓			✓
Sudden lane change left	[50]			✓	✓					✓
Lane change right	[50]				✓		✓			✓
	[36]	✓		✓			✓			✓
Sudden lane change right	[50]				✓					✓
Lane	[36]	✓		✓			✓			✓
Keeping	[25]	✓	✓				✓			✓
	[26]		✓				✓			✓
Anger	[41]	✓					✓			✓
	[51]	✓					✓			✓
Fatigue	[46]				✓		✓			✓
	[49]			✓			✓			✓
Sensation seeking	[41]	✓					✓			✓
	[51]	✓						✓		✓
The big five factors	[41]	✓					✓			✓

aVarious Attitudes: rear-end events, lane change events, inattention, drowsiness, distraction-related events, levels of risky behavior, lane boundary exceeding, lateral or longitudinal maneuvers, etc

6 Conclusion

In this paper, a literature review of the field of driving behavior on the basis of the psychophysical state and the behavioral operations of the driver is presented. An observation-based classification for driving type studies is provided with reference to the objective and subjective data corpus. We further propose two unconventional taxonomies: the first one addresses measurement types surveys to make the distinction between intrusive possibly disturbing experiments, and non-intrusive ones which are much more appealing to drivers for their naturalness, while the second classifies findings from the existing literature according to detection and prediction-based driving behavior models in view of the lack of underlying motives behind monitoring the driver's state and actions whether it is a detective model or a predictive one. Despite the fact that the expression "prediction" is used, it does not necessarily mean that the study forecasts a particular state or maneuver.

To synthesize, the reviewed research demonstrates a thorough understanding of driving behavioral indicators and psychophysical measures and their implications for traffic safety metrics which necessitates consideration of the relationship between the nature of the conducted study, the assessment factors and the clarity of determined motives. Current ongoing work is investigating the next stage of the proposed review including data corpus characteristics and a comprehensive machine learning techniques analysis.

Acknowledgements. This research received funding from the Moroccan Ministry of Equipment, Transport and Logistics and was supported by the Moroccan National Center for Scientific and Technical Research (CNRST).

References

1. World Health Organization, WHO | Road Safety: http://www.who.int/features/factfiles/roadsafety/en/ (2015)
2. Ministry of Equipment: Transport and Logistics - Morocco, 2017. [Ministère de l'Équipement, du Transport et de la Logistique - Maroc]. http://www.equipement.gov.ma/routier/Transport-Routier/Securiteroutiere/Pages/Strategie-Nationale-de-la-securite-routiere-2017-20261009-7462.aspx. Accessed 24 Apr 2018
3. Sabey, B.E., Taylor, H.: The known risks we run: the highway. Soc. Risk Assess. 43–70 (1980)
4. Evans, L.: Comment: the dominant role of driver behavior in traffic safety. Am. J. Public Health **86**(6), 784–786 (1996)
5. Jacobé de Naurois, C., Bourdin, C., Stratulat, A., Diaz, E., Vercher, J.L.: Detection and prediction of driver drowsiness using artificial neural network models. Accid. Anal. Prev., pp. 0–1. October, 2017
6. Yang, L., Ma, R., Zhang, H.M., Guan, W., Jiang, S.: Driving behavior recognition using EEG data from a simulated car-following experiment. Accid. Anal. Prev., pp. 1–11. October, 2017
7. Nederhof, A.: Methods of coping with social desirability bias: a review. Eur. J. Soc. Psychol. **15**, 263–280 (1985)

8. Paulhus, D.L.: Measurement and control of response bias. Meas. Personal. Soc. Psychol. Attitudes, 17–59 (1991)
9. Kang, H.B.: Various approaches for driver and driving behavior monitoring: a review. In: Proceedings of the IEEE International Conference on Computer Vision, pp. 616–623 (2013)
10. Barkley, R.A.: Driving impairments in teens and adults with attention-deficit/ hyperactivity disorder. Psychiatr. Clin. North Am. **27**(2), 233–260 (2004)
11. Michon John, A.: Dealing with danger. Gend. Technol. Dev. **10**(2), 191–210 (1979)
12. Ranney, T.A.: Models of driving behavior: a review of their evolution. Accid. Anal. Prev. **26** (6), 733–750 (1994)
13. Toledo, T.: Driving behaviour: models and challenges. Transp. Rev. **27**(1), 65–84 (2007)
14. Doshi, A., Trivedi, M.M.: Tactical Driver Behavior Prediction and Intent Inference : A Review, pp. 1892–1897 (2011)
15. Sagberg, F., Selpi, Bianchi Piccinini, G.F., Engström, J.: A review of research on driving styles and road safety. Hum. Factors **57**(7), 1248–1275 (2015)
16. Chhabre, R., Verma, S., Krishna, R.: A survey on driver behavior detection techniques for intelligent transportation systems. Cloud Comput. Data Sci. Eng. Conflu. **7**, 36–41 (2017)
17. Dahlen, E.R., Martin, R.C., Ragan, K., Kuhlman, M.M.: Driving anger, sensation seeking, impulsiveness, and boredom proneness in the prediction of unsafe driving. Accid. Anal. Prev. **37**(2), 341–348 (2005)
18. Kacprzyk, J.: Advances in Intelligent and Soft Computing (2002)
19. Neale, V.L., Klauer, S.G., Knipling, R.R., Dingus, T.A., Holbrook, G.T., Petersen, A.: The 100 car naturalistic driving study Phase I—experimental design. In: US DOT, Natl. Highw. Traffic Saf. Adm., no. December, 2002
20. Dingus, T.A., et al.: The 100-Car naturalistic driving study Phase II—results of the 100-Car field experiment. In: Dot Hs 810 593, no. April, p. No. HS-810 593 (2006)
21. Dingus, T.A., et al.: Naturalistic Driving Study: Technical Coordination and Quality Control (2015)
22. Bifulco, G.N., Galante, F., Pariota, L., Russo Spena, M., Del Gais, P.: Data collection for traffic and drivers' behaviour studies: a large-scale survey. Procedia Soc. Behav. Sci. **111**, 721–730 (2014)
23. Bifulco, G.N., Galante, F., Pariota, L., Russo-Spena, M.: Identification of driving behaviors with computer-aided tools. In: Proc. - UKSim-AMSS 6th Eur. Model. Symp. EMS 2012, pp. 331–336 (2012)
24. Wu, J., Xu, H.: Driver behavior analysis for right-turn drivers at signalized intersections using SHRP 2 naturalistic driving study data. J. Safety Res. **63**, 177–185 (2017)
25. Ghasemzadeh, A., Ahmed, M.M.: Utilizing naturalistic driving data for in-depth analysis of driver lane-keeping behavior in rain: non-parametric MARS and parametric logistic regression modeling approaches. In: Transp. Res. Part C Emerg. Technol., vol. 90, pp. 379–392 (2018)
26. Precht, L., Keinath, A., Krems, J.F.: Effects of driving anger on driver behavior—results from naturalistic driving data. Transp. Res. Part F Traffic Psychol. Behav. **45**, 75–92 (2017)
27. Bryman, A.: Research Methods and Organization Studies, vol. 20 (2005)
28. Saiprasert, C., Pholprasit, T., Thajchayapong, S.: Detection of driving events using sensory data on smartphone. Int. J. Intell. Transp. Syst. Res. **15**(1), 17–28 (2017)
29. Bahadoor, K., Hosein, P.: Application for the Detection of Dangerous Driving and an Associated Gamification Framework (2016)
30. Hori, C., Watanabe, S., Hori, T., Harsham, B.A., Hershey, J.R.: Driver Confusion Status Detection Using Recurrent Neural Networks Mitsubishi Electric Research Laboratories, Mitsubishi Electric Corporation Information Technology R & D Center (2016)

31. Kaiseler, M., Cunha, J.P., Cunha, P.S., Member, S.: A Mobile Sensing Approach to Stress Detection and Memory Activation for Public Bus Drivers A Mobile Sensing Approach to Stress Detection and Memory Activation for Public Bus Drivers, vol. 16, pp. 3294–3303 (2015)

32. Munoz-Organero, M., Corcoba-Magana, V.: Predicting upcoming values of stress while driving. IEEE Trans. Intell. Transp. Syst. 18(7), 1802–1811 (2017)

33. NIST/SEMATECH, "NIST/SEMATECH e-Handbook of Statistical Methods,". [Online]. Available: http://www.itl.nist.gov/div898/handbook/ (2012). Accessed 08 Apr 2018

34. Wang, J., Xu, W., Gong, Y.: Real-time driving danger-level prediction. Eng. Appl. Artif. Intell. 23(8), 1247–1254 (2010)

35. McDonald, A.D., Lee, J.D., Schwarz, C., Brown, T.L.: A contextual and temporal algorithm for driver drowsiness detection. Accid. Anal. Prev. 113, 25–37 (2018)

36. Kim, I.-H., Bong, J.-H., Park, J., Park, S.: Prediction of driver's intention of lane change by augmenting sensor information using machine learning techniques. Sensors 17(6), 1350 (2017)

37. Kaurin, A., Sauerberger, K.S., Funder, D.C.: Associations Between Informant Ratings of Personality Disorder Traits, Self-reports of Personality, and Directly Observed Behavior, vol. 49, pp. 1–72 (2017)

38. Hatfield, J., Williamson, A., Kehoe, E.J., Prabhakharan, P.: An examination of the relationship between measures of impulsivity and risky simulated driving amongst young drivers. Accid. Anal. Prev. 103, 37–43 (2017)

39. Golding, J.F.: Motion sickness susceptibility questionnaire revised and its relationship to other forms of sickness. Brain Res. Bull. 47(5), 507–516 (1998)

40. Horne, J.A., Östberg, O.: A self-assessment questionnaire to determine morningness-eveningness in human circadian rhythms. Int. J. Chronobiol. 4. Gordon and Breach Science Pub Ltd, Östberg, O.: Department of Human Work Sciences, University of Lulea, Lulea, Sweden, S-95187, 97–110 (1976)

41. Dahlen, E.R., White, R.P.: The Big Five factors, sensation seeking, and driving anger in the prediction of unsafe driving. Pers. Individ. Dif. 41(5), 903–915 (2006)

42. Goldberg, L.R.: A broad-bandwidth, public domain, personality inventory measuring the lower-level facets of several five-factor models. Pers. Psychol. Eur. 7, 7–28 (1999)

43. Deffenbacher, J.L., Huff, M.E., Lynch, R.S., Oetting, E.R., Salvatore, N.F.: Characteristics and treatment of high-anger drivers. J. Couns. Psychol. 47(1), 5–17 (2000)

44. Zuckerman, M.: Behavioral Expressions and Biosocial Bases of Sensation Seeking. Cambridge University Press, New York, NY, US (1994)

45. Deffenbacher, J.L., Oetting, E.R., Lynch, R.S.: Development of a driving anger scale. Psychol. Rep. 74(1), 83–91 (1994)

46. Li, Z., Chen, L., Peng, J., Wu, Y.: Automatic detection of driver fatigue using driving operation information for transportation safety. Sensors 17(6) (2017) (Switzerland)

47. Ragab, A., Craye, C., Kamel, M.S., Fakhri, K.: A visual-based driver distraction recognition and detection using random forest. Lect. Notes Comput. Sci. (Including Subser. Lect. Notes Artif. Intell. Lect. Notes Bioinformatics) 8814, 256–265 (2014)

48. Culig, J., Leppee, M.: From Morisky to Hill-bone; self-reports scales for measuring adherence to medication. Coll. Antropol. 38(1), 55–62 (2014)

49. Ji, Q., Zhu, Z., Lan, P.: Real-time nonintrusive monitoring and prediction of driver fatigue. IEEE Trans. Veh. Technol. 53(4), 1052–1068 (2004)

50. Pholprasit, T., Choochaiwattana, W., Saiprasert, C.: A comparison of driving behaviour prediction algorithm using multi-sensory data on a smartphone. In: 2015 IEEE/ACIS 16th International Conference on Software Engineering, Artificial Intelligence Networking and Parallel/Distributed Computing SNPD 2015 - Proc. (2015)

51. Delhomme, P., Chaurand, N., Paran, F.: Personality predictors of speeding in young drivers: anger vs. sensation seeking. Transp. Res. Part F Traffic Psychol. Behav. **15**(6), 654–666 (2012)
52. Podsakoff, P.M., MacKenzie, S.B., Podsakoff, N.P.: Sources of method bias in social science research and recommendations on how to control it. Annu. Rev. Psychol. **63**(1), 539–569 (2012)

An Efficient Model of Text Categorization Based on Feature Selection and Random Forests: Case for Business Documents

Fatima-Ezzahra Lagrari[1(✉)], Houssaine Ziyati[2], and Youssfi El Kettani[1]

[1] Department of mathematics, Ibn Tofail University, Kenitra, Morocco
Fatima.ezzahra.lagrari@gmail.com, Kettani.y@gmail.com
[2] Department of Computer Science, High School of Technology, Casablanca, Morocco
ziyati@gmail.com

Abstract. Huge amount of information on the internet is saved as text documents that are not classified, therefore the remaining issue is the recognition and classification of these text documents into the corresponding categories. Such text categorization task requires the use of feature selection techniques in order to reduce dimensionality which could enhance the models selectivity, accuracy and robustness. The present paper proposes a text categorization model based on feature selection using genetic algorithm and random forest method. The proposed approach has been tested on a publicly available dataset of business documents and the results show a classification accuracy of about 98.7% which outperforms other techniques tested on the same dataset.

Keywords: Feature selection · Genetic algorithm · Text mining · Random forests · Business documents

1 Introduction

We live in a universe where information has a great value. The huge growth of big data and resources available online challenges us to analyze them manually. This drive us to look for tools that can help to search, filter and manage these resources. Among these tools, text mining analysis has gained more importance in dealing with availability and the growing number of electronic documents [1].

Commonly, text mining techniques also known as text datamining or knowledge discovery from textual databases [2], include : categorization, summarization, topic detection, concept extraction, retrieval, clustering. Each of these techniques can be used in finding relevant information from a collection of documents.

Most of the available resources contain unstructured or semi-structured information from diverse domains such as: internet, biological databases, news articles, digital libraries, online forums, electronic mails, blog repositories [3]. Therefore, the union of natural language processing, data mining and machine learning techniques are highly needed in this context to classify and discover patterns

© Springer Nature Switzerland AG 2019
M. Ezziyyani (Ed.): AI2SD 2018, AISC 915, pp. 465–476, 2019.
https://doi.org/10.1007/978-3-030-11928-7_42

from textual information (text documents) [1]. In order to correctly present and classify these documents, other aspects have to be taken into consideration such as proper annotation of the documents, appropriate document representation and dimensionality reduction [4].

Documents are generally represented as bag-of-words, where each distinct term present in a document collection is considered as a separate dimension (feature). Hence, a document is represented by a multi-dimensional feature vectors where each dimension corresponds to a weighted value of the term within the document collection [5]. In practice, the number of irrelevant and interdependent features is very large that slows down the process of features analysis and model training which may have influence on the results, this is known as curse of dimensionality [6]. Therefore, one of the most important steps to face text categorization is to deal with the high dimensionality of the feature space.

The idea is to select a discriminative subset of features without sacrificing performance [7]. Dimension reduction methods can be classified as feature extraction [8] and feature selection. The feature extraction methods also known as feature construction methods transform a high dimensional feature space into a distinct low dimensional feature space through a combination or transformation of the original feature space. Feature selection methods also called variable selection concern the process of selecting a subset of relevant features to be used in the classification [9].

There are three general approaches for feature selection:

- **Filter approach** assess the relevance of features by looking only at the intrinsic properties of the data [10], without the use of a learning algorithm in the selection stage.
- **Wrapper approach** perform a search in the space of feature subsets and evaluate each one by training and testing a specific classification model; hence wrappers are tailored to a specific learning algorithm, and may achieve better performance than filters approaches, but at the price of a greater computational cost [11].
- **Embedded approach** leverages the internal parameters of a classification algorithm to select relevant features, often providing a good trade-off between computational cost and performance [12].

Many contributions have been done for solving text categorization problem. Zhou et al. [13] achieved a good classification accuracy on CNAE9 dataset by using latent factors extracted by probability latent semantic analysis in order to reduce dimensionality, they designed a new text classifier called LF-SVM for text categorization and compare their results with other existing classification models. Mahrooghy et al. [14] used filter based feature selection genetic algorithm (FFSGA) to find an optimal set of features where redundant and irrelevant features are deleted. To evaluate feature subset, they employed entropy index fitness function. Results indicates that feature selection technique improves the score by 7% and also reduce the dimensionality. A dimension reduction method for gene selection was proposed in [15] for gene selection. They integrate maximum relevance minimum redundancy (MRMR) with Genetic Algorithm (GA) to create an informative gene subset. They firstly apply MRMR to filter out the noisy and redundant genes from high dimensional gene space and then employ GA to select a subset of relevant discriminative features. The authors use support vector machine (SVM) and naive bayes (NB) classifiers to evaluate fitness of the selected genes. The experimental results illustrate that their method is able to select smallest gene subset that achieves the highest classification accuracy. [15] proposes a new feature selection and dimensionality reduction technique coupled with SIMCA method for the classification of CNAE9 text documents. The results are compared to classification and dimensionality reduction work done on the same dataset in literature. VSC-SIMCA shows best performance compared to other different techniques, not only in the amount of dimensionality reduction (60% less variables) but also achieved high classification rate of 95.34%.

A large variety of feature selection techniques are available in the literature. In this work we have adopted the wrapper approach by using Genetic Algorithm (GA) [16] and random forest algorithm for the classification of business documents. The proposed approach is inspired by the work in [17].

The paper is organized as follows: the next section gives insight about the different used techniques and the proposed approach then the used dataset and the experimental results are given after, finally the last section concludes the paper.

2   Proposed Approach

The proposed approach combines genetic algorithm, gradient boosting machine, recursive partitioning and random forest methods which will be explained in what follows.

2.1   Feature Selection Using Genetic Algorithm (GA)

Feature selection is the task of discovering the most relevant variables for a predictive model. Its a method that is used to identify and delete useless, irrelevant and redundant features that do not contribute or diminish the performance of the predictive model. Feature selection is considered as a combinatorial problem of optimization. An exhaustive selection of variables would evaluate various combinations (2^N, where N is the number of features). This process needs many computational work and if the number of variables is large it becomes inapplicable. Hence, we require brilliant methods that permit to perform feature selection practically. Genetic algorithm is considered as one of the most advanced algorithms for feature selection which is a stochastic method for optimization based on the process of natural genetics and biological evolution. In our work, we have used feature selection based on genetic algorithms to optimize the performance, by selecting the most relevant features [5].

The Genetic algorithm is an adaptive heuristic search algorithm inspired by the laws of natural selection and genetics. Genetic algorithm (GA) are receiving increasing application in a variety of search and optimization problems. Due to its advantages, it has been widely used as an effective tool for feature selection in text categorization. The goal of our study is to apply Genetic Algorithms (GA) as a feature selection method to select a best feature subset and to integrate these best features to recognize patterns. Genetic algorithm technique requires that the set of decision variables should be represented by a coded string of finite length [18]: a point in the search space is represented by a finite sequence of 0s and 1s, called a chromosome, a bit value of 1 in the chromosome means that the corresponding feature is included in the specified subset, and a value of 0 indicates that the corresponding feature is not included in the subset.

Genetic algorithms are dissimilar to conventional optimization and search procedures [10], they are probabilistic and not deterministic. The probability of survival is proportional to the chromosomes fitness value. as well as it works with a coding of solution set, not the solutions themselves. The quality of possible solutions is evaluated by a fitness function. Also, GA searches from a population of solutions, not a single solution. Basically, the initial population is randomly generated by three operators: selection, crossover, and mutation. The selection operator selects elites to send automatically to next generation. The crossover operator haphazardly exchanges a part of chromosomes between two chosen parents to generate offspring chromosomes. Finally, the mutation operator randomly alters a bit in chromosomes [16].

2.1.1   Encoding: The decision variables of a problem are ordinarily encoded into a limited length string, the variable could be a binary string or a list of integers.

2.1.2   Selection: The selection operator basically works at the level of chromosomes. The quality of each individual relies on its fitness. Fitness value can be defined by an objective function or by a subjective judgment particular to the problem. Since generations pass, the individuals of the population should get closer and closer to the solution (i.e. fitter). Classification accuracy and feature cost are the two key factors used to design a fitness function. The test accuracy measures the number of examples that are correctly classified [17]. Therefore, the individual who has high classification accuracy and low total feature cost produces a high fitness value. The individual with high fitness value has high probability to be selected to the next generation. The solution with high accuracy and fewer features will get a greater quality function value.

2.1.3   Cross-over: The crossover operator is a genetic operator that combines (exchange) two individuals (parents) in order to generate a new individual (offspring). The goal behind crossover is that the offspring could be better than both of the parents if it inherit the best characteristics from each of the parents [18].

2.1.4   Mutation: Mutation is considered as the modification of the value of each 'gene' of a solution with some probability pm (the mutation probability). The idea of mutation is the restoration of lost or unexplored genetic material in the population to prevent the premature convergence of the GA to suboptimal solution [18].

The whole fitness assignment, selection, recombination and mutation process is repeated until a stopping criterion is satisfied. Each generation is likely to be more adapted to the environment than the old one. Algorithm 1 shows the pseudo-code of the genetic algorithm.

Algorithm 1: A genetic algorithm pseudo code

Input: Determine randomly the initial population of individuals
Output: Evaluate the fitness of individuals
while *not stop criteria* **do**
> Select the best individuals to be used by the genetic operators;
> Generate new individuals to be used by the genetic operators;
> Evaluate the fitness of the individuals;
> Replace the worst individuals of the population by the best new individuals;

2.2   Pattern Recognition: Classification

Pattern recognition is the assignment of a label to a given input value. An example of pattern recognition is classification. Classification is considered as a supervised learning instance, where a training set of properly identified observations is available. The classification process consists on identifying (which group of categories an observation belongs to). In our work we use three classifiers: Random forest (RF), Gradient boosting machine (GBM) and Recursive partitioning (Rpart) model combined all together to produce a better prediction.

2.2.1   Random Forests (RF): is an ensemble learning method for classification and regression which consists of many individual trees. The RF algorithm chooses the individual classification with the most votes where each tree votes on an overall classification for the given set of data. In fact, each decision tree is built from a random subset of the training dataset using replacement in performing this sampling. In building each decision tree, a model based on a different random subset of the training dataset and a random subset of the available variables is used to choose how best to partition the dataset at each node [3]. Each decision tree is built to its maximum size, with no pruning performed. Random forests constructs aggregated predictions of the trees (majority votes for classification, average for regression) .The class label l of a case y is predicted by the following equation through majority voting:

$$l(y) = \arg\max c(\sum_{n=1}^{N} \mathbf{I}hn(y) = c))$$

There are two sources of randomness in the random forest method: random training set (bootstrap) and random selection of attributes. Using a random selection of attributes for dividing each node provide favorable error rates and are more robust with respect to noise. These attributes form nodes using standard tree building methods. Diversity is obtained by randomly choosing attributes at each node of a tree and using attributes that provide the highest level of learning. Each tree is developed at maximum without pruning until no more nodes can be created due to loss of information. Each individual tree receives an equal vote and the subsequent version of the random forest allows a weighted and un-weighted vote [3].

The RF algorithm calculates the out of bag error. The average misclassification for the entire forest is called as out of bag error, which serves to predict classifier performance without involving the test sample or cross-validation. The random forest error (out-of-bag) relies on the strength of the individual trees in the forest and the relation between them. With fewer attributes used for division, the correlation between two trees decreases and the trees strength decreases too [3]. Two factors that have a reverse effect on random forest error rates: a lower correlation increases the error rate while less strength decreases the error rate.

2.2.2   Gradient Boosting Machine (GBM): is a prediction algorithm which stems from the machine learning literature, and is based on the idea of creating an accurate learner by combining many so called "weak learners" [19]. Since its inception in 1990 (Freund, 1995; Freund & Schapire, 1996; Schapire, 1990), boosting has attracted a considerable amount of attention, it can be used for both regression and classification problems due to its excellent prediction performance over a wide range of applications in both the machine learning and statistics literatures. In gradient boosting machines, the learning procedure constantly fits new models to provide a more accurate estimate of the response variable. The main idea behind this algorithm is to construct the new base-learners to be maximally correlated with the negative gradient of the loss function, related with the whole ensemble. The loss functions applied can be arbitrary, but to give a better intuition, if the error function is the classic squared-error loss, the learning procedure would result in consecutive error-fitting.

Lets consider the dataset $(x, y)N_{i=1}$, where $x = (x_1, x_d)$ refers to the explanatory input variables and y to the corresponding labels of the response variable. The goal is to reconstruct the unknown functional dependence $x \rightarrow f \rightarrow y$ with our estimate $\widehat{f}$ such that some specified loss function $\Psi(y, f)$ is minimized:

$$\widehat{f}(x) = y$$
$$\widehat{f}(x) = \arg\min_{f(x)} \Psi(y, f(x))$$

In general, the choice of the loss function is up to the researcher, with both a rich variety of loss functions derived so far and with the possibility of implementing one's own task-specific loss. This high flexibility makes the GBMs highly customizable to any particular data-driven task. It introduces a lot of freedom into the model design thus making the choice of the most appropriate loss function a matter of trial and error. However, boosting algorithms are relatively simple to implement, which allows one to experiment with different model designs.

Finally we can formulate the complete form of the gradient boosting algorithm, as originally proposed by Friedman (2001) as shown below.

Algorithm 2: Fridman's gradient boosting algorithm

Input:
- input data (x, y)
- number of iterations M
- choice of the loss-function W
- choice of the base-learner model h

initialize f with a constant ;
for $i=1$ *to* M **do**

> compute the negative gradient $g_t(x)$;
> fit a new base learner function $h(x, \theta_t)$;
> find the best gradient descent step-size $\rho - t$;
>
> $$\rho = argmin_\rho \sum_{i=1}^{N} \Psi[y_i, \widehat{f}_{t-1}(x_i) + \rho h(x_i, \theta_t)]$$
>
> update the function estimate;
>
> $$\widehat{f}_t \leftarrow \widehat{f}_{t-1} + \rho_t h(x, \theta_t)$$

2.2.3 Recursive Partitioning (Rpart):

Recursive partitioning methods have become popular and largely used techniques for non-parametric regression and classification in various scientific domains. Particularly random forests, that can deal with great numbers of predictor variables even in complex interactions, it has been applied successfully in genetics, clinical medicine and bioinformatics within the past few years [20]. Examples of non-parametric approach are classification and regression trees. Their characteristic is that the feature space, i.e. the space spanned by all predictor variables, is recursively partitioned into a set of rectangular areas, the partition is created in a way that observations with same response values are grouped. After the partition is finished, a constant value of the response variable is predicted within each area. The recursive partitioning process is described below.

Algorithm 3: Recursive Partitioning process

Input: Take all the data

Consider all possible values of all variables

Select the variable/value ($x = t1$) that produces the "greatest" separation in the target

if $x \leq t1$ **then** send the data point to the left **else** send the data point to the right Repeat the same process on these two nodes.

---

3   Proposed Model

Since the application concern text categorization and since the features to be used in the training phase are words, the first step was the application of the genetic algorithm in order to reduce dimensionality and use only relevant features and this by using Random Forest in order to asses fitness function of individuals. Such reduction of dimensions leads to significant reduction in the complexity of the model and optimize the computational burden for classifying future samples. Second step is building our classification model based on Gradient boosting machines (GBM), Random forest (RF) and Recursive partitioning (Rpart). The flowchart of the proposed model is depicted in Fig.1.

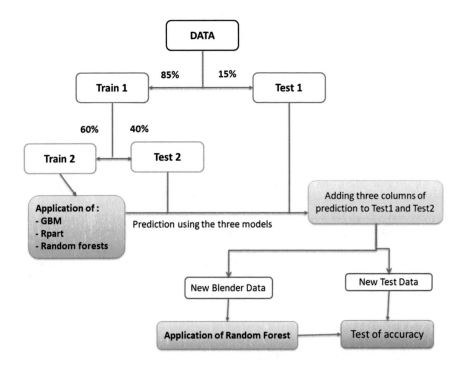

Fig. 1. Flowchart of the proposed classification framework

The different steps are described below:

1. Partitioning data into training 1 and testing 1 data sets (selected sub-sets).
2. Partitioning the training 1 data into training 2 data and testing 2 data.
3. Applying the three followed models on the training 2 subset:
   - First model: Gradient boosting machines (GBM).
   - Second model: Recursive partitioning (Rpart).
   - Third model: Random forest (RF).
4. We do predictions in test 2 and test 1 data.
5. We obtain new variables (predictors) that we add to test 1 and test 2 data.
6. Application of random forest model on the New Blender data.
7. We do prediction of the class of each document in new Test Data.
8. Test of accuracy.

4   Experiments

The aim of the experiment is to create a classification model for text documents that minimizes the number of variables while maximizing the models classification performance. Genetic algorithms coupled with random forests technique as a classifier enabled us to achieve that aim.

The data set under consideration 'CNAE-9', provided by (Bache & Lichman, 2013), was used to create and test the model. The dataset contains 1080 documents of free text business descriptions of Brazilian companies categorized into a subset of 9 categories cataloged in a table called National Classification of Economic Activities (CNAE). The original texts were pre-processed to obtain the current data set as follows: (i) only letters were kept; (ii) then, prepositions were removed from the texts; (iii) Next, the words were transformed to their canonical form; and (iv) finally, each document was represented as a vector, where the weight of each word is its frequency in the document.

The dataset is composed of 856 variables (words) and 1080 documents of nine classes [21]. The data set is highly sparse (99.22% of the matrix is filled with zeros). The documents were divided into two data sets : Training set with 727 documents and Testing set with 129 documents.

In this paper, we have proposed a predictive model for recognition of text documents based on feature selection using genetic algorithm to reduce dimensionality feature space followed by class prediction model (RF) for classification of text documents. In feature selection step, GA has selected 757 features between 856 with 10 fold cross validation using random forest technique to evaluate fitness function. After the selection of features, we have trained our model with the new subset using random forest model.

The following plot shows the average internal accuracy estimates (training set) as well as the average external estimates (testing set) calculated from the 50 out of sample predictions i.e. 10 cross validation repeated 5 times. Each two points in a generation correspond to the measurements of best selected model (Fig. 2).

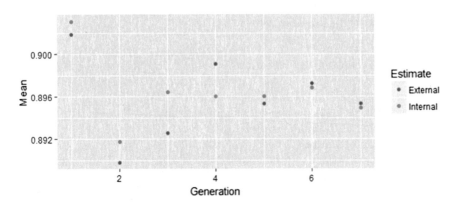

Fig. 2. Feature selection using genetic algorithm

Many performance measures can be used like Precision, sensitivity, specificity, recall and f-measurement. In this work, we used the accuracy, which is computed as follows :

$$Accuracy = \frac{N}{T}$$

Where N is the number of correctly classified cases and T is the total number of cases.

As stated in [17], using K nearest neighbors (KNN) the accuracy of 92.78% stabilizes when the number of dimensions reaches 100 (above this value the accuracy doesnt change). We compare the classification accuracy of our model with results published in Ahmed Abdelfattsah Saleh [22] and Xiaofei Zhou et al. [13].

Table 1 shows the proposed model compared to some of the best methods in the literature.

Table 1. Comparative study of the classification rates obtained after applying variables selection using GA and classification techniques on CNAE dataset

Methods	Number of selected features	Pattern recognition models	Classification Rate (%)
Proposed model	757	Random forests GBM RPART	98.7
VSC_SIMCA [22]	55	PCA	95.34
Feature extraction using PLSA model [13]	Unknown	Latent factor, SVM	95.19

5   Conclusion

Our method was applied on the data set 'CNAE-9', for classification of text documents belonging to 9 different classes. A classification accuracy of 98.7% was achieved for a number of selected features equal to 757, which is to our knowledge the best accuracy achieved so far. As future work we will investigates semantics aspects and enhance the current approach in order to reduce more the number of selected features.

References

1. Khan, A., Baharudin, B., Lee, L.H., Khan, K.: A review of machine learning algorithms for text-documents classification. J. Adv. Inf. Technol. **1**(1) (2010)
2. Navathe, S.B., Ramez, E.: Data warehousing and data mining. In: Fundamentals of Database Systems, pp. 841–872 (2000)
3. Rostami, M., Ayat, S.S., Attarzadeh, I., Saghari, F.: Proposing a method to classify texts using data mining. J. Adv. Comput. Res. **6**(4), 125–137 (2015)
4. Dasgupta, A., Drineas, P., Harb, B., Josifovski, V., Mahoney, M.W.: Feature selection methods for text classification. In: Proceedings of the 13th ACM SIGKDD International Conference on Knowledge Discovery and Data Mining, pp. 230–239. ACM (2007)
5. Mary, A., Madhavi, S.D.: Using Dimensionality Reduction Methods in Text Clustering (2015)
6. Chen, H., Jiang, W., Li, C., Li, R.: A heuristic feature selection approach for text categorization by using chaos optimization and genetic algorithm. Mathematical problems in Engineering (2013)
7. Bharti, K.K., Singh, P.K.: Hybrid dimension reduction by integrating feature selection with feature extraction method for text clustering. Expert Syst. Appl. **42**(6), 3105–3114 (2015)
8. Wang, X., Paliwal, K.K.: Feature extraction and dimensionality reduction algorithms and their applications in vowel recognition. Pattern Recogn. **36**(10), 2429–2439 (2003)
9. Roweis, S.T., Saul, L.K.: Nonlinear dimensionality reduction by locally linear embedding. Science **290**(5500), 2323–2326 (2000)
10. Goldberg, D.E.: Genetic algorithms in search. Optim. Mach, Learn (1989)
11. Guyon, I., Elisseeff, A.: An introduction to variable and feature selection. J. Mach. Learn. Res. **3**, 1157–1182 (2003)
12. Ma, S., Huang, J.: Penalized feature selection and classification in bioinformatics. Briefings Bioinform. **9**(5), 392–403 (2008)
13. Zhou, X., Guo, L., Liu, P., Liu, Y.: Latent factor svm for text categorization. In: 2014 IEEE International Conference on Data Mining Workshop (ICDMW), pp. 105–110. IEEE (2014)
14. Mahrooghy, M., Younan, N.H., Anantharaj, V.G., Aanstoos, J., Yarahmadian, S.: On the use of the genetic algorithm filter-based feature selection technique for satellite precipitation estimation. IEEE Geosci. Remote Sens. Lett. **9**(5), 963 (2012)
15. El Akadi, A., Amine, A., El Ouardighi, A., Aboutajdine, D.: A two-stage gene selection scheme utilizing mrmr filter and ga wrapper. Knowl. Inf. Syst. **26**(3), 487–500 (2011)

16. Aalaei, S., Shahraki, H., Rowhanimanesh, A., Eslami, S.: Feature selection using genetic algorithm for breast cancer diagnosis: experiment on three different datasets. Iran. J. Basic Med. Sci. **19**(5), 476 (2016)

17. Ciarelli, P.M., Oliveira, E.: Agglomeration and elimination of terms for dimensionality reduction. In: ISDA'09. Ninth International Conference on Intelligent Systems Design and Applications, pp. 547–552. IEEE (2009)

18. Abuiziah, I., Shakarneh, N.: A review of genetic algorithm optimization: operations and applications to water pipeline systems. Int. J. Math. Comput. Phys. Electr. Comput. Eng. **7**(12), 341–347 (2013)

19. Freund, Y., Schapire, R.E., et al.: Experiments with a new boosting algorithm. In: Icml, vol. 96, pp. 148–156. Citeseer (1996)

20. Strobl, C., Malley, J., Tutz, G.: An introduction to recursive partitioning: rationale, application, and characteristics of classification and regression trees, bagging, and random forests. Psychol. Methods **14**(4), 323 (2009)

21. Morgon, R., do Lago Pereira, S.: Evolutionary learning of concepts. J. Comput. Commun. **2**(08), 76 (2014)

22. Saleh, A.A., Weigang, L., et al.: A new variables selection and dimensionality reduction technique coupled with simca method for the classification of text documents. In: Proceedings of the MakeLearn and TIIM Joint International Conference, Make Learn and TIIM, pp. 583–591 (2015)

Association Rules Mining Method of Big Data for E-Learning Recommendation Engine

Karim Dahdouh[1]($\boxtimes$), Ahmed Dakkak[1], Lahcen Oughdir[1], and Abdelali Ibriz[2]

[1] Engineering Sciences Laboratory, FPT, Sidi Mohamed Ben Abdellah University, Taza, Morocco
karim.dahdoh@gmail.com
[2] High School of Technology, Sidi Mohamed Ben Abdellah University, Fez, Morocco

Abstract. Today, recommender systems are increasingly used due to its success in several areas such as e-commerce, tourism, social networks, and e-learning. Indeed, most of the computing environment for human learning, especially the online learning platforms have a very large number of learners' profiles, thousands of courses, and various educational resources. However, students often face many challenges, such as the absence of a real solution of recommendation to orientate them to take more appropriate learning materials. In this article, we develop a recommendation engine for the e-learning platform in order to help learners to easily find the most proper pedagogical resources without any search effort. It aims to discover relationships between student's courses activities through the association rules mining method. We also focus on the analysis of past historical data of the courses enrollments or log data. The article discusses particularly the frequent itemsets concept to determine the interesting rules among objects in the transaction database. Then, we use the extracted rules to find the list of suitable courses according to the learner's behaviors and preferences. Next, we implement our system using Apriori algorithm and R, which is efficient big data analysis language and environment, on data collected from ESTenligne [ESTenLigne project is supported by the EST Network of Morocco and the Eomed association (http://www.eomed.org)] platform database of High school of Technology of Fez. Finally, the experimental results prove the effectiveness and reliability of the proposed system to increase the quality of student's decision, guide them during the learning process and provide targeted online learning courses to meet the needs of the learners.

Keywords: Online learning · E-learning · Recommendation system · Big data · Association rules · Apriori algorithm · R environment

1 Introduction

The computing environment for human learning is changing rapidly, due to the emergence of new information and communication technology such as the big data [1] and cloud computing [2]. Furthermore, learning methods are changing every day.

© Springer Nature Switzerland AG 2019
M. Ezziyyani (Ed.): AI2SD 2018, AISC 915, pp. 477–491, 2019.
https://doi.org/10.1007/978-3-030-11928-7_43

Therefore, e-learning systems need to develop more techniques and tools to meet the increased needs of millions of learners around the world.

This article exposes a recommendation system applied in the online learning environment in order to be able to provide personalized courses and guide students to take more suitable courses. For example, emailing or sending notifications through the user interface of distance learning platform, to students who follow courses in a specific field and recommend the suitable educational resources that are likely to be interesting for them. Also, learners can be guided to enroll in the latest courses in their interest areas based on historical data of all users over a large dataset of courses enrollments.

In this article, we are interested in improving learning platforms through building a recommender system. Our system uses association rules method for to finding similarities in courses enrollments. It aims to extract more interesting relationships between learners' behaviors. Thus, discovering association rules enables us to target students who learn two or more courses together, i.e. finding a list of frequent courses enrollments to determine those that are more likely chosen by the learners. So, based on the discovered patterns, we can guide students to take specific courses. The pedagogical team can also improve the quality of non-frequent courses or create new ones.

The rest of the article is organized as follows: In Sect. 2, we present a state of the art of recommendation system for e-learning environment. In Sect. 3, we introduce the basic concepts of the association rules technique and then we give a detailed description of Apriori algorithm. In Sect. 4, we implement the course recommendation system using data from ESTenLigne platform and R Studio as an integrated development environment (IDE). For making the experimental results clear and easy to understand, we use arulesViz [3] package which provides rich set of powerful data visualization techniques for association rules.

2   Related Work

To help the human mind in its selection process, several recommender systems have emerged in the last decade of the twentieth century. In the literature, we find three basic approaches, namely collaborative filtering [4], Content-based filtering [5], and in addition, there are hybrid recommender systems [6], combining the two types of filtering. The method used in this article is part of the recommender systems based on collaborative filtering, of which there is no analysis of the subject or content of objects to recommend. This type of system is very effective in the case where the content of the objects is complex, e.g. pedagogical resource.

Many research works have been conducted in the field of distance learning in higher education using big data techniques including machine learning methods. There are a lot of applications of these techniques. Particularly, recommendation system which is used in many areas such as basket analysis (Amazon), social networks (LinkedIn, Twitter, ect.), government, education, etc.

Mihai [7] proposed the prototype of a recommendation system based on association rules for the distributed learning management system. The article uses distributed data mining algorithms and data obtained from Learning Management Systems (LMS) database in order to identify strong correlations between sets of courses followed by students. It also gives a brief description of the architecture and methodology of course recommendation system without providing an implementation of the proposed architecture.

Jooa et al. [8] focused on implementing recommendation system using association rules and collaborative filtering. The proposed system uses the distance data from Global Positioning System (GPS) to recommend products that customers are likely to purchase based on their preferences.

Hrženjak et al. [9] applied association rules technique in learning management system of the Rijeka University. They use students from MudRi e-learning database, which is based on the Moodle open source software. Then, they apply Apriori algorithm for finding connections between various actions. They find that students have better success in the course when they are using videos course. Also, they identify which lessons seem to have a greater connection to the final grades.

Sunita et al. [10] provided an approach for course recommendation system based on the combination of clustering and association rules techniques. In order to find useful pattern over Moodle (Modular Object-Oriented Dynamic Learning Environment) database. They used the open data source data mining tool, called Weka, to implement the proposed system for extracting the list of relevant courses to the learner, based on the choice of other learners for a specific collection of courses.

To overcome the limitations of the existing systems, such as provide a real implementation of the recommendation system in the field of education that ensures the relevancy of the recommended courses to the learner's requirements. In addition, our system aims to enhance the efficiency and reliability of the existing system through the integration of R environment. This article presents a smart courses recommendation system using association rules method and the big data analysis technology with R programming language. Moreover, the system presented in this article uses many data visualization techniques which aim to communicate and visualize clearly the hidden patterns over a large dataset of historical data of courses enrollments.

3   Method

In this section, we focus on the basic concepts of association rules used for developing the proposed courses recommender system. Then we present Apriori algorithm which is used to find the more strong relationships between itemsets in a transaction database, based on frequent itemsets that satisfy the minimum support and confidence thresholds.

3.1   Association Rules Method

Association rules is an unsupervised learning method that is widely used in many fields including recommendation engines, retail analysis of the transaction, and clickstream analysis across web pages [11]. It aims to find hidden patterns in large amounts of data, in the form of interesting rules. In other words, its goal is to discover groups of items that appear frequently together in enrolments made by learners.

The term Association rules are often referred to as Market Basket Analysis application. Because the first time used was in 1993 by Agrawal et al. [12] in order to find useful relationships between items through a large database of customer transactions. Each transaction consists of items purchased by a customer. For detecting all significant connections between items bought by a customer over a period of time not necessarily consist of items bought together at the same time [12].

In general, the commendation systems consist of three principle steps; first, collect data from large transaction database; second, find similarities between users behavior's, according to more frequent item set, and finally, recommend more suitable items for users.

Considering $C = \{c_1, c_2, c_3, \ldots, c_n\}$ a set of all items or courses enrollments stored in the database and $L = \{l_1, l_2, l_3, \ldots, l_n\}$ a set of learner profiles. Each learner l_i enrolls into k courses, where k is a subset of courses chosen from set of items C. In association rules, we define a rule as an implication of $\Rightarrow Y$, Where $X, Y \subseteq C$ (X and Y are sets of courses) and $X \cap Y = \emptyset$, which means when course X followed by the learner l_i, course Y is likely followed as well with a high probability. The set of attributes X is called antecedent or left-hand-side (LHS) of the rule; the set of attributes Y is called consequent or right-hand-side (RHS) of the rule [12].

Generally, The association rules technique produce a large number of rules $X \Rightarrow Y$, but to select interesting rules from the set of all generated rules, there are two important measures to determine the quality of an association rule, the most known are minimum thresholds of support and confidence.

The support is the percentage (%) of transactions in the dataset that contain the itemset X while confidence is defined as the percentage (%) of transactions that contain X, which also contain Y. The formal definition of the confidence is: $\text{conf}(X \Rightarrow Y) = \frac{\text{supp}(X \cup Y)}{\text{supp}(X)}$. Therefore, a strength association rule $X \Rightarrow Y$ should satisfy: $\text{supp}(X \cup Y) \geq \sigma$ and $\text{conf}(X \Rightarrow Y) \geq \delta$, where σ and δ are the minimum support and minimum confidence, respectively.

In the context of our research, we apply association rules technique in the online learning. Accordingly, a transaction in our case is represented by student's profile. Similarly, items are replaced by courses followed by a given student during the learning process. So, we can define the support and confidence respectively as follows:

$$\text{supp}(X \Rightarrow Y) = \frac{\text{number of learners following X and Y courses}}{\text{total number of learner enrollments in database}} \tag{1}$$

$$\text{conf}(X \Rightarrow Y) = \frac{\text{number of learners following X and Y courses}}{\text{number of learners profiles following X courses}} \tag{2}$$

Support is the first one which is defined as the percentage of transactions that contain X, It means, support is an indication of how frequently the itemset appears in the database. On the other hand, confidence is defined as the percentage (%) of transactions (students profiles) that follow X, which also follow Y.

3.2   Apriori Algorithm

There are several algorithms for implementing association rules method to extract interesting relationships between variables or items in a large database, through finding more frequent itemsets. Apriori is the most popular and simplest algorithm. It has been implemented in several languages including R, Java, C/C++, Python, etc. Other relative algorithms such as FP-growth and MAFIA (Maximal Frequent Itemset Algorithm) are also available. Furthermore, Apriori is the most popular algorithm and easy to implement. It identifies the frequent items in the database and extends them to larger and larger itemsets as long as those itemsets appear sufficiently often in the dataset [13]. The key property of Apriori is: "If an itemset is frequent, then all its subsets items will be frequent." i.e. any subset of a frequent itemset must be frequent.

Figure 1 describes the template of Apriori algorithm. In the beginning, the algorithm simply counts item occurrences in order to determine the large 1-items. Second step consists of these phases. First, the large itemsets L_{k-1} are used to generate the candidate itemsets C_k. Next, the database is scanned and the support of candidates in C_k is calculated, i.e. increment the count of all candidates that are contained in a given transaction t. After, the support of each candidate k-itemset is compared with sup_{min}. The k-itemset is frequent only if it has the support greater than user-specified minimum support sup_{min}. The next step is identifying all rules having confidence greater or equal to the user-specified minimum confidence, i.e. The algorithm deletes all rules not satisfy the condition of $conf_{min}$ [12, 15].

Apriori algorithm template

k-itemsets	An itemset having k items
C_k	Set of candidate k-itemsets (potentially large itemsets), which each member of this set has two fields: itemset and support count.
L_k	Set of frequent items of size k.
sup_{min}	User-specified minimum support
$conf_{min}$	User-specified minimum confidence

1) $L_1 = \{$large 1-itemsets$\}$
2) **for** (k=2 ; L_{k-1} !=∅; k++) **do begin**
3) C_k = apriori-gen(L_{k-1}); // generate new candidates from L_{k-1} [14]
4) **for each** transaction t ∈ D **do begin**
5) C_t = subset(C_k, t); // candidates contained in t
6) **for each** candidates c ∈ C_t **do begin**
7) c.count++; //increment the count of all candidates that are contained in the transaction t
8) **end**
9) $L_k = \{$c ∈ C_k | c. count ≥ $sup_{min}\}$ //candidates in C_k with minimum support
10) **end**
11) **return** $\cup_k L_k$

Fig. 1. Apriori algorithm template

Figure 2 shows the flow chart of this algorithm that represents its workflow which includes: counts item occurrences from the dataset. Then, the candidates' itemsets generation process checks the support and of each itemset with the user-specified minimum support threshold, and minimum confidence. Finally, use the frequent itemsets to determine more interesting association rules between items in large database transactions.

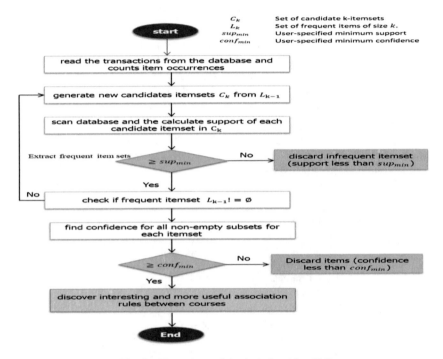

Fig. 2. Flow chart of Apriori algorithm [16]

4   E-Learning Recommendation Engine

4.1   System Architecture

The proposed courses recommendation system consists of two roles which are learners and teachers or pedagogical team. It has the following components: online learning platform and MySQL database server that stores and manages data produced by learner's interactions during the learning session including courses enrollments, learner's behavior, etc. There is also R environment to develop, execute, and test association rule method. Furthermore, the architecture describes different steps including data discovery, modeling, processing, and data visualization in order to efficiently finding useful rules between all courses enrollments.

Figure 3 illustrates the global architecture of the implemented system. The historical data of courses enrollments are integrated into R environment using RMySQL

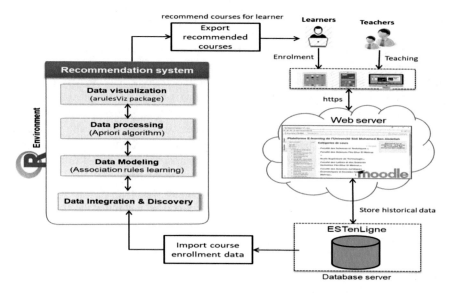

Fig. 3. Courses recommendation engine architecture

driver to connect to the database server. The course recommendation system workflow consists of these steps:

- Importing historical data from the ESTenLigne database.
- Data discovery including data integration, collection, aggregation and exploration.
- Data modeling using the association rules method.
- Data processing by running Apriori algorithm.
- Data visualization through the use of arulesViz visualization techniques [3].
- Exporting list of recommended courses.

After building and executing of our recommendation system, we have in output the more useful rules; it means the list of recommended courses.

4.2 ESTenLigne Project

The present work is a part of the ESTenLigne project, which is the result of several years of experience for developing e-learning in the Sidi Mohamed Ben Abdellah University of Fez. It was started since 2012 by the EST network of Morocco. It aims the development of distance education based on new information and communication technologies through the implementation of open, adapted and scalable online learning platform, and taking into account the dimensions of exchange, sharing and mutualization of pedagogical resources [17, 18].

Several works have been done as part of this project including the training of experts across e-learning in the context of the Coselearn I project, the, and teacher training through Franco-Moroccan EST[1] and IUT[2] cooperation [18, 19]. Furthermore, there are some researches that have been done around this project such as the analysis of the use of educational resources where the objective was to analyze the use peda-gogical resources in some courses namely the algorithmic course [20]. Also, a case study for collaboration analysis of online course based on activity theory [21].

However, in ESTenLigne platform, we have never worked on systems of recom-mendation, due to its important role as a support to orientate students. Especially, most of the learners in this platform are new graduates who have just come to integrate higher education and who need a system to help them to target the relevant courses to follow during their learning process. In fact, the students have a lot of difficulties and are lost in the diversity of educational resources, particularly the large number of available courses. This requires the adaptation of the teaching to meet the needs of students. To solve these problems, we develop a course recommendation system to promote learning to learners through creating a smart solution. It is able to generate the most appropriate courses automatically based on historical data of learner's activities.

4.3   Dataset Structure

The ESTenLigne project is based on LMS Moodle [22]. Indeed, it is an open source learning management system. It uses a relational database which has around 250 tables. We focus only on student's enrollments into courses. Especially, we focus on the tables that represent the information we need to implement our recommendation system based on association rules technique. In general, Our solution collect data from four tables. First, there is mdl_user that gives information about student's profile. Second, all user enrollments have record into mdl_user_enrolments table. Third, mdl_enrol table con-tains data of courses enrollments. For the same course, there can be different enrollment start and end dates. Some students may require a course for one period of time but other users may want to enroll in the same course for a different period of time. Fourth, mdl_course table stores all the details of the courses that are uploaded on the learning management system. It stores the names of the course, category, full name, short name, summary, time created, time modified etc. [23].

4.4   Courses Recommender System Flow Chart

The Flow chart illustrated in Fig. 4, shows the dynamic aspects of our system. It describes a series of actions or activities performed by different actors.

In the beginning, learners should create an account through page registration. After the login into ESTenLigne platform, learner's login name and password is verified. If it is valid then the student can access a set of courses available in the dataset. After browsing these courses, Learners will choose the courses in which he is interested. The data of learner enrollments, during the learning session, are stored in ESTenLigne database. Next, we collect appropriate data from historical data. Then, we prepare those

---

[1] http://www.iut.fr.

[2] http://www.est-usmba.ac.ma.

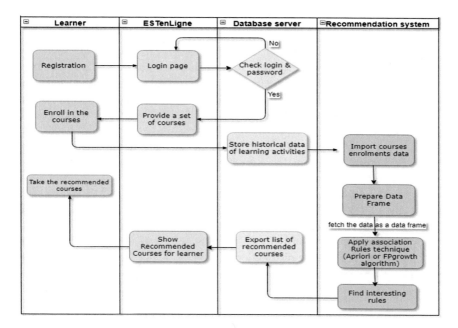

Fig. 4. Flow chart of courses recommendation system

data in the form of data frame. Indeed, the courses enrollments that belong to each learner are aggregated into a single vector as an array of enrollments. Afterward, we use R environment to apply Association rules techniques. The result Apriori algorithm, according to support and confidence specified values, is a catalog of interesting correlations between courses. The next step consists of exporting the list of recommended courses to ESTenLigne database. Finally, we can display the result of recommendation system to the learner in order to guide and suggest them more relevant courses.

5 Experiments and Results

5.1 Experiments

To evaluate the effectiveness of the courses recommendation system presented in this article, we have conducted many experiments on 1218 students from the high school of technology (EST) of Fez. 859 of them enroll in at least one course and 359 have never followed any course. So, we concentrate just on students who have course enrollments. The proposed system recommends the suitable courses for students among 153 courses. In addition, some of these courses may not follow by students. We consider only the set of courses which have been opted by the students.

In order to test and validate the proposed system, we choose R Studio as an integrated development environment (IDE). It is a powerful big data tool for the advanced statistical analysis. It provides a rich set of high-level packages for statistical purpose. It also allows flexible graphical options that enable different data visualization techniques.

To prepare the required data, before launching the execution of our system, we collect data from ESTenLigne database. To do that, we develop a SQL query to extract a list of courses followed by all learners. Indeed, we focus essentially on four tables includes mdl_user, mdl_user_enrolments, mdl_enrol and mdl_course. To do this task efficiently, we integrated RMySQL package in R Studio to easily connect and execute SQL statements.

Then, we need to record courses by student id (user_id), so the individual courses followed by a given learner are aggregated into a single record as a vector of courses. Next, we convert the grouped data into the optimized object (S4) for running the Apriori algorithm. After we execute SQL query though RMySQL tool and create the group of courses for each student, we obtain a collection of courses order by learner identifier (user_id) which represent the input data of Apriori algorithm.

In order to present the items frequency visually, we use itemFrequencyPlot function of arules package. The relative distribution of the most frequent courses enrollments in our database transaction is illustrated in Fig. 5.

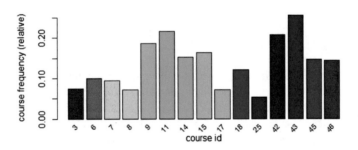

Fig. 5. Relative frequency distribution of courses enrollments

The result in the histogram shows the fifteen courses in our dataset with at least 5 percent support. The top course studied was course number 43 with 219 enrollments of 2553 transactions in ESTenLigne database.

The next step consists of running Apriori algorithm on data captured in data discovery phase. For this purpose, we use arules package [24] which implements the Apriori and Eclat algorithms. At first, we specify the minimum support and confidence threshold, respectively, to find more strong relationships between courses enrollments. The number of interesting association rules changes according to the value of support and confidence and the database size. In order to find more interesting roles, we use the minimum support threshold of 5% and we set 50% as a minimum confidence threshold. Finally, we can run Apriori algorithm as shown in Fig. 6.

```
Apriori
Parameter specification:
confidence minval smax arem  aval originalSupport maxtime sup-
port minlen maxlen target ext
  0.5    0.1 1 none FALSE   TRUE   5 0.05   1  10   rules FALSE
Algorithmic control:
 filter tree heap memopt load sort verbose
   0.1 TRUE TRUE  FALSE TRUE    2     TRUE
Absolute minimum support count: 42
set item appearances ...[0 item(s)] done [0.00s].
set transactions ...[144 item(s), 859 transaction(s)] done
[0.00s].
sorting and recoding items ... [15 item(s)] done [0.00s].
creating transaction tree ... done [0.00s].
checking subsets of size 1 2 3 done [0.00s].
writing ... [23 rule(s)] done [0.00s].
creating S4 object  ... done [0.00s].
```

Fig. 6. The experimental results of Apriori algorithm

5.2 Results

The result of running Apriori algorithm is a set of 23 rules which satisfy the minimum support and confidence thresholds. The top 10 useful rules ordered by the confidence measure are illustrated in Table 1.

Table 1. Confidence and support results

Rule	lhs		rhs	Confidence	Support
[1]	{11,46}	⇒	{45}	1.0000000	0.06519208
[2]	{11,45}	⇒	{46}	0.9824561	0.06519208
[3]	{46}	⇒	{45}	0.9593496	0.13736903
[4]	{15,46}	⇒	{45}	0.9387755	0.05355064
[5]	{15,45}	⇒	{46}	0.9387755	0.05355064
[6]	{45}	⇒	{46}	0.9365079	0.13736903
[7]	{6,7}	⇒	{18}	0.8518519	0.05355064
[8]	{6,18}	⇒	{7}	0.8363636	0.05355064
[9]	{7}	⇒	{18}	0.8024691	0.07566938
[10]	{7,18}	⇒	{6}	0.7076923	0.05355064

According to the obtained results of support and confidence; as we can see from the experimental results in Table 1, the association between courses {11 and 46} and {45} has the highest confidence; also the association between courses {7 and 18} and {6} are the lowest. Based on the calculated values of support and confidence, it is clear which courses are more likely followed by learners and we can determine the suitable course to recommend for each learner. For example, the rule 1 {11, 46} ⇒ {45} has the highest confidence, so our system recommend course 45 to students who enroll into courses {11 and 46}. According to Table 1, the efficiency of rule 1 is 100% because there are 56 students who enroll into courses {11 and 46} where 56 among them enroll also into course {45}. For course rule 2, there are 57 students in historical data of learners enrollments who take both of courses {11 and 45}, 56 among them follow course {46} in subsequent courses, so the efficiency of the rule 1 is 98%. So the system recommends the course {46} to students who enrolled in courses {11 and 45}. With regard to rule 3, there are 123 learners enroll into course {46}, because a high proportion (118 learners) of them enroll also into course {45} in subsequent courses, the efficiency of rule 3 is 95%, so the system recommends the course {45} to students who enrolled in course {46}, and so on. For the top 10 rules, we notice that the values of confidence are between 0.707(70.7%) and 1.00 (100%), which prove that we have obtained good results. Thus, we can conclude that the proposed course recommendation system provides the more appropriate courses according to the historical data of students' activities, especially courses enrolments.

5.3   Data Visualization

In order to view more clearly the results of the conducted experiments, we use R-extension Package arulesViz [3] which is an advanced technique for visualizing the strong relationships between courses.

A straight-forward visualization of association rules is to use a scatter plot (Fig. 7) using support and confidence on the axes. In addition, a third measure (lift) is used as the color of the points.

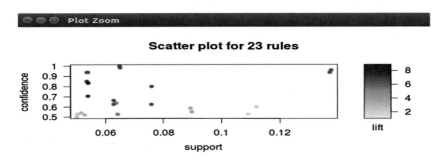

Fig. 7. Scatter plot visualization

Figure 8 illustrates very clearly the 10 interesting rules using graph-based techniques. Indeed, It visualizes association rules using vertices and edges where vertices typically represent item(course) or itemset (set of courses) and edges indicate a relationship in rules. As we can see from rule 1 from the graph in Fig. 8 students who enroll into course {Arch-Norm-Réseaux and Ing-sys-Info} enroll also in {Réseaux-Info} course.

Another technique to represent the strong rules is grouped matrix (Fig. 9) that is capable to analyze large rule sets [3]. Indeed, this technique gives us the possibility to select and zoom interesting relationship between courses.

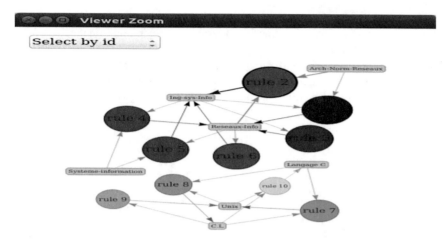

Fig. 8. Graph-based visualization with rules as vertices

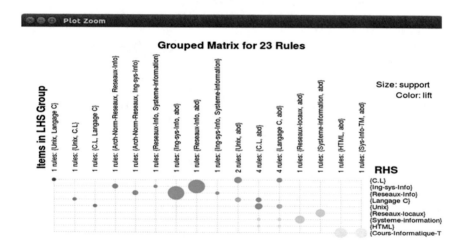

Fig. 9. Grouped matrix-based visualization for 23 rules

6   Conclusion and Future Work

In this article, we have presented a course recommendation system for e-learning platform. It aims to help students decide which courses are the most suitable to study through the finding of all interesting relationships between courses enrollments over the database transactions. We used association rules as a method and Apriori algorithm for implementing the business logic of our system. We collected historical data of students' activities from e-learning platform of High school of Technology of Fez. Then, we build our solution using the open source software R Studio for data discovering, modeling, processing, and visualization through arulesViz [3] package. The results of the Experiments prove the effectiveness and reliability of the course recommendation system for providing targeted online learning able to guide and orientate students to take the convenient courses.

Our future research will be focused on how we could apply this work in a distributed environment through the integration of more big data technologies, especially Hadoop ecosystem and Spark framework.

References

1. Dahdouh, K., Dakkak, A., Oughdir, L., Messaoudi, F.: Big data for online learning systems. Educ. Inf. Technol., mai 2018
2. Dahdouh, K., Dakak, A., Oughdir, L.: Integration of the cloud environment in E-Learning systems. Trans. Mach. Learn. Artif. Intell. 5(4) (2017)
3. Hahsler, M. Chelluboina, S.: Visualizing Association Rules: Introduction to the R-extension Package arulesViz (2018)
4. Linden, G., Smith, B., York, J.: Amazon.com recommendations: item-to-item collaborative filtering. IEEE Internet Comput. 7(1), 76–80 (2003)
5. Balabanović, M., Shoham, Y.: Fab: content-based, collaborative recommendation. Commun. ACM 40(3), 66–72 (1997)
6. Good, N., et al.: Combining Collaborative Filtering with Personal Agents for Better Recommendations, p. 8 (1999)
7. Mihai, G.: Recommendation system based on association rules for distributed E-Learning management systems. ACTA Univ. Cibiniensis 67(1) (2015)
8. Jooa, J., Bangb, S., Parka, G.: Implementation of a recommendation system using association rules and collaborative filtering. Procedia Comput. Sci. 91, 944–952 (2016)
9. Hrženjak, M.P., Matetić, M., Bakarić: Mining Association Rules in Learning Management Systems (2015)
10. Aher, S.B., Lobo, L.M.R.J.: Combination of machine learning algorithms for recommendation of courses in E-Learning System based on historical data. Knowl. Based Syst. 51, 1–14 (2013)
11. Larose, D.T., Larose, C.D.: Data Mining and Predictive Analytics, 2nd edition. Wiley, Hoboken (2015)
12. Agrawal, R., Imielinski, T., Swami, A.: Mining Association Rules between Sets of Items in Large Databases (1993)
13. Kumbhare, T.A., Chobe, S.V.: An overview of association rule mining algorithms. Int. J. Comput. Sci. Inf. Technol. 5(1), 927–930 (2014)
14. Agrawal, R., Srikant, R.: Fast Algorithms for Mining Association Rules (1994)
15. Agrawal, R., Srikant, R.: Fast Algorithms for Mining Association Rules in Datamining. In: Proceedings of the 20th VLDB Conference Santiago Chile, vol. 2, p. 13–24 (1994)
16. Mittal, M., Singh, J., Aggarwal, A., Kumari, K., Yadav, M.: Ordering policy for imperfect quality itemsets using cross selling effects. Int. J. Model. Optim. 4(1), 25–30 (2014)
17. Ibriz, A.: Une Démarche Innovante de Conduite de Projet Elearning: C.D.I.O . 2ème Congrès International du Génie Industriel et du Management des Systèmes (CIGIMS) (2015)
18. Ibriz, A., Safouane, A.: L'Innovation Pédagogique dans les EST du Maroc : Le Model et la Conduite d'un cas réussi à travers le Projet ESTenLigne (2014)
19. Oughdir, L., Ibriz, A., Harti, M.: Modélisation de l'apprenant dans le cadre d'un environnement d'apprentissage en ligne. TELECO2011 & 7ème JFMMA Mars 16–18, 2011 – Tanger MAROC (2011)

20. Benslimane, M., Ouazzani, K., Tmimi, M., Berrada, M.: Proposal of an Approach of Online Course Design and Implementation: A Case Study of an Algorithmic Course, vol. 7, p. 7 (2016)
21. Ibriz, A., Benslimane, M., Ouazzani, K.: Didactics in Online Learning Technical Courses: A Case Study Based on Activity Theory, vol. 7, p. 6 (2016)
22. Moodle - Open-source learning platform | Moodle.org. [En ligne]. Disponible sur: https://moodle.org/. [Consulté le: 03-avr-2018]
23. Garg, A.: SCORM Based Learning Management System For Online Training. Kansas State University, Manhattan, Kansas (2012)
24. Hahsler, M.: Rules-Mining Association Rules and Frequent Itemsets with R. Engineering Management, Information, and Systems Lyle School of Engineering Southern Methodist University, Apr 2018

Optimal Placement of Wind and Solar Generation Units in Medium and Low Voltage Distribution Systems

Saad Ouali[✉] and Abdeljabbar Cherkaoui

Laboratory of Innovative Technologies (LTI), National School of Applied Sciences, Abdelmalek Esaadi University, Tangier, Morocco
{saad.oualil,cherkaoui.lti}@gmail.com

Abstract. In Medium and Low voltage electrical distribution systems, the introduction of distributed generation, from renewable energy sources, such as Solar and Wind units, had negatively influences their voltage plan, and increment the losses level. The active and reactive power produced and consumed by those distributed generations had change the ordinary operation of the classical radial distribution networks. In this paper an analysis approach for choosing the optimal placement of wind and solar generation units is proposed to identify the parts of the network with the important capacity to receive distributed generation without producing significant impact on the voltage plan, and the part of the network where connecting even DG with small capacity may lead to major impact on the network voltage and may cause the destruction of the voltage plan, with several voltage drops and rises. The main aim of this paper is to understand how the connection of a DG in any part of the network can influence the voltage magnitude in each network point, and choosing the less influence part of the network as optimal placement for future DG units. A case study is presented, in the IEEE 33-bus system, the results obtained had allowed to divide the network point in three categories, and identifying the optimal placements to connect a wind or a solar generation unit.

Keywords: Wind and solar generation units · Radial distribution system · Power flow summation · Distributed generation · Voltage control · Renewable energy

1   Introduction

By connecting distributed generation to the existing medium voltage distribution networks, many technical, economic and environmental benefits could be provided for customers and utilities. In several studies [1, 2], the main obstacles for interconnecting a large amounts of distributed generation units, is reported as steady state voltage rise and drops.

Unlike transmission systems, the conductors used in sub-transmission are characterized by high R/X ratio. Studies have estimated that 13% of total electricity generation is wasted at the distribution level. The R/X high ratio leads also to poor

© Springer Nature Switzerland AG 2019
M. Ezziyyani (Ed.): AI2SD 2018, AISC 915, pp. 492–503, 2019.
https://doi.org/10.1007/978-3-030-11928-7_44

convergence characteristics of the classical methods used for network analysis, such as: Newton-Raphson, Gauss-Seidel, and Fast-Decoupled methods.

With no generation units connected to the distribution system, voltage profile decreases along the feeder, depending on the impedance of lines, as a consequence, the biggest voltage drop happen at the end of the feeder.

Medium and low voltage distribution systems are designed and calibrated for a passif use, with unidirectional power flow from the MV/LV substation for the low voltage systems, or from the HV/MV substation in medium voltage systems to the end of the line. The penetration of distributed generators in distribution systems will challenge the correct functioning of those systems. Unfortunately, the classical models designed for high voltage network analysis, such as Newton-Raphson, Gauss-Seidel or Fast-Decoupled power flow are not adequate to distribution network.

References [2, 3] report a comparative study of the most used algorithms, the power summation methods seems to be the best choice, thanks to its robustness and convergence properties.

A voltage control strategy is a challenging task due to the non-linear relationship between the active/reactive power and voltage magnitude. The implantation of such control will avoid disconnection of distributed production units and will increase the active power production [4].

In literature, we can identify four approaches used to control voltage plan of distribution systems with the presence of distributed generation: Control of active power generated by DGs, the control of reactive power produced or consumed by DGs, Capacity banks or FACTs, the use of the on-line tap changing installed on the HV/MV transformer, and the network reinforcement.

The scientific contribution of this paper is state in the frame of voltage profile improvement by the help of the control of the active power produced by the new DG, The proposed control is made by adjusting and choosing a best placement that minimize the impacts of DGs on the voltage system.

In this paper, an analysis method, to minimize the impact of active and reactive on the voltage plan of radial systems, is presented. The results obtained from the proposed method are useful for voltage control and loss reduction.

The main aim of this paper is to conceive a tool able to quantify the impact of adding or eliminating a distributed generation unit, or changing the topology configuration of the network. This tool can be used directly as a decision support tool for utilities in cases of having several possibilities for choosing the connection of a new distributed generation.

In what follows, we present the relationship between voltage magnitude, feeder characteristics and active/reactive power, and to mitigate the impact of distributed generation on network voltage in Sect. 2. Next in Sect. 3 we provide the theoretical foundation of the proposed mathematic analysis method of the impact of variation in active and reactive power on the voltage plan of radial distribution networks, in Sect. 4 we present a case study of the proposed method with the real medium voltage distribution system, in Sect. 5 we discuss the results obtained from the case study.

2 Steady State Voltage Plan and Distributed Generation

Considering the electrical network shown in Fig. 1.

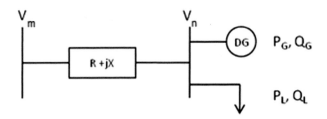

Fig. 1. Electrical system with DG

The power between the node "m" and "n" is:

$$S_m = P_m + jQ_m = (P_m + jQ_m) - (P_m + jQ_m) \tag{1}$$

It can also be expressed as:

$$S_m = V_m \cdot I_{mn}^* \tag{2}$$

The current Imn between the nodes "m" and "n":

$$I_{mn} = \frac{P_m - j \cdot Q_m}{V_m^*} \tag{3}$$

The relationship between the voltage of node "m" can be obtained from Eqs. (1) to (3):

$$V_m = V_n + Z \cdot I_{mn} = V_n + (R + jX)(P_m - jQ_m)/V_m^* \tag{4}$$

$$V_m = V_n + (P_m \cdot R + Q_m \cdot X)/V_m^* + j(P_m \cdot X - Q_m \cdot R)/V_m^* \tag{5}$$

Considering the diagram phasor in Fig. 2:

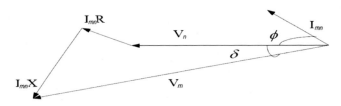

Fig. 2. Phasor diagram

$$V_m \cdot \sin \delta = (P_m \cdot X - Q_n \cdot R)/V_n \tag{6}$$

Since the voltage angle δ is very small, the term $(P_m \cdot X - Q_n \cdot R)/V_n$ can be neglected, and the Eq. (5) become:

$$V_m = V_n + (P_m \cdot R + Q_m \cdot X)/V_m^* \tag{7}$$

And the voltage difference between the nodes "m" and "n" can be expressed as:

$$\Delta V = (P_m \cdot R + Q_m \cdot X)/V_m^* \tag{9}$$

With the presence of a distributed generation unit in the node "m":

$$P_m = P_L - P_n \text{ and } Q_m = Q_L \pm Q_n \tag{10}$$

So, the voltage difference between the nodes "m" and "n", with the presence of a distributed generation unit in the node "m":

$$\Delta V = [((P_L - P_n) \cdot R + (Q_L \pm Q_n) \cdot X)]/V_m^* \tag{11}$$

The active power produced by distributed generation unit increase the voltage, whereas the reactive power can further increase or reduce it depending on the type of DG.

These outcomes, in combination with the distribution network characteristics (R/X) and load profile, determine whether the voltage plan.

3 Proposed Mathematic Analysis for Optimal Placement of Distributed Generation

Changes in voltage are related to changes in active power (P) and reactive power (Q) by the partial differential equation:

$$\begin{bmatrix} \Delta V \\ \Delta \delta \end{bmatrix} = \begin{bmatrix} \frac{\partial V}{\partial P} & \frac{\partial V}{\partial Q} \\ \frac{\partial \delta}{\partial Q} & \frac{\partial \delta}{\partial Q} \end{bmatrix} \times \begin{bmatrix} \Delta P \\ \Delta Q \end{bmatrix} \tag{12}$$

Let's consider [S] a column vectors of complex power of power nodes, the dimension of [S] is (m $\times$ 1):

$$[S] = [V] * [I^*] = [P] + j[Q] \tag{13}$$

where [P] and [Q] are the column vectors, dimension (m $\times$ 1), whose elements are, respectively, the node active and reactive powers.

The complex conjugate of [S] is given by:

$$[S] = [V] * [I] = [P] - j[Q] \tag{14}$$

The column vector of current at each node:

$$[I] = \frac{[P] - j[Q]}{[V^*]} \tag{15}$$

The current at each node is often called the current injections, and the current between two node is called the branch current, the relationship between the bus current injections and branch current can be obtained by applying Kirchhoff's current law. The branch currents can then be formulated as functions of equivalent current injections.

Let's consider a 7 nodes radial system, as example to illustrate the proposed method, as shown in Fig. 3.

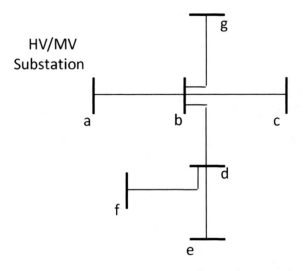

Fig. 3. Single line diagram of a radial distribution network

By applying Kirchhoff's current law, the branch currents ka, kb, kc, kd, ke, kf and kg can be expressed by equivalent current injections as:

$$k_a = I_b + I_c + I_d + I_e + I_f + I_g \tag{16.1}$$

$$k_b = I_c \tag{16.2}$$

$$k_c = I_e + I_f \tag{16.3}$$

$$k_d = I_e \tag{16.4}$$

$$k_e = I_f \tag{16.5}$$

$$k_e = I_f \tag{16.6}$$

$$k_f = I_g \tag{16.7}$$

The relationship between the current of each node or the bus current injections and branch currents can be obtained from Eq. (16):

$$
\begin{bmatrix} k_a \\ k_b \\ k_c \\ k_d \\ k_e \\ k_f \end{bmatrix} =
\begin{bmatrix}
1 & 1 & 1 & 1 & 1 & 1 \\
0 & 1 & 0 & 0 & 0 & 0 \\
0 & 0 & 1 & 1 & 1 & 0 \\
0 & 0 & 0 & 1 & 0 & 0 \\
0 & 0 & 0 & 0 & 1 & 0 \\
0 & 0 & 0 & 0 & 0 & 1
\end{bmatrix}
\begin{bmatrix} I_b \\ I_c \\ I_d \\ I_e \\ I_f \\ I_g \end{bmatrix}
\tag{17}
$$

The relationship between branch currents and bus voltages can be obtained as follows:

$$V_b = V_a - J_a Z_{ab} \tag{18.1}$$

$$V_c = V_b - J_b Z_{bc} \tag{18.2}$$

$$V_d = V_b - J_c Z_{bd} \tag{18.3}$$

$$V_e = V_d - J_d Z_{de} \tag{18.4}$$

$$V_f = V_d - J_e Z_{df} \tag{18.5}$$

$$V_g = V_b - J_f Z_{bg} \tag{18.6}$$

Substituting (18.1) and into (18.6), the Eq. (18.6) can be written as:

$$V_g = V_a - J_a Z_{ab} - J_b Z_{bc} - J_f Z_{bf} \tag{19}$$

Let's apply the same substituting to the other nodes; therefore the relationship between branch currents and bus voltages can be expressed as:

$$
\begin{bmatrix} V_a \\ V_a \\ V_a \\ V_a \\ V_a \\ V_a \end{bmatrix} -
\begin{bmatrix} V_b \\ V_c \\ V_d \\ V_e \\ V_f \\ V_g \end{bmatrix} =
\begin{bmatrix}
Z_{ab} & 0 & 0 & 0 & 0 & 0 \\
Z_{ab} & Z_{bc} & 0 & 0 & 0 & 0 \\
Z_{ab} & 0 & Z_{cd} & 0 & 0 & 0 \\
Z_{ab} & 0 & Z_{cd} & Z_{de} & 0 & 0 \\
Z_{ab} & 0 & Z_{cd} & 0 & Z_{ef} & 0 \\
Z_{ab} & 0 & 0 & 0 & 0 & Z_{fg}
\end{bmatrix}
\begin{bmatrix} J_a \\ J_b \\ J_c \\ J_d \\ J_e \\ J_f \end{bmatrix}
\tag{20}
$$

the relationship between bus current injections and bus voltages can be expressed as:

$$[\Delta V] = [DLF][I] \tag{21}$$

where DLF is a multiplication matrix of BCBV and BIBC matrices

Let's consider two matrices [R] and [X] as:

$$[R] = real([Z]) \quad and \quad [X] = im([Z]) \tag{22}$$

The elements (xy) of the matrix [R] are the sum of the impedance of the branches in which both Px + 1 and Py + 1 flow. For instance, in order to obtain the element (3, 2) of [R].

$$[V] = [V_{substation}] - ([R] + j[X]) * \left(\frac{[P] - j[Q]}{[V^*]} \right) \tag{23}$$

Equation (23) can be simplified considering the hypotheses below (commonly accepted in distribution networks analysis) [5]:

The phase difference between node voltages is negligible and, as a consequence, if phasor V1 is chosen on the real axis, only the real part of voltage [V] = real[V] is considered.

Constant current models are considered for loads (node powers are referred to system nominal voltage instead of actual node voltage).

Equations (23) can be written as:

$$[V] = [V_{Substation}] - ([R] + j[X]) * \left(\frac{[P] - j[Q]}{V_{nom}} \right) \tag{24}$$

For a node x:

$$V_i = V_0 - \frac{1}{V_{nom}} \left(\sum R_{ij}P_j + \sum X_{ij}Q_j \right) \tag{25}$$

From Eq. (25), the voltage of node x depend on the active and reactive power injections or consumed of all node networks.

As the substation node is the slack bus, its voltage is always constant.

$$\begin{cases} \frac{\partial V_x}{\partial P_y} = -\frac{1}{V_{nom}} R_{xy} \\ \frac{\partial V_x}{\partial Q_y} = -\frac{1}{V_{nom}} X_{xy} \end{cases} \tag{26}$$

The total differential of function Vx is:

$$dV_x = \sum \frac{\partial V_x}{\partial P_y} dP_y + \sum \frac{\partial V_x}{\partial Q_y} dQ_y \tag{27}$$

Considering all network nodes:

$$
\begin{bmatrix} dV_a \\ \cdots \\ dV_m \end{bmatrix} = \begin{bmatrix} \frac{\partial V_a}{\partial P_a} & \cdots & \frac{\partial V_n}{\partial P_a} & \frac{\partial V_a}{\partial Q_a} & \cdots & \frac{\partial V_m}{\partial Q_a} \\ \cdots & \cdots & \cdots & \cdots & \cdots & \cdots \\ \frac{\partial V_a}{\partial P_m} & \cdots & \frac{\partial V_m}{\partial P_m} & \frac{\partial V_a}{\partial Q_m} & \cdots & \frac{\partial V_m}{\partial Q_m} \end{bmatrix} \times \begin{bmatrix} dP_a \\ \cdots \\ dP_m \\ dQ_a \\ \cdots \\ dQ_m \end{bmatrix} \quad (28)
$$

In the next section a case study is proposed, in which is possible to evaluate and mitigate the impact of each possible placement for a new distributed generation. An optimal placement is chosen in a way to have the less sensitivity influence value on the system performance.

4 Case Study

As provided in Sect. 3, the voltage of a node "x", depends on the powers injected or absorbed at the other network nodes:

$$
V_x = V_x(P_a, P_b, \ldots, P_m, Q_a, Q_b, \ldots, Q_m) \quad (29)
$$

The proposed mathematic method is tested in this section with a medium voltage network of 33 bus, as shown in Fig. 4, the topology characteristics of the network is presented in Table 1 [6].

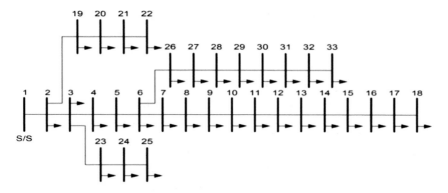

Fig. 4. Single phase diagram of IEEE 33-bus distribution system

From a Line Data, that indicates the resistance and reactance of each branches, and the topological structure of the network, The BIBC and BCBV matrices are developed and the DLF matrix is calculated as the multiplication of the matrices BIBC and BCBV.

The value of the maximum sensitivity for each busbar are computed and presented at Table 1,

Those most critical busbars are recorded at nodes: 1, 2 3 4 5 19; 19; 20; 22 and 23 which represent the ends of the network branches and the most distance nodes from the substation. Further, it can be easily highlighted that the greater the node distances from the origin, the higher the voltage sensitivity.

Table 1. IEEE 33-bus network characteristics and sensitivity values

Branch number	Sending bus	Receiving bus	R	X	Sp	Sq
1	1	2	0.0922	0.047	−0.0922	−0.047
2	2	3	0.493	0.2511	−0.5852	−0.2981
3	3	4	0.366	0.1844	−0.9512	−0.4825
4	4	5	0.3811	0.1941	−1.3323	−0.6766
5	5	6	0.819	0.707	−2.1513	−1.3836
6	6	7	0.1872	0.6188	−2.3385	−2.0024
7	7	8	0.7114	0.2351	−3.0499	−2.2375
8	8	9	1.03	0.74	−4.0799	−2.9775
9	9	10	1.044	0.74	−5.1239	−3.7175
10	10	11	0.1966	0.065	−5.3205	−3.7825
11	11	12	0.3744	0.1238	−5.6949	−3.9063
12	12	13	1.468	1.155	−7.1629	−5.0613
13	13	14	0.5416	0.7129	−7.7045	−5.7742
14	14	15	0.591	0.526	−8.2955	−6.3002
15	15	16	0.7463	0.545	−9.0418	−6.8452
16	16	17	1.289	1.721	−10.3308	−8.5662
17	17	18	0.732	0.574	−11.0628	−9.1402
18	2	19	0.164	0.1565	−0.2562	−0.2035
19	19	20	1.5402	1.3554	−1.7964	−1.5589
20	20	21	0.4095	0.4784	−2.2059	−2.0373
21	21	22	0.7089	0.9373	−2.9148	−2.9746
22	3	23	0.4512	0.3083	−1.0364	−0.6064
23	23	24	0.898	0.7091	−1.9344	−1.3155
24	24	25	0.896	0.7011	−2.8304	−2.0166
25	6	26	0.203	0.1034	−2.3543	−1.487
26	26	27	0.2842	0.1447	−2.6385	−1.6317
27	27	28	1.059	0.9337	−3.6975	−2.5654
28	28	29	0.8042	0.7006	−4.5017	−3.266
29	29	30	0.5075	0.2585	−5.0092	−3.5245
30	30	31	0.9744	0.963	−5.9836	−4.4875
31	31	32	0.3105	0.3619	−6.2941	−4.8494
32	32	33	0.341	0.5302	−6.6351	−5.3796

Figure 7, gives a representation of the parts of the network most influenced by the variation of active power of the three level of network busbar are presented. In green the best placement of connecting a new DG, in Black the second level to connect a DG, and the parts of the networks in red are to avoid.

We can also observe that each generation influence the most at its nearest nodes, and the influence of different DGs active power variation is the same at the nodes located in the same trajectory from the connection point of the DG to the substation (Figs. 5 and 6).

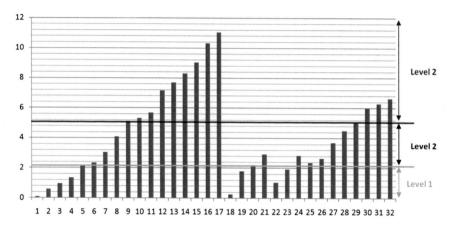

Fig. 5. Sensitivity of the variation of active generation power and the three levels of DG placement

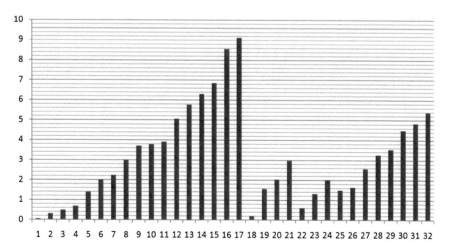

Fig. 6. Sensitivity of the variation of reactive generation power

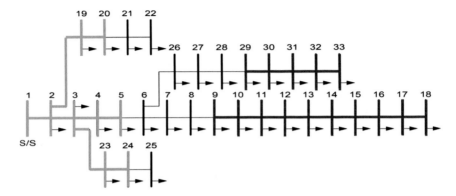

Fig. 7. The three level of the IEEE 33-bus network placement

In Fig. 7, a graphical representation is given, to compare the influence of the connecting point, we can distinguish clearly the three levels in green, black and red.

Figure 7, gives an immediate perception of DG locations and how changing the connection point may reduce their impact on voltage plan of the network, such graphical representation is useful to get the most optimal parts to connect a distributed generation and must critical parts of the network where a the same distributed generation may destroy the voltage plan of the network, if it is connect it in the red parts of the network shown in Fig. 7.

5   Conclusions

A analytical method to choose the best location for DG units that has the less impacts on the voltage plan of radial distribution networks. This method is based on the voltage sensitivity analysis to the with respect to the conductor network characteristics, The proposed method is developed based on the exploitation of the radial structure of medium voltage distribution system, and the backward/forward sweep concept, and the power summation approach

As shown in this paper, the selection of the connection point of distributed generation is critical, and may increase or decrease the impacts on the voltage plan, with the same DG size, an optimal placement may allow the integration of the DG with no significant impacts on the voltage plan, however, not paying attention to the choice of the connection may bring major impacts on the system voltage.

The limitation of the proposed approach is that it is only applicable for radial distribution systems, with a static-constantly topology, the proposed approach is not effective for meshed or weakly meshed networks with variable topologies.

References

1. Shivarudraswamy, R., Gaonkar, D.N.: Coordinated voltage control using multiple regulators in distribution system with distributed generators. In: World Academy of Science, Engineering and Technology, International Journal of Electrical, Computer, Energetic, Electronic and Communication Engineering, vol. 5, no.2 (2011)
2. Ouali, S., Cherkaoui, A.: Load flow analysis for moroccan medium voltage distribution system. In: Conférence Internationale en Automatique & Traitement de Signal (ATS-2018), Proceedings of Engineering and Technology – PET, vol. 36, pp. 10–16
3. Mokhtari, G., Ghosh, A., Nourbakhsh, G., Ledwich, G.: Smart robust resources control in LV network to deal with voltage rise issue. IEEE Trans. Sustain. Energy 4(4), 1043–1050 (2013)
4. Conti, S., Raiti, S., Vagliasindi, G.: Voltage sensitivity analysis in radial MV distribution networks using constant current model. In: IEEE International Symposium Industrial Electronics (ISIE), Nov 2010
5. Conti, S., Greco, A.M., Raiti, S.: Voltage sensitivity analysis in MV distribution networks. In: The 6th WSEAS/IASME International Conference on Electric Power Systems, High Voltages, Electric Machines, Tenerife, Spain, 16–18 Dec 2006
6. Stagg, G.W.: El-Abiad, A.H.: Computer Methods in Power System Analysis, McGraw Hill (1968)

Three-Dimensional Micro-Computed Tomographic Study of Porous Bioceramics Using an Adaptive Method Based on Mathematical Morphological Operation

M. Ezzahmouly[1(⊠)], A. ELmoutaouakkil[1], M. Ed-dhahraouy[1],
H. Khallok[2], E. Gourri[2], K. Karim[3], and Z. Hatim[2]

[1] LAROSERI, Computer Science Department, Chouaïb Doukkali University,
El-jadida, Morocco
ezzahmoulymnl@gmail.com
[2] Electrochemical and Biomaterials Team, Chemistry Department,
Chouaïb Doukkali University, El-jadida, Morocco
[3] LIIAN, Department of Computer Science, Sidi Mohamed Ben Abdellah
University, Fez, Morocco

Abstract. Porous Calcium-hydroxyapatite $(Ca_{10}(PO_4)_6(OH)_2)$ ceramics are used for bone repair. Numerous clinical studies have demonstrated the influence of size, number and pore shape of calcium-phosphate ceramics on the bone re-colonisation process. The objective of this study is to determine the microstructure, the morphological characteristics and classes of pores of the prepared hydroxyapatite (HAP) bioceramics using an adaptive method based on mathematical morphological operation. The study was carried out using X-ray micro tomography (μCT) images. The traditional method of openings alone presents limitation of calculation and not sufficient to achieve our objective. The proposed method allowed us to extract local characteristics and calculate precisely the morphological parameters while preserving the original volume of pores. The number and classes of pores with their size were calculated. The efficiency of the method is clearly demonstrated through the different reports and measurements generated. The proposed method can have interesting applications in the characterization of porous materials used in the medical field or in other sectors.

Keywords: Biomaterials · Microstructural analysis · Image processing · Morphological operations

1 Introduction

At present, calcium-hydroxyapatite $((Ca_{10}(PO_4)_6(OH)_2$: HAP), ceramics are very attractive biomaterials as bone substitute due to their excellent biocompatibility, bioactivity and osteoconduction properties [1–3].

Depending on the desired application, these biomaterials exist in several porous forms as granules or blocks [4, 5]. Volume porosity and pore size affect the ability of the scaffold to promote vascularization, cells proliferation and in vivo osteoconduction.

M. Ezziyyani (Ed.): AI2SD 2018, AISC 915, pp. 504–513, 2019.
https://doi.org/10.1007/978-3-030-11928-7_45

It has been established that pore sizes of at least 40 μm are required for bone ingrowth, whereas interconnected pores larger than 100 μm in diameter are required to promote the integration of the implant. Characterization of the porous architecture of scaffolds is essential in predicting their performance in vivo [6]. Several processing methods have recently been used for porosity study. However, many of them can't be used to quantify the closed porosity, inaccessible by external agents (mercury, nitrogen, argon...).

To exploit and evaluate the porous microstructure from μCT images, several image-processing methods should be exploited and adapted efficiently depending on the desired information. Image processing is then a crucial step in the quantification of porous structures.

Imaging technique usually uses mathematical morphology, which enables selective enhancement of target pores. Mathematical morphology applies shape information to image processing [7]. It operates by series of morphological operations, which use small structuring elements (typically, a single structuring element is used). The structuring element acts as a moving probe that samples each pixel of the image [8]. Since the structuring element moves across the image, some intricate images may not be properly processed. Consequently, an artifact in the shape of structuring elements may be generated at the object periphery or squarely the periphery shape changes. Another issue is the separation of connected pores while preserving the irregular shape of the initial pore. The use of the traditional method leads to loose small connected pores, which causes the deformation of the original shape of the pore. Therefore a bad quantitate porosity study is generated. Those drawbacks are especially serious problems, since pores in biomaterial samples consist of delicate structural features.

To overcome those problems, an adaptive method based on the mathematical morphological algorithm is proposed in order to efficiently segment and characterize the porosity structure.

Porous calcium-hydroxyapatite ceramics prepared from cement paste was used and the microstructure of ceramics was examined by μCT.

The proposed method is used for local features extraction and calculation of morphological parameters while preserving the original volume of pores. The method is subjectively and quantitatively evaluated using different computed phantoms and its efficiency is demonstrated through the different reports and measurements generated.

2 Materials and Methods

2.1 Porous Calcium-Hydroxyapatite Ceramics

Porous calcium-Hydroxyapatite ceramics Hydroxyapatite Ceramic ($Ca_{10}(PO_4)_6(OH)_2$: HAP) was prepared from cement paste according to the method described by Lacout et al. [9] with some modifications. All of the used reagents are of analytical grade.

The cement was prepared by mixing tetracalcium calcium powder ($Ca_4(PO_4)_2O$) with aqueous solution of phosphoric acid (H_3PO_4), calcium chloride ($CaCl_2$, $2H_2O$) and lactic acid ($C_3H_6O_3$). The molar ratio Ca/P of mixture was 1.667 (molar ratio of the stoichiometric hydroxyapatite) and the liquid (L) to solid (S) ratio (L/S) according to 0.55 ml g^{-1}. The mixture was done manually in a mortar with a pestle for 2 min.

In order to produce the pores in the prepared block, hydrogen peroxide (H_2O_2, 30% (w/w)) was mixed with the fresh material paste allowing the pores interconnection formed by the gases when escaping.

Cement pellets were prepared by filling cylindrical silicone mold with the prepared paste. The parts were then placed in water at 80 °C for 24 h. After drying, pellets are demolded and calcined at 1200 °C for 3 h. Photography of Fig. 1 shows the microstructure of prepared porous ceramic.

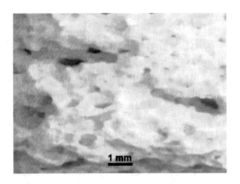

Fig. 1. Photography of porous calcium-hydroxyapatite ceramic

2.2 Image Techniques—X-Ray Microtomography

Microtomography uses X-rays to create cross-sections of a physical object that can be used to reconstitute a virtual model without destroying the original object [10].

The Beer-Lambert law is the linear relationship between absorbance and concentration of an absorbing species. Figure 2 illustrates the principle of tomography.

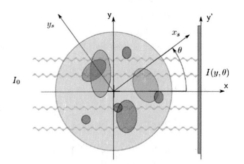

Fig. 2. Illustrated principle of tomography

The exponential attenuation law of Lambert-Beer is represented by Eq. (1)

$$I = I_0 exp(-\mu x) \tag{1}$$

I-intensity of light. μ-the linear attenuation coefficient [11].

Image reconstruction is the phase in which the scan data set is processed to produce an image:

- The scan data phase produces a data set, named sinogram.
- Filtered back projection is the reconstruction method used in μCT.
- The image reconstruction phase produces an image from the scan data set by the process of filtered back projection [12].

The calcium-hydroxyapatite ceramic was submitted to a computed microtomograph (μCT) using a high-resolution device (EasyTom XL duo (2 sources)). The pixel size was determined at 10.38 μm under the following conditions: 90 kV, 111 mA. About 1331 cuts were generated. The reconstructed images were processed with XAct (RX solution) software.

2.3   Image Processing Method

Description of the Method

The objective of our work is to carry out a qualitative and quantitative evaluation of the porous microstructure of HAP ceramic using μCT images.

An accurate method is proposed to characterize pores and separate them at the same time. The method makes it possible to easily calculate many quantitative measurements, in particular those that provide information on the connection and the size distribution of the pores.

To realize those tasks, an adaptive method based on the morphological operation algorithm is proposed. The traditional method of openings alone is not sufficient to achieve our objective. It presents incorrect separations of the pores, imprecise volumes of each pore and therefore a limitation of calculations.

The proposed method lets us to calculate precisely a specific porosity and define classes of pores.

We proceed first by the preprocessing step applied on μCT images. Figure 3 shows a μCT slice image of prepared ceramic.

Using the classical thresholding, it is useful to be able to separate out the regions of the image corresponding to pores in which we are interested, from the regions of the image that correspond to the rest of sample and the background. However, it does not allow separating pores between them depending on their size.

Generally, Erosion and dilation are used to characterize morphological features and particle distributions.

Erosion reduces the size of the pores by eroding its outline and dilation by dilating its outline, with a predefined structure element. Erosion followed by dilation is called opening.

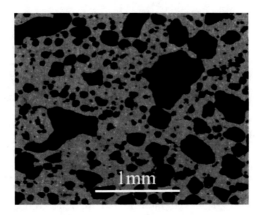

Fig. 3. Tomographic slice image of HAP bioceramic

– Erosion of an image I by the structure element H is given by the set operation

$$I \ominus H = \{p \in Z2|(p+q) \in I, \text{for every } q \in H\} \quad (2)$$

– Dilation of an image I by the structure element H is given by the set operation

$$I \oplus H = \{(p+q)|p \in I, q \in H\} \quad (3)$$

Holes in the foreground that are smaller than H will be filled [13].

Erosion and dilation are mathematical morphology tools that process images based usually on shapes and most commonly change them. Those operations affect directly the efficiency of pores measurements especially those with irregular shape.

For an efficient porosity study, it is useful to separate the pores from one another and label them. This allows us to calculate many parameters mainly the volume, the apparent perimeter and the surface contact.

Moreover, the traditional method based on openings alone is inappropriate for an efficient quantitative analysis. This approach does not take into account convexity hypotheses on the forms encountered and does not divide them to achieve a distribution of the separated pores.

To surpass those limits, a method based on the use of morphological operations is proposed. Successive openings operations are computed with structuring element increasing in diameter to make the particles disappear progressively. The difference between the images before and after an opening, corresponds to the total volume of the particles disappeared.

After obtaining the subtracted image containing the elements of the size corresponding to the structuring element, the volume and the contact area of the isolated elements are calculated with the original element. This calculation is done via a voxel path in the subtracted image. Neighboring voxels of components are compared; a voxel having different gray level value neighbors in the original image; it is indeed a contact surface.

A component may be connected with more than one other component. The method allows us to calculate for each component, the number of contacts (Nsc) with other interfaces.

After those operations, the small elements and the corners belonging to the pore, which are found in the reference image, disappear.

The old method considers them as distinct components, but the originality of our method is that it does not take them into account on the basis of a geometric criterion. The contact surface, the number of contact surfaces with the other elements, and the total and specific pore volume will be calculated.

Since the structuring element of the traditional method moves across the image, some intricate images may not be properly processed. Consequently, an artifact in the shape of structural elements may be generated at the object periphery or squarely the periphery shape changes that leads also directly to a bad quantitative study. To overcome this, the analyses are carried out on the contact surface; if it is larger than the surface area of the subtracted element, the element is left with its original structure otherwise, it is not taken into account in the calculation of the porosity. We then solve the problem of small connected structures considered as a single pore which disappears after the opening. Figure 4 illustrates the flowchart of the proposed method to calculate porosity parameters.

2.4 Error Estimation

To evaluate the accuracy of our method, the absolute error value of the conventional opening method and the proposed one was calculated and then the Mean Absolute Error (MAE) value was determined [14].

Absolute error (*e*) is the difference between the measured value and the actual value. It is one way to consider error when measuring the accuracy of values.

$$e = x_o - x \tag{4}$$

where e—the absolute error (the difference, or change, in the measured and actual value), x_o—the measured value, and x—the actual value.

Mean absolute error (**MAE**) is a measure of difference between two variables. It is expressed as

$$MAE = \sum_{i=1}^{n} |e_i|/n \tag{5}$$

where n—number of variables.

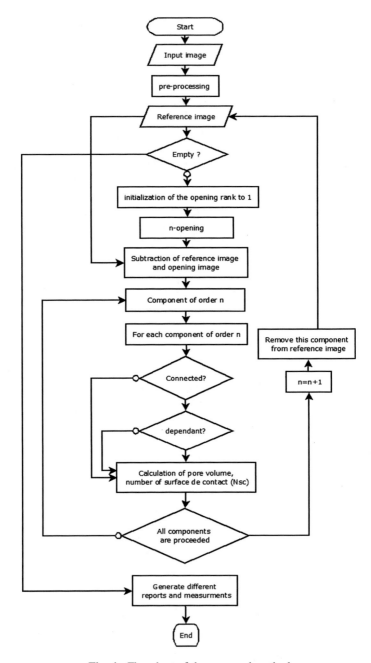

Fig. 4. Flowchart of the proposed method

3 Results and Discussion

3.1 Application of the Proposed Method on the Tomographic Images

After applying the filtering processing, the proposed method is applied on the X-ray μCT images.

With all the described tools in materials and methods section applied on our μCT images sample, the distribution of pores with their size volume is obtained (Table 1).

Table 1. Number and size distribution of pores

Pore size (μm)	$r \leq 50$	$50 \leq r \leq 100$	$100 \leq r$
Number of pores (Nb)	8350	1460	752
Number of pores (%)	79	13	7
Porosity (%)	$\Phi = 83$		

The porosity achieved is about (Φ) (%) 83% which is almost in line with the overall porosity of the sample, estimated from the apparent density data, (Φ) (%) 80%.

The results reveal that bioceramics have a high volume of porosity (83%) with a high interconnectivity.

The radius variation obtained by the proposed method shows a random distribution of pores inside and on the surface of the ceramic and a wide size variation of pores.

3.2 Comparison Between Conventional and the Proposed Method on the Tomographic Images

To know how reliable our method is, the error calculation method was chosen using Eqs. 4 and 5. The results are summarized in Table 2. The manual method was chosen as a reference method for the error calculation.

Table 2. MAE value of the conventional and the proposed method for the number of components

	Conventional method	Proposed method
Mean Absolute Error (MAE)	172	18

For a low MAE value, the reliability of the method increases. Compared to the high error value of the traditional method, the error value of the proposed one does not really affect the general statistics. The difference observed in the proposed method is due to the preprocessing step. The result shows that our method gives close outcomes to the real structure.

The proposed method makes it possible to determine the micro and macro porosity and to define with precision the percentage of each class of pores and it helps as well to determine the range of pores sought in such materials.

4   Conclusion

This study concerns the microstructural characterization of porous calcium phosphate bioceramics using an adaptive method based on the mathematical morphological algorithm.

The proposed method is used for the separation of the holes, classification and calculation of pore volumes by performing series of openings. This method specifically takes into account, during the computation, the original shape of the structures contrary to the traditional one. Hence, the error calculation caused by the changes of the shape at the component periphery, the problem of the separation of connected pores and the preservation of the irregular shape of the initial pore have been overcame.

The effectiveness and usefulness of the method were demonstrated by its application to µCT images. The good performance of the proposed method was demonstrated by comparing the structure distribution on images with the conventional one. This method allows us to have accurate quantitative information of the porous microstructure of ceramic demonstrated through the low error value compared to the conventional one. The results of this work show that the proposed method can have interesting applications in the characterization of porous materials used in the medical field or in other sectors such as molten metal filtration, catalysis, refractory insulation, and hot gas filtration.

Acknowledgements. The authors thank Pr R. Brahmi, Pr A. ElAlbani and M. A. Mazurier of University of Poitiers for assistance with µCT technique and providing µCT images. We gratefully acknowledge support from the CNRST Morocco (National Center of Scientific and Technique Research).

References

1. LeGeros, R.Z.: Properties of osteoconductive biomaterials: calcium phosphates. Clin. Orthop. **395**, 81–98 (2002)
2. Bohner, M.: Resorbable biomaterials as bone graft substitutes panel. Materialstoday **13**, 24–30 (2010)
3. Yan, X., Yu, C., Zhou, X., Tang, J., Zhao, D.: Highly ordered mesoporous bioactive glasses with superior in vitro bone-forming bioactivities. Angew. Chem. Int. Ed. Engl. **43**, 5980–5984 (2004)
4. Erlind, P., Lait Kostantinos, B., Gaspare, P., Gianluca, T., Guido, M.: Nano-hydroxyapatite and its applications in preventive, restorative and regenerative dentistry: a review of literature. Ann. Stomatol. **5**(3), 108–114 (2014)
5. Mueller, B.: Antibacterial active open-porous hydroxyapatite/lysozyme scaffolds suitable as bone graft and depot for localized drug delivery. J. Biomater. Appl. **31**, 1123–1134 (2017)
6. Gauthier, O., Bouler, J.M., Aguado, E., Pilet, P., Daculsi, G.: Macroporous biphasic calcium phosphate ceramics: influence of macropore diameter and macroporosity percentage on bone ingrowth. Biomaterials **19**, 133–139 (1998)
7. Serra, J.: Image Analysis and Mathematical Morphology. Academic Press, London (1982)
8. Dougherty, E.R., Lotufo, R.A.: Hands on Morphological Image Processing. SPIE Publications (2003)

9. Lacout, J.L., Hatim, Z., Botton, M.F.: Patent US 6521264 B1 (2003)
10. Kalender, W.A.: Computed Tomography: Fundamentals, System Technology, Image, Quality, Applications. Wiley, New Jersey (2005)
11. Maire, E., Buffière, J., Salvo, L., Blandin, J.J., Ludwig, W., Létang, J.M.: On the application of X-ray microtomography in the field of materials science. Adv. Eng. Mater. **3**, 539–546 (2001)
12. Mortele, K.J., McTavish, J., Ros, P.: Current techniques of computed tomography; Helical CT, Multidetector CT, and 3D reconstruction. Hepatic Imaging Interv. **6**, 29–52 (2002)
13. Hjam, H., Ronse, C.: The algebraic basis of mathematical morphology I. Dilations and erosions. Comput. Vis. Graph. Image Process. **50**, 245–295 (1990)
14. Willmott, C.J., Matsuura, K.: Advantages of the mean absolute error (MAE) over the root mean square error (RMSE) in assessing average model performance. Clim. Res. **30**, 79–82 (2003)

Towards an Improvement of the Software Documentation Using a Traceability Approach

Othmane Rahmaoui(✉)(ID), Kamal Souali(ID), and Mohammed Ouzzif

ESTC, Labo RITM, ENSEM CED, University Hassan II, Casablanca, Morocco
{othmane.rahmaoui,kml.souali,ouzzif}@gmail.com

Abstract. Today traceability is a buzz word and it used in several domains like healthcare, food industry and transportation sectors. In Information Technology (IT), traceability plays a very important role and it can be defined in various ways, depending on the environment and the process under consideration. Traceability is one of the essential activities of good software development lifecycle because it helps to reduce the effort required to determine the impacts of requested changes. Software Documentation plays also a very important role in the Software Engineering and without it, it is hard to maintain any software project and every new project we will reinvent the wheel. In this work, we propose a new approach to improve the software documentation with data traceability management.

Keywords: Traceability · Software documentation · Trace · Data traceability

1 Introduction

The traceability is the ability to trace all stages of its manufacture, as well as the source of all its components. The traceability of a product makes it possible, for example, to find the suppliers of the raw materials, the different places where the product has been stored, the manipulations and equipment used in its manufacture, etc. The goal of the traceability is to be able to monitor a product and evaluate its quality. But it's not just about finding the failing item; it is also important to know the products that make up this element and the operations that have been carried out on these products. This method has several interests: to rectify the conformity of the product as quickly as possible and to manage the resulting consequences; establish a complete product analysis and be able to decide corrective actions; integrate prevention into the design and production of relevant elements; sue a producer who has caused serious damage to customers or their property [1]. At the IT level and especially at the level of a software project, each project manager wants the requirements to be known at the beginning but the reality is that the needs are always very late and they change regularly throughout the project. This is why the agile method today is more and more important hence the importance of using a traceability management to get an idea of all the changes made to the artifacts such as the source code, models or tests. A good documentation management of a software project involves developing a document of all specifications for developers and testers as well as a technical document for internal users or a manual for

M. Ezziyyani (Ed.): AI2SD 2018, AISC 915, pp. 514–525, 2019.
https://doi.org/10.1007/978-3-030-11928-7_46

end users to help them to understand the features. It plays a very important role for software engineers and for users (Technical and end users).

For technical users, a specification document is used to evaluate the work of the programmers as well as the testers. this document must have several elements; information about files and databases created by the development team, functions and programs with an explanation of each treatment done, how variables and constants are used and finally the overall structure of the program with a documentation in the source code to explain the role of functions, sub-programs, variables and constants.

For end users, functional reasons need to be considered in order to document the use of the application and to reduce the costs of technical support. The documentation must be explanatory with an interface design in a simple way and if a screen of the application requires complex documentation is better to change the design of the screen with something more intuitive [2].

2 State of the Art and Existing Work

2.1 State of the Art

Traceability can provide many benefits in terms of impact and added value to the companies that implement it. The traceability between artifacts in a software project currently interested many research communities and software engineering. Software documentation is a basic component of the software development process and it is very important in all the phases of a software system life cycle. In 2005, Andrian Marcus & al. presented an approach for the semi-automatic recovery of the traceability link between the software documentation and the source code, based on information retrieval techniques to extract and to analyze the semantic information of the source code and the associated documentation [3]. This approach consists in using a semantic indexing technique for retrieving information from the documentation and the source code, the latter method was also proposed by Maletico'01 [4] and Marcus'01 [5] in 2001, but Andrian'05 [3] used other information to define measures of similarity between the elements of the documentation (expressed in natural language) and the components of the software system. The methodology is based on the extraction, analysis and representation of comments and identifiers of the source code. The approach has several advantages, one of the most important is its flexibility of use determined by the fact that the methodology does not rely on a predefined vocabulary or grammar for the documentation and the source code, without forgetting the fact to reduce the costs of link recovery. In 2008, a new method used the example of collaborative writing (CW) in software product line (SPL) engineering domain has been presented by Lago et al. [6]. There are three SPL engineering traceability issues that have been presented by them which are traceability links between feature and structural models, traceability links between SPL level and product level models and lastly traceability links between generic and concrete structural models. The description of each issue is in Table 1. present the framework of the tracing which is shown in Fig. 1, the tracing is done from feature model to structural model (a1 and b2) and from SPL level to Product level (a2 and b1).

Table 1. Description of SPL engineering traceability issues

Issue	Description
1	Clear documentation of the dependency between feature model of SPL and products
2	The documentation of where SPL commonality is realized in the different products
3	Documentation of the generic models embodied by the concrete structural solutions develops for the product line

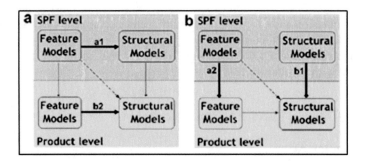

Fig. 1. a Traceability links between feature and structural models and **b** traceability links between SPL level and product level models

On March 2012, Azram and Atan [7] presented a traceability method to facilitate in tracing of the software documentation based on [6] research. Based on the issues, they proposed the traceability metrics and attributes that are significant to verify and validate the tracing result. The proposed metrics are shown in Table 2 while the attributes are shown in Table 3. They take the concept of the tracing from the framework and modify it to suit for Software Engineering Documentation. The modified framework is shown in Fig. 2. From the modified framework, the tracing is done from Document 1 to Document 2, Document 2 to Document 3 and Document 1 to Document 3.

Table 2. Description of SPL engineering traceability issues

Metric	Description
Dependency	Dependency of keyword from one document to another
Commonality	Similarity of keyword within a document or from one document to another
Structural solution	Standard documentation followed

Table 3. The proposed attributes

Attribute	Description
Number of document used	Total number of document used for tracing
Number of document linked	Total number of document that linked with one another
Dependency of document	Percentage of dependency between documents
Number of keyword used	Total number of keyword used for tracing
Number of common keyword	Total number of common keyword used in each document
Keyword linked	Percentage of keyword that linked between documents
Categorization of document	Type of document
Scope of document	Total range cover by document following standard documentation
Document compliance	Document compliance percentage following standard documentation

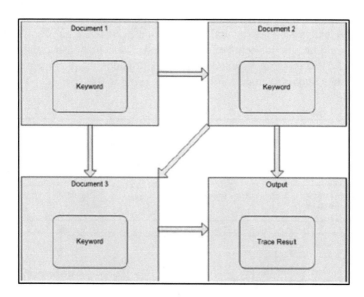

Fig. 2. The modified framework

In 2013, Dasgupta et al. [8] proposed a novel approach for expanding corpora with relevant documentation that is obtained using external function call documentation and sets of relevant words, which it implemented in TraceLab. This last is a software infrastructure designed to address the issue related to the reproducibility of experiments (i.e., lack of implementation, implementation details, datasets, etc.) in software engineering (SE) research. TraceLab was funded by the National Science Foundation and was developed at DePaul University in collaboration with Kent State University, University of Kentucky, and the College of William and Mary. Since its introduction,

TraceLab has already been successfully used in several projects. TraceLab provides a set of predefined components (i.e., tools that are commonly used in SE techniques and approaches, such as data importers, pre-processors, Information Retrieval (IR) approaches, state of the art Traceability Link (TL) recovery techniques, etc.), as well as a development kit which includes the guidelines and support for creating custom components. These components can be assembled to create experiments, which can be executed alongside other SE techniques, on the same datasets, and their results can be compared to determine which technique produces the best results using standard metrics (e.g., precision, recall, etc.), as well as statistical tests. In addition, the newly created experiments, which are fully reproducible, are shared with the community in order to facilitate the creation of new techniques (based on the existing one) and the comparison of new techniques against existing ones.

In the context of ERP (Enterprise Resource Planning), the relevance of the software documentation is even more important due to the complexity of such a kind of software systems and the strategic role they have within operative organizations. On November 2017, Aversano et al. [9] are presenting a framework for evaluating the quality of the documentation of ERP (Enterprise Resource Planning) Open Source Software system. They are focusing on the evaluation of the quality of the various types of documents that may be useful for understanding a software artifact. It mainly considers the user point of view, analyses both structural and content aspects that a good software system document should include for being effectively used. The content aspects are defined by considering the ERP system context and all the information the documentation of such a kind of system should include for successfully using it (Fig. 3).

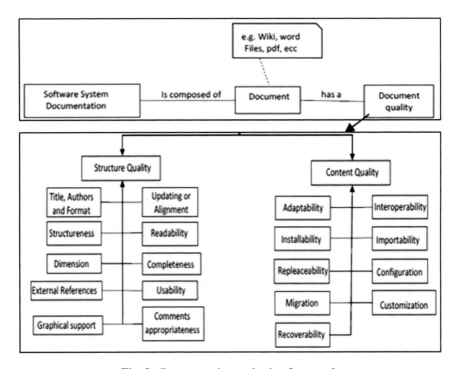

Fig. 3. Documentation evaluation framework

2.2 Existing Work

The previous research in [8], the researchers have made a mix of two approaches to increase the accuracy of the traceability links (TLs), the first one allows to increase the precision of information retrieval approaches (IR) where there are quite a few approaches based on syntagmatic associations, that are used in several techniques to calculate traceability links such as a Vector Space Model (VSM) where artifacts are represented as vectors of words, by expanding the vocabulary of artifacts using related words. The second approach allows the use of Application Programming Interface (API) Calls to compute the similarities between requirements and software artifacts with a higher degree of precession. The main problem with VSM is that different programmers can use the same words to describe different requirements (synonymy), as well as use different words to describe the same requirements (polysemy), which is why developers who participate in Projects must use consistent vocabulary to write code and documentation. This will help improve the traceability of API calls and keywords at the source code level, requirements documents and artifacts as well as external sources of information. That's why they called the proposed method ENTRANCE; for ENhancing TRAceability usiNg Calls API and reElevent woRds and the following Fig. 4 shows its implementation on TraceLab.

TraceLab already implements a set of IR approaches, which will be described briefly as independent variables for our experimental design. In the context of ENTRANCER, these techniques take as input a corpus of documents (i.e., the target artifacts) and a set of queries (i.e., the source artifacts) and compute the textual similarities between the source and target artifacts;

- The vector space model (VSM) procedure can be divided into three stages. The first stage is the document indexing where content bearing terms are extracted from the document text. The second stage is the weighting of the indexed terms to enhance retrieval of document relevant to the user. The last stage ranks the document with respect to the query according to a similarity measure.
- Latent semantic indexing (LSI), sometimes referred to as latent semantic analysis, is a mathematical method developed in the late 1980s to improve the accuracy of information retrieval. It uses a technique called singular value decomposition (SVD) to scan unstructured data within documents and identify relationships between the concepts contained therein.
- Jensen-Shannon (JS) is a recent IR technique that represents each artifact of the corpus as a probability distribution of the terms occurring in the artifact. The probability distribution is based on the weight assigned to each term for that particular artifact. The similarities between two software artifacts (i.e., two probability distributions), are measured using an entropy-based metric, called the Jensen-Shannon Divergence.
- Latent Dirichlet Allocation (LDA), It's a way of automatically discovering topics that these sentences contain. For example, given these sentences and asked for 2 topics, LDA might produce something like:
  - Sentences 1 and 2: 100% Topic A
  - Sentences 3 and 4: 100% Topic B

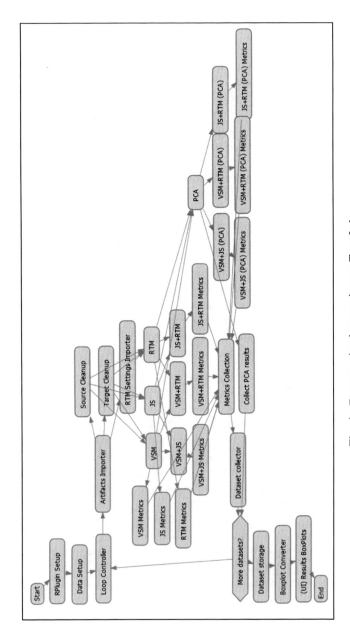

Fig. 4. Entrancer implementation on TraceLab

- Sentence 5: 60% Topic A, 40% Topic B
- Topic A: 30% broccoli, 15% bananas, 10% breakfast, 10% munching, ... (at which point, you could interpret topic A to be about food)
- Topic B: 20% chinchillas, 20% kittens, 20% cute, 15% hamster, ... (at which point, you could interpret topic B to be about cute animals)

• The Relational Topic Model (RTM) is a hierarchical probabilistic model that generalizes LDA, it is a model of documents and the links between them. For each pair of documents, the RTM models their link as a binary random variable that is conditioned on their contents.

• The Principal Component Analysis (PCA) can be used to determine various orthogonal dimensions (called principal components) present in the data. These principal components also quantify the variability found in the data.

ENTRANCER experimented with three Java applications and by using it the precision of recovering traceability links was increased by up to 31% in the best case and by approximately 9% on average.

In the research [9], a framework for evaluating the documentation of a software project has been proposed (Fig. 3), the documentation is composed of several documents of different types (API, WIKI, Comments and code) it is why steps need to be taken in a consensual way to make the documentation more understandable and well structured.

3 The Proposed Work

Our method is based on the previous researches works [8] and [9], by proposing the hybrid of enhancing software traceability and analysis of the documentation of software project, because it will be possible to increase the precision of computing traceability links (TLs) and also to evaluate the software project documentation with a quality model (the documentation structure and the content of documents).

3.1 Overview of the Proposed Approach

The use of relevant external documentation to expand the corpus of different artifacts can lead to discover more TLs with a higher degree of accuracy. For example, if a requirement specifies that cryptographic services should be used to protect information, and a module in an application uses encryption, then these requirement and software artifacts are relevant to a certain degree, hence the importance of improving the quality of textual information in requirements and artifacts in order to allow the good recovery of information and TLS. The calculation of traces between different artifacts saves costs and improves various software maintenance efforts and if some traces are wrong, the validation of these traces requires a significant investment, hence the importance of using a system document evaluation. The quality of each document must be analyzed and evaluated according to two aspects; the quality of the structure and the quality of the content. The following figure shows the schematization of our approach in order to introduce a complete system for the improvement of the documentation while using the traceability and the analysis of the data in order to control the processes throughout the software project (Fig. 5).

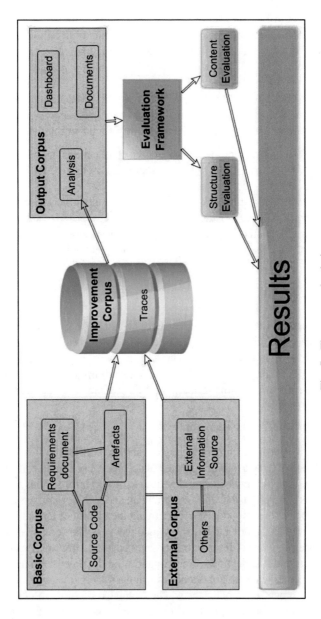

Fig. 5. The proposed solution

Content Quality:

- Title, Authors, and Format, have been consider as general information regarding the document.
- Structureness: regarding the textual documentation and aiming at evaluating the quality of the actual structure in terms of number of chapters, sections, sub-sections nesting, document length, and density of tables and figures. A good structure and organization of the document helps to consult it.
- Dimension: to analyses the length of the document sentences: sentences that are too long express text that is too difficult to be understood, and sentences too short may not exhaustively express a concept. Cuts asserted that over the whole document, average sentence length should be 15-20 word.
- External references: to understand if references to documents external to the documentation or to source code exist to better support the comprehension of software engineers and users.
- Graphical Support: to verify the availability of visual aids (figures and tables) facilitating the understand ability of the text. The citations of the visual aids within the text and existence of clear captions are verified. It may occur that figures or tables not included in the document are indexed.
- Updating or alignment: to verify whether the documentation is updated with reference to the project release it refers to.
- Readability: to examine if the sentences express clear and understandable concepts. The index score ranges from 0 to 100 and a value equal to 50 is considered adequate; while higher scores refers to material that is easier to read and lower marks indicate documents that are more difficult to read.
- Completeness: to evaluate the completeness level of the documentation with reference to the source code; in particular, these quality indicator checks whether the documentation describes the entire source code items (packages, classes, methods).
- Usability: concerning API and Wiki and assessing the organization from a usability point of view. Aspects that will be investigated are the fragmentation of the concepts within web pages, and the size of the Java Doc and Wiki.
- Comments appropriateness: to estimate the density of comments in the code. A high density of comments helps the developer in the comprehension of source code.

Structure Quality:

- Adaptability: to evaluate if in the documentation adequately indicates the supported operating system and database management systems.
- Installability: to verify whether the documentation adequately describes the installation process.
- Replaceability: to evaluate is a description exists in the documentation with reference to the possibility of replacing the software system with a different one.
- Migration: to verify whether the documentation adequately describes the migration process referring the generated reports.
- Recoverability: to evaluate if the functionality for the transactions management are adequately described in the documentation.

- Interoperability: to evaluate how the documentation discusses the web-services support.
- Importability: to evaluate if the documentation adequately describes the formats for importing data.
- Configuration: to analyze if the software system configuration functionality, such as Wizard, charts of accounts, supported languages, tax category management, Multicurrency coverage, setup, are well described.
- Customization: to verify if the customization functionality regarding the full system, user interface, workflows and reports is adequately described.

4   Example and Results

In this section, we took into consideration an application for stock management that was developed by students at the end of studies project level. In order to evaluate the documents made throughout the project, we propose an example of evaluation of these documents considering that we already have a vision on the traces and the links between the corpora.

- Specifications report SR1
- Design and modelling report DM1
- Development Guide DG1
- User Guide UG1 (Table 4).

Table 4. Example of the evaluation of the documentation structure

	Stock management project			
	SR1	DM1	DG1	UG1
Title and authors				
%Doc with title	100	100	100	100
%Doc with authors	0	0	50	100
Structureness	60	80	80	100
%Doc with paragraphs				
Dimension	10,156	11,259	14,523	18,114
Doc Dimension				
External references				
%Doc with external links	0	30	80	80
%Doc referring source code	0	0	0	0
Graphical support				
% Doc with figures	0	60	70	90
%Doc with tables	10	0	20	0
%Doc with diagrams	0	80	20	0
Updating	60	50	10	5
% Updated Doc				
Readability	15	8	9	8
AVG sentences length				

5   Conclusion and Future Work

The traceability allows in real time to provide at any time, proofs of the conformity of a product, the elements which compose it and its origin. Traceability has become one of interest topics in software engineering research.

Software engineering is a field that allows applying several approaches to design, operate and maintain software systems and the study of all the activities involved in the realization of high-performance information systems. Over the years, there have been major changes in the type of software systems developed; however, traceability is one of the essential activities of good software development lifecycle because it helps to reduce the effort required to determine the impacts of requested changes.

In this paper, we are proposing a hybrid of two approaches that can be used to improve the quality of software documentation project by using data traceability management.

In our future work, we aim to experiment our approach on a real software project in order to study the benefits of using it and to generalize it throughout the development of a software system while making it automatic and intelligent.

References

1. Souali, K., Rahmaoui, O., Ouzzif, M.: An overview of traceability: Definitions and techniques. In: CIST 2016, pp. 789–793
2. da Silva, W.M.C., de Sousa, R., da Mata, D.Q., Araújo, A.P.F., Holanda, M., dos Santos, G. D.: Software documentation quality: a case study for the software documentation of SIGEPE. In: 2015 10th Iberian Conference on Information Systems and Technologies (CISTI)
3. Marcus, A., Meletic, J., Sergeyev, A.: Refining traceability links between code and software documents. Int. J. Soft. Eng. Knowl. Eng. **15**, 811 (2005)
4. Maletic, J.I., Marcus, A.: Supporting program comprehension using semantic and structural information. In: Proceedings of 23rd International Conference on Software Engineering (ICSE'01), pp. 103–112. Toronto, Ontario, Canada, 12–19 May (2001)
5. Marcus, A., Maletic, J.I.: Identification of high-level clones in source code. In: Proceedings of Automated Software Engine (ASE'01), pp. 107–114. San Diego, CA, 26–29 November (2001)
6. Lago, P., Muccini, H., Vliet, H.V.: A scoped approach to traceability management. J. Syst. Softw. **82**, 168–182 (2008)
7. Azram, N.A., Atan, R.: Traceability method for software engineering documentation. IJCSI Int. J. Comput. Sci. **9**(2), No. 2 (2012)
8. Dasgupta, T., Grechanik, M., Moritz, E., Dit, B., Poshyvanyk, D.: Enhancing software traceability by automatically expanding corpora with relevant documentation. In: 2013 IEEE International Conference on Software Maintenance
9. Aversano, L., Guardabascio, D., Tortorella, M.: Analysis of the documentation of ERP software projects. In: CENTERIS—International Conference on ENTERprise Information Systems/ProjMAN—International Conference on Project MANagement/HCist—International Conference on Health and Social Care Information Systems and Technologies, CENTERIS/ProjMAN/HCist 2017, Barcelona, Spain, 8–10 November 2017

Vanishing Point Detection Under Foggy Weather with Edge-Based Approach

Salma Alami[(⊠)] and Abdelhak Ezzine

Laboratory of Information and Communication Technology LabTIC, National
School of Applied Sciences ENSAT, University Abdelmalek Essaadi UAE,
Tanger, Morocco
alami.salmaa@gmail.com

Abstract. Vanishing Point detection is one of the vision-based approaches
used for autonomous vehicles and Driver Assistance Systems DAS. It is prin-
cipally useful for detecting the road needed in vehicle navigation and tracking.
Like other methods based on vision, the vanishing point detection approach is
deeply sensitive to the presence of bad weather as fog. In this paper, we present
an efficient edge-based approach for detecting the vanishing point of road scene
under foggy weather based on a combination of an adaptive Canny method for
edge detection, and the Hough Transform for straight line extraction. The
optimal vanishing point is estimated by applying a k-mean clustering on the
candidate points obtained by the straight lines intersection. We tested our
approach on 731 real and synthetic images, where the experimental results show
that the proposed approach for detecting the vanishing point under foggy
weather gives good results.

Keywords: Vanishing point detection · Edge-based · Bad weather · Fog ·
Driver assistance

1 Introduction

Recently vision-based methods are increasingly used in Driver Assistance Systems
(DAS) and autonomous vehicles. They offer large information about the vehicle
environment, such as the road, the weather, the vehicles and obstacles movements and
positions. While there are various methods to detect the road, many of them used the
vanishing point [1–4]. Furthermore, the vanishing point can be also used for camera
calibration [5–7], road tracking [8], lane detection [9] and weather detection [10, 11].
Thus, the vanishing point, must be detected efficiently and quickly to be integrated in
DAS and intelligent vehicles under any driving condition. In addition, the approaches
relaying on vision sensors, like the vanishing point detection, are very sensitive to
weather conditions as fog, in which presence, the high frequencies of the images are
degraded. In case those methods have not been adapted to the foggy weather, their
robustness may be reduced or lost.

Widely, the methods for detecting the vanishing point are classified into three main
categories. The two most used categories are based either on texture [4, 12–14] or on
edges [8, 9, 15–17], while the last one is based on prior information [18]. Although the

© Springer Nature Switzerland AG 2019
M. Ezziyyani (Ed.): AI2SD 2018, AISC 915, pp. 526–536, 2019.
https://doi.org/10.1007/978-3-030-11928-7_47

texture-based methods present robust detection, they remain challenging in the computational time. On the other hand, the edge-based methods require less computational time, but still challenging, whether in detecting the right edges or in the vanishing point voting. Yet, almost all works for detecting vanishing point do not discuss this situation, nor take into consideration the presence of foggy weather.

In this paper, we present an approach that gives compromising results to detect efficiently the vanishing point under foggy weather. We used the Canny Parameter Free presented by Lu et al. [19] to detect the edges, and then we extract the straight lines by using Hough method. We compute the VP candidates from the intersection of the relevant lines. Finally, we process to a k-mean clustering to estimate the optimal VP. We adopt an edge-based method, as it requires less computational time.

This paper is organized as follows: Sect. 2 presents the previous vanishing point detection methods. The proposed approach is presented in Sect. 3. Then in Sect. 4, experimental results are provided to show the accuracy of the proposed method. Finally, we conclude in Sect. 5.

2 Related Work

In the real world, the vanishing point is defined as the intersection of the scene parallel lines. By applying edge based approaches [8, 9, 15–17], the vanishing point is generally estimated by the intersection of the relevant scene straight lines such as lane marking, road or buildings borders. At the beginning, the picture edges are determined and the straight lines are extracted. Then, the optimal VP is selected from the straight lines intersection with various techniques.

In the work of Nieto et al. [15, 16], the lanes marking were firstly extracted, and then fitted with straight lines by applying the Hough Transform method. Next, the VP was obtained by resolving the VP candidates equations system obtained from the straight lines intersection. In the end, the final position of the vanishing point is stabilized by applying a temporal low pass filter. To detect the lane marking, Nieto et al. presented two approaches. The first approach [16] is reflected in segmenting the picture with the image gray-level histogram followed by frequencies filtering. In the second work [15], an edge map is computed with the steerable filter bank. However, the steerable filter needs more computational time, moreover, the robustness of edge detection depends of the number of orientations used for the filter bank.

On the other hand, papers like [8] and [17] compute at first the image contrast and the edges by applying a Canny filter with a constant and manual thresholds. In [17], the straight line segments are then estimated by clustering the local orientation of the pixels contrast. To keep only relevant lines needed for computing the VP, the authors filter and weight the lines based on some criterion including the line length and orientation, and the distance between the end-point of the line and the VP computed in the previous frame. The candidate points are then computed from the intersection of the left and right lines. Each point will have a weight obtained from the intersected lines. Finally, the optimal VP is selected depending on its weight. As for Yuan et al. [9], they use the adaptive Canny filter proposed by Sun [20]. The straight lines are then obtained by applying the probabilistic Hough transform combined with an edge gradient orientation constraint. Finally, the optimal VP is estimated based on the position of the vanishing point in the previous frame. Despite, this method gives good results; it needs prior information about the VP, which may affect the exact estimation of the current VP.

Nonetheless, due to the fog veil and scattering, the high frequencies of the images are reduced. Consequently, these methods might fail or loose robustness by applying frequency and intensity filtering without taking into consideration the foggy weather. Moreover, using constant thresholds for Canny filter is not suitable for autonomous navigation. As well, the choice of Canny adaptive threshold method should be appropriate in the presence of fog.

3 Method

Similar to the edge-based methods for detecting the vanishing point (VP), our proposed approach involves three main steps: edge detection, straight lines extraction and intersection and finally the optimal vanishing point selection.

Concerning the edge detection, varied approaches have been proposed to detect the edge defined as an intensity sharp change occurring to contiguous pixels. Yet, the Canny operator [21] is considered to be the most accurate method reducing the number of false edge response.

The Canny filter consists in computing the image gradient, then suppressing the false edge responses by applying a non-maximum suppression. Thereafter, false edges are deleted if the pixel gradient is lower than a given low threshold. In the other case, the edges are kept if the pixel gradient is higher than a given high threshold. Otherwise, the edges are called weak. However, the choice of these two thresholds remains a challenging task due to the driving conditions. Setting a high value for the maximum threshold can lead to missing important edges. As well as setting very low threshold leads to detecting noisy edges. Moreover, it is more appropriate to have adaptive thresholds for pictures acquired with camera-embedded vehicles.

To our knowledge, there are two methods for computing adaptively the Canny thresholds without any prior parameters. The first one cited in [22], is based on the Otsu thresholding [23]. The second method called the Canny Parameter Free [19] employs statistics combined with observations on human vision perception. We note that, although those methods give good results, none of them had been tested under foggy condition.

The Otsu thresholding is known to be more robust when used in scenes with separated background and foreground. Still, we tested it with our images and get an unsatisfactory outcome (Figs. 4 and 5), hence, we withdraw this method.

We designate the Canny Parameter Free (CannyPF) method for detecting the edges. We recall that the CannyPF is based on probability integrated with psychological observations of the human perception known as the Helmholtz principle [24]. Authors of [19] present an approach called Canny Parameter Free that computes adaptively the low and high Canny thresholds. The Helmholtz principle assumes that a geometric structure is perceived by chance and have no meaning, if it occurs many times in a random situation. Edges are one of the geometric structures detected by Helmholtz principle [25]. Based on this principle, an edge is called meaningful, if its number of occurrence is very small in a random situation. Namely, the edge did not appear by chance or just by randomness, but there were some common features that allowed grouping it as a geometric structure based on the Gestalts theory.

After detecting the edges, we extract straight lines from the edge map with the Hough Transform method, a classical algorithm widely used for extracting straight lines. The Hough Transform approach consists in transforming the image space into a parametric space. Such as, the pixel coordinates in the Hough Transform accumulator HT_{acc} correspond to the image straight lines having as equation $y = mx + b$ (Fig. 1). The transformation of the image space into the HT_{acc} is computed with Eq. (1).

$$\rho = x.\cos\theta + y.\sin\theta \qquad (1)$$

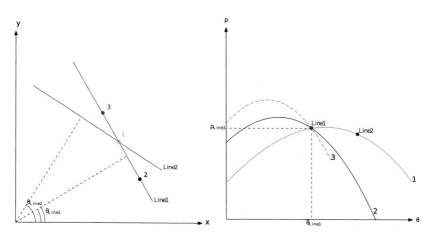

Fig. 1. Representation of straight lines in the image space (left) and in the Hough parametric space (right)

With (x, y) the coordinates of 2D image pixels and (ρ, θ) the coordinates in the Hough Transform space called HT_{acc}.

Thus, the maximums peaks on the Hough Transform accumulator HT_{acc} will correspond to the straight lines containing the greatest amount of pixels. The highest is the value of $HT_{acc}(\rho, \theta)$, the more points belong to the straight line having as equation $y = mx + b$.

Accordingly, to extract relevant lines needed to compute the VP, we select the N highest local maximums on the HT_{acc}. We head to compute the local maximums instead of the maximums peaks to avoid the extraction of close lines; we also exclude the horizontal and vertical lines. The size of the local window is set to 5 × 5. While the choice of N the number of local maximums remains challenging, we proceed to compare the accuracy of the proposed method by varying the value of N. In fact, setting a high number for N could detect false lines, while assigning a low value could miss important lines and thereby reduce the detection accuracy.

To select an adequate and relevant number of N lines, we computed the accuracy of the proposed method for N varying from two to 10. As can be seen in Fig. 2, the lowest accuracy is obtained from the lowest and highest value of N, namely 2 and 10.

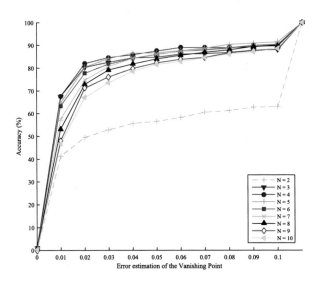

Fig. 2. Comparison of the vanishing point accuracy by setting different values of N. With N, the number of the highest local maximums selected from the Hough transform accumulator

We choose an optimal value N equal to 5, where we get good accuracy for our different types of data containing different kinds of fog.

Generally, outdoor scenes contain more than one vanishing point, depending on the scene structure. In the case of driving assistance systems, the considered vanishing point is interpreted as the point where the road converges due to the perspective projection. Meanwhile, the VP is represented in the image space as the intersection of the world parallel lines. However, the intersection of those lines does not reproduce a unique VP but a set of points. Namely, having N lines reproduce $\sum(N - i)$ intersections. With i varying from one to $N - 1$. Later, we called the intersection points, the vanishing point candidates V_c.

After obtaining the V_c, we proceed to measure the optimal VP designated as the centroid of the closest points based on the Euclidean distance. Nonetheless, some false intersections V_c lead to an inaccurate position of the centroid.

Hence, we kept the closest V_c and neglected the far ones by applying a k-mean clustering. The k-mean aims to regroup points into k clusters, where each point belongs to the cluster with the nearest mean, such as the squared error is minimized. Afterwards, we set k = 2 to produce two clusters. The first cluster contains the nearest points that vote for the optimal VP. While the second one regroups the aberrant points. Figure 3 shows an example of the obtained V_c regrouped into two clusters. Once we obtain the cluster with the nearest points, we assign the final VP as the centroid of this cluster.

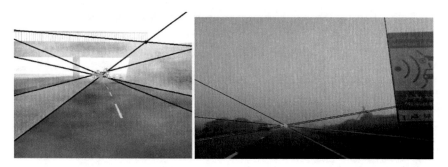

Fig. 3. The vanishing point candidates grouped into two clusters with k-mean clustering. The cluster with red circle grouped the aberrant points. The other cluster contains the candidates voting for the optimal VP

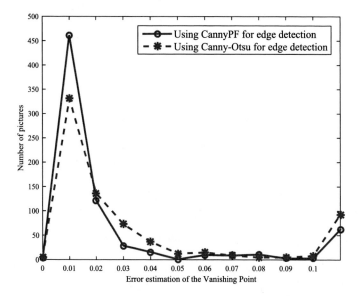

Fig. 4. Comparison of the vanishing point estimation error obtained by using Canny-Otsu and CannyPF for the edge detection step

An example containing the three main steps for computing the vanishing point under the foggy weather is shown in Fig. 6.

4 Results and Discussion

The vanishing point detection approach was tested on 731 real and synthetic pictures with road fog. 316 of the pictures are synthetic images taken from FRIDA [26] and FRIDA2 [27] database. Such as, the images contain four types of synthetic fog: homogeneous (U), heterogeneous (K), cloudy homogeneous (L) and cloudy

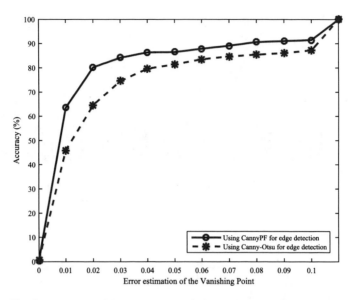

Fig. 5. Accuracy of detecting the vanishing point under foggy weather

heterogeneous fog (M). In addition, two videos named Video1 and Video2 were taken with a mobile on the Moroccan highways during different daytime and different fog density (average and dense fog respectively). The rest of the real images are gathered in Data1 including some pictures from the internet and others taken with our mobile under foggy weather and under different driving time of the day.

4.1   Error of Estimation and Accuracy

To evaluate this approach, we measure with Eq. (2) the accuracy by computing the normal Euclidean distance between the ground truth and the estimated vanishing point. We called it later the error of estimation δ. The vanishing point is well estimated when δ is close to 0. Figure 4 shows the set of images that have voted for each error estimation bin value. It also contains a comparison between the error estimation obtained by using Canny-Otsu and CannyPF for the edge detection.

$$\delta = \frac{\left\| \hat{V} - V_{gt} \right\|}{diagonal(I)} \qquad (2)$$

With $\hat{V}$ the estimated vanishing point, V_{gt} the ground truth and *diagonal(I)* the diagonal length of the image. The ground truth of the vanishing point was set manually.

The error estimation of the vanishing point δ for each data is grouped in Table 1. The overall mean of δ by using this approach is equal to 0.0355, which fit in the interval of the other methods detecting VP without taking into consideration the presence of fog. In [28], δ for 600 images taken into clear weather is equal to 0.0471.

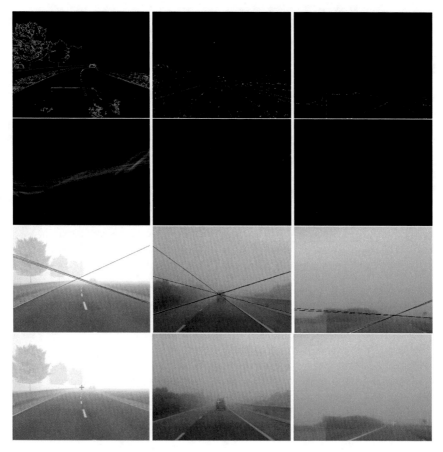

Fig. 6. Steps for detecting the vanishing point applied to a synthetic picture from FRIDA (left) and a real picture (middle and right). From top to bottom: edge detection step, Hough transform accumulator, extracted straight lines and detection of the optimal vanishing point

Table 1. The error estimation of the vanishing point

	Data1	Data2	Video2	FRIDA and FRIDA2				Overall
				U	K	L	M	
δ	0.0135	0.0099	0.0071	0.0706	0.0665	0.0766	0.0665	0.0355

While in [4] and [12], it is respectively equal to 0.0507 and 0.036 for over 1000 and 500 images taken under clear weather.

In previous works, where general road images were taken under clear weather, the accuracy for detecting the VP reaches 90% in [13] for a δ higher than 0.1. In our case, despite the presence of fog, Fig. 5 shows that our accuracy reaches 90% with an error of estimation above 0.07. Figure 5 displays the accuracy of the vanishing point detection under foggy weather by using the Canny Parameter Free method for edge detection.

4.2 Time of Execution

We tested the proposed approach using an i7 laptop 2.5Ghz CPU and 8G of memory. The code was developed with C++ and OpenCV library.

The average execution time of the different phases for detecting the vanishing point is shown in Table 2. Where phase (a), (b) and (c) are successively the edge detection, lines extraction and intersection and finally the optimal VP estimation by k-mean clustering.

Table 2. Total and phases execution time for the proposed approach

	Data1	Video1	Video2	FRIDA	FRIDA2	Overall mean
(a)	0.2458	0.2909	0.2879	0.0423	0.0426	0.1778
(b)	0.5882	0.9162	0.4506	0.7642	0.5793	0.6221
(c)	0.0002	0.0003	0.0002	0.0004	0.0003	0.0003
Total time	0.8718	1.2986	0.7828	0.7863	0.6077	0.826

The mean of the total execution time of the proposed approach is 0.826 s, which is far to meet the real-time system requirement. Nevertheless, the time of execution of phase (b) taking the greatest amount of time, might be increasingly reduced by optimizing the algorithm and the implementation of the Hough Transform, the line extraction and intersection. Thus, the proposed approach can reach the real-time constraint to be integrated in driving autonomous systems.

5 Conclusion

In this paper, we have presented an efficient approach for detecting the vanishing point (VP) in road images containing different types of fog. First, the edges are detected using the Canny Parameter Free method. Then, the straight lines are extracted from the edges by the Hough Transform. Thereafter, the vanishing point candidates are generated by the intersection of the straight lines. Finally, a k-mean clustering is applied to the vanishing point candidates in order to keep only the closest points, such as their centroid represents the final optimal VP. Results show that the proposed approach gives good accuracy for detecting the vanishing point and overtaken the limits of the bad weather driving condition. It also can meet the DAS real-time acquirement, only by optimizing the implementation of the Hough Transform method.

References

1. Kong, H., Audibert, J.Y., Ponce, J.: General road detection from a single image. IEEE Trans. Image Process. **19**, 2211–2220 (2010)
2. Wu, Q., Zhang, W., Kumar, B.V.K.V.: Example-based clear path detection assisted by vanishing point estimation. In: 2011 IEEE International Conference on Robotics and Automation, pp. 1615–1620. IEEE, Shanghai, China (2011)
3. Alvarez, J.M., López, A.M., Gevers, T., Lumbreras, F.: Combining priors, appearance, and context for road detection. In: IEEE Transactions on Intelligent Transportation Systems, vol. 15, pp. 1168–1178. IEEE (2014)
4. Bui, T.H., Saitoh, T., Nobuyama, E.: Vanishing point-based road detection for general road images. IEICE Trans. Inf. Syst. **E97.D**, 618–621 (2014)
5. Caprile, B., Torre, V.: Using vanishing points for camera calibration. Int. J. Comput. Vision **4**, 127–139 (1990)
6. Li, B., Peng, K., Ying, X., Zha, H.: Simultaneous vanishing point detection and camera calibration from single images. In: Bebis G., et al. (eds) Advances in Visual Computing. ISVC 2010. LNCS, vol 6454, pp. 151–160. Springer, Heidelberg (2010)
7. Song, H., Gao, Y., Chen, Y.: Traffic meteorological visibility estimation based on homogenous area extraction. Int. J. Comput. Appl. Technol. **48**, 36 (2013)
8. Wang, Y., Teoh, E., Shen, D.: Lane detection and tracking using B-snake. Image Vis. Comput. **22**, 269–280 (2004)
9. Yuan, J., Tang, S., Pan, X., Zhang, H.: A robust vanishing point estimation method for lane detection. In: Proceedings of the 33rd Chinese Control Conference, pp. 4887–4892. IEEE (2014)
10. Bronte, S., Bergasa, L.M., Alcantarilla, P.F.: Fog detection system based on computer vision techniques. In: 12th International IEEE Conference on Intelligent Transportation Systems, pp. 1–6. IEEE (2009)
11. Alami, S., Ezzine, A., Elhassouni, F.: Local fog detection based on saturation and RGB-correlation. In: 13th International Conference on Computer Graphics, Imaging and Visualization CGiV, pp. 1–5. IEEE (2016)
12. Moghadam, P., Starzyk, J., Wijesoma, W.S.: Fast vanishing-point detection in unstructured environments. IEEE Trans. Image Process. **21**, 425–430 (2012)
13. Kong, H., Sarma, S.E., Tang, F.: Generalizing Laplacian of Gaussian filters for vanishing-point detection. IEEE Trans. Intell. Transp. Syst. **14**, 408–418 (2013)
14. Fan, X., Deng, C., Rehman, Y., Shin, H.: Fast road vanishing point detection based on modified adaptive soft voting. In: The Seventh International Conferences on Pervasive Patterns and Applications, pp. 50–54. Nice, France (2015)
15. Nieto, M., Salgado, L., Jaureguizar, F., Cabrera, J.: Stabilization of inverse perspective mapping images based on robust vanishing point estimation. In: 2007 Intelligent Vehicles Symposium, pp. 315–320. IEEE (2007)
16. Nieto, M., Salgado, L.: Real-time vanishing point estimation in road sequences using adaptive steerable filter banks. In: Blanc-Talon, J., Philips, W., Popescu, D., Scheunders, P. (eds.) Advanced Concepts for Intelligent Vision Systems, ACIVS 2007. LNCS, vol. 4678, pp. 840–848. Springer, Berlin, Heidelberg (2007)
17. Suttorp, T., Bucher, T.: Robust vanishing point estimation for driver assistance. In: IEEE Intelligent Transportation Systems Conference, pp. 1550–1555. IEEE, Toronto, Canada (2006)

18. Wu, Q., Zhang, W., Chen, T., Kumar, B.V.K.V.: Prior-based vanishing point estimation through global perspective structure matching. In: 2010 IEEE International Conference on Acoustics, Speech and Signal Processing, pp. 2110–2113. IEEE, Dallas, TX, USA (2010)

19. Lu, X., Yao, J., Li, K., Li, L.: Cannylines : A parameter-free line segment detector. In: 2015 IEEE International Conference on Image Processing (ICIP), pp. 507–511. IEEE, Quebec City, QC, Canada (2015)

20. Sun, T., Tang, S., Wang, J., Zhang, W.: A robust lane detection method for autonomous car-like robot. In: 2013 Fourth International Conference on Intelligent Control and Information Processing (ICICIP), pp. 373–378. IEEE, Beijing, China (2013)

21. Canny, J.: A Computational approach to edge detection. IEEE Trans. Pattern Anal. Mach. Intell. **PAMI-8**, 679–698 (1986)

22. Huo, Y., Wei, G., Zhang, Y., Wu, L.: An adaptive threshold for the Canny operator of edge detection. In: 2010 International Conference on Image Analysis and Signal Processing, pp. 371–374. IEEE (2010)

23. Otsu, N.: A threshold selection method from gray-level histograms. IEEE Trans. Syst., Man, and Cybern. **9**, 62–66 (1979)

24. Desolneux, A., Moisan, L., Morel, J.-M.: From Gestalt Theory to Image Analysis. Springer, New York (2008)

25. Desolneux, A., Moisan, L., Morel, J.-M.: Edge detection by Helmholtz principle. J. Math. Imaging Vis. **14**(3), 271–284 (2001)

26. Tarel, J.-P., Hautière, N., Cord, A., Gruyer, D., Halmaoui, H.: Improved visibility of road scene images under heterogeneous fog. In: 2010 IEEE Intelligent Vehicles Symposium, pp. 478–485. IEEE, San Diego, CA (2010)

27. Tarel, J.-P., Hautière, N., Caraffa, L., Cord, A., Halmaoui, H., Gruyer, D.: Vision enhancement in homogeneous and heterogeneous fog. IEEE Intell. Transp. Syst. Mag. **4**, 6–20 (2012)

28. Wu, Z., Fu, W., Xue, R., Wang, W.: A novel line space voting method for vanishing-point detection of general road images. Sensors **16**, 948 (2016)

Latency Over Software Defined Network

Souad Faid[✉] and Mohamed Moughit

Mobility and Modeling IR2M Laboratory, University Hassan 1, Settat, Morocco
faidsouad28@gmail.com

Abstract. Telecom operators are always looking to optimize the deployed resources while ensuring the satisfaction of their customers, supporting end-to-end Quality of Service (QoS) in existing network architectures is an ongoing problem. Software SDN is the evolving network concept, which makes possible the automation of control and services development. Its main advantages are the centralized global network view, programmability, and separation management of the data plane as well as the control plane. These features have got attention of researchers to improve the QoS of today's various network applications. We aim to make a picture of QOS based on OpenFlow for SDN networks. The main goal of this paper is to present a comparison of SDN and Hardware Defined Network (HDN) in terms of QoS metrics like latency by using a POX Controller.

Keywords: Quality of service (QOS) · SDN · HDN · POX controller · OpenFlow

1 Introduction

SDN is today recognized as an architecture to open the network to applications. This includes the following two components:

– Allow applications to schedule the network to speed up deployment;
– Allow the network to better identify the transported applications in order to better manage them. The SDN Controller allows SDN users to gain a central look at the entire network.

2 Hardware Defined Network

Traditional networks are the most dominant networks until the arrival of the SDN solution, indeed the main characteristic is the coupling of the control plan and that of the data (Figs. 1 and 2).

The main difference between traditional networks resides in the technique of packets processing that transits the network, in fact just the first packet that takes a long time since it is sent to the controller in order to store the necessary information so that

© Springer Nature Switzerland AG 2019
M. Ezziyyani (Ed.): AI2SD 2018, AISC 915, pp. 537–544, 2019.
https://doi.org/10.1007/978-3-030-11928-7_48

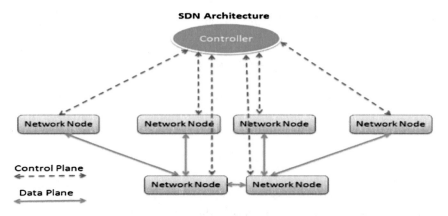

Fig. 1. SDN architecture

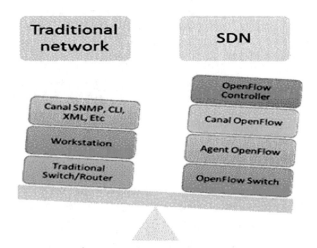

Fig. 2. Comparison between SDN and traditional networks

the other packets Belonging to the same frame will be processed with minimal time, in this way, we will compare the latency over SDN & HDN in order to prove the benefit of SDN technology.

3 State of the Art of the Quality of Service

In the current context, Quality of Service has become a determining factor for telecommunication operators who have therefore found that the quality of their services must be constantly monitored on the one hand to determine the state of their infrastructure and on the other to improve their competitiveness.

To simplify and facilitate the understanding and implementation of a simple quality of service approach, the following principles are defined:

- The quality of service concerns only the set of properties, characteristics and parameters that can be selected, measured and compared with limit values (threshold value).
- Evaluation of quality of service can reduce some essential quality characteristics. It is not necessary to define and measure each property of the service devices.

To meet the demand for quality of service flows, several management mechanisms have been proposed in the literature.

3.1   Quality of Service Definition

In recent decades, the management of quality of service in computer networks has been a major challenge for network operators due to the increasing demands of a wide range of applications. QoS is defined as the capacity of a network to carry the packet flow satisfactorily according to the requirements of the users. Indeed, to every application is associated a requirement related to the manipulation of the traffic in the network. A set of quality of service mechanisms has been specified to meet this demand. These mechanisms are based on the idea of measuring, improving and limiting prior guarantee of network performance. This property is particularly indispensable for the transmission of multimedia content [1].

3.2   Quality of Service Metrics

Quality of Service expresses the level of quality relative to the native metrics of the network, its ability to provide a service.

The effective management of QoS, as a major challenge for service providers, is based on a set of qualitative parameters. The quantitative parameters express the level of quality relative to the network, such as the end-to-end packet routing time. The most important metrics of QoS in IP networks are as follows:

- The transit delay: it represents the time interval required to transmit a data packet from the source to the destination.
- The flow: this parameter designates the amount of information that the application carries over a given time interval.
- Packet loss rate: this parameter indicates the probability that the data does not reach its destination.
- The jitter: this parameter designates the latency variation of the packets. The network must respect this parameter when transmitting voice and video conferencing.

3.3   Latency Management

Latency is the time required to deliver a packet across a network. Latency may be measured by different methods and it may be impacted by any network element like workstation, WAN links, routers, LAN... and ultimately it may be limited, for large networks, by the speed of light.

A low latency network is a network in which the design of the hardware, systems and protocols are geared towards minimizing the time taken to move units of data between any two points on that network (Fig. 3).

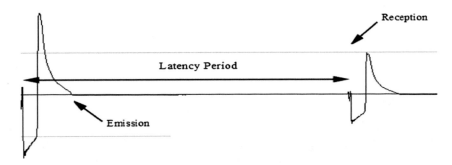

Fig. 3. Latency period

4   Latency Evaluation Benchmark Report

4.1   Hardware Defined Network

In traditional networks, quality of service is assessed through latency & throughput. The main objective of the SDN is to improve the quality of service by reducing latency and increasing the rate that is required in converged networks, which is not the case in HDN networks. To compare the performance of the two SDN & HDN solutions, emulation for SDN will be done using Mininet, for HDN, the emulator used is GNS3 [2].

GNS3 is a graphical network simulator that allows us to create complex network topologies and simulate them in different ways. A simple schema is designed, after executing a ping we can see the latency for all the packets belonging to the ping (Fig. 4).

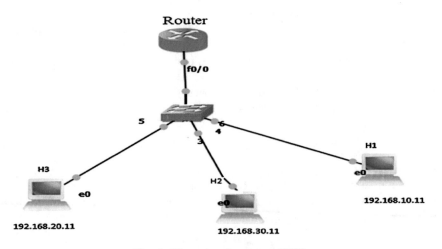

Fig. 4. Network scheme over GNS3

Analysis

- The latency for every packet from H1 to H3 is either same or more as observed in Fig. 5.

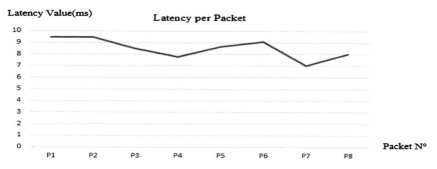

Fig. 5. Latency for HDN emulated on GNS3

- When the first packet from the source arrives to the switch, this latter registers in its MAC table; the MAC and IP address of the source host corresponding to the port at which the packet arrives.
- The switch checks its MAC table for the destination address in the MAC table. Since this is the first packet and there is no entry for the address, the switch forwards the packet to the router for the routing decisions.
- The router makes the routing decisions and sends the routing decision entry to switch. The switch forwards the packet accordingly and flushes the entry.

This process repeats for every packet that arrives consecutively to the switch leading to high latency of every packet [3].

4.2 Software Defined Network

The software defined networking (SDN) control system significantly reduces the time taken to execute the control loop. The POX controller standard provides multi-vendor, scalable, low latency monitoring of the entire network, server and application infrastructure. The OpenFlow protocol provides a fast, programmatic means for the controller to re-configuring forwarding in the network devices, significantly reducing the configuration delay.

Mininet is a network emulation platform used to test SDN applications based on virtualization concepts. It can support different types of topologies. Here we will show the configurations that will be useful for SDN technology test. Mininet creates virtual networks as shown in Fig. 6 [4].

The controller chosen is POX controller [5]. Once the network is created, the controller has to be instantiated. This controller is a remote controller on the IP address 192.168.3.50 over port 6633. The controller is up and now connected to the Open Flow

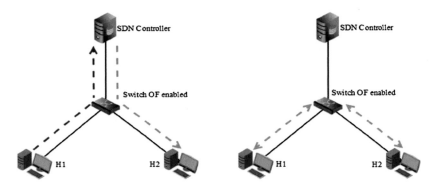

Fig. 6. Packets treatment by the switches OpenFlow-enabled

switch, which is on IP address 192.168.3.32. The virtual hosts H1, H2 and H3 that are created are connected to the Open Flow switch via virtual Ethernet links.

In order to determine the latency of packets in SDN, a ping test from H1 to H2 is conducted as shown in Fig. 7.

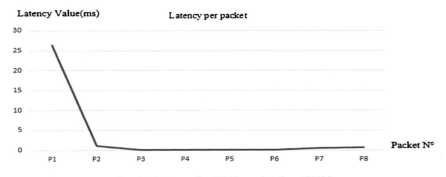

Fig. 7. Latency for HDN emulated on GNS3

Analysis

- We see from Fig. 7, the first packet takes 26.4 ms, i.e. more time compared to the consecutive packets. All the consecutive packets take very less time compared to the first packet.
- The reason for first packet to take longer time is, the routing decision happens only for first packet. Once the controller inserts the flow rule for the first packet, the switch buffers the flow rule in its flow table for 30 s.
- The consecutive packets are forwarded by the switch without contacting the controller for the routing decision.
- After 30 s, the buffer is timed out and the flow table is cleared. Again the same procedure repeats.

5 Comparison of the Packet Flow in HDN and SDN

The centralized controller in the SDN architecture can be programmed by using a high-level languages, in this way we can implement different ways in order to improve QOS [6].

The programmability of the SDN controller is not only a principle as a single programmable entity, it combined with its network visibility results in efficient and agile deployment of network topologies. Software Defined Networking is expected to have several business benefits compared to HDN as noted in Table 1 [7].

Table 1. Summarizes the HDN and SDN packet flow

Packet no.	HDN	SDN
1	Packet originating from H1 arrives to switch port	Packet originating from H1 arrives to switch port
2	The switch sends the packet to the router for routing decision	Switch checks for a flow rule corresponding to the packet in its flow table. If there is no entry, the packet is forwarded to controller
3	The routing decision from router is received and the switch just forwards the packet correspondingly	The flow rule is inserted in the openFlow switch by the controller. The switch buffers this entry for further communication
4	The consecutive packet is again sent to the router for routing decision	All the consecutive packets are forwarded based on the flow table entry until the buffer time expires
5	Packet sent to router again	
6	Packet sent to router again	
⋮	⋮	⋮
N	Packet sent to router again	The buffer time is out and the packet will be sent to controller

6 Conclusion

SDN is a modern technology that eliminates complexity network and control dynamically the whole by handling (QOS) management using high-level language and APIs. QOS management allows a global monitoring for entire network, this by different methods such as: provisioning, operating, monitoring, optimizing, and managing: faults, configuration, Accounting, Performance, and security in a different environments.

SDN promises to transform traditional networks include their static nature into flexible, scalable, programmable platforms with the intelligence to allocate resources automatically and this guaranteed end-to end QOS management. With its many benefits, SDN is the actual way to become the new approach for a current scalable networks.

Finally, notice that SDN is a tool. The research community can use this tool to create new innovative services and applications.

References

1. Wang, G., Eugene Ng, T.S., Shaikh, A.: Programming your network at run-time for big data applications. In: HotSDN'12, pp. 10–80, 13 Aug 2012, Helsinki, Finland
2. Wang, S.-Y., Chou, C.-L., Yang, C.-M.: Estinet openflow network simulator and emulator. Commun. Mag. IEEE **51**(9), 110–117 (2013)
3. Gudipati, A., Perry, D., Li, L.E., Katti, S.: SoftRAN: software definedradio access network. In: Proceedings of ACM HotSDN, 2013
4. Jin, X., Li, L., Vanbever, L., Rexford, J.: SoftCell: scalable and flexible cellular core network architecture. In: Proceedings of ACM CoNEXT, 2013
5. ONF: SDN architecture overview v 1.0. Updated white paper on "network functions virtualisation", 20 Dec 2013
6. Mckeown, N., Anderson, T., BalaKrishnan, H., Parulkar, G., Peterson, L., Rexford, J., Shenker, S., Turner, J.: Openflow: enabling innovation in campus networks. ACM SIGCOMM Comput. Commun. Rev. **38**(2), 69–74 (2008)
7. Heresy, N.: The Scaling Implications of SDN. Network Heresy, pp. 13–30, 12 April 2016

Symmetry Group of Heat Transfer Flow in a Porous Medium

Tarik Amtout[✉], Mustapha Er-Riani, and Mustapha el Jarroudi

Department of Mathematics, Faculty of Sciences and Techniques, LMA,
BP 416, ancienne route de l'aéroport, km 10 Ziaten, 90000 Tangier, Morocco
tareqfstt@gmail.com
erriani@yahoo.fr
eljarroudi@hotmail.com

Abstract. In this paper, the symmetry group is performed for the heat transfer flow in a porous medium, this flow is described by coupled partial differential equations. Thanks to the method of the symmetry group, the symmetries of the coupled equations are given. The similarity variables and reduction equations generated from the symmetry transformations are provided. Such similarity reductions are computed and exact solutions are given such solutions are important in engineering applications and on the theory of nonlinear science.

Keywords: Symmetry group · Nonlinear partial differential equations · Computer-algebra · Heat transfer · Porous medium

1 Introduction

In recent years, one of the basic tools available to the engineering is approximate methods such as finite differences, finite element,..., have been developed considerably for nonlinear partial differential equations. These methods require a great amount of time and memory due to the discretization and usually the effect of round-off error causes loss of accuracy in the results. So recently considerable attention has been directed toward analytical solutions of nonlinear partial differential equations and one of the most famous methods is a symmetry group also called Lie group theory due to Sophus Lie is the first who developed and applied this theory to solve differential equations in the 19th century.

His approach has made a fundamental contribution to the study of the solvability of ordinary differential equations and the search for particular solutions to partial differential equations. One of Lie's strong ideas was to consider the transformations that constitute a continuous dependent group of one or more parameters and to show that these transformations are perfectly characterized by their linear part. The symmetry group of a system of differential equations or partial derivatives, we mean linear or nonlinear transformations that maps a solution of this system to another. It is a method that requires only algebraic calculations whose main difficulty is the size which grows rapidly with the number of independent variables, dependent variables and equations studied.

© Springer Nature Switzerland AG 2019
M. Ezziyyani (Ed.): AI2SD 2018, AISC 915, pp. 545–557, 2019.
https://doi.org/10.1007/978-3-030-11928-7_49

Although all the building blocks of the theory and its effective application were posited from the beginning of the century, the application to partial differential equations dates back only to the 1950s. Since then, the study of symmetry groups of PDEs has been reintroduced and applied to different equations of physics thanks to the school under the leadership of Olver [8], Ovsiannikov [9], Ames [1], Birkhoff [4] and Stephani [10] participated in the renewed interest in theory and its applications.

For the large applications of this theory in engineering and physics [1], we applied the symmetry group to study the heat transfer and fluid flow in porous medium that involves several applications in several engineering fields. For example:

- Combustion processes and conversion methods.
- Insulation of buildings and equipment, mechanical devices.
- Energy storage, geothermal reservoirs, nuclear waste disposal and chemical reactor engineering.

Among the works that have used the symmetry groups in a porous medium, we can mention, Lee et al. [6], they have investigated by the simplified Lie group analysis namely scaling group of the natural convection heat transfer flow past an inclined plate embedded in a fluid saturated porous medium. Afify et al. [3], they have used a scaling group of transformations to obtain the reduction equations and are then solved numerically a steady two-dimensional double-diffusive free convection boundary layer flow in a porous medium.

In the work published by Amtout et al. [2] have performed a preliminary group classification of equations governing the flow of a thermodependent fluid in a porous medium and they demonstrate that the form of arbitrary functions admits an extension of this algebra. Based on this paper [2] and taking the two arbitrary functions, thermal conductivity and viscosity as constant, the symmetry group governing the heat transfer is determined.

The outline of this work is as follows: In Sect. 2, we give a brief description of the symmetry group method. In the third Sect. 3 we give the governing equations relating to the heat transfer in a porous medium and the problem is formulated as a system of coupled partial differential equations. Section 4 is devoted to computing the symmetry group and determining the vector generators. In the last Sect. 5 we deal with similarity transformations of equations using symmetry group and provide all possible reductions equations with their exact solutions if it is possible.

2 Brief Description of Symmetry Group Method

The method see([8] and [10]) of calculating the symmetry groups is based on the prolongation of a vector field. We consider the nth order differential equation in p independent variables $x = (x_1, \ldots, x_p)$ and q dependent variables $u = (u_1, \ldots, u_q)$

$$\Delta\left(x, u^{(n)}\right) = \Delta_i\left(x, u^{(n)}\right) ,$$

where $u^{(n)}$ are all nth order partial derivatives of u with respect to x.
Consider the continuous transformation group G of one-parameter in x and u,

$$\bar{x}_i = X_i\,(x, u, \epsilon)\ for\ 1 \leq i \leq p\,,$$
$$\bar{u}_j = U_j\,(x, u, \epsilon)\ for\ 1 \leq j \leq q\,.$$

The research groups of symmetry of a system of differential equations of nth order locally solvable and of maximal rank are done by the following steps:

– In the first step we must calculate the prolongation $Pr^{(n)}\mathbf{V}\,(\Delta)$ for a generator

$$\mathbf{V} = \sum_{i=1}^{p} X_i\,(x, u)\, \frac{\partial}{\partial x_i} + \sum_{j=1}^{q} U_j\,(x, u)\, \frac{\partial}{\partial u^j}\,,$$

a priori unknown.
The prolongation formula is given by:

$$Pr^{(k)}\mathbf{V} = \mathbf{V} + \sum_{\substack{j=1 \\ 1 \leq |\mu| \leq k}}^{p} U^{j,\mu} \frac{\partial}{\partial u_\mu^j}\,,$$

where $U^{j,\mu}$ is given by

$$U^{j,\mu} = D_\mu \left(U^j - \sum_{i=1}^{p} X_i u_{\delta(i)}^j \right) + \sum_{i=1}^{p} X_i U_{\mu+\delta(i)}^j\,.$$

The continuous transformation group G associated with the generator $\mathbf{V}$ is a symmetry group for the differential system if and only if

$$Pr^{(n)}\mathbf{V}\,(\Delta) = 0\quad \text{wherever}\quad \Delta = 0\,.$$

– In the second step it must then express higher order derivatives based on derivatives of lower order taking into account the system $\Delta = 0$.
– In the third step by injecting the derivative in the condition of invariance $Pr^{(n)}\mathbf{V}\,(\Delta)$ we obtain the determining equations.
– In the last step it must be solved the determining equations.

The use of a symbolic system is essential since the resolution and the manipulation of the determining equations by hand is tedious, so we had forced ourselves to use systems of symbolic computation, several programs were developed, these last years, which allow the resolution of these systems, among these programs we can mention: Desolv [5] developed by Carminati et al., this program contains some routines which will automatically generate and attempt to integrate the determining equations for the Lie symmetries of differential equations.

3   Mathematical Formulation

We consider the flow of Newtonian fluid through a porous medium [7], governed by the equations:

$$\nabla . \mathbf{v} = 0 \, , \tag{1}$$

$$\mathbf{v} = -\frac{K}{\mu} \nabla . p \, , \tag{2}$$

$$\nabla T . \mathbf{v} = \nabla . (\alpha \nabla T) \, , \tag{3}$$

where $\mathbf{v}$ is the vector de Darcy velocity and K is the permeability of the porous medium. The dependent variables $p(x, y)$ and $T(x, y)$ are the pressure and temperature field respectively. The independent variables x and y are the Cartesian coordinates, α and μ are the thermal conductivity and viscosity parameters respectively. Recall that the permeability measures the ability of a porous material to allow the fluids to move through it. K depends only on the geometry of the medium and not on the characteristics of the fluid. In the following, K is assumed to be constant.

Henceforth, the continuity equation (3) become

$$\frac{\partial u}{\partial x} + \frac{\partial v}{\partial y} = 0 \, . \tag{4}$$

Using (2), the fluid velocity in x and y directions are respectively

– **Velocity in horizontal direction:**

$$u = -\frac{K}{\mu} \frac{\partial p}{\partial x} \, . \tag{5}$$

– **Velocity in vertical direction:**

$$v = -\frac{K}{\mu} \left(\frac{\partial p}{\partial y} + \rho g \right) \, . \tag{6}$$

The variation of density with respect to temperature can be described by Boussinesq approximation as

$$\rho = \rho_\infty \left(1 - \beta_T (T - T_\infty) \right) \, , \tag{7}$$

where ρ_∞ is the fluid density at some reference temperature T_∞ and the β_T is the coefficient of thermal expansion.

The above equations have pressure terms in the respective direction in order to facilitate the solution, these terms can be eliminated by mathematical operations.

Differentiating equation (5) with respect to y yields

$$\frac{\partial u}{\partial y} = -\frac{K}{\mu}\frac{\partial^2 p}{\partial x \partial y} .$$ (8)

Similarly differentiating equation (6) with respect to x after incorporating Boussinesq approximation result

$$\frac{\partial v}{\partial x} = -\frac{K}{\mu}\left(\frac{\partial^2 p}{\partial x \partial y} - \rho_\infty \beta_T g \frac{\partial T}{\partial x}\right) .$$ (9)

Eliminating pressure from Eqs. (8) and (9) gives

$$\frac{\partial v}{\partial x} - \frac{\partial u}{\partial y} = \frac{gK\beta}{\nu}\frac{\partial T}{\partial x} ,$$ (10)

where $\nu = \frac{\mu}{\rho_\infty}$ and $\beta = \beta_T g$.

The energy equation (3) in (x, y) is given as

$$u\frac{\partial T}{\partial x} + v\frac{\partial T}{\partial y} = \alpha\left(\frac{\partial^2 T}{\partial x^2} + \frac{\partial^2 T}{\partial y^2}\right) .$$ (11)

The continuity equation (4) can be satisfied automatically by introducing the stream function ψ as

$$u = \frac{\partial \psi}{\partial y} ,$$ (12)

$$v = -\frac{\partial \psi}{\partial x} .$$ (13)

Equations (10) and (11) are the two governing partial differential equations in dimensional form with many variables. These equations can be non-dimensioned to reduce the number of variables and thus facilitate the solution.

The following non dimensional parameters are used to convert the above equations into a non dimensional form $\tilde{x} = \frac{x}{L}$, $\tilde{y} = \frac{y}{L}$, $\tilde{\psi} = \frac{\psi}{\alpha}$, $\tilde{\theta} = \frac{T-T_\infty}{T_w - T_\infty}$, $R_a = \frac{g\beta_T(T_w - T_\infty)KL}{\nu\alpha}$, where R_a is the Rayleigh number, which describes the relationship between momentum diffusivity and thermal conductivity.

Substitution of these relations into (10) and (11) and taken into account (12) and (13), we give raises to the following non-dimensional equations after dropping tildes.

$$\frac{\partial^2 \psi}{\partial x^2} + \frac{\partial^2 \psi}{\partial y^2} = -R_a \frac{\partial \theta}{\partial x} ,$$ (14)

$$\frac{\partial \psi}{\partial y}\frac{\partial \theta}{\partial x} - \frac{\partial \psi}{\partial x}\frac{\partial \theta}{\partial y} = \frac{\partial^2 \theta}{\partial x^2} + \frac{\partial^2 \theta}{\partial y^2} .$$ (15)

Equations (14) and (15) are two coupled partial differential equations as change of a variable in one equation affect the other equation.

4 Symmetry Groups

In this section, we perform the classical Lie group method of (14)–(15). Consider a one-parameter Lie group of infinitesimal transformations acting on the independent and dependent variables of the system (14)–(15),

$$x \rightarrow x + \epsilon \xi_1 (x, y, \psi, \theta) \ ,$$

$$y \rightarrow y + \epsilon \xi_2 (x, y, \psi, \theta) \ ,$$

$$\psi \rightarrow \psi + \epsilon \eta_1 (x, y, \psi, \theta) \ ,$$

$$\theta \rightarrow \theta + \epsilon \eta_2 (x, y, \psi, \theta) \ ,$$

(16)

with a small parameter $\epsilon \ll 1$ and where ξ_1, ξ_2 and η_1, η_2 are the unknowns infinitesimals functions of the transformations for the independent and dependent variables, respectively.

The infinitesimal generator $\mathbf{V}$ associated with the above group of transformations can be written as

$$\mathbf{V} = \xi_1 (x, y, \psi, \theta) \frac{\partial}{\partial x} + \xi_2 (x, y, \psi, \theta) \frac{\partial}{\partial y}$$

$$+ \eta_1 (x, y, \psi, \theta) \frac{\partial}{\partial \psi} + \eta_2 (x, y, \psi, \theta) \frac{\partial}{\partial \theta} \ .$$

(17)

We then set

$$\Delta_1 = \frac{\partial^2 \psi}{\partial x^2} + \frac{\partial^2 \psi}{\partial y^2} + R_a \frac{\partial \theta}{\partial x} \ ,$$

(18)

$$\Delta_2 = \frac{\partial^2 \theta}{\partial x^2} + \frac{\partial^2 \theta}{\partial y^2} - \frac{\partial \psi}{\partial y} \frac{\partial \theta}{\partial x} + \frac{\partial \psi}{\partial x} \frac{\partial \theta}{\partial y} \ .$$

(19)

The generator (17) generates a one-parameter symmetry group of Eqs. (18)–(19), if and only if the invariance conditions holds, since the system has at most second-order derivatives, we prolong the infinitesimal generator $\mathbf{V}$ to the second order in the following form

$$Pr^{(2)} \mathbf{V} (\Delta_i) |_{\Delta_i = 0} = 0; \ \text{for } i = 1, 2 \ .$$

(20)

We act on (18)–(19) with the second prolongation of the operator $\mathbf{V}$ and this is given by

$$Pr^{(2)} (\mathbf{V}) = \mathbf{V} + \varsigma_1^x \frac{\partial}{\partial \psi_x} + \varsigma_1^y \frac{\partial}{\partial \psi_y} + \varsigma_2^x \frac{\partial}{\partial \theta_x} + \varsigma_2^y \frac{\partial}{\partial \theta_y}$$

$$+ \varsigma_1^{xx} \frac{\partial}{\partial \psi_{xx}} + \varsigma_1^{yy} \frac{\partial}{\partial \psi_{yy}} + \varsigma_2^{xx} \frac{\partial}{\partial \theta_{xx}} + \varsigma_2^{yy} \frac{\partial}{\partial \theta_{yy}} \ ,$$

where the coefficient functions of the extended infinitesimals ς_j^i, $i = x, y$; $j = 1, 2$, are explicitly given by

$$\varsigma_1^x = D_x(\eta_1) - \psi_x D_x(\xi_1) - \psi_y D_x(\xi_2) ,$$

$$\varsigma_1^y = D_y(\eta_1) - \psi_x D_y(\xi_1) - \psi_y D_y(\xi_2) ,$$

$$\varsigma_2^x = D_x(\eta_2) - \theta_x D_x(\xi_1) - \theta_y D_x(\xi_2) ,$$

$$\varsigma_2^y = D_y(\eta_2) - \theta_x D_y(\xi_1) - \theta_y D_y(\xi_2) ,$$

$$\varsigma_1^{xx} = D_x(\varsigma_1^x) - \psi_{xx} D_x(\xi_1) - \psi_{xy} D_x(\xi_2) ,$$

$$\varsigma_1^{yy} = D_y(\varsigma_1^y) - \psi_{xy} D_y(\xi_1) - \psi_{yy} D_y(\xi_2) ,$$

$$\varsigma_2^{xx} = D_x(\varsigma_2^x) - \theta_{xx} D_x(\xi_1) - \theta_{xy} D_x(\xi_2) ,$$

$$\varsigma_2^{yy} = D_y(\varsigma_2^y) - \theta_{xy} D_y(\xi_1) - \theta_{yy} D_y(\xi_2) ,$$

The total derivative operators are defined as

$$D_x = \frac{\partial}{\partial x} + \psi_x \frac{\partial}{\partial \psi} + \psi_{xx} \frac{\partial}{\partial \psi_x} + \theta_x \frac{\partial}{\partial \theta} + \theta_{xx} \frac{\partial}{\partial \theta_x} + \psi_{xy} \frac{\partial}{\partial \psi_y} + \theta_{xy} \frac{\partial}{\partial \theta_y} .$$

$$D_y = \frac{\partial}{\partial y} + \psi_y \frac{\partial}{\partial \psi} + \psi_{yy} \frac{\partial}{\partial \psi_y} + \theta_y \frac{\partial}{\partial \theta} + \theta_{yy} \frac{\partial}{\partial \theta_y} + \psi_{xy} \frac{\partial}{\partial \psi_x} + \theta_{xy} \frac{\partial}{\partial \theta_x} .$$

The employment of the second prolongation $Pr^{(2)}$ onto (18) and (19) yields the following determining equations

$$\varsigma_1^{xx} + \varsigma_1^{yy} + R_a \varsigma_2^x = 0 ,$$

$$\varsigma_2^{xx} + \varsigma_2^{yy} - \theta_x \varsigma_1^y + \theta_y \varsigma_1^x = 0 . \tag{21}$$

The invariance condition (21) results in an over-determined linear system of determining equations for the coefficients ξ_1, ξ_2, η_1 and η_2. Manipulation of these determining equations is very tedious. In order to decrease the number of calculations, we take advantage of a computer algebra system to solve these set of over-determining equations.

Thus, we have obtained the following determining equations:

$$\frac{\partial}{\partial\theta}\xi_1 = 0\,, \qquad \frac{\partial}{\partial\psi}\xi_1 = 0\,, \quad \frac{\partial}{\partial x}\xi_1 = -\frac{\partial}{\partial\theta}\eta_2\,,$$

$$\frac{\partial}{\partial\theta}\xi_2 = 0\,, \qquad \frac{\partial}{\partial\psi}\xi_2 = 0\,, \quad \frac{\partial}{\partial x}\xi_2 = 0\,,$$

$$\frac{\partial}{\partial y}\xi_2 = -\frac{\partial}{\partial\theta}\eta_2\,, \quad \frac{\partial}{\partial\psi}\eta_2 = 0\,, \quad \frac{\partial}{\partial x}\eta_2 = 0\,,$$

$$\frac{\partial}{\partial y}\eta_2 = 0\,, \qquad \frac{\partial^2}{\partial\theta^2}\eta_2 = 0\,, \quad \frac{\partial}{\partial\theta}\eta_1 = 0\,,$$

$$\frac{\partial}{\partial\psi}\eta_1 = 0\,, \qquad \frac{\partial}{\partial x}\eta_1 = 0\,, \quad \frac{\partial}{\partial y}\eta_1 = 0\,.$$

Solving the above equations, we obtain

$$\xi_1 = -c_1 x + c_4\,, \quad \xi_2 = -c_1 y + c_5\,,$$

$$\eta_1 = c_3\,, \qquad\qquad \eta_2 = c_1\theta + c_2\,,$$

where c_i for $i = 1,\ldots,5$ are arbitrary constants.

Thus the Lie algebra of infinitesimal symmetries of (18)–(19) is spanned by the following linearly independent vector generators

$$\mathbf{V_1} = -x\frac{\partial}{\partial x} - y\frac{\partial}{\partial y} + \theta\frac{\partial}{\partial\theta}\,, \quad \mathbf{V_2} = \frac{\partial}{\partial\theta}\,, \mathbf{V_3} = \frac{\partial}{\partial\psi}\,, \quad \mathbf{V_4} = \frac{\partial}{\partial x}\,, \quad \mathbf{V_5} = \frac{\partial}{\partial y}\,.$$

It is easy to verify that $\{\mathbf{V}_1, \mathbf{V}_2, \mathbf{V}_3, \mathbf{V}_4, \mathbf{V}_5\}$ is closed under the Lie bracket $[\ ,\ ]$.

In fact, we have

Table 1. Commutations relations for the Lie algebra $\{\mathbf{V}_i\}$ for $i = 1,\ldots,5$

$[\ ,\ ]$	$\mathbf{V}_1$	$\mathbf{V}_2$	$\mathbf{V}_3$	$\mathbf{V}_4$	$\mathbf{V}_5$
$\mathbf{V}_1$	0	$-\mathbf{V}_2$	0	$\mathbf{V}_4$	$\mathbf{V}_5$
$\mathbf{V}_2$	$\mathbf{V}_2$	0	0	0	0
$\mathbf{V}_3$	0	0	0	0	0
$\mathbf{V}_4$	$-\mathbf{V}_4$	0	0	0	0
$\mathbf{V}_5$	$-\mathbf{V}_5$	0	0	0	0

In Table 1, we see that the Lie bracket is skew symmetric that is, $[\mathbf{V}_i, \mathbf{V}_j] = -[\mathbf{V}_j, \mathbf{V}_i]$ for any two Lie algebra vector $\mathbf{V}_i$ and $\mathbf{V}_j$ and the diagonal elements are all zero.

Thus, the corresponding one-parameter groups G_i generated by the $\mathbf{V}_i$, $(i = 1, \ldots, 5)$, are computed by solving the Lie equations

$$\frac{d\bar{x}}{d\epsilon} = \xi_1\left(\bar{x}, \bar{y}, \bar{\psi}, \bar{\theta}\right) \ , \quad \frac{d\bar{y}}{d\epsilon} = \xi_2\left(\bar{x}, \bar{y}, \bar{\psi}, \bar{\theta}\right) \ ,$$

$$\frac{d\bar{\psi}}{d\epsilon} = \eta_1\left(\bar{x}, \bar{y}, \bar{\psi}, \bar{\theta}\right) \ , \quad \frac{d\bar{\theta}}{d\epsilon} = \eta_2\left(\bar{x}, \bar{y}, \bar{\psi}, \bar{\theta}\right) \ ,$$

Subject to the initial conditions

$$\bar{x}|_{\epsilon=0} = x \ , \quad \bar{y}|_{\epsilon=0} = y \ ,$$

$$\bar{\psi}|_{\epsilon=0} = \psi \ , \quad \bar{\theta}|_{\epsilon=0} = \theta \ .$$

By solving this system of ordinary differential equations, we obtain the following groups of symmetry generated by $\mathbf{V}_i$ for $i = 1, \ldots, 5$:

$$G_1 : \quad (x, y, \psi, \theta) \rightarrow (e^{-\epsilon}x, e^{-\epsilon}y, \psi, e^{\epsilon}\theta) \ ,$$

$$G_2 : \quad (x, y, \psi, \theta) \rightarrow (x, y, \psi, \theta + \epsilon) \ ,$$

$$G_3 : \quad (x, y, \psi, \theta) \rightarrow (x, y, \psi + \epsilon, \theta) \ ,$$

$$G_4 : \quad (x, y, \psi, \theta) \rightarrow (x + \epsilon, y, \psi, \theta) \ ,$$

$$G_5 : \quad (x, y, \psi, \theta) \rightarrow (x, y + \epsilon, \psi, \theta) \ ,$$

where ϵ is any real number.

We can see that G_1 is a scaling transformation, G_2 is a dependent variable translation, G_3 is a dependent variable translation, G_4 is a space translation along the coordinate x and G_5 is a space translation along the coordinate y.

5   Similarity Transformations and Exact Solutions

In the preceding section, we obtained the symmetry groups of (18)–(19). Now we will consider the exact solutions of this coupled system of equations based on the symmetry group. Since each G_i $(i = 1, \ldots, 5)$ is a one-parameter group, it implies that if $\psi = f(x, y)$ and $\theta = g(x, y)$ is the known solutions of (18)–(19), then by using the above groups G_i $(i = 1, \ldots, 5)$, the corresponding new solutions $\psi^{(i)}$ and $\theta^{(i)}$ $(i = 1, \ldots, 5)$ can be obtained respectively as follows:

$$\psi^{(1)} = f(e^{-\epsilon}x, e^{-\epsilon}y) \ , \quad \theta^{(1)} = e^{\epsilon}g(e^{-\epsilon}x, e^{-\epsilon}y) \ ,$$

$$\psi^{(2)} = f(x, y) \ , \quad \theta^{(2)} = g(x, y) + \epsilon \ ,$$

$$\psi^{(3)} = f(x, y) + \epsilon \ , \quad \theta^{(3)} = g(x, y) \ ,$$

$$\psi^{(4)} = f(x + \epsilon, y) \ , \quad \theta^{(4)} = g(x + \epsilon, y) \ ,$$

$$\psi^{(5)} = f(x, y + \epsilon) \ , \quad \theta^{(5)} = g(x, y + \epsilon) \ ,$$

where ϵ is any real number.

In the following, we derive symmetry reductions of (14)–(15) associated with the vector generators V_i $(i = 1, \ldots, 5)$, by using similarity variables and we will calculate the reduced equation and determining exact solutions if it is possible.

We distinguish the following cases.

Reduction with V_1: In this case, the corresponding characteristic system is given by

$$\frac{dx}{-x} = \frac{dy}{-y} = \frac{d\psi}{0} = \frac{d\theta}{\theta} . \tag{22}$$

Solving (22) lead to the invariants

$$I_1 = \frac{y}{x} , \quad I_2 = \psi , \quad I_3 = x\theta .$$

Therefore, the invariant solutions takes the form

$$F(r) = \psi, \quad G(r) = x\theta , \tag{23}$$

where $r = \frac{y}{x}$ is the similarity variable.

Substituting (23) into (14)–(15), we obtain the following ordinary differential equations:

$$\left(1 + r^2\right) F''(r) + 2rF'(r) - R_a \left(G(r) + G'(r)\right) = 0 ,$$

$$\left(1 + r^2\right) G''(r) + 4rG'(r) + 2G(r) + F'(r) G(r) = 0 .$$

Here $'$ prime denotes differentiation with respect to r.

By using the similarity transformations, we switched from an EDP system to a lower order system. We can also for boundary conditions solve the reduced equations by a numerical or analytical methods.

Reduction with V_2: In this case, the corresponding characteristic system is given by

$$\frac{dx}{0} = \frac{dy}{0} = \frac{d\psi}{0} = \frac{d\theta}{1} . \tag{24}$$

Solving (24) lead to the invariants

$$I_1 = x , \quad I_2 = y , \quad I_3 = \psi , \quad I_4 = \theta .$$

Therefore, the invariant solutions takes the form

$$F(r_1, r_2) = \psi , \quad G(r_1, r_2) = \theta , \tag{25}$$

where $r_1 = x$ and $r_2 = y$ are the similarity variables.

Substituting (25) into (14)–(15), we obtain the following equations:

$$\frac{\partial^2 F}{\partial r_1^2} + \frac{\partial^2 F}{\partial r_2^2} + R_a \frac{\partial G}{\partial r_1} = 0 .$$

$$\frac{\partial^2 G}{\partial r_1^2} + \frac{\partial^2 G}{\partial r_2^2} - \frac{\partial F}{\partial r_2} \frac{\partial G}{\partial r_1} + \frac{\partial F}{\partial r_1} \frac{\partial G}{\partial r_2} = 0 .$$

Reduction with $\mathbf{V}_3$: In this case, the corresponding characteristic system is given by

$$\frac{dx}{0} = \frac{dy}{0} = \frac{d\psi}{1} = \frac{d\theta}{0} . \tag{26}$$

Solving (26) lead to the invariants

$$I_1 = x , \quad I_2 = y , \quad I_3 = \psi , \quad I_4 = \theta .$$

Therefore, the invariant solutions takes the form

$$F(r_1, r_2) = \psi , \quad G(r_1, r_2) = \theta , \tag{27}$$

where $r_1 = x$ and $r_2 = y$ are the similarity variables.

Substituting (27) into (14)–(15), we obtain the following equations:

$$\frac{\partial^2 F}{\partial r_1^2} + \frac{\partial^2 F}{\partial r_2^2} + R_a \frac{\partial G}{\partial r_1} = 0 .$$

$$\frac{\partial^2 G}{\partial r_1^2} + \frac{\partial^2 G}{\partial r_2^2} - \frac{\partial F}{\partial r_2} \frac{\partial G}{\partial r_1} + \frac{\partial F}{\partial r_1} \frac{\partial G}{\partial r_2} = 0 .$$

Reduction with $\mathbf{V}_4$: In this case, the corresponding characteristic system is given by

$$\frac{dx}{1} = \frac{dy}{0} = \frac{d\psi}{0} = \frac{d\theta}{0} . \tag{28}$$

Solving (28) lead to the invariants

$$I_1 = y , \quad I_2 = \psi , \quad I_3 = \theta .$$

Therefore, the invariant solutions takes the form

$$F(r) = \psi , \quad G(r) = \theta , \tag{29}$$

where $r = y$ is the similarity variable.

Substituting (29) into (14)–(15), we obtain the following ordinary differential equations:

$$F''(r) = 0 ,$$

$$G''(r) = 0 .$$

In this case, we obtain the following exact solutions by integration.

$$\psi(y) = c_1 y + c_2 ,$$

$$\theta(y) = c_1 y + c_2 ,$$

where c_1 and c_2 are arbitrary constants.

Reduction with $\mathbf{V}_5$: In this case, the corresponding characteristic system is given by

$$\frac{dx}{0} = \frac{dy}{1} = \frac{d\psi}{0} = \frac{d\theta}{0} . \tag{30}$$

Solving (30) lead to the invariants

$$I_1 = x , \quad I_2 = \psi , \quad I_3 = \theta .$$

Therefore, the invariant solutions takes the form

$$F(r) = \psi , \qquad G(r) = \theta , \tag{31}$$

where $r = x$ is the similarity variable.

Substituting (31) into (14)–(15), we obtain the following ordinary differential equations:

$$F''(r) + R_a G'(r) = 0 .$$

$$G''(r) = 0 .$$

As the previous example Case.4, the exact solutions are found by integration.

$$\psi(x) = -\tfrac{1}{2} c_3 R_a x^2 - R_a c_4 x + c_1 x + c_2 ,$$

$$\theta(x) = c_3 x + c_4 ,$$

where c_1, c_2, c_3 and c_4 are arbitrary constants.

6   Conclusion

We have calculated the symmetry group for heat transfer in a porous medium and we have searched the algebraic structure of the governing equations. And we have reduced partial differential equations to ordinary differential equations, for the giving boundary conditions the reduced equations can be solved numerically or analytically or the similarity solutions can serve as benchmarks in the design, accuracy testing, and comparison of numerical algorithms. It can be seen that the symmetry group is an effective method for studying coupled nonlinear partial differential equations.

References

1. Ames, W.F.: Nonlinear Partial Differential Equations in Engineering, vol. 18, 1st edn. Academic Press (1965)
2. Amtout, T., Er-Riani, M., El Jarroudi, M., Cheikhi, A.: Preliminary group classification for the flow of a thermodependent fluid in porous medium. Int. J. Nonlin. Mech. **104**, 19–27 (2018)
3. Afify, A.A., Uddinc, Md.J.: Lie symmetry analysis of a double-diffusive free convective slip flow with a convective boundary condition past a radiating vertical surface embedded in a porous medium. J. Appl. Mech. Tech. Phys. **5**(57), 925–936 (2016)
4. Birkhoff, G.: Hydrodynamics. Princeton University Press (1960)

5. Carminati, J., Vu, K.: Symbolic computation and differential equations: Lie symmetries. J. Symb. Comput. **29**, 95–116 (2000)
6. Lee, J., Kandaswamy, P., Bhuvaneswari, M., Sivasankaran, S.: Lie group analysis of radiation natural convection heat transfer past an inclined porous surface. J. Mech. Sci. Technol. **22**, 1779–1784 (2008)
7. Nield, D.A., Bejan, A.: Convection in Porous Media, 4th edn. Springer (2013)
8. Olver, P.J.: Applications of Lie Groups to Differential Equations, 2nd edn. Springer (1993)
9. Ovsiannikov, L.V.: Group Analysis of Differential Equations, 1st edn. Academic Press (1982)
10. Stephani, H.: Differential Equations: Their Solution Using Symmetries, 1st edn. Cambridge University Press (1989)

Using Fractal Dimension to Check Similarity Between Mandelbrot and Julia Sets in Misiurewicz Points

Ouahiba Boussoufi[✉], Kaoutar Lamrini Uahabi,
and Mohamed Atounti

Laboratory of Applied Mathematics and Information (MASI), Multidisciplinary
Faculty of Nador, University Mohammed First, Oujda, Morocco
ouahibabsf@gmail.com, lamrinika@yahoo.fr,
atounti@hotmail.fr

Abstract. Checking the similarity of some Julia sets and Mandelbrot sub areas
in Misiurewicz points by calculating their fractal dimension is the main purpose
of this paper. MATLAB programs are used to generate the Julia sets images that
match the Misiurewicz points; these images are the entry to the FracLac software.
Using this software we were able to find different measurements that characterize
those fractals in textures and other features. We are actually focusing on fractal
dimension and the error calculated by the software. When performing the given
equation of regression or the logarithmic slope of an image, a Box Counting
method is applied to the entire image, and the chosen features (grid design,
scaling method, number of grid positions…) are available in a FracLac Program,
then we attempt to prepare the appropriate settings to get the best performance of
the software. Finally, a comparison is done for each image corresponding to the
area (boundary) where the Misiurewicz point is located.

Keywords: Box counting · FracLac · Fractal dimension

1 Introduction

This paper is about a comparison between fractal dimension of Mandelbrot set and that
of Julia sets in Misiurewicz points using FracLac software. In order to calculate each
fractal dimension, we use MATLAB software to generate some images associating to
each parameter c (by varying a parameter c).

First, we introduce Julia and Fatou sets, then that of Mandelbrot. Second, we define
what is Misiurewicz point where we are going to calculate a fractal dimension for each
image associated with a given value of that point. Finally, we summarize what we
obtained as tables to both sets and discuss found results.

1.1 Julia and Fatou Sets

In the plane of complex numbers, we can obtain Julia set [1] by a simple iteration from
the polynomial:

© Springer Nature Switzerland AG 2019
M. Ezziyyani (Ed.): AI2SD 2018, AISC 915, pp. 558–566, 2019.
https://doi.org/10.1007/978-3-030-11928-7_50

$$z_{n+1} = z_n^2 + c \tag{1}$$

For a fixed value of c, the behavior of the sequence is evaluated.

The point's z for which the sequence is bounded form the set of filled Julia associated with the point c. The Julia set denoted by J_c is the boundary of the previous set while the interior is called Fatou set [2].

In [3], we can find the three definitions below:

The filled in Julia set of the function f is defined as

$$K(f) = \{z \in C : f^k(z) \to \infty\} \tag{2}$$

The Julia set of the function f is defined to be the boundary of

$$K(f) \text{ i.e. } J(f) = \partial K(f) \tag{3}$$

The Fatou set of f is defined to be the complement of K (f) i.e.

$$F(f) = \mathbb{C} \backslash K(f) \tag{4}$$

In some cases, the points are gathered in a single connected surface, whereas for other values of c it is formed of isolated points and we say that the set is non-connected [4].

The Julia set is a disconnected set if, and only if, the iteration of the critical point 0 leads to infinity (in absolute value) [5].

The Julia set is one piece (connected) if, and only if, the iteration of the critical point 0 is bounded. E.g. of this case (see Fig. 1) [5].

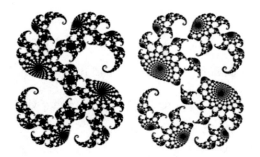

Fig. 1. A connected and disconnected Julia set

For our study we are interesting in the connected case of Julia set because it is the one who is contained in Mandelbrot set, which makes the comparison appropriate if not disconnected Julia set escape to infinity.

1.2   Mandelbrot Set

There are as many sets of Julia as there are complex numbers, Mandelbrot who had discovered this set, studied Julia's sets, that leads him to create the set: $M = \{c \in \mathbb{C} :$ Jc is connected$\}$ [6].

The Mandelbrot set can be generated using the same polynomial (1). This time, we set the point $z_0 = 0$ and evaluating the behavior of the sequence of iterations for each number c of the plane. If the sequence is bounded, point c is part of M. Moreover, the position of a parameter gives us some properties of its associated Julia sets. In [4], Douady and Hubbard gave him the Mandelbrot set name.

We can understand the similarity of Julia sets and Mandelbrot set in neighborhood of some points that are called Misiurewicz points.

1.3   Misiurewicz Points

Misiurewicz points constitute infinity of points that lie within the boundary of the Mandelbrot set where Julia sets are asymptotically self-similar with the Mandelbrot set [2]. This means that if the parameter c is a Misiurewicz point then the Julia set and the Mandelbrot set have the same shape except some rotation and scaling. They are parameters values where the critical orbits are strictly preperiodic [5]. A parameter c is a Misiurewicz point M_{k,n} if it satisfies the equations [7]:

$$f_c^{(k)}(z_{cr}) = f_c^{(k+n)}(z_{cr}) \tag{5}$$

And

$$f_c^{(k-1)}(z_{cr}) \neq f_c^{(k+n-1)}(z_{cr}) \tag{6}$$

So:

$$M_{k,n} = c : f_c^{(k)}(z_{cr}) = f_c^{(k+n)}(z_{cr}) \tag{7}$$

where, z_{cr} is a critical point of f_c, k and n are positive integers and f_c^k denotes the kth iterate of f_c.

Douady and Habbard [8, 9] proved that for c, a Misiurewicz point,

1. 0 and then c is eventually repulsive periodic
2. $K_c = J_c$ i.e. K_c has no interior

1.4   Similarity at Misiurewicz Point

If we take the Misiurewicz point $y = -0.1011 + 0.9563i$ we will find the both Julia set and Mandelbrot set almost identical [5] as shown in Fig. 2.

Near Misiurewicz points, [5] a copies of Mandelbrot set are revealed which explain the fact of self similarity of this set and the same thing for julia sets; the thing that couldn't be since both sets are expected to be closely similar, yet this similarity is thwarted by the results found on this work,

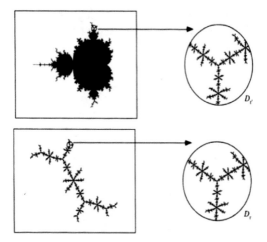

Fig. 2. Mandelbrot set for c = ɣ (top) and Julia set for c = ɣ(bottom)

2 Pretreatment and Preliminary Results

2.1 FracLac

FracLac [10] delivers a measure of complexity—a fractal dimension—called the box counting fractal dimension or D_B. It is measured from the ratio of increasing detail with increasing scale (ε). The ratio quantifies the increase in detail with increasing magnification or resolution seen in fractals but also in microscopy. The basic technique for calculating the D_B used in FracLac [10] is called box counting. The D_B is the slope of the regression line for the log-log plot of box size (or scale) and count from a box counting scan [11].

Some preparations are required on ImageJ and most image processing software can convert images to black and white, before a fractal dimension will be calculated. So, we convert the Julia sets **(matching each time to a specific Misiurewicz Points)** on binary image as shown below (Figures).

Why Binary image? The Image Type (binary or grayscale) affects how fractal dimensions are calculated. To summarize, a box counting fractal dimension (DB) is a scaling rule inferred from the relationship between the number of parts (N) counted in some pattern and the relative size (f) of the measuring thing used to count them. For instance, if we measured a line using a ruler the same length as the line then measured it again using a ruler 1/3 that length, f would be 1/3 since we multiplied the original pattern's size by 1/3 to get the measuring device's size. The general equation of a dimensional scaling rule is: $N = f^{-D}$.

The method used to calculate a fractal dimension is Box counting scaling which is based on the concept of 'covering' the binary image whether of fixed scaled box or scaling grid which is called overlapping scan. Here, both methods of Box counting are used to cover the image. Each method is characterized by a box size. The size of boxes necessary to cover the image is determined on function of the size of image.

Standard Error. The standard error for the regression line is the value which appears beside each fractal dimension in the results table.

How is the standard error calculated?

$$SE = \sqrt{\frac{\sum C^2 - b \sum C - m \sum SC}{n - 2}} \qquad (8)$$

S is the logarithm of scale or size, C is the logarithm of count, n is the number of sizes, b is the y-intercept of the regression line and m is the slope of the regression line.

How is the slope of the regression line calculated?

The slope of the regression line, used for calculating the D_B, is:

$$m = -\frac{n \sum SC - \sum S \sum C}{n \sum S^2 - (\sum S)^2} \qquad (9)$$

S is the logarithm of scale or size, C is the logarithm of count, n is the number of sizes, slope of the regression line.

How is the Y-intercept of the regression line calculated?

$$y\,int = \frac{\sum C - m \sum S}{n} \qquad (10)$$

S is the logarithm of scale or size, C is the logarithm of count, n is the number of sizes; m is the slope of the regression line [9].

2.2 Creating of Julia Sets at Misiurewics Points

See Figs. 3, 4, 5 and 6.

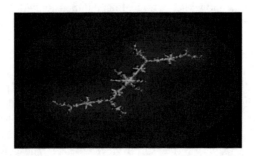

Fig. 3. Julia set associated to c = −0.10114 − 0.9563i

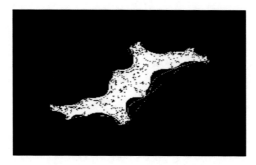

Fig. 4. Binary Julia set associated to c = −0.10114 − 0.9563i

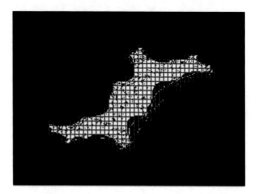

Fig. 5. Julia set associated to c = −0.10114 − 0.9563i covered with BC Method

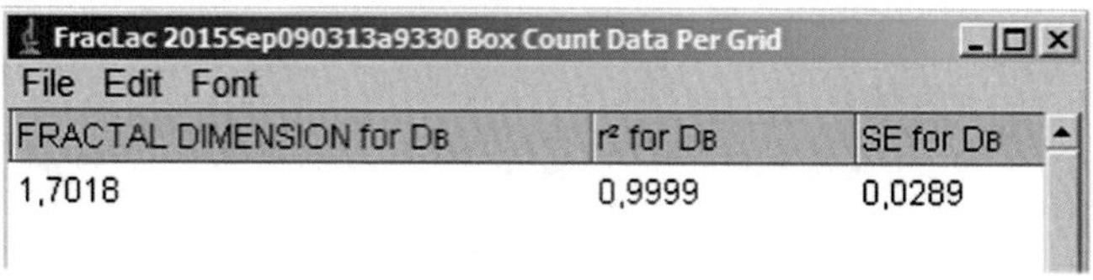

FracLac 2015Sep090313a9330 Box Count Data Per Grid		_ □ ×
File Edit Font		
FRACTAL DIMENSION for D$_B$	r² for D$_B$	SE for D$_B$
1,7018	0,9999	0,0289

Fig. 6. Fractal dimension obtained by FracLac of Julia set associated at c = −0.10114 − 0.9563i

2.3 Mandelbrot Set at Misiurewicz Points

See Figs. 7, 8 and 9.

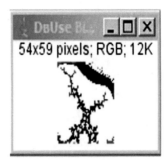

Fig. 7. Sub Area at Mandelbrot set in c = −0.10114 − 0.9563i

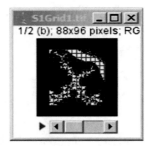

Fig. 8. Sub-Area of Mandelbrot set, c = −0.1011 4 − 0.9563i covered with BC method

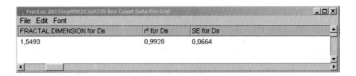

Fig. 9. Fractal dimension obtained by FracLac (using BC method) of Mandelbrot set associated with c = −0.10114 − 0.9563i

3 Results

See Tables 1 and 2.

Table 1. Summary of the calculated fractal dimension of Julia sets

Value of parameter c (Julia)	Fractal dimension D_B	Error calculated SE
−0.10114 − 0.9563i	1.7018	0.0289
−0.75	1.8167	0.0571
+0.25	1.7807	0.1324
−0.743643887037 + 0.131825904205330i	1.6482	0.0472
−0.74364386269 + 0.13182590271i	1.466	0.0442
+0.437089746625744 − 0.3440458692654341i	1.5299	0.0673

Table 2. Summary of the calculated fractal dimension of Mandelbrot sub areas

Value of parameter c (Mandelbrot)	Fractal dimension D_B	Error calculated SE
−0.10114 − 0.9563i	1.5493	0.0664
−0.75	1.6518	0.1028
+0.25	1.6184	0.0599
−0.743643887037 + 0.131825904205330i	1.7574	0.078
−0.74364386269 + 0.13182590271i	1.7682	0.0689
+0.437089746625744 − 0.3440458692654341i	1.6592	0.0586

4   Discussion

The main objective of this section is to give interpretations of the results found.

A fractal dimension is a ratio providing a statistical index of complexity comparing how detail in a pattern (strictly speaking, a fractal pattern) changes with the scale at which it is measured. Among the techniques discussed by Mandelbrot [12] the box counting method is also found like the most adapted for the estimation of fractal dimension; so we intended to use this technique in order to calculate a fractal dimension of each case of Julia and Mandelbrot sets associated each time to a specific value of a parameter c which consists on Misiurewicz point.

In Tables 1 and 2 we see that at c = −0.10114 − 0.9563i we have D_B = 1.5493 of Mandelbrot set and D_B = 1.7018 of Julia set, that differences of all D_B calculated here reflect how much the irregularity is between the same area (Misiurewicz point) which is considered as the area of similarity [13] of Julia and Mandelbrot sets, even the place where Julia is on the border of Mandelbrot set.

Since the Mandelbrot set is the connected Julia sets for each c in $\mathbb{C}$ that's prove that when we are chosen parameters c as Misiurewicz points that is for to be the Julia sets in the boundary of Mandelbrot set, i.e. when Julia sets and Mandelbrot are similar and their fractal dimension is equal to 2, as found in [14]. However the results above show that the Fractal Dimensions are not equal and couldn't be the same e.g. once the Julia set Fig. 3 at **c = −0.10114 − 0.9563i** is connected and Mandelbrot set at the same c form an island Fig. 7. In fact, it is in the particular case of fractal sets with strict auto-similarity [15], as the Sierpinski gasket, that all definitions of fractal dimension give identical results.

Our results can be interpreted as follows:

The difference seen between the two sets in the boundary of Mandelbrot set, where the Misiurewicz points are located, reveals that it is conceivable that these sub-sets should follow up some normalization and transformation to have equal dimension fractal.

Such normalization could give rise to drastic change of the both sets, the thing that could affect the integrity of the sets, we can in future work study this case and see the possible changes.

5 Conclusion

In the present paper, we performed a statistical analysis of most widespread Misiurewicz points that give a similar set of both Julia and Mandelbrot, in order to calculate their fractal dimension. We also proceed to show the difference between the two sets even in the boundary where the sets are supposed to have the same fractal dimension. We wish to find other properties of Misiurewicz points, which may be useful in this comparison.

References

1. Les fractales: Art, Nature et Modélisation, Tangente Hors-série no. 8, Editions Pôles (2004)
2. Milnor, J.: Self-similarity and hairiness in the Mandelbrot set. Comput. Geom. Topol. **114**, 211–257 (1989)
3. Fraser, J.: An Introduction to Julia Sets (2009)
4. Lajoie, J.: La géométrie fractale. Diss. Université du Québec à Trois-Rivières (2006)
5. Falconer, K.J.: Fractal Geometry: Mathematical Foundations and Applications, 2nd edn. Wiley, England (2004)
6. Peitgen, H.-O., Jürgens, H., Saupe, D.: Chaos and Fractals: New Frontiers of Science, 2nd edn. Springer, Science & Business Media, Verlag, New York (2006)
7. Lei, T.: Voisinages connexes des points de Misiurewicz. Annales de l'institut Fourier **42**(4), 707–735 (1992)
8. Douady, A., Hubbard, J.H.: Itération des pôlynomes quadratiques complexes. CRAS Paris **294**, 123–126 (1982)
9. Douady, A., Hubbard, J.H.: Etude dynamique des polynômes complexes. Part II. Publication mathématique d'Orsay, 85–02 (1985)
10. Fraclac Homepage: https://imagej.nih.gov/ij/plugins/fraclac/fraclac.html. Last accessed 23 July 2018
11. Karperien, A.: FracLac for ImageJ. http://rsb.info.nih.gov/ij/plugins/fraclac/FLHelp/Introduction.htm (1999–2013)
12. Mandelbrot, B.B., Pignoni, R.: The Fractal Geometry of Nature. Revised and enlarged ed. WH freeman and Co, New York (1983)
13. Lei, T.: Similarity between the Mandelbrot set and Julia sets. Commun. Math. Phys. **134**(3), 587–617 (1990)
14. Shishikura, M.: The Hausdorff dimension of the boundary of the Mandelbrot set and Julia sets. Ann. Math. **147**(2), 225–267 (1998)
15. Bézivin, J.-P.: on the Julia and Fatou sets of ultrametric entire functions. Annals de l'institut Fourier **51**(6), 1635–1661 (2001)

IoT Data-Based Architecture on OpenStack for Smart City

Chaimaa Ait Belahsen[✉], Abdelouahid Lyhyaoui,
and Nadia Boufardi

LTI Laboratory, National School of Applied Sciences,
Abdelmalek Essaadi University, BP 1818, Tangier, Morocco
{chaimaa.belahsen.cb,lyhyaoui,nadiabufardi}@gmail.com

Abstract. The integration of the Internet of things (IoT) with the power of Cloud Computing and the Big Data insight to build a Smart City is absolutely the main aim of this Article. From the point of view of most governments, adopting a Smart City concept in their cities by implementing Big Data applications, offers the potential for cities to obtain and reach the required level of development and sustainability. Cloud computing and IoT are two distinct technologies having wide applications in human life. Their acquisition and use are extremely pervasive, making them the future of the internet. Therefore, in this article we propose an IoT detailed, scalable and secured architecture on OpenStack: an open source platform for establishing public and private clouds, for the IoT data management, analyzing and processing from a raw data to an insight. Tangier as a fast-growing population city attending in 2017, 1 million people, will be our goal for implementing our smart applications by collecting from sensors enclosed to its infrastructure the data to treat. For this, we will use sensors deployment including smart parking, smart home, smart weather and water sensors… We are proposing an efficient and scalable architecture which gather all the IoT on the cloud workflow important components.

Keywords: Big data · Smart city · IoT · Cloud computing · OpenStack · Hadoop · Spark

1 Introduction

In 2010, the World Health Organization published a projection that urban population will almost double from 3.4 billion in 2009 to 6.4 billion in 2050. Modern cities are facing a critical growth and development. The use of technology and planning to re-think problems in cities, to become more effective in handling operations [1]. A Smart City invests in Information and Communications Technology (ICT) to invest in appropriate public service and transportation, to ensure sustainable socio-economic development, furthermore enhance the quality-of-life and intelligent management of natural resources [2]. This Article reviews the power and potentials of combining the IoT with cloud using Big Data technologies which drive a city to be smart. In the IoT, all that is real becomes virtual: each person and thing has a locatable, addressable, and readable counterpart in the Internet. Objects can produce and consume services and

© Springer Nature Switzerland AG 2019
M. Ezziyyani (Ed.): AI2SD 2018, AISC 915, pp. 567–577, 2019.
https://doi.org/10.1007/978-3-030-11928-7_51

collaborate with other counterparts toward a common goal. Cloud computing considered as a practice using the network for computing and remoting servers hosted on the Internet to store, manage, and process data. Cloud and IoT are two distinct technologies of the future internet which are included already in our daily life. Big Data is defined as a large and unstructured set of data coming from everywhere: sensors used for gathering climate information, posts to social media sites, digital pictures and videos... Integrating IoT with cloud services to get real-time city data and then processing such big amount of data in an efficient way to establish a Smart City, is a challenging task. The idea is to start by investigating the visibility of the city by gathering data from all networks, devices, sensors enclosed in its infrastructure, then it comes the role of the Big Data computing and advanced Big data analytics to make the collected data valuable, such as passing the data by different processing stages. Through this research, a Multi-Level IoT in the cloud architecture is proposed based on OpenStack components. Our proposed architecture is describing the IoT indispensable layers and OpenStack services integrated in each IoT layer.

The research done by [3], discusses the IoT layers from perception to business, and the issues and challenges faced while integrating the IoT with cloud computing, while [4] have presented a platform based on Cloud Computing for management of mobile and wearable healthcare sensors for Smart healthcare, since healthcare applications generate a vast amount of data. On the other hand, [5] are discussing the needs for integrating the cloud and IoT under the name CloudIoT, and they have too talked about the challenges deriving from such integration. The authors in [6] are examining the benefits of the IoT and Cloud integration, also discussing the security challenges encountered. Conversely, the paper in [7] is presenting the OpenStack conceptual architecture where it describes the component on this architecture dividing them depending to their characteristics as computing, networking, storing, shared and supporting services. Stack4thing is a proposed framework by [8] for sensing-and-actuation-as-a-Service, considered as an IoT framework based on OpenStack aiming to integrate the IoT with the cloud. By assembling all these information, we can distinguish that each paper from above is treating a specific part in the IoT merged with the cloud.

From here the idea has come to propose an architecture which gathers all the points discussed below, from raw data to smart applications with each step well-detailed, integrating in parallel OpenStack adequate to our needs services. Along with our architecture, an important part which is the cloud of things Life-cycle data security as an important step, that is mostly not included in specific case proposed architectures. Our paper is dealing with the Big Data management collected from everywhere and everything any time using OpenStack as an open-source cloud, proving its advantages compared to others. Instead of offering separated parts to assemble, we would present an all in one architecture with each layer and stage described, such a conceptual proposition will help us in our future research to make the realization and development easily.

The paper is organized as follow: Sect. 2 reviews the concept of Big Data and IoT for building a smart city and presenting the cloud computing current definition and services. Furthermore, it compares IoT cloud platforms. While the Sect. 3 is proposing the IoT platform architecture on OpenStack by describing each one of its layers.

This article contribution, approach and challenges are discussed in Sect. 4. To sum up Sect. 5 gives some conclusions and an outlook of our future work in this area.

2 Big Data and IoT Concept for Smart City

Recently more objects and devices are now connected to the internet. They have a locatable, addressable, and readable counterpart in the Internet, transmit information they gather back for treatment and analysis. Two terms have been widely getting more attention: Big Data and the IoT, despite the difference between them, they depend to each other. This is possible thanks to intense interactions among objects, which collaborate for offering complex services using IoT in smart cities systems and enhancing all things to be interconnected each other's. Hence this fact is resulting in the overwhelming amount of the Big Data, by analyzing such huge quantity based on the user choices and needs, so then the cities would become even smarter. Figure 1 shows the relationship between Big Data and Smart City using the cloud. It starts from the generation of all the huge amount of data collected and ends up by using these obtained data to afford information to get the smart cities applications enhanced. The Big Data systems will deal with the data by storing it processing and mining the applications information in an intelligent and efficient way. From here the big data and IoT are used together, therefore large amounts of information can be gathered and studied to see where improvements can be made.

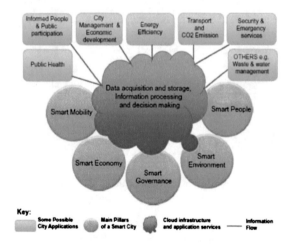

Fig. 1. Using the cloud to store data generated from different components of a smart city [9]

The smart applications presented in Fig. 1 are considered as nowadays trend, we are defining the benefits of some of them detailed as follow: Smart Energy system which has the vision of the smart grid and smart metering system is combining the traditional power grid, renewable energy, and the IT technologies. The smart grid uses smart meters, sensors and analytics to manage and automate the flow of information and energy between the utility and the consumers [10]. Smart Weather and Water, most world water flood damage is due to the lack of technology use thus, the use of smart weather and water are very important and indispensable for predicting insights [11]. Smart Environment as ubiquitous sensing and intelligent climate management are jointly applied in smart environment applications, we can monitor waste gas, greenhouse gas, city noise, air and water pollution, forest conditions, and so on, to afford intelligent and sustainable development [12]. Smart Transportation and Traffic, since the city infrastructure is growing, Intelligent transportation systems will be the perfect solution. By using smart technologies such as IoT that visualize all the transportation network items and use Big Data platforms to understand the behavior of the movements, we will be able then to extract values that help decision making, to achieve more vehicles but less traffic [13].

2.1 Cloud Computing Services

Cloud computing is a general term for the delivery of hosted services over the internet, it is defined as computing paradigm, where many systems are connected in public or private network, in order to provide a scalable dynamic infrastructure for Big data (Fig. 2).

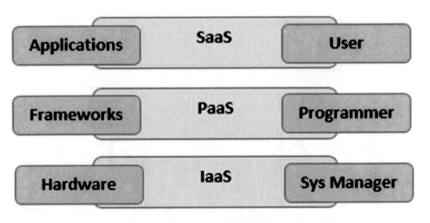

Fig. 2. A conceptual view of cloud computing [14]

Cloud is offering services which can be grouped into three categories: First, Software as a Service (SaaS) which is a software distribution model, where the end user can get services as a highly scalable internet-based application hosted on the cloud, since SaaS applications are delivered over the internet, users can access them from any internet-enabled device and location. Comparing with conventional software, SaaS applications are hosted at the service network provider, delivered as a web application, and serve as services for multiple tenants. Second, the Platform as a Service (PaaS) where the end user is free to build his own applications, benefiting from the PaaS service as a software or development environment. It provides a predefined combination of OS and applications servers such as LAMP platform, Google's App etc. The PaaS are used for designing, developing, building and testing applications by the infrastructure of the cloud. Finally, the Infrastructure as a Service (IaaS) which is providing virtualized computing capabilities, resources and storage as services over the network, its role is monitoring and managing remote datacenter infrastructures, end user can purchase IaaS based on consumption instead of hardware. IaaS provides something much disparate than the earlier two cloud services. IaaS broadens your existing hardware and incorporates it into your local resources. You can obtain whole network segments that run in the cloud. You may include hard drive storage, servers, routers, and switches to your network and allow them to run completely in the cloud.

2.2 Comparison of IoT Cloud Platforms

As discussed in the previous section, Cloud Computing is the most discussed topics in the IT's world nowadays, since it provides an efficient service, scalable infrastructure, high performance, an important and secure data storage. By using cloud services companies, we can eliminate the hazards and costs involved with the installation and management of traditional IT infrastructure. Nevertheless, choosing the suitable and adequate to our needs, cloud computing platform is a confusing and hard step. Hence after looking for the top systems available, we present in the current section a comparison of some IoT cloud platform depending on our features requirements of Cloud Management Platforms (CMPs) such as Eucalyptus, CloudStack, OpenStack, and OpenNebula. They can be used to deploy and manage instances of virtual machines either on local physical resources or on external public clouds.

Eucalyptus is an open-source cloud computing framework that provides VM and user data storage, VM scheduling, administrative interfaces, construction of virtual networks, and cloud computing user interfaces, designed to be user-friendly from the standpoint of installation, with no need for customized or dedicated resources. It is highly modular, and interfaces easily with industry-standard, and third-party communication mechanisms. Its external interface is based on the API developed by Amazon. Eucalyptus is unique among the open-source IaaS solutions such as OpenStack, OpenNebula, Nimbus and Proxmox by isolating network traffic and allowing clusters of users to appear as belonging to the same Local Area Network (LAN) [15].

Another well-known platform is OpenStack which is an open-source developed in 2010 as a joint project of Rackspace Hosting and NASA. It is a kind of platform deployed in companies all over the world employing distributed architectures measured in petabytes and is massively scalable up to 1 million physical machines, 60 million virtual machines, and billions of stored objects. It aims to build a hosting architecture with massive scalability while remaining open-source and free from the constraints of proprietary technologies [16]. We can distinguish another platform called Apache CloudStack is an open-source from Apache Software Foundation (ASF) which is used for the creation, management, and deployment of IaaS clouds, and large networks of VMs, as well as it provides a highly scalable IaaS cloud computing platform [18].

Overall, contributions from the open-source community come from a wide range of organizations for OpenStack while contributions for Eucalyptus and OpenNebula come from a small number of organizations, indicating that the OpenStack project has the largest and most active community both in terms of number of members and development activity [19]. Another reason for adopting OpenStack is that it supports different hypervisors (Xen, VMware or kernel-based virtual machine [KVM] for instance) and several virtualization technologies (such as bare metal or high-performance computing). OpenStack controls large pools of compute, storage and networking resources throughout a datacenter. Its services communicate each other, and responsible for the various functions expected from virtualization and cloud management software. Hence, we are proposing an architecture of the IoT platform on OpenStack by integrating the OpenStack services with the IoT layers in the next section.

3   A Proposed IoT Platform Architecture on OpenStack

IoT devices are inherently connected, for that we need a reference architecture for scalability and flexibility in storage, compute and network levels to deal with the 3Vs of Big Data: Volume, Velocity, and Variety, therefore, Cloud is the efficient and best solution. The architecture in Fig. 3 is presenting some specific IoT requirements:

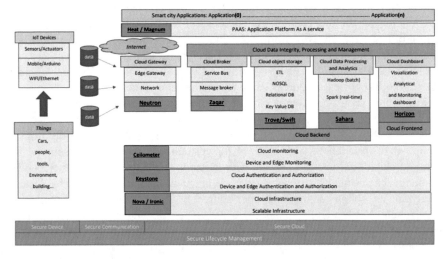

Fig. 3. IoT and OpenStack integration architecture

3.1   Device and Edge Management

Sensors collect data from the environment, which convert physical phenomenon into an electrical impulse that can be interpreted to determine a reading. While the actuator takes electrical input and turns it into physical action. In this infrastructure sensors will collect information, transfer it through Edge gateways which aggregate these data, translate it between sensors protocols and process it before sending it to the cloud. After a decision making the actuator gets back a response to offer an action. The interaction between the sensors, devices and actuators with the cloud is happening thanks to the internet, here comes the OpenStack Neutron service [20]. This service runs on the network node to service the Networking API and its extensions. It also enforces the network model and IP addressing of each port. The neutron-server requires indirect access to a persistent database. This is accomplished through plugins, which communicate with the database using AMQP (Advanced Message Queuing Protocol) ....

3.2 Platform Management

The scalable architecture presented is computed by the OpenStack service Nova [21], the compute component enables the provisioning and management of CPU resources to the users. The compute resources are accessed on demand, in a scalable manner. Users can create and manage compute specific or storage-specific Virtual Machines (VMs) in a need-based manner.

Various fixed configuration for VMs in form of flavors are available. Users can select the desired flavor and operating system and can have a running machine without acquiring the actual physical hardware. Elastic scalability and the ability to deploy in a cloud infrastructure are essential, for that our architecture offers an authentication mechanism which is applied to verify the identities of a service provider and a requester after a successful authentication, there is also the authorization mechanism which should control access rights of resource requesters. *Keystone* is present in this level as OpenStack Identity service that manages user databases and analysis of system architecture to understand the working principle. Keystone [22] provides a central directory of users mapped to the OpenStack services they can access. It acts as a common authentication system across the cloud. On the other hand, *Ceilometer* [23] is a data collection service that provides the ability to normalize and transform data across all current OpenStack core components, used to provide customer billing, resource tracking, and alarming capabilities across all OpenStack core components. We have applied it in our architecture as a cloud monitoring service which is the process of evaluating, monitoring, and managing cloud-based services, applications and infrastructure. The relationship between the cloud services and the cloud end-users is managed and negotiated by an entity called: Cloud broker, considered as a third-party brokerage-as-a-service advanced in our cloud platform architecture, for facilitating the encryption, deduplication and transfer of the end-user's data to the cloud. The OpenStack messaging component *Zaqar* [24] is defined in our architecture as it is a multi-tenant cloud messaging and notification service for web and mobile developers to surface events to end users. Then for our large-scale data management and processing, Big Data and cloud computing are used in our proposed architecture and aims to satisfy our system requirements. In one hand, by dealing with hundreds of petabytes of heterogenous data which will be generated and processed for future usage, the key advantage of smart city applications is that they generate large volumes of data in a variety of formats and from many sectors. To ensure proper and useful utilization of this data in smart city applications, it is important to have suitable and effective big data management tools in place. Big data management includes development and execution of architectures, policies, practices and procedures that properly manage the full data lifecycle needs throughout its use in smart city applications. We proceed with this data on the Cloud using both big data PaaS and IaaS. We are using in this layer *Trove*, [25] as a database as a service which provides relational and nonrelational database engines, allows users to manage relational database services in an OpenStack environment easily. In the same layer we can distinguish the cloud object storage for storing our data as discrete objects identified by their unique address in applications side, the well-known OpenStack component adequate to this method is *Swift* [26]. OpenStack Object Storage is a scalable redundant storage system, and is widely used for such purposes, it is one of the main components of the OpenStack software package. Although Swift has become extremely popular in recent times, its proxy server-based design limits the overall throughput and scalability of the cluster. Additionally, the Stream computing is supporting the prediction, thus making decision in real-time, it is used in the high-speed data environment to provide real-time analytics for detecting insights and relevant data that can be recognized and acted upon at an instant's sign, for that there is many frameworks of Big Data which deal with the real-time processing. Spark Streaming is becoming the platform of choice to implement data processing and analytics solutions for real-time data received from IoT and sensors. For Batch Computing system, Hadoop is the most widely implemented in Big Data environment. Hadoop is an open-source apache project, works by parallelizing the processing of the data across computing nodes for the sake of dealing with the large data volumes in the minimum time possible, it has a main and important component, [27] Hadoop Distributed File System (HDFS): which is a data service for managing files in Big Data environments. In HDFS, the data files that needs to be processed are broken into blocks that sizes are between 64 and 128 MB and distributes across nodes. The OpenStack *Sahara* [28] aims to provide users with a simple means to provision Hadoop, Spark, and Storm clusters by specifying several parameters such as the framework version, cluster topology, hardware node details and more. After a user fills in all the parameters, Sahara deploys the cluster in a few minutes. Also, it provides means to scale an already provisioned cluster by adding or removing worker nodes on demand.

To complete our cloud architecture, we should integrate the visualization layer, where all data is visualized in web portal via some statistical graphics, and information graphics, for providing us with a complete and Smart visualization and manipulation to observe the behavior of many things and gain important insights. OpenStack Dashboard *Horizon* is the canonical implementation of OpenStack's Dashboard, which provides a web-based user interface to OpenStack services including Nova, Swift, Keystone [29]. Furthermore, it provides administrators and users with a graphical interface to access, provision, and automate deployment of cloud-based resources.

For our cloud PaaS, we propose to integrate the OpenStack Heat: a service to orchestrate composite cloud applications using a declarative template format through an OpenStack-native REST API. It provides a template-based orchestration for describing a cloud application by executing appropriate OpenStack API calls to generate running cloud applications [30]. Magnum is an OpenStack project which offers container orchestration engines for deploying and managing containers as first-class resources in OpenStack [31]. Magnum uses Heat to orchestrate an OS image which contains Docker and Kubernetes and runs that image in either virtual machines or bare metal in a cluster configuration.

3.3 Security

The security of data is also a challenging task in both client and server sides, since many IoT devices have limited amounts of storage, memory and processing capability. The security approaches that rely heavily on encryption are not a good fit for these constrained devices, because they are not capable of performing complex encryption and decryption quickly enough to be able to transmit data securely in real-time.

4 Discussion

As seen in our proposed architecture, the integration of cloud and IoT, is dealing with a global usage and management of applications, and infrastructure. The architecture is handling thoroughly all cloud of things components and steps.

This integration has many benefits related to communication, storage and processing. The cloud is an optimal and economical solution for connecting and managing all the applications transmitted through the IoT. Furthermore, the cloud provides unlimited virtual processing capabilities and on-demand usage option, which will absolutely handle the limited processing capabilities of the IoT. As the IoT is generating a huge amount of non-structured data, the cloud is the most effective solution to deal with it.

Nevertheless, it is not going to be that easy to make everything a part of IoT and having all resources available through OpenStack. This combination is facing many challenges, we cite among them the high consummation of power due to sensor networks and connectivity with the cloud. Besides, the extensive heterogeneity of devices, platforms, operating systems, and services used for the new created applications also is considered as a big issue, especially when end-users adopt multi-Cloud approaches. Additionally, our architecture is a complex system requiring a security and privacy controls in each stage of this system life-cycle. Hence, we added the secure life-cycle management layer, being indispensable and best practice in the whole architecture, as some security related software's like firewalls, intrusion detectors and surveillance mechanisms.

The raw data gathering from devices should be done depending on our needs related to the smart application we would like to create. These devices will constantly generate huge amount of data which could be a user personal data. This triggers the necessity of devices' security to take care of the user privacy. Through the internet, the communication between the things and cloud should be done in a secure way too, once in the cloud the data is not a security risk-free, whereas a secure cloud is primary to assure the protection of our data in all over our architecture layers. Treating it in a scalable way, retrieving from it the values for predicting smartly how the applications would be with insights and cognizance.

5 Conclusions and Future Work

This paper discusses the Integration of the IoT with the cloud computing, for enhanced and more useful service for the end-users, to use resources efficiently. Since the IoT has limited capabilities as we have discussed in this paper in terms of processing and storage. This is related to performance security, privacy and more. The Cloud and IoT, we have proposed are more beneficial for deploying smart applications, hence these applications can be boosted in cloud of things combination. The architecture we have presented is showing how cloud services could be developed and puzzled in an IoT layers aiming to make smart applications data useful. In fact, no standard architecture is available, our study contributes by proposing a reference architecture. Thereafter more investigation will be done in the future in order to start the realization and installation of OpenStack environment based on our proposed architecture.

Since we have focused on security in the cloud of things architecture as a critical and important fact to handle, we are aiming to concentrate on the security of data from collection to insights in more detailed way in each cloud of things layer, consequently the end-user's privacy. Moreover, we will concentrate on the Sahara OpenStack component by installing Hadoop framework and developing our application, all these challenges have been left for the future too.

References

1. https://www.seventhgenerationadvisors.org/smart-cities
2. Khan, Z., Anjum, A., Kiani, S.L.: Cloud based big data analytics for smart future cities. In Proceedings of the 2013 IEEE/ACM 6th International Conference on Utility and Cloud Computing, pp. 381–386. IEEE Computer Society (2013)
3. Aazam, M., Khan, I., Abdullah, A., Huh, E.: Cloud of things: integrating internet of things and cloud computing and the issues involved. In: Proceedings of 2014 11th International Bhurban Conference on Applied Sciences & Technology (IBCAST) Islamabad, Pakistan 14–18 Jan 2014
4. Doukas, C., Maglogiannis, I.: Bringing IoT and cloud computing towards pervasive healthcare. In: Proceedings of 2012 Sixth International Conference on Innovative Mobile and Internet Services in Ubiquitous Computing
5. Botta, A., Donata, W., Persico, V., Pescape, A.: On the integration of cloud computing and internet of things. In: 2014 International Conference on Future Internet of Things and Cloud
6. Stergiou, C., Psannis, K.E., Kim, B.-G., Gupta, B.: Secure integration of IoT and cloud computing, Future Gener. Comput. Syst. (2016)
7. Rosado, T., Bernardino, J.: An overview of Openstack architecture. Comput. Syst Implement. (2014)
8. Longo, F., Bruneo, D., Distefano, S., Merlino, G., Puliafito, A.: Stack4Things: an OpenStack-based framework for IoT. In: Proceedings of 2015 3rd International Conference on Future Internet of Things and Cloud
9. Liu, X., Heller, A., Nielsen, P.S.: Research data management for smart cities (In submission to Journal of Information Management)
10. Kehoe, M., Cosgrove, M., De Gennaro, S., et al.: A foundation for understanding ibm smarter cities

11. Mazhar Rathore, M.: IoT-based smart city development using big data analytical approach. In: IEEE, Daegu, Korea, 2016
12. Zanella, A., Bui, N., Castellani, A., Vangelista, L., Zorzi, M.: Internet of things for smart cities. IEEE Internet of Things J. **1**(1), 22–32 (2014)
13. Alshawish, R.A., Alfagih S.A.M., Musbah, M.S.: Big data applications in smart cities. In: IEEE, Benghazi, Libya, 2016
14. Rompante Cunha, C., Paulo Morais, E., Paulo Sousa, J., Pedro Gomes, J.: The role of cloud computing in the development of information systems for SMEs. J. Cloud Comput. **2017**. Doi:10.5171/2017.736545
15. Nurmi, D., Wolski, R., Grzegorcyzk, C., Obertelli, G., Soman, S., Youseff, L., Zagorodnov, D.: The eucalyptus open-source cloud-computing system, cluster computing and the grid, 2009. In: 9th IEEE/ACM International Symposium, pp. 124–131, May 2009
16. Sefraoui, O., Aissaoui M., Eleuldj, M.: OpenStack: toward an open-source solution for cloud computing. Int. J. Comput. Appl. **55**(03) (2012)
17. Kumar, R., Jain, K., Maharwal, H., Jain N., Dadhich, A.: Apache CloudStack: open source infrastructure as a service cloud computing platform. In: Proceedings of the International Journal of Advancement in Engineering Technology, Management & Applied Science, pp. 111–116 (2014)
18. Siddharth, J., Kumar, R., Kumar S., Anamika, A comparative study for cloud computing platform on open source software. ABHIYANTRIKI—An Int. J. Eng. Technol. **1**(2), 28–35 (2014)
19. Ismaeel, S., Miri, A., Chourishi D., Dibaj, R.: Open source cloud management platforms: a review. In: Cyber Security and Cloud Computing (CSCloud), 2015 IEEE 2nd International Conference, pp. 470–475, Nov 2015
20. https://docs.openstack.org/security-guide/networking/architecture.html
21. P. Jain, A. Datt, A. Goel, S.C. Gupta, Cloud Service Orchestration based Architecture of OpenStack Nova and Swift, 2016 Intl. Conference on Advances in Computing, Communications and Informatics (ICACCI), Sept 21–24, 2016, Jaipur, India
22. Khan, R.H, Ylitalo, J., Ahmed, A.S.: OpenID authentication as a service in OpenStack. In: 2011 7th International Conference on Information Assurance and Security (IAS). pp. 372–377 IEEE, 2011
23. https://docs.openstack.org/ceilometer
24. https://docs.openstack.org/zaqar
25. Kumar, R., Gupta, N., Charu, S., Jain, K., Jangir, S.K.: Open source solution for cloud computing platform using OpenStack. Int. J. Comput. Sci. Mobile Comput. **3**(5), 89–98 (2014)
26. Gugnani, S., Lu, X., Panda, D.K.: Swift-X: accelerating OpenStack swift with RDMA for building an efficient HPC cloud. In: 2017 17th IEEE/ACM International Symposium on Cluster, Cloud and Grid Computing
27. Zikopoulos, P., Eaton C., et al.: Understanding Big Data: Analytics for Enterprise Class Hadoop and Streaming Data. McGraw-Hill Osborne Media (2011)
28. https://docs.openstack.org/sahara
29. https://docs.openstack.org/horizon
30. https://docs.openstack.org/heat
31. https://docs.openstack.org/magnum

Data Mining Dynamic Hybrid Model for Logistic Supplying Chain: Assortment Setting in Fast Fashion Retail

Naila Fares[1]([⊠]), Maria Lebbar[1,2], Najiba Sbihi[1],
and Anas El Boukhari El Mamoun[3]

[1] Ecole Mohammadia d'Ingénieurs, Rabat, Morocco
naila.fares@gmail.com, lebbar@enim.ac.ma, sbihi@emi.ac.ma
[2] Ecole Nationale Supérieure des Mines de Rabat, Rabat, Morocco
[3] Nutek Startup Company, Tangier, Morocco
anb.elboukhari@gmail.com

Abstract. Data science tools have been used in many fields as effective techniques for data analysis. Artificial intelligence, machine learning and data mining made the buzz on both industrial and scientific communities, pushing the researchers to look for the potential value added they might have by using the tool. Fast fashion retailers joined the vague too, but still have many untapped fields to work on. In this paper, we work on the assortment problem for a worldwide fast fashion retailer, who sells a large quantity of products, with a wide range of models and different regions of sales. Every region has its own features in term of habits, clothing choices and trends, thus the retailer uncertainty to dispatch its inventory in an optimal way, as to meet the expectations of the customers, building the consumers loyalty and maximize the sales. The proposed procedure is programmed with Python and orange software, and then tested with data instances, inspired from real cases.

Keywords: Fast fashion retail · Supply chain · Assortment problem · Data mining · K-means clustering · Classification · Data science · Dynamic model

1 Introduction

Orders, shipping, processing orders and payment arrangement delays, errors, miscommunications [1] are some of the main reasons of long supply chain lead times. From suppliers until final customers, every single delay in the chain might impact the further processes progress and then the final product/service delivery, especially if the delay was not managed smartly.

In this context, assortment problem is a challenging issue in fast fashion retail. Which products are sold together in each store? How should we organize the shipment contents in term of assortment so that the customer finds the set of products needed as per its profile? We propose a data mining hybrid model, in order to answer these questions.

© Springer Nature Switzerland AG 2019
M. Ezziyyani (Ed.): AI2SD 2018, AISC 915, pp. 578–585, 2019.
https://doi.org/10.1007/978-3-030-11928-7_52

The hybrid procedure will let to sort out the data analysis of sales and customers choices, and translate it into customer profile definition of each store. Our goal is to help the decision maker afterwards to allocate the suitable assortment set for each point of sales.

We test the model with data inspired from real cases, and we analyze the results given. The analysis allows us to trace the guidelines for retailer's decision makers. The application is supported by a graphic interface, letting the retailer to use it as an interface to sort out the hidden sides of its data.

The model is programmed with Python and uses machine learning modules for data analysis. We present the value added of this work according to the previous researches in the fast fashion field, as we explore so far the expected benefit that the model will provide to the fast fashion retailers.

In the next sections, our problematic work frame is detailed. After a literature review, the problem statement and the proposed model are described. The model validation is explored, followed by the model discussion. Finally, future perspectives of the work are presented.

2   Literature Review

The assortment optimization problem is a classical problem in retail. It was analyzed and solved through different disciplines.

A shelf space allocation model was first implemented in order to make the assortment homogenous with the shelf space constraint [2]. Static and dynamic models were developed afterwards: Van Ryzin & Mahajan (1999) same as Smith & Agrawal (2000) worked on static models with a stochastic demand [3], Kök et al. (2008) presents a good literature survey on this field [4]; dynamic approaches were published in order to meet the dynamic feature of the market, as per learning customers' tastes [5].

The dynamic features was treated first with stochastic model and dynamic programs of operation research, and lately machine learning and data science tools took the lead, as analysis data tools, due to the performance they demonstrate.

Managing the product complexity level, and its relationship with the assortment was discussed [6] in previous papers, as per the assortment pricing impact on customer choices [7], but none of them was applied on fast fashion retail.

Recent works use the multi-nominal logit model (MNL) and nested logit model [8] for dynamic assortment optimization, and self classifier for fashion design [9].

When we talk about assortment models dedicated for fast fashion retail application, few works were done in this field, as cited above.

To the best of our knowledge, no study was reported in the literature, applying data mining tools for the assortment problematic, in fast fashion field. Hence, our contribution in the presented research is investigating this potential combination.

3 Problem Statement

Our article is dealing with the assortment problem in fast fashion retail: the purpose of this study is to propose a novel hybrid approach, for fast fashion retailers, in order to define the suitable assortment for each point of sales in the network; whether it is a local or a worldwide network.

The framework is presented for a worldwide retailer that displays a wide range of diversified products, and needs to decide on the optimized distribution arrangement.

4 The Suggested Model

Key input data to an assortment definition model is the sales data. The features of each store are defined among the analysis and exploration of data, as an important raw material to work on.

In our approach, we use the K-means clustering method and hierarchical classification in order to cluster the dresses models. The model is coded with python, using libraries from scikit-learn. The visualization is enhanced with Orange: on open source software for machine learning and data mining visualization.

The k-means method is joined with the predict method of scikit-learn [10]. The predict module provides the nearest cluster of the centers, for hidden data.

5 The Model Validation

The model is programmed with Python, and in order to test it, we used a data inspired from real cases.

The data set is about dress selling, from an open data sets repository called UCI machine learning [11] (see extracts in Tables 1 and 2).

It contains several attribute information about the dresses, such as size, season, style, fabric, pattern type… and sales data of a specified period.

The data is not a time series data, since sales dates are picked up differently.

6 Experimental Results and Model Discussion

We suppose that we have to define the assortment of 30 dresses, divided into 7 groups. We set the number of clusters to 7 by choosing the model selections.

All the attributes data, except the dress ID, were given as input data to the algorithm. The customer ID was excluded since it is the attribute to work on. The program exports the results in an external csv file. A screenshot of the results' extract is described in Fig. 1.

The hierarchical classification of the same set of 30 dresses gave us the bellow results (Fig. 2):

Table 1. Extract of data: sales data on date basis

Dress_ID	29/8/2013	31/8/2013	09/02/2013	09/04/2013	09/06/2013	09/08/2013	09/10/2013
1006032852	2114	2274	2491	2660	2727	2887	2930
1212192089	151	275	570	750	813	1066	1164
1190380701	6	7	7	7	8	8	9
966005983	1005	1128	1326	1455	1507	1621	1637
876339541	996	1175	1304	1396	1432	1559	1570
1068332458	4	5	11	13	13	13	16
1220707172	45	61	131	165	176	209	216
1219677488	4	13	55	73	76	89	94
1113094204	5	6	10	12	13	15	16
985292672	9	11	12	12	12	12	12
1117293701	15	28	42	49	49	55	56
898481530	23	38	54	59	65	72	77
957723897	1235	1333	1471	1568	1602	1722	1756
749031896	2498	2545	2627	2656	2669	2738	2769
1055411544	22	28	40	43	44	45	45

Table 2. Extract of data: sales data on attributes basis

Dress_ID	Style	Price	Rating	Size	Season	Neck line	Sleeve length	Waiseline	Material	Fabric type	Decoration	Pattern type
1006032852	Classic	Low	4.6	M	Summer	O-neck	Sleevless	Empire	Null	Chiffon	Ruffles	Animal
1212192089	Casual	Low	0	L	Summer	O-neck	Petal	Natural	Microfiber	Null	Ruffles	Animal
1190380701	Vintage	High	0	L	Automn	O-neck	Full	Natural	Polyster	Null	Null	Print
966005983	Brief	Average	4.6	L	Spring	O-neck	Full	Natural	Silk	Chiffon	Embroidary	Print
876339541	cute	Low	4.5	M	Summer	O-neck	Butterfly	Natural	Chiffonfabric	Chiffon	Bow	Dot
1068332458	Bohemian	Low	0	M	Summer	V-neck	Sleevless	Empire	Null	Null	Null	Print
1220707172	Casual	Average	0	XL	Summer	O-neck	Full	Null	Cotton	Null	Null	Solid
1219677488	Novelty	Average	0	Free	Automn	O-neck	Short	Natural	Polyster	Broadcloth	Lace	Null
1113094204	Flare	Average	0	Free	Spring	V-neck	Short	Empire	Cotton	Broadcloth	Beading	Solid
985292672	Bohemian	Low	0	Free	Summer	V-neck	Sleevless	Natural	Nylon	Chiffon	Null	Null
1117293701	Party	Average	5	Free	Summer	O-neck	Full	Natural	Polyster	Broadcloth	Lace	Solid
898481530	Flare	Average	0	Free	Spring	V-neck	Short	Null	Nylon	Null	Null	Animal
957723897	Classic	Low	4.7	M	Winter	O-neck	Threequarter	Null	Null	Chiffon	Lace	Print
749031896	Vintage	Average	4.8	M	Summer	O-neck	Short	Empire	Cotton	Jersey	Null	Animal
1055411544	Casual	Low	5	M	Summer	Boat-neck	Short	Null	Cotton	Null	Sashes	Solid

Dress_ID	Cluster KMeans
1006032852	3.0
1212192089	6.0
1190380701	5.0
966005983	4.0
876339541	0.0
1068332458	5.0
1220707172	1.0
1219677488	5.0
1113094204	5.0
985292672	5.0
1117293701	5.0
898481530	5.0
957723897	0.0
749031896	3.0
1055411544	5.0
1162628131	5.0
624314841	0.0
830467746	5.0
840857118	5.0
1113221101	1.0
861754372	1.0
856178100	4.0
1122989777	1.0
840516484	0.0

Fig. 1. K-means clustering results

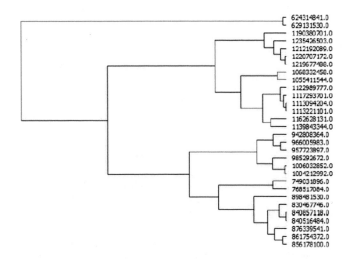

Fig. 2. Hierarchical classification results

The product features are described by: price, components, model... and the sales on date basis. Taking all these attributes in consideration for clustering, means that all the criteria, which defines the model and influences the customer choice, defines the assortment clusters of dresses.

The 2 algorithms gave similar ID dresses approximation in most cases, but some differences between the 2 approaches exist for some models. However, the 2 algorithms are completing each other.

The K-means help the decision maker to have a general idea about the assortment components, taking into consideration the limitation of packages to be shipped.

While the hierarchical classification, goes through the detailed models approximations, above several levels: for instance, if we could not ship the 1190380701, 1235426503, 1212192089, 1220707172 and 1219677488 models together, at least the 2 last models should be sent together, since they are highly collated.

Finally, the assortment setting is based on the cluster definition. In term of each store trend, the joined choices, and the customer profiles. The algorithms help the decision maker to join the models, but the final setting is finalized according to the existing inventory and the eventual additional constraints.

7   Conclusion and Perspectives

The present work was a contribution in assortment setting for fast fashion retail field. It presents a novelty in terms of the bellow points:

- It is a contribution in measuring the data mining tools, applied to fast fashion retail application: in fact few papers were published in this specific challenging section of fashion.
- It is a hybrid model, dynamically analyzed, responding to the continuous market injection of new items.

That model is useful for in-season assortment decisions, as per the dynamic requested changes in fast fashion assortments.

Future works might focus on the capsule networks, and the products assortment modeling on their basis for assortment recognition.

References

1. http://www.mhlnews.com/global-supply-chain/reduce-lead-time-your-global-supply-chain-lean-thinking
2. Bultez, A., Naert, P.: SH. ARP: shelf allocation for retailers' profit. Mark. Sci. **7**(3), 211–231 (1988)
3. Caro, F., Gallien, J.: Dynamic assortment with demand learning for seasonal consumer goods. Manage. Sci. **53**(2), 276–292 (2007)
4. Caro, F., Martínez-de-Albéniz, V., Rusmevichientong, P.: The assortment packing problem: multiperiod assortment planning for short-lived products. Manage. Sci. **60**(11), 2701–2721 (2014)
5. Ulu, C., Honhon, D., Alptekinoğlu, A.: Learning consumer tastes through dynamic assortments. Oper. Res. **60**(4), 833–849 (2012)
6. Sardar, S., Lee, Y.H.: Analysis of product complexity considering disruption cost in fast fashion supply chain. Math. Prob. Eng. **2015** (2015)

7. Choi, C., Mattila, A.S., Upneja. A.: The effect of assortment pricing on choice and satisfaction: the moderating role of consumer characteristics. Cornell Hosp. Q. **59**(1) (2018)
8. Chen, X., Wang, Y., Zhou, Y.: Dynamic assortment planning without utility parameter estimation (March 2, 2018). Available at SSRN: https://ssrn.com/abstract=3133401 or http://dx.doi.org/10.2139/ssrn.3133401
9. Vincent, O.R., et al.: A self-adaptive k-means classifier for business incentive in a fashion design environment. Appl. Comput. Inf. **14**(1), 88–97 (2018)
10. http://scikit-learn.org
11. https://archive.ics.uci.ed

A Customer Profiling' Machine Learning Approach, for In-store Sales in Fast Fashion

Naila Fares[1]([⊠]), Maria Lebbar[1,2], and Najiba Sbihi[1]

[1] Ecole Mohammadia d'Ingénieurs, Rabat, Morocco
naila.fares@gmail.com, lebbar@enim.ac.ma,
sbihi@emi.ac.ma
[2] Ecole Nationale Supérieure des Mines de Rabat, Rabat, Morocco

Abstract. In the last few decades, fast fashion retailers competitiveness is highly increasing, to get the market shares. With few historical data, the data analysis is a real challenge in this field. From the other hand, the customer service focus is a must, since the expectations of consumers are extremely selective. In this context, data science and machine learning tools are the latest trend in big data analysis, with short calculation time, that attract leader from many sectors to test their abilities in problem solving. This paper is a contribution to a machine learning based procedure, for customer profiling in fast fashion retail. It helps to build linking rules, of customers and their choices. Results will be a support in customer assistance, for increasing the in store sales basket size.

Keywords: Fast fashion · Retail · Supply chain · Customer profiling · Machine learning · In store sales

1 Introduction

Fast fashion, and the according evolution from 2 terms calendar to fast consumption [1] is a challenging field.

Where customers are expecting to get the latest trends, at affordable prices, with a dynamic assortment change, understanding the customer need is a must, in order to get his loyalty.

We start by a literature review, followed by the problem statement and the proposed model. The model validation and discussion are explored, before concluding with future perspectives.

2 Literature Review

Applications of the customer profiling on hotels in tourism sector [2], for Targeted advertisement based on user history [3], are some of the recent works of customer segmentations applications.

According to the methods used: customer maps, combined to system and computer method programmed [4] were explored lately as tools for customer segmentation.

© Springer Nature Switzerland AG 2019
M. Ezziyyani (Ed.): AI2SD 2018, AISC 915, pp. 586–591, 2019.
https://doi.org/10.1007/978-3-030-11928-7_53

For the machine learning tools applied to this problematic, namely the combination between time series and clustering, a recent work [5] proposed a combined model. It presents the consumer clustering problem as a multi-instance clustering problem and applies a multi-instance clustering algorithm to solve it.

Previous works joined the clustering to the time series data [6], but it was for only k-medoids algorithm utilization.

While some recent works focused on: the investigation of information and new technologies on fashion, from customers point of view [7]; the impact of seasonality demand learning on customer choices [8]; and a larger study of the customer behavior influencing factors is developed, in a specific case study [9], but none was specifically dedicated to the fast fashion field of fashion retail.

Our work is an extension of [10] where the authors focused on customer relationship and customer profiling.

The main problem in that paper [10], is how to better choose the marketing strategy, by using the Customer Relationship Management (CRM). Data of customers' sales is clustered and analyzed by using K-means, decision tree and Radio Frequency Monetary (RFM). They found as a result characteristics and recommendations for customer relationship, as per CRM basics. The study is done in medium industrial companies work frame.

To the best of our knowledge, the proposed procedure of segmentation was not treated in this manner in the literature, applied to fast fashion retail sector.

3   Problem Statement

We focus on an international fast fashion retailer, which stores network is worldwide. Each store has its own features, in term of basket size, as per the customer profile (educational, financial, cultural...).

The main objective of this work is to increase the basket size and the customer loyalty. Actions will be taken as recommendations for in-store sales, and in-store flow supply chain decisions.

4   The Proposed Model

4.1   Overall Proposed Scheme

The model is inspired from e-commerce customer segmentation and profiling; in this field, intelligent systems behind the customer interface analyze the previous purchased products, or even the ones that were checked before and seems that the customer is interested in. This analysis led the system to suggest to the customer:

1. Seasonality modeling: weather, trendy fashion, special events...have an extremely high impact on fast fashion retail sales. We have limited sales data and short period of products life cycle, but we can divide the sales period on season's units. The first step in our analysis is to define the seasonality segmentation in order to set the features of each season.

2. Definition of customer profiling of each season: at this stage we define the potential consumer expected category on a season basis. This segmentation is based on many features according to the season characterization.
3. Basket learning of each profile on season basis: choices of customer purchasing are analyzed. Further sales actions are recommended.

The figure bellow describes the 3 steps scheme (Fig. 1).

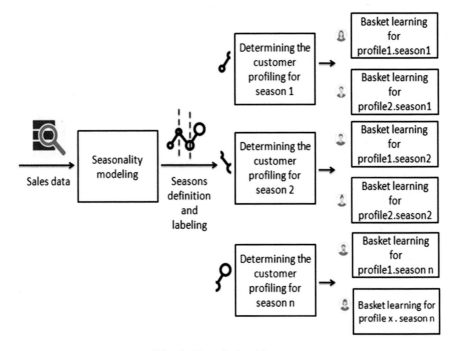

Fig. 1. Overall algorithm steps

For instance, after the 1st step of seasonality modeling, we might find 3 seasons: summer, back to school and national holidays.

For summer, we might have 2 kinds of customer profiles that we find thanks to the 2nd step segmentation on attributes basis: tourists (they speak foreign languages and are from other cities or other countries), and local customers (we recognize them with their clothing and dialect pronunciation).

With the sales supporting team, we define visual features of each profile, for each season. This visual recognition might be couples with some questions, to unhide the personal characteristic of the customer (introvert vs extrovert, accept sales support and supplementary products suggestion, or prefers to establish the shopping experience alone…).

Thanks to these visual recognition techniques, the identification of the customer profile is done according to the visual features, and then the sales actions will be done accordingly, as per the related season.

4.2   Algorithm Procedure

In this section, we will develop the proposed algorithm procedure. It is described as bellow:

(1) Data preparation for seasonality analysis
(2) Data decomposition according to the seasonality (ARIMA, time series…)
(3) Getting the seasons segmentation
(4) For each season:
   (a) Data preparation (missing data elimination, defining training and testing data…)
   (b) Data normalization
   (c) Defining the optimal number of clusters
   (d) Executing the clustering through (hierarchical, density-based, prototype-based, spectral)
   (e) Calculation of indexes
   (f) Defining the best clustering segmentation
   (g) Validation of the clusters with sales team and operations team.

The level of data affinity is at product group basis, and store basis.

5   The Model Validation

The model validation necessitates both sales data, and field data from stores and points of sales. It necessitates a field application, in order to gather the customer characteristics, which will be a pillar in clusters classification.

The source of sales data might be the ERP (Enterprise Resource Planning), or any managing IT system of sales. While the source of the field data, is done according to the continuous observations, from sales advisors and management teams; where linking are established, between the customer behaviors, buying needs and personal characterizations.

However, the effectiveness of each tool used, is demonstrated in the machine learning literature, as high and effective tools [11–13]. The validation with real data will aim to measure the performance related to fast fashion retail.

Future works might focus on a real application, with real instances, or inspired from real ones.

6   Model Discussion

The value added of our work is that:

- It defines the customer profiling for each season, since seasonality is a very specific feature of fast fashion.
- It supports the in store customer service through machine learning tools, at operation level and through the visible recognition of the customer profile.

- It includes with the machine learning algorithm the human expertise, for setting the categories: the retailer experience is used for both setting and after executing the algorithm; the clusters setting are dynamically validated with the retailer experience.
- Recently, fast fashion retailers are adding the e-commerce module to their sales units, more and more. The model might be helpful in associating the store sales rules to the online ones, but by ignoring the visual recognition attributes.

It is both art and science; a machine learning procedure combined with a customer personal feature study, in order to get a better draw of customer definition.

Concerning the related time to achieve the analysis, the first part of seasonality analysis might be the most complicated or time consuming. It might be done on country basis instead of store basis, for an international retailer, since the common seasonality season for a single country (holidays, festivals…).

7   Conclusion and Perspectives

In this paper we propose a machine learning based procedure, mixed with field human profile recognition, for customer profiling. Our main goal is to increase the basket size, and the customer loyalty, in fast fashion retail field.

Output of this work, are recommendation given to retailers, in order to take in-store sales actions, and recommendations for sales supporting.

In next papers, our perspective is to work on real data cases, and eventually including the sale season effect on the customers 'clusters definition.

References

1. Heuer, M., Becker-Leifhold, C.: Eco-Friendly and Fair: Fast Fashion and Consumer Behaviour (2018)
2. Talón-Ballestero, P., et al.: Using big data from customer relationship management information systems to determine the client profile in the hotel sector. Tour. Manag. **68**, 187–197 (2018)
3. Alsina, T., et al. Targeting customer segments. US Patent No. 9,881,320. 30 Jan 2018
4. Lederman, R.D., McFaddin, H.S., Narayanaswami, C.: US Patent Application No. 15/282,703 (2018)
5. Gómez-Boix, Alejandro, Arco, Leticia, Nowé, Ann: Consumer Segmentation Through Multi-instance Clustering Time-Series Energy Data from Smart Meters, pp. 117–136. Soft Computing for Sustainability Science. Springer, Cham (2018)
6. Jalab, H.A., Shaygan, M.A., Jalali, A.: A hybrid algorithm for clustering of time series data based on affinity search technique. Sci. World J. **2014**, 562194 (2014)
7. Amendola, Carlo, Calabrese, Mario, Caputo, Francesco: Fashion companies and customer satisfaction: a relation mediated by information and communication technologies. J. Retail. Consum. Serv. **43**, 251–257 (2018)
8. Aviv, Y., Wei, M.M., Zhang, F.: Responsive pricing of fashion products: the effects of demand learning and strategic consumer behavior (March 27, 2018). Available at SSRN: https://ssrn.com/abstract=3150571 or http://dx.doi.org/10.2139/ssrn.3150571

9. Dayana, S., Quan, S.Z.: Research and analysis on the influencing factors of the purchase decision of the consumers of fast fashion goods in Kazakhstan. Int. J. Bus. Manag. **13**(5), 37 (2018)
10. Maryani, I., Riana, D.: Clustering and profiling of customers using RFM for customer relationship management recommendations. In: 2017 5th International Conference on Cyber and IT Service Management (CITSM), IEEE, 2017
11. Erel, I., Stern, L.H., Tan, C., Weisbach, M.S.: Selecting Directors Using Machine Learning (No. w24435). National Bureau of Economic Research (2018)
12. Erel, I., Stern, L.H., Tan, C., Weisbach, M.S.: Selecting Directors Using Machine Learning (No. w24435). National Bureau of Economic Research2018))
13. Alsina, E.F., Chica, M., Trawiński, K., Regattieri, A.: On the use of machine learning methods to predict component reliability from data-driven industrial case studies. The Int. J. Adv. Manuf. Technol. **94**(5–8), 2419–2433 (2018)

Topic Hierarchies for Knowledge Capitalization using Hierarchical Dirichlet Processes in Big Data Context

Badr Hirchoua[1(✉)], Brahim Ouhbi[1], and Bouchra Frikh[2]

[1] National Higher School of Arts and Crafts (ENSAM), Industrial Engineering and Productivity Department, Moulay Ismal University (UMI), Meknes, Morocco
Badr.hirchoua@gmail.com, ouhbib@yahoo.co.uk
[2] Higher School of Technology (EST), Computer Science Department, Sidi Mohamed Ben Abdellah University (USMBA), Fez, Morocco
bfrikh@yahoo.com

Abstract. Intelligent Technologies and research results from the field of knowledge management, have steadily and progressively improved knowledge quality, over the course of the last decades, especially in the current industrial context. The companies consider the knowledge as an important strategic resource for innovation. This paper focus on the problem of learning topic hierarchies from knowledge. The aim targeted is to respond to knowledge capitalization issues in big data context, by proposing a Knowledge capitalization system as an adaptive intelligent technique. This system acts on top of a big data platform, and runs on large scale globally to constitute a robust intelligent knowledge capitalization paradigm, with a clear separation of concerns. The architecture considers a batch processing as a preparation stage which starts by extracting hidden topics, by means of the HLDA in order to handle the complexity of multi knowledge domains, and to keep the semantic relations between knowledge entities. The hierarchical mechanism gives an effective and flexible way to store and analyses the knowledge. As a result, the time responding is obtained of high quality, and with the best precision, in comparison with the systems which uses LSA and LDA approach as a preparation stage.

Keywords: Knowledge capitalization · Data intelligence · Topic modeling · Machine learning · Big data computing

1 Introduction

Big Data is a new term used to identify the datasets that are of large size and have greater complexity. It has become an indispensable part of every economy, industry, organization, business function and individual. There are many misunderstandings about big data and it is known that there are at least 43 different definitions [1]. The data which contains valuable knowledge, is moving too fast,

© Springer Nature Switzerland AG 2019
M. Ezziyyani (Ed.): AI2SD 2018, AISC 915, pp. 592–608, 2019.
https://doi.org/10.1007/978-3-030-11928-7_54

it is too big and does not fit the structure of traditional database architectures. To gain value from this data, an alternative way to process it must be chosen. Big Data is much different from the classical data by the well-known five V's that characterize it:

1. Volume: the amount of data is measured in exabyte and zettabytes.
2. Variety: data comes from different sources.
3. Velocity: the streaming of data.
4. Variability: there are changes in the structure of data and how users want to interpret it.
5. Value: business value that gives organization a compelling advantage, and opportunities.

Making sense of large amounts of disorganized information, which is spread across wide swaths of an organization, has always been the defining challenge of knowledge management. Capitalization of knowledge takes place when it (knowledge) generates an added value. The generation of the value should be 'direct' and not correlated to any domain. Knowledge management (KM) is the process of identifying, capturing, organizing, and disseminating the intellectual assets, which is critical to the organization's long-term performance. Traditional KM systems have many limitations, and a new generation of KM systems should offer the following capabilities in the era of big data: it should create personalized experiences, track different multiple sources, move and reposition knowledge from different sources, and provide real-time on-demand knowledge, enable the KM system to be seamless and interoperable, and to have realistic connectivity that reduces costs, improves quality, and derives greater productivity, also helps in decision making area.

Determining the knowledge requirements and obtaining pertinent, consistent, and up-to-date knowledge across a large company, is a complex process. It is necessary in the KM field, to identify what knowledge is imperative to an organization. Identifying crucial knowledge aims to define, locate, characterize, and classify knowledge to be capitalized. "Knowledge capitalization" refers to a process through which a knowledge is managed, and can then be adapted, improved, adopted by other systems and up-scaled, leading to a greater impact in future uses. Thus, knowledge capitalization is a process, by which "a knowledge" in general or within a context is described and analyzed, identified, shared and used to improve the quality of knowledge. Capitalizing on big data era becomes a necessity, especially when it offers responses to many faced challenges like: duplication detection from large knowledge datasets, keeping the semantic relations between different knowledge concepts, and time response for a given request. In order to solve these challenges, a new collective control knowledge capitalization system has been developed, which concerned by designing strategies using distributed environment. The aim is to achieve a global control objective through this environment, by using topic modeling [2] especially by using hierarchical Latent Dirichlet Allocation (HLDA) [3] model and comparing it with the most known ones latent semantic analysis (LSA) [4] and latent dirichlet allocation (LDA) [5].

Topic models are widely used to uncover the latent semantic structure, from large corpus. The approach is based on the idea that the knowledge bases are a mixture of topics, where each topic is deduced according to a probability distribution of words. For a given knowledge base, after identifying the distribution of words, a clustering of words is done. These techniques, based on HLDA , have been growing for various applications. Using HLDA in big data systems, has many benefits, it offers-Parallel knowledge loading, and the distributed computing and storage. Being able to use the extracted knowledge in an intelligent way, is the aim targeted by knowledge capitalization. In this work, there has been an implementation of a retrieval mechanism on a top of prepared hierarchical knowledge graph, which is based on coherence computation. So in order to achieve this goal, a comparison of results with LSA and LDA has been done.

The remainder of this paper is organized as follows: Section 2 discusses some of the related research efforts and highlights them, Sect. 3 provides the preliminaries of our research on topic modeling approach, the coherence measure used, and the global vision of LSA, LDA and the HLDA approaches. The proposed architecture for our system is described in Sect. 4. Section 5 is devoted to the experiments and results. Finally, Sect. 6 presents the conclusion and future works.

2   Related Work

Knowledge Capitalization is an active process of capturing knowledge assets and making them actionable to support workers at the time of need when they are performing a task. This process adds value to organizations knowledge and expertise to produce higher revenue, profits and overall organization value. Typical results include more effective marketing, efficient distribution, smarter products and services that better serve customers, greater understanding of market forces, and more accurate revenue and profit predictions. The capitalization process does not depend on knowledge domain especially in big data context, it's a generative process, which can be applied to capitalize on equipment data and models as discussed in [6], also to the effects of capitalization on travel memories, and the influence of listener responsiveness on tourists destination examined in [7]. Capitalizing on knowledge, which is presented in [8] and accumulated in trustworthy relationships, increases the reliability, breadth and depth of tacit and codified knowledge available to an organization; thus, it improves the organization innovative performance.

Reference [9] presents an ontological framework dedicated to taking full advantage of already implemented educational analyses. The goal is to empower both expert and non-expert analysis stakeholders with the possibility to be involved in the elaboration of analysis processes and their reuse in different contexts, by improving both human and machine understanding of these analyses. This possibility is known as the capitalisation of analysis processes of learning traces. Authors in [10] analyze how knowledge-based practices adopted by innovation intermediaries enable them to generate value for themselves when collaborating with clients. The obtained results indicate that by capitalizing on existing knowledge vested in employees and collaborators as well as understanding and shaping the knowledge base of the innovation ecosystem, innovation intermediaries generate internal value from their involvement in collaborative innovation, which range from different financial to non-financial types of value.

The work [11] identifies two important problems, along with using topic models, in qualitative studies (opinion analysis and media studies): lack of a good quality metric, that closely matches human judgment in understanding topics, and the need to indicate specific subtopics, that a specific qualitative study may be most interested in mining. They propose an interval semi-supervised approach, where certain predefined sets of keywords (that define the topics researchers are interested in), are restricted to specific intervals of topic assignments. The contribution of [12] aims to enable better decision-making, by gathering, representing and modeling the linkages of integrating the available knowledge obtained by various research. This is achieved by conducting a systematic review of contributions and gathering the information into a database, and organizing that information in a mind-map. As an example, they showed how a Bayesian Network model and scenarios can be built using the mind-map and database information. They evinced how gathering information into mind-maps works as a first step to the creation of a unified knowledge base, while Bayesian Network models allow for a better management of data uncertainty, commonly associated with the representation of complex models. Thus, this contribution shows how available knowledge can be linked to improve the understanding of complex issues.

Reference [13] provides a comprehensive overview of the broad area of semantic search on knowledge bases. In a nutshell, semantic search refer to various parts of the search process: understanding the query, understanding the data (instead of just searching it for such matches), or representing knowledge in a suitable way for meaningful retrieval. The work is classified according to two dimensions: the type of data (text, knowledge bases, and combinations of these) and the kind of search (keyword, structured, natural language). Another important aspect in the semantic search is the entity disambiguation, that maps ambiguous terms in natural language text to its entities in a knowledge base. It finds its application in the extraction of structured data in RDF (Resource Description Framework) from textual documents, equally in facilitating artificial intelligence applications.

Authors in [14], propose a framework, which is initially, generates semantic embedding entity automatically, by given one or multiple knowledge bases. Then the system collectively links the input to an entity in a knowledge base with a graph based approach. An effective graphical model is applied, in order to perform collective entity disambiguation, by using the probabilistic approach proposed in [15].

3   Preliminaries

3.1   Topic Modeling

Topic modeling, as described in [5,16] is a text processing technique that determines themes within a collection of texts, using statistical analysis. While there is a broad and evolving range of available techniques, most of them produce results of a similar form: topics are represented by sets of commonly occurring words, allowing documents to be assigned to topics, by considering the words they contain. Most topic modeling techniques are probabilistic, creating weighted assignments of words to topics, by using the most representative approaches probabilistic latent semantic analysis (PLSA [17]), LDA [5] and HLDA [3].

The effort of mining the semantic structure in a text collection can be dated from latent semantic analysis (LSA) [4], which employs the singular value decomposition, to project documents into a lower dimensional space, called latent semantic space. PLSA [17] improves LSA with a sound probabilistic model, based on a mixture decomposition derived from a latent class model. In PLSA, a document is represented as a mixture of topics, while a topic is a probability distribution over words. LDA model inherits the notion of PLSA, but it employs an extra generative process on the topic proportion of each document and models the whole corpus via a hierarchical Bayesian framework [18]. In fact, PLSA turns out to be a special case of LDA with a uniform Dirichlet prior in a maximum posteriori model [19], while LDA has a better ability of modeling large-scale documents for its well-defined a-priori model. Many variants and extensions of the standard LDA model have been proposed, which can be found in the survey presented in [20]. The hierarchical dirichlet processes (HDP) is an extension of LDA, designed to address the case where the number of mixture components (the number of "topics" in document-modeling terms) is not known a priori. Using LDA for document modeling, one treats each "topic" as a distribution of words in some known vocabulary. For each document a mixture of topics is drawn from a Dirichlet distribution, and then each word in the document is an independent draw from that mixture. For HDP (applied to document modeling), one also uses a Dirichlet process to capture the uncertainty in the number of topics. So a common base distribution is selected which represents the countably-infinite set of possible topics for the corpus, and then the finite distribution of topics for each document is sampled from this base distribution. As far, HDP has the advantage that the maximum number of topics can be unbounded and learned from the data rather than specified in advance.

3.2   Topic Coherence

The state of the art in terms of topic coherence are the intrinsic measure UMass [21] and the extrinsic measure UCI, both based on the same high level idea. Both measure compute the sum (Eq. 1) of pairwise scores (Eq. 2) on the words $w_i, \ldots, w_n$, which is used to describe the topic K, usually the top n words by frequency $p(w|k)$.

$$Coherence = \sum_{i<j} score(w_i, w_j), \tag{1}$$

The UMass measure introduced by Mimno in [21] is used in this work. The topic is generally represented as a list of the most probable words for that topic, $D(w_i)$ is defined as the count of documents containing the word w_i, $D(w_i, w_j)$ the count of documents containing both words w_i and w_j, and D the total number or documents in the corpus. The corpus used to compute the counts is specified in a subscript of symbol D.

The UMass measure uses the following equation as pairwise score function:

$$score_{UMass}(w_i, w_j) = \log \frac{D(w_i, w_j) + 1}{D(w_i)} \tag{2}$$

which is the empirical conditional log-probability (Eq. 3) smoothed by adding one to $D(w_i, w_j)$.

$$\log p(w_j|w_i) = \log \frac{p(w_i, w_j)}{p(w_j)} \tag{3}$$

The score function is not symmetric as it is an increasing function of the empirical probability $p(w_j|w_i)$, where w_i is more common than w_j, words being ordered by decreasing frequency $p(w|k)$. So this score measures how much, within the words used to describe a topic, a common word is in average a good predictor for a less common word.

3.3 Latent Semantic Analysis

Latent Semantic Analysis (LSA), created a high dimensional, spatial representation of a corpus and allowed texts to be compared geometrically. A significant part of its processing is a type of principle components analysis called singular value decomposition (SVD) which compresses a large amount of co-occurrence information into a much smaller space. This compression step is somewhat similar to the common feature of neural network systems where a large number of inputs is connected to a fairly small number of hidden layer nodes. If there are too many nodes, a network will memorize the training set, miss the generalities in the data, and consequently perform poorly on a test set. The input for LSA is a large amount of data. The corpus is turned into a co-occurrence matrix of terms by documents or knowledge in our case. SVD computes an approximation of this data structure of an arbitrary rank K. It has been claimed that this compression step captures regularities in the patterns of co-occurrence across terms and across documents, and furthermore, that these regularities are related to the semantic structure of the terms and documents.

3.4 Latent Dirichlet Allocation

LDA uses two probability distributions. The first one is the probability distribution over words in the same topic and the second one, is the probability distribution over topics in the document. In other words, the LDA model represents documents as mixtures of topics that split out words with certain probabilities. It assumes that documents are produced using the following LDA algorithm:

- Decide on the number N of words the document will have (according to a Poisson distribution).
- Choose a topic mixture for the document (according to a Dirichlet distribution over a fixed set of K topics).
- Generate each word w_i in the document by:
  • Picking a topic (according to the multinomial distribution that was sampled above).
  • Using the topic to generate the word itself (according to the topic's multinomial distribution).

The generative process of LDA can be seen as follow:

- For each document w in a corpus D:
  • Choose N ∼ Poisson (ξ).
  • Choose θ ∼ Dir(α).
  • For each one of the N words $w_{(n)}$:
    Choose a topic $z_{(n)}$ ∼ Mult(θ).
    Choose a word $w_{(n)}$ from p($w_{(n)}/z_{(n)}$, β), a multinomial probability conditioned on the topic $z_{(n)}$.

Several simplifying assumptions are made in this basic model. First, the dimensionality k of the Dirichlet distribution (and thus the dimensionality of the topic variable z) is assumed known and fixed. Second, the word probabilities are parameterized by a k × V matrix Where $\beta_{(ij)}$= p(w^j = $1/z^i$ = 1), which for now is treated as a fixed quantity that is to be estimated. Finally, the Poisson assumption is not critical to anything that follows and more realistic document length distributions can be used as needed. Furthermore, note that N is independent of all the other data generating variables (θ and z).

Given the parameters α and β, the joint distribution of a topic mixture θ, a set of topics Z, and a set of N words w is:

$$p(\theta, z, w/\alpha, \beta) = p(\theta/\alpha) \prod_{n=1}^{N} p(z_n/\theta)p(w_n/z_n, \beta), \tag{4}$$

and the marginal distribution of a document is :

$$p(w/\alpha, \beta) = \int p(\theta/\alpha)(\prod_{n=1}^{N} \sum_{z_n} p(Z_n/\theta)p(W_n/z_n, \beta))d\theta \tag{5}$$

3.5 Hierarchical Latent Dirichlet Allocation

The Dirichlet process (DP) and the DP mixture model are mainstays of non parametric Bayesian statistics.

The definition of DPs is given as follow:

Let (Θ, B) be a measurable space, with G_0 a probability measure on the space, and let α_0 be a positive real number. A Dirichlet process is the distribution of a random probability measure G over (Θ, B) such that, for any finite partition $(A_1, \ldots, A_r)$ of Θ, the random vector $(G(A_1), \ldots, G(A_r))$ is distributed as a finite-dimensional Dirichlet distribution:

$$(G(A_1), \ldots, G(A_r)) \sim Dir(\alpha_0 G_0(A_1), \ldots, \alpha_0 G_0(A_r)). \tag{6}$$

$G \sim DP(\alpha_0, G_0)$ is written, in the case of a random probability measure distributed according to a DP, it is called G_0, the base measure of G, and α_0 the concentration parameter.

The DP can be used in the mixture model setting in the following way: consider a set of data, x $= (x_1, \ldots, x_n)$, assumed exchangeable. Given a draw $G \sim DP(\alpha_0, G_0)$, independently draw n latent factors from G: $\phi_i \sim G$. Then, for each $i = 1, \ldots, n$, draw $x_i \sim F(\phi_i)$, for a distribution F. This setup is referred to as a DP mixture model. If the factors ϕ_i were all distinct, then this setup would yield an (uninteresting) mixture model with n components. In fact, the DP exhibits an important clustering property, such that the draws ϕ_i are generally not distinct. Rather, the number of distinct values grows as $O(log_n)$, and it is this that defines the random number of mixture components.

One of the most significant conceptual and practical tools in the Bayesian paradigm is the notion of a hierarchical model. Hierarchical models has the following general setting: For J groups of data, each consisting of n_j data points $(x_{j1}, \ldots, x_{jn_j})$. The data points in each group are exchangeable, and are modeled with a mixture model. While each mixture model has mixing proportions specific to the group, sharing the same set of mixture components is required for different groups. While different groups have different characteristics given by a different combination of mixing proportions, using the same set of mixture components allows statistical strength to be shared across groups, and allows generalization to new groups.

The HDP is a non parametric prior, which allows the mixture models to share components. It is a distribution over a set of random probability measures over (Θ, B): one probability measure G_j for each group j, and a global probability measure G_0. The global measure G_0 is distributed as $DP(\gamma, H)$, with H the base measure and γ the concentration parameter, while each G_j is conditionally independent given G_0, with distribution $G_j \sim DP(\alpha_0, G_0)$. To complete the description of the HDP mixture model, each x_{ji} is associated with a factor ϕ_{ji}, with distributions given by $F(\phi_{ji})$ and G_j respectively.

HLDA uses a stochastic process called nested Chinese Restaurant Process (nCRP) [22]). to set a prior probability over the various topic hierarchies that can be inferred from the document corpus. NCRP is used to arrive at a generative process that is assumed to have generated the document corpus, based on a latent topic hierarchy. The hierarchy is characterized as a multi-way tree that comprises a set of nodes representing topics and each topic is a distribution over a set of words. Each path in the multi-way tree from the root to a leaf node is supposed to contain a set of hierarchically related topics with the generic topics near the top and concrete topics near the bottom levels of the tree [22]. nCRP allocates every document to one of the paths in the tree, after which it picks a topic in the path according to the GEM distribution over the topics in the path. A word for the document is picked according to the word distribution of the topic drawn from the GEM distribution. This probabilistic generative process has to be backtracked to infer the latent topic hierarchy underlying the document corpus.

Finally, topic inference is done through approximation methods that determines the posterior distribution over the topic hierarchies, levels in the hierarchy and the mapping of documents to topic proportions, using a sampling technique called 'Collapsed Gibbs Sampling' [23]. Typically topic inference is iterative in nature that requires repeatedly sampling latent parameters given the document corpus and other fixed latent parameters in the current sampling iteration [22]. Even after marginalizing out latent variables that are not of significant interest, the topic inference is known to be a computationally intensive process, due to the large number of sampling iterations before convergence and a handful of relevant latent variables.

4   The Proposed System

Knowledge capitalization is a new mechanism that can be applied to classical context systems, except for next generation systems, which will take it into account at the first time. For this aim, The proposed approach starts from the existing knowledge bases stored in distributed sites. Indeed, a distributed algorithm has been designed using HLDA for knowledge streams. This algorithm partitioned the knowledge sets across separate processors and inference is accomplished in a distributed and parallel way (using Apache spark as a container). In this algorithm, processors concurrently perform HLDA model over local site followed by a global update of the hierarchical topic model in the other sites. Hence, this mechanism is the main key to separate different knowledge bases by topics, and preparing knowledge for use.

In this paper, a new approach is proposed using the idea of managing the existing knowledge before using it. The aim is handling the big data challenges, by changing the whole knowledge bases structure, and keeping semantic relationships between different knowledge entities. In this sens, the three first Vs in big data are handled:

- Volume: starting from the idea that correlated knowledge remains in the same site; a distributed storage is used.
- Variety: unifying the knowledge representation (OWL format is used).
- Velocity: a kernel module is proposed to handle the preparation stage, which is the most important component in the framework.

Thus, before searching for knowledge, it's obligatory to find its location, first. This process, unlike in traditional contexts, proves to be unreliable in big data context, due to the additional time required to respond to a user request. For this aim, the focus was on the step of building the intelligent system in order to use the capitalized knowledge so as to avoid the problem of using it.

Knowledge management system is concerned with creating, using, identifying, capturing, and organizing knowledge. For this reason, the final step in traditional KM systems is always knowledge discovery. In big data context, the whole process is changing due to the following two major challenges: the huge volume, and the streams of knowledge. To overtake this issue, a new approach based on three components is proposed: batch processing, real time processing, and the service layer.

This system offers several axes, which connects workers to the knowledge they need at any time, when they are performing a task, making a decision, or solving a problem. Workers have immediate access to the knowledge they need so they can act on it when they need it. The system presents strengths keys by using Topic modeling to get the big picture of what is in the knowledge bases, and to eliminate the redundant knowledge. The HLDA algorithm, keep the semantic relationship between different entities. This approach can act on a top of any knowledge management system, due to the power of processing techniques (batch processing and real time processing). The big data context have come up with multiple issues to deal with. A distributed storage for the huge volume of knowledge is proposed, and also a OWL format to cut with the variety of knowledge, without forgetting the real time processing for the velocity of new knowledge.

This system has some limitations that should be taken into account in the next version. Communication between different sites is needed, in order to minimize the time consumed during knowledge streams update and storage. The storage limitation is an important issue, since knowledge that is received every second, cannot be stored infinitely. There is a possibility that knowledge update can cut with the two first limitations: minimizing the storage space as well as modifying the existing knowledge.

4.1   Batch processing system

Batch processing is an efficient way of processing high/large volumes of data. It is processed, especially where a group of transactions is collected over a period of time. In this process, at first, data is collected, entered and processed. Afterwards, it produces batch results.

Batch processing access to all data. It might compute something big and complex. Generally, it is very concerned with throughput. Rather than the latency of individual components of the computation. Batch processing has latency measured in minutes or more. Fig 1 describes the different components of our system's batch processing:

1. Knowledge preparation: in this step, the knowledge bases are prepared by dividing the knowledge bases into smaller groups and save them into different sites.

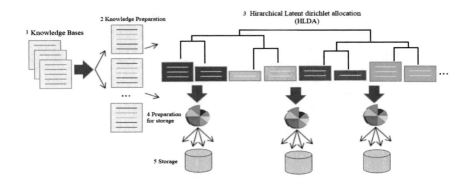

Fig. 1. The system's batch processing

2. build the hierarchical HLDA model: The existing algorithms for HLDA are not efficient in big data context, which have limited the evaluation at a small-scale and made HLDA not applicable in practice. To scale up HLDA, a distributed hierarchical topic modeling using HLDA is used. For this aim, the beginning was building a model base on a small number of groups. For the rest of groups, the previous module is just updated. The focus is on updating each previous model and passed it to the next site to update it, using the new knowledge. In the final site, the global module and the global dictionary are obtained, containing the entire set of features.
3. preparation for storage: The storage parameters are fixed (the number of available sites and the number of topics by site).
4. Storage: As a final result, only the correlated topics are stored, in every distributed site.

4.2   Real time processing system

Real-Time Processing involves continuous input, process, and output of data. Hence, it processes in a short period of time. In big data context, knowledge comes in streams (so fast), this is the reason behind using the abstraction levels mechanism for real time processing as shown in Fig 2. The Master site have to manage the different procedures as follow:

1. In the first step, The knowledge streams are received, then they are queued for processing.
2. Prepare the knowledge by dividing it into a knowledge groups.
3. In every distributed site and for the new knowledge streams:
   (a) calculate the coherence between the new knowledge and the stored one.
   (b) choose the site that present a higher coherence.
   (c) for the chosen site : calculate the coherence to each knowledge slots stored in this site to fuse the new knowledge with the most correlated one.
4. Store the new knowledge in the suitable correlated site, precisely with the chosen place (most correlated topic).

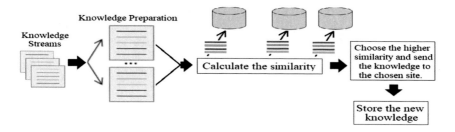

Fig. 2. Knowledge updating using new knowledge streaming

4.3 Knowledge retrieval service

The Knowledge retrieval service offered by the system is based on coherence computing (Fig 3):

1. When the system receives a request, an agent in the master site preprocesses it by extracting key words.
2. Based on these keywords, the system search for correlated topics. In other words, the same principle is used as the real time processing step in order to get the higher coherence.
3. The final step is concerned by seeking the answer from the correlated topics from the chosen site.

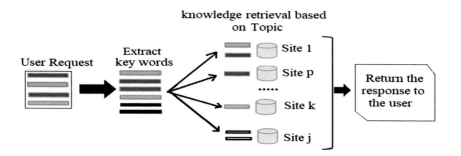

Fig. 3. Knowledge retrieval system

5   Experimental Evaluation

5.1   Knowledge Bases

In this study, different real-world datasets are used, such as Mesh, NIF-FUNCTION, and GEN ontologies, which contains more than five million triples. An explanatory summary of knowledge bases appears in Table 1.

Table 1. Summary of Knowledge bases

Knowledge base	Number of triples
Mesh	1,262,119
NIF-FUNCTION	124,337
Gen	1,618,739
Other OWL files	1,456,980

The initial point of every knowledge capitalization process is the knowledge bases. The ontology representation has been chosen as the main knowledge base representation. This representation, which is considered as the most used format especially in big data context, offers the facility to build and process knowledge, as well as the ability to keep the semantic relations between different entities.

5.2   Discussion of Experimental Results

The performance of a system is measured by the number of offered services. Topic modeling approaches are typically evaluated by measuring performance on some secondary tasks, such as classification, clustering, or knowledge retrieval.

To test the global system performances, a handling of the main critical issue in big data is chosen: the value. In other words, getting the correct value from the huge volume of knowledge in due time. With the aim of establishing a link between traditional uses of knowledge bases and the proposed framework, the dedicated time has been measured in order to get the response for different requests.

To put the system under evaluation, different requests have been used (relying on concepts from different knowledge bases). The first request type consists of seeking knowledge that doesn't exist in the knowledge bases. The second type looks into knowledge within different knowledge bases, which is omnipresent in several distributed sites.

Capitalizing on existing knowledge base using HLDA, minimize the risk of failure and increase their ability to generate new knowledge by combining existing knowledge bases. In practice, for the used knowledge-based, knowledge capitalization was found to influence positively on big data value creation. This highlights the need for capitalizing proven and established knowledge. The results revealed that the proposed system using HLDA outperforms the others systems in terms of response time as well as its ability to return direct (correlated) and indirect (less correlation) related knowledge. Table 2 shows the results of this use case. Ten different requests from different types are compared. The HLDA presents the best results for all requests, followed by LDA, LSA, and by the system without any knowledge capitalization mechanism. The three models presents a stability of time responding, also require a batch step for preparation; however, for real-time process, the HLDA offers the best combination between the update number through knowledge streams, and the update speed. In addition to that,

Table 2. Necessary time for request responding based on request type

Requests	Ordinal system (s)	LSA (s)	LDA (s)	HLDA (s)
Request 1	26	0.49	0.45	0.059
Request 2	27.12	0.45	0.43	0.065
Request 3	28.34	0.45	0.45	0.065
Request 4	29.15	0.47	0.46	0.059
Request 5	30.98	0.46	0.45	0.061
Request 6	34.04	0.47	0.46	0.058
Request 7	35.45	0.47	0.47	0.065
Request 8	37.97	0.47	0.46	0.065
Request 9	40.75	0.46	0.46	0.064
Request 10	43.81	0.46	0.46	0.064

the HLDA represents the best deal handling distributed computing issues (site down issue). Thus, the storage strategy offers more advantages than the LDA and LSA, taking into consideration that the topics are represented as hierarchical tree. So in terms of storage, the topics combination storage is obtained by just dividing the number of topics by the number of available sites. Moreover, unlike the LDA and LSA approaches, in the HLDA, the clustering step is omitted.

Understanding that extracting keywords from the request, with taking into account the topic mixture of the existing knowledge, which influences how topics are composed, can lead to a great results; however, since topics are not fixed because of real time processing, the most correlated and relevant knowledge should be returned to the user.

The precision is about returning the exactly correct value, with the higher scores. In other words, the keywords, which are used into the request must contribute to the construction of the topic positively.

To understand the theoretical and practical value of the precision, a very long request is used. It contains twenty three concepts, and it's very correlated to topic id_0. Table 3 shows the precision for each used approach: HLDA response correctly, with a high precision by just returning the topic id_0. The contribution of request keywords to the topic id_0 in the positive direction using HLDA is 0.91. On the other hand, LSA gives also the higher score to topic id_0, in comparison with other models, but it returns other less correlated knowledge even those who are contributing negatively to the topic. The positive and the negative values indicate the contribution of request keywords to the topic id_0 in both directions (positive and negative). Moreover, LSA requires a response filter in order to precise the response to the user request. In other words, it eliminates the less correlated knowledge; however, that demands much time, and more resources. On the contrary, the LDA returns the topic id_0 but not in the first place; it is given with the lowest score 0.08.

Table 3. Comparing the response precision

Approach	Topic Id	Coherence score
HLDA	0	0.917583
LSA	0	1
	8	0.999978
	1	0.805581
	3	0.288206
	5	0.033806
	6	−0.000121
	2	−0.098400
	9	−0.456703
LDA	5	0.283462
	7	0.263599
	8	0.113564
	0	0.082229
	9	0.078572

6   Conclusion

Knowledge extraction is one of the most important challenges in big data context; hence, for more effectiveness and usefulness of discovered knowledge, there is a great need of a knowledge capitalization system allowing easy access and sharing. In this paper, a new approach has been proposed, taking into consideration the context of big data. This approach is based on a clear idea, which aims to find only the related knowledge in every distributed site that can be achieved via a distributed topic modeling, precisely by using the HLDA as the preparation stage also as a flexible storing mechanism. As a result, the access to the desired knowledge is very quick, and very precise. Our system outperforms the traditional knowledge search algorithms, which have no knowledge capitalization system, also systems that are using the LSA and LDA as a preparation stage approach. In addition, it serves to keep the semantic relations between entities, and merge different knowledge bases without any redundant entities. As a future work, different knowledge representations will be used, and the system will be tested with different kinds of knowledge bases, by taking into account the cost, time response, and effectiveness of stored knowledge.

References

1. Huang, T., Lan, L., Fang, X., An, P., Min, J., Wang, F.: Promises and challenges of big data computing in health sciences. Big Data Res. **2**(1), 2–11 (2015)
2. Davenport, T.H., Patil, D.: Data scientist. Harvard Bus. Rev. **90**(5), 70–76 (2012)

3. Griffiths, T.L., Jordan, M.I., Tenenbaum, J.B., Blei, D.M.: Hierarchical topic models and the nested Chinese restaurant process. In: Advances in Neural Information Processing Systems, pp. 17–24 (2004)
4. Deerwester, S., Dumais, S.T., Furnas, G.W., Landauer, T.K., Harshman, R.: Indexing by latent semantic analysis. J. Am. Soc. Inf. Sci. **41**(6), 391 (1990)
5. Blei, D.M., Ng, A.Y., Jordan, M.I.: Latent dirichlet allocation. J. Mach. Learn. Res. **3**, 993–1022 (2003)
6. Garcia, G., Roser, X.: Enhancing integrated design model–based process and engineering tool environment: towards an integration of functional analysis, operational analysis and knowledge capitalisation into co-engineering practices. In: Concurrent Engineering, 1063293X17737357 (2016)
7. Tung, V.W.S., Cheung, C., Law, R.: Does the listener matter? the effects of capitalization on storytellers evaluations of travel memories. J. Travel Res. **0047287517729759**, (2017)
8. Martín-de Castro, G.: Knowledge management and innovation in knowledge-based and high-tech industrial markets: the role of openness and absorptive capacity. Ind. Mark. Manag. **47**, 143–146 (2015)
9. Lebis, A., Lefevre, M., Luengo, V., Guin, N.: Capitalisation of analysis processes: enabling reproducibility, openness and adaptability thanks to narration. In: Proceedings of the 8th International Conference on Learning Analytics and Knowledge. ACM, pp. 245–254 (2018)
10. De Silva, M., Howells, J., Meyer, M.: Innovation intermediaries and collaboration: knowledge-based practices and internal value creation. Res. Policy **47**(1), 70–87 (2018)
11. Nikolenko, S.I., Koltcov, S., Koltsova, O.: Topic modelling for qualitative studies. J. Inf. Sci. **43**(1), 88–102 (2017)
12. Pascual, M., Miñana, E.P., Giacomello, E.: Integrating knowledge on biodiversity and ecosystem services: mind-mapping and bayesian network modelling. Ecosyst. Serv. **17**, 112–122 (2016)
13. Bast, H., Buchhold, B., Haussmann, E., et al.: Semantic search on text and knowledge bases. Found. Trends® Inf. Retrieval **10**(2–3), 119–271 (2016)
14. Zwicklbauer, S., Seifert, C., Granitzer, M.: Doser-a knowledge-base-agnostic framework for entity disambiguation using semantic embeddings. In: International Semantic Web Conference. Springer, pp. 182–198 (2016)
15. Ganea, O.E., Ganea, M., Lucchi, A., Eickhoff, C., Hofmann, T.: Probabilistic bag-of-hyperlinks model for entity linking. In: Proceedings of the 25th International Conference on World Wide Web, International World Wide Web Conferences Steering Committee, pp. 927–938 (2016)
16. Wang, C., Blei, D.M.: Collaborative topic modeling for recommending scientific articles. In: Proceedings of the 17th ACM SIGKDD International Conference on Knowledge Discovery and Data Mining. KDD'11. ACM, New York, NY, USA, pp. 448–456 (2011)
17. Hofmann, T.: Probabilistic latent semantic indexing. In: Proceedings of the 22nd Annual International ACM SIGIR Conference on Research and Development in Information Retrieval. ACM, pp. 50–57 (1999)
18. Berger, J.B.M.B.J., Dawid, A., Smith, D.H.A., West, M.: Hierarchical Bayesian models for applications in information retrieval. In: Bayesian Statistics 7: Proceedings of the Seventh Valencia International Meeting, p. 25. Oxford University Press (2003)

19. Girolami, M., Kabán, A.: On an equivalence between PLSI and LDA. In: Proceedings of the 26th Annual International ACM SIGIR Conference on Research and Development in Information Retrieval. SIGIR'03, pp. 433–434. ACM, New York, NY, USA (2003)
20. Blei, D.M.: Probabilistic topic models. Commun. ACM **55**(4), 77–84 (2012)
21. Mimno, D., Wallach, H.M., Talley, E., Leenders, M., McCallum, A.: Optimizing semantic coherence in topic models. In: Proceedings of the Conference on Empirical Methods in Natural Language Processing, Association for Computational Linguistics, pp. 262–272 (2011)
22. Blei, D.M., Griffiths, T.L., Jordan, M.I.: The nested Chinese restaurant process and Bayesian nonparametric inference of topic hierarchies. J. ACM (JACM) **57**(2), 7 (2010)
23. Andrieu, C., de Freitas, N., Doucet, A., Jordan, M.I.: An introduction to MCMC for machine learning. Mach. Learn. **50**(1), 5–43 (2003)

Urban Parks Spatial Distribution Analysis and Assessment Using GIS and Citizen Survey in Tangier City, Morocco (2015 Situation)

Abdelilah Azyat[1]([⊠]), Naoufal Raissouni[2], Nizar Ben Achhab[1], Assad Chahboun[1], Mohamed Lahraoua[1], Ikram Elmaghnougi[3], Boutaina Sebbah[3], and Imane Alaoui Ismaili[1]

[1] Remote Sensing & Geographic Information System (RS&GIS), Reseach Laboratory, Remote Sensing & GIS Unit, National Engineering School for Applied Sciences of Tangier, University Abdelmalek Essaadi, Tangier, Morocco
{azyat.ensat,world.nizar}@gmail.com,
{chahboun_asaad,m_lahraoua}@yahoo.fr
[2] Remote Sensing & Geographic Information System (RS&GIS), Reseach Laboratory, National Engineering School for Applied Sciences of Tetuan, University Abdelmalek Essaadi, Tetuan, Morocco
raissouni.naoufal@gmail.com
[3] Faculty of Sciences and Technology of Tangier, University of Abdelmalek Essaadi, Tangier, Morocco
ikram_br_19@hotmail.fr, boutainasebbah@gmail.com

Abstract. In the last years, the city of Tangier (northern Morocco) has faced tremendous growth pressure. Actually, it is considered as one of the most densely populated cities with a density of 930 inhabitants per km^2. This strong demographic pressure has contributed to the increase of urbanization rate up to 60.3% compared to 55.1% nationally. In the present paper, based on Geographical Information System (GIS) technics, the proximity of four Tangiers' commons; Tanger, Boukhalef, Charf and Benimakada, to urban parks is analyzed. First, the spatial distribution of these urban parks is studied in terms of efficiency level referring to three indices (i.e., Park Area per Capita, PAC, Park Area Ratio, PAR, and Population Ratio, PR). Second, assessment of the population satisfaction and needs is carried out through both face-to-face and online citizen survey questionnaire. Accordingly, a total of 610 returns are collected from citizens of different commons. The outcomes highlight interesting points mainly the insistence and requirement for more urban parks. Finally, results show that public urban parks are not efficiently distributed in relation to residents and urban development. Some populations have access to urban parks, whereas more than half of the inhabitants were found to have limited access because of their dispersed and inconvenient spatial distribution. PAC values corresponding to Tanger, Boukhalef, Charf and Benimakada commons were determined to be 6.08, 2.07, 0.61 and 0.08 m^2, respectively. Therefore, Charf and Benimakada commons show to be the most affected commons.

Keywords: Urban parks · GIS · Spatial distribution analysis · Accessibility · Citizen survey

© Springer Nature Switzerland AG 2019
M. Ezziyyani (Ed.): AI2SD 2018, AISC 915, pp. 609–621, 2019.
https://doi.org/10.1007/978-3-030-11928-7_55

1 Introduction

Rapid urbanization has converted more than half of the world's population to urban dwellers during the past few decades. This wave of rural-to-urban migration will continue into the future with an estimated 66% of the world population living in urban areas by 2050 [1–3]. Indeed, this urbanization phenomenon has influences, such as urban changes and development which have some environmental impacts on Urban Green Spaces (UGS) and biodiversity. The loss or degradation of UGS may deprive the habitats for creatures, disrupt the structure and process of the urban ecosystem [4–6]. The influence of UGS in mitigating these negative effects has received considerable interest amongst scientists and urban planners [7, 8]. Over the last decade, there has been a shift in the health agenda towards promoting healthy lifestyle behavior and choices. The UGS can play a vital role in enhancing health and being-well [9, 10].

There is a lack of information concerning Urban Parks (UP); their distribution, their size, and the local regulations to establish them. According to the last census on 2014, Tangier city (northern Morocco) has about one million of population and tends to be densely built [11]. It suffers from a shortage of UGS and playing areas. The problem is that the open spaces are converted to built-up with a minimum percentage for green parks. The reason is that many Tangier commons and urban subdivisions consists often of house lots, and planning policies assign land use to residential, industrial and commercial purposes [12]. As a result, every piece of land was exploited to construct buildings, streets and sidewalks.

Citizen survey about urban green parks and open spaces should be evaluated in the spatial and environmental planning process. Natural spaces play an important role to decrease stresses and are considered as restful spaces, particularly for overwhelmed people. Thus, such parks integration in urban landscape is becoming a necessity for a healthier environment [12].

UGS can be defined as range of parks, street trees, urban agriculture, residential laws and roof gardens [13–16]. They are indispensable infrastructure in cities and can provide urban residents many essential benefits. They play a crucial role in cleaning the air, adjusting the microclimate [17, 18], eliminating noise, beautifying the surroundings [19] and maintaining biodiversity [20, 21]. In addition, preventing soil erosion [22], absorbing rainwater and pollutants, improving self-esteem and mood personal health, well-being [23, 24] and social cohesion as well [25]. On the other hand, they provide considerable socioeconomic benefits [26–28]. Hence, their spatial distribution should be established using scientific methods and according to international standards. This paper aims to study and assess the spatial distribution of public UP in Tangier city and their sufficiency to the population. These UP were analyzed using two methods: GIS-based analysis and social assessment of the study area using an urban population survey. In this study, green parks spatial examination is performed in terms of three indices (i.e., Park Area per Capita, PAC, Park Area Ratio, PAR and Population Ratio, PR); in order to list these parks regarding the number, size, areas, services and inhabitants proportion. This spatial distribution was compared to the international standards that form the modern urbanization background over many countries. Furthermore, determining the degree of population's benefits, an investigation instrument was utilized targeting the community assessment of UP. The findings of this research indicated that some populations have access to UP, whilst more than half of inhabitants were found to have limited access to UP in the city, and their spatial distribution was dispersed, inconvenient and inequity.

2 Methods

2.1 Study Area

The study was carried out in the city of Tangier in the north of Morocco (Fig. 1). Nationally, it is the third major city, located at 35.76° N, 5.80° W. Geographically, it is a connection point between the Mediterranean sea and Atlantic ocean. Such strategic position has made it an important location for ancient civilizations [29]. The city integrates three industrial zones and two free zones (the Tangier Free Zone (TFZ), about 500 hectares, and the Platform Industrial Motor Jouamaa that is developed on a 300 hectares) [30]. In the last decade, the city witnesses a big development whether urban, industrial, commercial, infrastructural and population density. Therefore, more demands will be in public services, specifically for UP. In other word, an increase in green parks infrastructure is becoming a necessity to improve people's life conditions by designing a relevant distribution, also creating and maintaining all types of green parks serving residents.

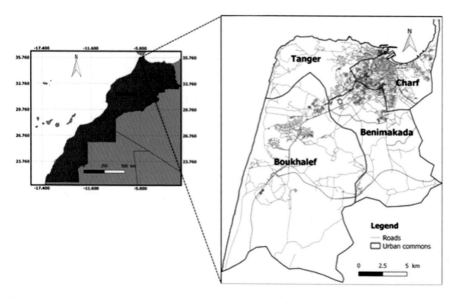

Fig. 1. Study area; Tangier city localization (northern Morocco) located at 35°.76' N, 5°.80' W coordinates. Legend: roads, communs (Tanger, Boukhalef, Charf and Benimakada)

In the last years, the city of Tangier has faced tremendous growth pressure. It is considered as one of the most densely populated areas in Morocco with a density of 930 inhabitants per km^2; this strong demographic pressure has contributed to raising the urbanization rate up to 60.3% compared to 55.1% nationally [30, 31]. According to the latest general census of the population in 2014, Tangier city has 971,553 inhabitants living in urban areas (in the 4 commons) [32]. The total surface of the study area is about 358.75 km^2. In Fig. 1, the study area comprises 4 urban commons (Tanger common, Benimakada assembled with Laaouama common, Charf-Mghogha and Charf-Souani commons which are assembled in Charf common, and Boukhalef added to Gueznaia common).

Tangier city is classified as the most expensive city in Morocco as an outcome of the high demand on jobs, services and residences. Consequently, land prices are in a permanent increase due to fast population growth. Therefore, the possibility of creating new parks is becoming very difficult.

2.2 Spatial Distribution of Urban Parks

Geographical Information System (GIS) is considered recently as a science, a technology and an industry. It provides a great number of geo-processing, analyses and management tools for spatial and non-spatial data [33]. Before many ages and nowadays, a number of studies have been realized in terms of UP location standards, location methods and relevance of their distribution and provision based on GIS technology. GIS has been widely used for analyzing the services of parks by studying their proximity, accessibility and size involves drawing lines around parks at a given distance [34].

With regard to measuring inhabitant's needs towards UP, researchers and planners have been implementing GIS for managing, planning and treating concerns of spatial distribution [35]. Thereby, lot of GIS-based researches have been adopted in order to analyze and assess green spaces and UP in different ways. For instance; (i) identifying green space ecological, recreational and aesthetic characteristics [36, 37], (ii) modeling planning scenarios to create new green parks within some neighborhoods [38], (iii) developing, linking and enhancing existing public UP in a process of planning [39], (iv) evaluating accessibility and equity to UP using the buffering method [40], (v) investigating whether populations have equal access to local parks or not [41–43] and (vi) studying the public parks distribution for identifying assemblies most in need to parks [37, 44].

2.3 Data Preparation Using GIS

Four steps are to follow: step 1: data collection, step 2: digitalization of the essential component of the city, step 3: areas calculation and step 4: buffering method application. Different thematic maps were established about buildings, roads, parks and open spaces using QGIS 2.8.2 open source software. Moreover, the spatial distribution (Fig. 2) study is performed. Calculation involving areas and UP indices was estimated to verify if the parks size and facilities are satisfying the inhabitants. To find out the served population, a buffer zone with a radius of 800 m was created for each park [35] (Fig. 3, see Sect. 3.1).

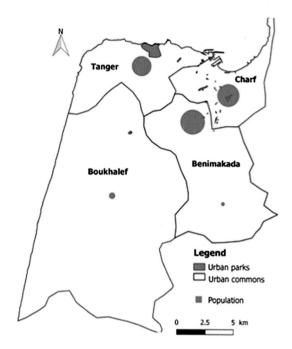

Fig. 2. Spatial distribution of urban public parks and population in the 4 commons

2.4   Urban Park Indices

Urbanization has effects on environmental components (e.g., biosphere, climate, rainfall runoff and green space diversity). In addition, many factors put on the biodiversity in urban areas, for instance, size, amount of parks, green space types, the use and spatial distribution of UP and others [35]. These changes are related to the nature and human activities. Certain indices are defined to evaluate the characteristics of UP. Our interest was mainly focused on green space diversity and specifically on UP spatial distribution. Thus, the objective was to answer the question: is this distribution sufficient and efficient or not over the city? For this, three indices have been considered: Park Area per Capita (PAC), Park Area Ratio (PR) and Population Ratio (PR) (Table 1). It should be noted that UP indices refer to the estimation of the sufficiency and the accessibility relative to population based on UP spatial distribution.

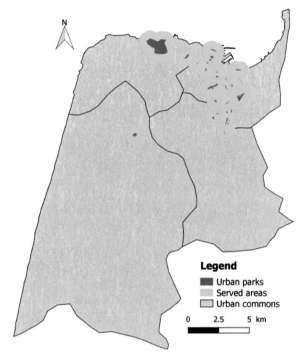

Fig. 3. The UP proximity to population for a distance of 800 m with the served areas

Table 1. UP standard indices in planning practices [5]. Park Area per Capita (PAC), Park Area Ratio (PR) and Population Ratio (PR)

Index	Formula	Description
PAC	$\dfrac{\text{total area of parks}}{\text{total population}}$	Represents the total area of parks devised on the total population (the amount of accessible urban park per capita)
PAR	$\dfrac{\text{area by parks}}{\text{Total area–park area}} \times 100$	The percentage of parks area within the area of analysis excluding park area
PR	$\dfrac{\text{population by park}}{\text{total population}} \times 100$	The percentage of population served by the parks in a common

3   Results and Discussion

3.1   Urban Parks Spatial Analysis

The UP spatial distribution study is analyzed by the GIS buffering tool with QGIS 2.8.2 software after catchment areas, road and building maps creation. The UP studied include neighborhood parks and one authority-managed natural park. The investigated distance parameter was set at 800 m [33], in order to check the accessibility of UP in Tangier city (see Fig. 3). Table 3 shows the number of existing parks, their area and ratio, children playground and sport facilities availability. The study area contains 22 UP having a total surface of 1.75 km^2. The majority of them concentrated in the Charf common in a number of 12 in different sizes, 6 from them without playgrounds and seven without sport facilities. In Tanger common five UP are defined including the natural one managed by the authority, one without sport facilities and two without children games. The less one is Boukhalef common with only two UP requiring sport facilities (Table 2).

The results show that the UP distribution over the city is inequity according to population distribution (whether in number, size or area). Consequently, not all residents have the sufficient accessibility. Especially, in Tanger, Benimakada and Boukhalef commons where urban public parks are insufficient and they do not respond to the growth and needs of these commons. We noticed that the majority of the population do not benefit from enjoying the existing parks for two reasons, either the parks are too far from where they live or they do not exist in their neighborhood at all. From Fig. 3, we remarked that the UPs are distributed without any regulations/standards, and their sizes do not follow any formulas. They are rare in some places.

3.2 Comparison of Urban Park Indices

In planning practices concerning UP, the current standards based on main indices have been applied (Table 3). Results of comparisons are expressed in terms of differences between commons. Table 3 shows that there is no similarity of tendency between indices. The higher PR is shown in the Benimakada common (39.75%), the lower one is in Boukhalef common (2.43%). However, in the terms of PAC and PAR indices, Tanger common shows a higher value of 6.08 m^2 and 2.06% respectively; whereas, the lowest value was recorded in Benimakada common with 0.08 m^2 for PAC and 0.03% for PAR.

Although, in the case of Charf common where appears the highest number of UP (12 parks), the PAC and PAR are lower than the Tanger common with only 5 parks (Table 3). This means that three elements are essential; size, location and distribution, which have a great impact on the accessibility of UP. Hence, it is important to take in consideration these elements when making parks arrangement and planning for having equally accessibility to all inhabitants. The three estimated indices gave a clear vision on how the UP are spatially distributed in relation with the population and the location, consequently, measuring the benefits to residents.

3.3 Citizen Assessment

As previously mentioned, a survey questionnaire to assess people's satisfaction towards UP in Tangier city has been realized. The questionnaire has been done during April, May and June 2015, including nine questions about gender, age, neighborhood and the existence/absence of urban green parks, with or without facilities/services (children games, playgrounds), the park availability within each neighborhood and the level of inhabitants' satisfaction. Table 4 provides the corresponding relevant demographic characteristics of respondents.

Table 2. Urban Parks (UP) properties; name, area, ratio, children playground and sport facilities for each common (Charf, Tanger, Boukhalef and Benimakada). Available (A), Not Available (NA)

Common	Urban Parks (UP)	Park Area (m²)	Park Ratio (%)	Children playground	Sport facilities
Charf	Jardin Route de Rabat	58,632	30.4	A	A
	JardinMoulay Youssef	32,426	16.8	NA	NA
	Jardin Badr	9110	4.7	NA	NA
	Jardin Ain ktiouet	11,942	6.2	A	NA
	Jardin Al Wilaya	4064	2.1	NA	NA
	Jardin de Tanja Balia	29,586	15.3	NA	A
	Parc Moulay Abdelaziz	1484	0.8	A	A
	Riad Tetouan	2915	1.5	NA	NA
	Jardin Dar Tounsi	6411	3.3	A	A
	Plasatoro	7097	3.7	NA	NA
	Nation Unies Garden	10,855	5.6	A	A
	Park Hay Benkirane	18,353	9.5	A	NA
Tanger	Parcs Achaba	87,069	5.9	A	A
	Jardin de La Mandoubia	22,798	1.5	A	A
	Jardin Iberia	4604	0.3	NA	NA
	Parc Rmilat	1,352,575	91.4	A	A
	Merkala	12,906	0.9	NA	A
Benimakada	Jardin Regaye	7714	24.5	NA	NA
	Jardin Gourziana	13,188	41.8	A	NA
	Jardin Beni Makada	10,643	33.7	A	NA
Boukhalef	Parcboukhalef1	43,953	89.8	A	NA
	Parc boukhalef2	4975	10.2	NA	NA

Four levels have been chosen to assess the UP's existence; high, moderate, low and non-existent. The low level was the more dominated in the four commons (Table 5); with 61% in the Charf, 51.90% in Tanger, 48.33% in Benimakada and 40% in Boukhalef. In the other side, the responds about the moderate confirmation of UP were 21, 19.50, 36.66 and 41.17% in Charf, Tanger, Benimakada and Boukhalef commons, respectively. While none of the surveyed people answered by high, except in Tanger (9.61%) and Boukhalef (8.23%) commons. This explained that this percentage was relative to inhabitants living near to UP.

Table 3. UP numbers and indices (Park Area per Capita, PAC (in m^2), Park Area Ratio, PAR (in %), Population Ratio, PR (in %)) for the four commons; Tanger, Boukhalef, Charf and Benimakada

Urban common	UP numbers	Total park area (m^2)	Population	PAC (m^2)	PAR (%)	PR (%)
Tanger	5	1,479,952	243,082	6.08	2.06	25.02
Boukhalef	2	48,928	23,601	2.07	0.03	2.43
Charf	12	192,875	318,679	0.61	0.65	32.61
Benimakada	3	31,545	386,191	0.08	0.03	39.75
Total	22	1,753,300	971,553			

Table 4. Demographic characteristics of the respondents

Demographic characteristics		Frequency	Percentage (%)
Gender	Male	203	33.3
	Female	407	66.7
Age	18–25	288	47.8
	25–45 years	162	26.6
	45 years and older	160	25.5
Common	Charf	202	33.1
	Tanger	145	23.7
	Benimakada	148	24.1
	Boukhalef	117	19,1

Table 5. Percentage of UP availability degree in Charf, Tanger, Benimakada and Boukhalef Commons

Items/value	Common				
		Charf	Tanger	Benimakada	Boukhalef
High	Citizen	0	14	0	9
	%	0	9.61	0	8.23
Moderate	Citizen	43	29	33	48
	%	21.40	19.50	36.66	41.17
Low	Citizen	124	74	44	47
	%	61.60	51.90	48.33	40
Non-existent	Citizen	35	28	13	13
	%	17	19.23	15	10.58

Additionally, 17, 19, 15 and 10.58% present the opinion of non-existent in the four commons successively cited above. It was found that the residents living far away from UP responded by unavailability of it in each neighborhood. Furthermore, the majority of people are least pleased for the actual situation of UP (Table 5). In other terms, they are unsatisfied on services provided by UP.

UP have great positive impacts on urban environment; improving health, reducing stress, they are important restful and recreation spaces. Undoubtedly, each neighbourhood should have an UP and creating new UP would be made a priority to residents.

However, on the one hand, comparing with the international standards [9, 35, 41] there was a difference concerning the UP amount in Tangier city. Besides, when we draw a parallel between the other cities, Tangier city is really far from the international regulations (Table 6). On the other hand, this study showed that Tangier population suffers from a shortage in urban green spaces. This was due to poor planning regulations system, ineffective preparation priorities, and misunderstanding of community needs.

Table 6. PAC and PAR indices comparison of urban parks in some world cities [45–48]

City	PAC (m^2)	PAR (%)	Date
Seoul	15	27	2015
Tokyo	3.4	5	2011
Nantes	57	6	2013
Austin	40.46	15	2015
London	29.73	5.77	2015
New Yourk	14.85	27	2010
Tangier	2.21	0.7	2015

In this study, focuses have been made on UP realized by common authorities including facilities, but urban natural parks and conservative spaces were not taken in account. Spatial analysis illustrated that urban parks spatial distribution was inefficient and insufficient in terms of size/area and number. It was found that facilities/services (e.g. playgrounds, games, seating, toilets) are minimal and not provided for all parks.

For citations of references, we prefer the use of square brackets and consecutive numbers.

Finally, to face the shortage of UP and associated services, this research suggests some recommendations such as: developing a strategy for protecting and improving UP effectively is a vital point to upgrade the Tangier city life quality. Also, UP distribution strategies for the development of parks, management, arrangement (location and size) and planning based on citizen's needs are required. Further, policies for stipulating more neighbourhood parks should be developed for these commons, particularly, Cherf, Benimakada and Boukhalef. Moreover, local government and authorities should take measures in order for designing, protecting, and building parks in Tangier city with suitable services based on set up rules can resolve the lack of UP.

4 Conclusions

The present study assessed the urban parks spatial distribution and their facilities in the one fastest growing Moroccan cities. The spatial distribution of UP was evaluated relatively to the population of residential areas using two methods; GIS-based approach within a distance of 800 m illustrating the number of parks accessible, and a questionnaire-based citizen survey in order to identify services, equity and to quantify the satisfaction of inhabitants. Three indices; park area per capita, park area ratio and population ratio have been calculated to measure the accessibility and the sufficiency relative to UP. The results have revealed three points: First, the number of parks is really insufficient and they distributed inconveniently in the four commons; Charf, Tanger, Benimakada and Boukhalef. The common of Benimakada is the more populated and only had 3 parks. Second, services not existed in all parks specifically, children playgrounds, toilets and sport facilities. Third, the park area per capita and park area ratio indices showed that the Charf (0.61 m^2 and 0.65%) and Benimakada (0.08 m^2 and 0.03%) commons had serious matter depending UP.

The respondents demonstrated that there are needs regarding the UP availability and they were unsatisfied and not all urban people benefit from UP accessibility. The utility of these approaches could help in the creation; identification, and sustainable management of urban green areas. In addition, these results have implications for managers and researchers for urban planning as to the best way to assess the citizen needs. Future work will compare these results with ones will obtain using network analysis taking in account the recent efforts realized by authorities to improve and create more urban green spaces.

References

1. World Urbanization Prospects: The 2014 Revision. Department of Economic and Social Affairs, Population Division. https://esa.un.org/unpd/wup/Publications/Files/WUP2014-Highlights.pdf. Last Accessed 05 June 2016
2. State of world population 2007: Unleashing the potential of urban growth. United Nations Population Fund. https://www.unfpa.org/sites/default/files/pub-pdf/695_filename_sowp2007_eng.pdf. Last Accessed 02 Sep 2016
3. Dong, W., Gregory, B., Yan, L.: The physical and non-physical factors that influence perceived access to urban parks. Landscape Urban Plann. **133**, 53–66 (2015)
4. Byomkesh, T., Nakagoshi, N., Dewan, A.M.: Urbanization and green space dynamics in Greater Dhaka. Bangladesh Landscape Ecol. Eng. **8**, 45–58 (2012)
5. Kyushik, O., Seunghyun, J.: Assessing the spatial distribution of urban parks using GIS. Landscape Urban Plann. **82**, 25–32 (2007). https://doi.org/10.1016/j.landurbplan.2007.01.014
6. Robert, D.B., Jennifer, V., Natasha, K., Sanda, L.: Designing urban parks that ameliorate the effects of climate change. Landscape Urban Plann. **138**, 118–131 (2015)
7. Heikki, S., Viljami, V., Anna, L.R., Arto, P., Vesa, Y.P.: Does urban vegetation mitigate air pollution in northern conditions? Environ. Pollut. **183**, 104–112 (2013)
8. Hadi, S.A., Nakagoshi, N.: Landscape ecology and urban biodiversity in tropical Indonesian cities. Landsc. Ecol. Eng. **7**(1), 33–43 (2011)

9. Nakagoshi, N., Watanabe, S., Kim, J.E.: Recovery of green resources in Hiroshima City after World War II. Landsc. Ecol. Eng. **2**, 111–118 (2006)
10. Alberti, M.: Urban patterns and ecosystem function. In: Advances in Urban Ecology: Integrating Humans and Ecological Processes in Urban Ecosystems. pp. 61–92. Springer, New York (2008)
11. HCP, RGPH 2014: Cartographie thématiques des données. http://rgph2014.hcp.ma/. Last Accessed 03 Feb 2016
12. Frischenbruder, M., Pellegrino, P.: Using greenways to reclaim nature in Brazilian cities. Landscape Urban Plann. **76**, 67–78 (2006)
13. Kong, F., Nakagoshi, N.: Spatial-temporal gradient analysis of urban green spaces in Jinan. China. Landscape Urban Plann. **78**, 147–164 (2006)
14. Wendy, Y.C., Jim, C.Y.: Assessment and valuation of the ecosystem services provided by urban forests. In: Margaret, M.C., Yong, C.S., Jianguo, W., editors. Ecology, Planning, and Management of Urban Forests, pp. 53–83. Springer, New York (2007)
15. Charlie, M.S., Andrew, B.: Perceptions and use of public green space is influenced by its relative abundance in two small towns in South Africa. Landscape Urban Plann. **113**, 104–112 (2013)
16. Nadja, K., Salman, Q., Dagmar, H.: Human–environment interactions in urban green spaces—a systematic review of contemporary issues and prospects for future research. Environ. Impact Assess. Rev. **50**, 25–34 (2015)
17. Jim, C.Y., Chen, S.S.: Comprehensive green space planning based on landscape ecology principles in compact Nanjing city. China. Landscape Urban Plann. **65**, 95–116 (2003)
18. Neema, A.O.: Multi-objective location modeling of urban parks and open spaces: Continuous optimization. Comput. Environ. Urban Syst. **34**, 359–376 (2010)
19. Richard, G.D., Olga, B., Richard, A.F., Jamie, T., Nicholas, B., Daniel, L., Philip, H.W., Kevin, J.G.: City-wide relationships between green spaces, urban land use and topography. Urban Ecosyst. **11**(3), 269–287 (2008)
20. Attwell, K.: Urban land resource and urban planting—case studies from Denmark. Landscape Urban Plann. **52**, 145–163 (2000)
21. Pham, D.U., Nobukazu, N.: Application of land suitability analysis and landscape ecology to urban green space planning in Hanoi, Vietnam. Urban For. Urban Greening **7**, 25–40 (2008)
22. Ashley, C.N., Wei, X., Jeff, Y., David, W.: Planning for multi-purpose greenways in Concord. North Carolina. Landscape Urban Plann. **68**, 271–287 (2004)
23. Tabassum, S., Sharmin, F.: Accessibility analysis of parks at urban neighborhood: the case of Dhaka. Asian J. Appl. Sci. Eng. **2**, 48–61 (2012)
24. Bolund, P., Hunhammar, S.: Ecosystem services in urban areas. Ecol. Econ. **29**, 293–301 (1999)
25. Gilbert, O.: The Ecology of Urban Habitats. Chapman & Hall, London (1989)
26. Korpela, K., Hartig, T.: Restorative qualities of favorite places. J. Environ. Psychol. **16**, 221–233 (1996)
27. Liisa, T., Kirsi, M., Jasper, S.: Tools for mapping social values of urban woodlands and other green spaces. Landscape and Urban Plann **79**, 5–19 (2007)
28. Julien, L.T., Fathallah, D., Lahoucine, A.: Urban mobility in Tangier metropolitan: evolutions and prospects, Plan bleu, Centre d'Activités Régionales, Sophia Antipolis (2009). http://planbleu.org/sites/default/files/publications/mob_urb_tanger_rapport2009_0.pdf. Last Accessed 20 Jan 2016
29. William, K.: State and Territorial Restructuring in the Globalizing City Region of Tangier (2010)
30. TFZ., Tanger Free Zone (2016). http://www.tangerfreezone.com/en/tanger-automotive-city. Last Accessed 03 Mar 2016

31. Khadija, A.: Les formations littorales quaternaires de la péninsule de Tanger (Maroc nord occidental): Lithostratigraphie, processus sédimentologiques, pétrologie et corrélations à l'échelle de la Méditerranée centre-occidentale. Ph. D. dissertation, Mohammed V University Rabat, Morocco (2009)

32. RGPH 2014. http://rgph2014.hcp.ma/downloads/Publications-RGPH-2014_t18649.html. Last Accessed 01 Feb 2016

33. Ahn, T.M., Choi, H.S., Kim, I.H., Cho, H.J.: A study on the method of measuring accessibility to urban open spaces. Landscape Architect. 18, 17–28 (1991)

34. Abdelilah, A., Naoufal, R.: Design and development of a mobile geographic information system platform (MGISP) based on GPS technology for spatial data acquisition, management and geovisualisation: multi-utilization interface. Ph. D. dissertation, UAE Univ., Tetuan, Morocco (2011)

35. Sarah, N.: Measuring the accessibility and equity of public parks: a case study using GIS. Managing Leisure 6, 201–219 (2001)

36. Salem, A.T.: Integration of GIS and perception assessment in the creation of needs-based urban parks in Ramallah. Palestine. J. Urbanism 7, 170–186 (2014)

37. Mahon, J.R., Miller, R.W.: Identifying high-value green space prior to land development. J. Arboric. 29, 25–33 (2003)

38. Herbst, H., Herbst, V.: The development of an evaluation method using a geographic information system to determine the importance of wasteland sites as urban wildlife areas. Landscape Urban Plann. 77(1–2), 178–195 (2006)

39. Randall, T.A., Churchill, C.J., Baetz, B.W.: A GIS-based decision support system for neighborhood greening. Environ. Plan. 30, 541–563 (2003)

40. Jim, C.Y., Chen, W.Y.: Perception and attitude of residents toward urban green spaces in Guangzhou (China). Environ. Manage. 38, 338–349 (2006)

41. Alexis, C., Chris, B., Edmund, G.: Using a GIS-based network analysis to determine urban green space accessibility for different ethnic and religious groups. Landscape Urban Plann. 86, 103–114 (2008)

42. Sarah, N., Shafer, C.S.: Measuring accessibility and equity in a local park system: the utility of geospatial technologies to park and recreation. J. Park Recreation Adm. 19, 102–124 (2001)

43. Stephan, P., Roland, E., Yvonne, G.: Modeling the environmental impacts of urban land use and land cover change—a study in Merseyside. UK. Landscape Urban Plann. 71, 295–310 (2005)

44. Talen, E., Anselin, L.: Assessing spatial equity: An evaluation of measures of accessibility to public playgrounds. Environ. Plann. A 7, 437–456 (1998)

45. Henri, M.: Creativity Takes Courage. World cities culture report (2015). http://www.worldcitiescultureforum.com/data/of-public-green-space-parks-and-gardens. Last Accessed 01 July 2016

46. Greenspace Information for Greater London CIC (2016). http://www.gigl.org.uk/our-data-holdings/keyfigures/. Last accessed 12 July 2016

47. Seoul, S.: Changes in Park & Green Space Policies in Seoul (2015). https://seoulsolution.kr/content/changes-park-green-space-policies-seoul?language=en. Last Accessed 11 Aug 2015

48. European Green Capital Award Nante. Green Urban Areas (2013). http://ec.europa.eu/environment/europeangreencapital/wp-content/uploads/2011/05/EGCNantesUKChap3-F.pdf. Last Accessed 15 Aug 2015

Amazigh POS Tagging Using TreeTagger:
A Language Independant Model

Samir Amri[✉] and Lahbib Zenkouar

ERSC Laboratory, EMI School, Med V University, Rabat, Morocco
amri.samir@gmail.com, zenkouar@emi.ac.ma

Abstract. Part of Speech (POS) tagging has high importance in the domain of Natural Language Processing (NLP). POS tagging determines grammatical category to any token, such as noun, verb, adjective, person, gender, etc. Some of the words are ambiguous in their categories and what tagging does is to clear of ambiguous word according to their context. Many taggers are designed with different approaches to reach high accuracy. In this paper we present a Machine Learning algorithm, which combines decision trees model and HMM model to tag Amazigh unknown words. In case of statistical methods such as TreeTagger, this will have added practical advantages also. This paper presents creation of a POS tagged corpus and evaluation of TreeTagger on Amazigh text. The results of experiments on Amazigh text show that TreeTagger provides overall tagging accuracy of 93.19%, specifically, 94.10% on known words and 70.29% on unknown words.

Keywords: POS tagging · TreeTagger · Amazigh · Corpus

1 Introduction

Part-of-Speech (POS) tagging is an essential step to achieve the most natural language processing applications because it identifies the grammatical category of words belong text. Thus, POS taggers are an import and module for large public applications such as questions-answering systems, information extraction, information retrieval, machine translation… They can be used in many other applications such as text-to-speech or like a pre-processor for a parser; the parser can do it better but more expensive. In this paper, we decided to focus on POS tagging for the Amazigh language. Currently, TreeTagger (hence fore TT) is one of the most popular and most widely used tools thanks to its speed, its independent architecture of languages, and the quality of obtaining results. Therefore, we sought to develop a settings file TT for Amazigh.

Our work involves the construction of the dataset and the input pre-processing in order to run the two main modules: training program and tagger itself. For this reason, this work is the part of the still scarce set of tools and resources available for Amazigh automatic processing. The rest of the paper is organized as follows. Sect. 2 puts the current article in context by overviewing related work. Sect. 3 describes the linguistic background of Amazigh language and presents the used Amazigh tagset and our training corpus. Experimental results are discussed in Sect. 4. Finally, we will report our conclusions and eventual future works in Sect. 5.

© Springer Nature Switzerland AG 2019
M. Ezziyyani (Ed.): AI2SD 2018, AISC 915, pp. 622–632, 2019.
https://doi.org/10.1007/978-3-030-11928-7_56

2 POS Tagging

Part-of-speech (POS) tagging is the process of assigning to each word in a sentence the proper POS tag in the context it appears. In general, a word can be classified into some POS classes. In a given context, however, there is a POS tag which is more appropriate than the others, and the task of a tagger is to find this tag. The input of a tagging algorithm is a string (usually a sentence) of words and a specific tagset. The output is a string in which each word is assigned with the most appropriate tag according to the context it appears in the sentence. The challenges in the POS tagging task are how to find POS tags of new words and how to disambiguate multi-sense words. Several methods have been proposed to deal with the POS tagging task in Amazigh.

They usually consider the task as a sequence labeling problem, and various kinds of learning models have been investigated.

2.1 POS Tagging Challenges

There are two challenges that we need to tackle to be able to predict part-of-speech tags. Some words can have different labels depending on their role in the sentence. For instance, "illi" in Amazigh is used as a verb (exist) (base form VB and present form VBP) and a as noun (NN) (daughter). The second problem is unseen words for which we don't know in advance their tags. For instance number are given the CD tag. But there is an infinity of numbers which are not in the training data.

Our classifier will have to learn to deal with both problems. In HMM taggers, this is generally handled by estimating the probability for a word to have a given tag (to help with the ambiguity problem) and the probability for a tag to be followed by another tag (to help with generalization on unseen words). We can do similarly by defining a feature for the current word and the associated tag, and a feature for the current tag given the previous tag.

2.2 Classification of POS Taggers

The importance of the problem focuses from the fact that the POS is one of the first stages in the process performed by various natural language related process. POS tagging is the commonest form of the corpus annotation. POS is mainly for information retrieval, text to speech, information extraction and linguistic research for corpora and for higher level NLP tasks like parsing, semantics, machine translation and many more. Pos tag gives some information about the sense of the word in the context of use. It is a non-trivial task [1]:

- Some words that occur in the lexicon or dictionary have more than one possible Part of Speech.—Some words are unknown.
- Tags are not well-defined. The approaches of POS tagging can be divided into three categories; rule based tagging, statistical tagging and hybrid tagging.

A set of hand written rules are applied along with it the contextual information is used to assign POS tags to words in the rule based POS [2]. The disadvantage of this system is that it doesn't work when the text is not known. The problem being that it cannot predict the appropriate text. Thus, in order to achieve higher efficiency and accuracy in this system, exhaustive set of hand coded rules should be used. Frequency and probability are included in the statistical approach.

The basic statistical approach works on the basis of the most frequently used tags for a specific word in the annotated training data and also this information is used to tag that word in the unannotated text. But the disadvantage of this system is that some sequences of tags can come up for sentences that are not correct according to the grammar rules of a certain language. Another approach is also there that is known as the hybrid approach. It may even perform better than statistical or rule based approaches. First of all the probabilistic features of the statistical method are used and then the set of hand coded language specific rules are applied in the hybrid approach.

In the area of POS tagging, many studies have been made. It reached excellent levels of performance through the use of discriminative models such as maximum entropy models [MaxEnt] [3–5], support vector machines [SVM] [6, 7] or Markov conditional fields [CRF] [8, 9]. Among stochastic models, bi-gram and tri-gram Hidden Markov Models (HMM) are quite popular. TNT [10] is a widely used stochastic trigram HMM tagger which uses a suffix analysis technique to estimate lexical probabilities for unknown tokens based on properties of the words in the training corpus which share the same suffix.

The development of a stochastic tagger requires large amount of annotated text. Stochastic taggers with more than 95% word-level accuracy have been developed for English, German and other European languages, for which large labeled data are available. Then decision trees have been used for POS tagging and parsing as in [11]. Decision tree induced from tagged corpora was used for part-of-speech disambiguation [12]. For Amazigh POS tagging, Outahajala et al. built a POS-tagger for Amazigh [13], as an under-resourced language. The data used to accomplish the work was manually collected and annotated. To help increase the performance of the tagger, they used machine learning techniques (SVM and CRF) and other resources or tools, such as dictionaries and word segmentation tools to process the text and extract features' sets consisting of lexical context and character n-grams. The corpus contained 20,000 tokens and was used to train their POS-tagger model. Therefore, there is a pressing necessity to develop an automatic Part-of-Speech tagger for Amazigh.

3   TreeTagger

One common technique for predicting part-of-speech tags is decision tree learning [14, 15]. A decision tree learner is a machine learning algorithm that sequentially partitions the training data set based on attribute values, recursively partitioning the data until all attributes at a node can be classified with the same value [16]. In the same line, TreeTagger is a system for tagging text with part-of-speech and lemma information. It was developed in the TC project at University of Stuttgart.

TreeTagger has been successfully used to tag German, English, French, Italian, Dutch, Spanish, Russian, etc. It is generally adaptable to other languages if a lexicon and a manually tagged training corpus are available. The heart of TreeTagger, as its name suggests, is « estimation of transition probabilities with a binary decision tree"

[15]. The initial stage of building the decision tree happens during the training phase. It will parse through the text and analyze trigrams, inserting each unigram into the tree. Probabilities for which tag to use are determined for a given node of the tree based on the information obtained from the two previous nodes (trigram). Once the tree is created, its nodes are pruned. If the information gain of a particular node is below a defined threshold, its children nodes are removed. Figure 1 represents a simplified version of a decision tree using an example of Amazigh sentence.

4   Linguistic Background

This section presents background knowledge related to this research. First, a short description of characteristics of words in Amazigh language is presented in Subsection A. Subsections B and C describe the Amazigh script and the transliteration system. A brief introduction to corpus and tagset used are presented in Sub-section D.

4.1   Amazigh Language

Amazighe language belongs to the Hamito-Semitic/"Afro-Asiatic" languages, with rich morphology [17]. In linguistic terms, the language is characterized by the proliferation of dialects due to historical, geographical and sociolinguistic factors. It is spoken in Morocco, Algeria, Tunisia, Libya, and Siwa (an Egyptian Oasis); it is also spoken by many other communities in parts of Niger and Mali. It is used by tens of millions of people in North Africa mainly for oral communication and has been introduced in mass media and in the educational system in collaboration with several ministries in Morocco. In Morocco Amazigh language uses different dialects in its standardization (Tachelhit, Tarifit and Tamazight). Amazigh NLP presents many challenges for researchers. Its major features are:

- It has its own script: the Tifinagh, which is written from left to right.
- It does not contain uppercase.
- Like other natural language, Amazigh presents for NLP ambiguities in grammar classes, named entities, meaning, etc. For example, grammatically; the word (illi) depending on the context can mean a noun in this sentence (tfulki illi: my daughter is beautiful) or a verb in this sentence (ur illi walou: there is nothing).
- As most languages whose research in NLP is new, Amazigh is not endowed with linguistic resources and NLP tools.
- Amazigh, like most of the languages which have only recently started being investigated for NLP, still suffers from the scarcity of language processing tools and resources.

4.2   Amazigh Script

Like any language that passes through oral to written mode, Amazigh language has been in need of a graphic system. In Morocco, the choice ultimately fell on Tifinaghefor technical, historical and symbolic reasons. Since the Royal declaration on

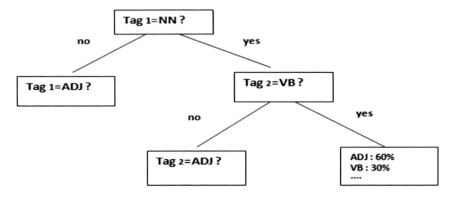

Fig. 1. A simplified decision tree from Amazigh text

2003, Tifinaghe has become the official graphic system for writing Amazigh. Thus, IRCAM has developed an alphabet system called Tifinaghe-IRCAM. This alphabet is based on a graphic system towards phonological tendency. This system does not retain all the phonetic realizations produced, but only those that are functional. It is written from left to right and contains 33 graphemes which correspond to:

- 27 consonants including: the labials (ⵛ, ⵀ, ⵞ), dentals (ⵜ, ⵏ, ⵟ, ⵟ, ⵍ, ⵔ, ⵇ, ⵥ), the alveolars (ⵙ, ⵅ, ⵣ, ⵥ), the palatals (ⵛ, ⵊ), the velar (ⴽ, ⵅ), the labiovelars (ⴽ ˮ, ⵅ ˮ), the uvulars (ⵕ, ⵅ, ⵖ), the pharyngeals (ⵄ, ⵂ) and the laryngeal (ⵁ);
- 2 semi-consonants: ⵢ and ⵓ;
- 4 vowels: three full vowels ⵄ, ⵉ, ⵊ and neutral vowel (or schwa) ⴻ.

4.3 Transliteration System

We have decided to use a specific writing system based on ASCII characters for technical reasons [6]. So, correspondences between the different writing systems and transliteration correspondences are shown in Table 1.

4.4 Corpus and Tagset

Amazigh Tagset
A tagset is a collection of labels which represent word classes. A coarse-grained tag set might only distinguish main word classes such as adjectives or verbs, while more fine-grained tagsets also make distinctions within the broad word classes, e.g. distinguishing between verbs in past and future tense. This is an important step for a lexical labeling work to be based on the word classes of language and shall reflect all morphosyntactic relationships words of the Amazigh corpus (Table 2).
Corpus
A corpus is a collection of language data that are selected and organized according to explicit linguistic criteria to serve as a sample of jobs determined a language. Generally, a corpus contains up few millions of words and can be lemmatized and annotated with information about the parts of speech. Among the corpus, there is the British

Table 1. Mapping from existing writing system and the chosen writing system

Tifinaghe Unicode		Transliteration		Chosen writing
Code	*Character*	*Latin*	*Arabic*	system
U+2D30	ⵀ	A	ا	A
U+2D31	ⴱ	B	ب	B
U+2D33	ⵅ	G	گ	G
U+2D33&U+2D6F	ⵅˮ	Gw	گ	Gw
U+2D37	ⴷ	D	د	D
U+2D39	ⴹ	ḍ	ض	D
U+2D3B	ⴻ	E		E
U+2D3C	ⴼ	F	ف	F
U+2D3D	ⴽ	K	ک	K
U+2D3D&+2D6F	ⴽˮ	Kw	گ+	Kw
U+2D40	ⵀ	H	ھ	H
U+2D43	ⴶ	ḥ	ح	H
U+2D44	ⵄ	E	ع	E
U+2D44	ⵅ	X	خ	X
U+2D45	ⵇ	Q	ق	Q
U+2D47	ⵉ	I	ي	I
U+2D47	ⵊ	J	ج	J
U+2D47	ⵍ	L	ل	L
U+2D47	ⵎ	M	م	M
U+2D47	ⵏ	N	ن	N
U+2D47	ⵓ	U	و	U
U+2D47	ⵔ	R	ر	R
U+2D47	ⵕ	ṛ	ر	R
U+2D47	ⵖ	Y	غ	G
U+2D47	ⵙ	S	س	S
U+2D47	ⵚ	ṣ	ص	S
U+2D47	ⵛ	C	ش	C
U+2D47	ⵜ	T	ت	T
U+2D47	ⵟ	ṭ	ط	T
U+2D47	ⵡ	W	و	W
U+2D47	ⵢ	Y	ي	Y
U+2D47	ⵣ	Z	ز	Z

National Corpus [18] (100 million words) and the American National Corpus [19] (20 million words).

A balanced corpus would provide a wide selection of different types of texts and from various sources such as newspapers, books, encyclopedias or the web. For the Moroccan Amazigh language, it was difficult to find ready-made resources. We can just mention the manually annotated corpus of Outahajala et al. [20, 21]. This corpus contains 20 k words using a tagset described in Table 3 that is why we decided to build our own corpus. In order to have a vocabulary sufficiently large, we took texts from the web sites of some Moroccan ministries, texts from IRCAM website[1] and from primary school textbooks...etc. We have collected these different resources; after that, we have cleaned them and convert them to text format especially UTF-8 Unicode.

---

[1] www.ircam.ma.

Table 2. Amazigh tag set

Tag	Attributes with the number of values
Noun	Gender(3), number(3), state(2), derivation(2), Sub classification POS (4), number(3), gender(3), person(3)
Verb	Gender(3), number(3), person(3), aspect(3), negation(2), form(2), derivation (2), voice(2)
Adjective	Gender(3), number(3), state(2), derivation(2), POS subclassification (3)
Pronoun	Gender(3), number(3), person(3), POS subclassification (7), deictic(3)
Determinant	Gender(3), number (3), Sub classification POS (11), deictic(3)
Adverb	Sub classification POS (6)
Preposition	Gender(3), number(3), person(3), number(3),gender(3)
Conjunction	POS subclassification(2)
Interjection	Interjection
Particle	POS subclassification (7)
Focalizer	Focalizer
Foreign word	POS subclassification (5), gender (3), number (3)
Punctuation	Type de la marque de ponctuation(16)

Table 3. Constituents of Amazigh corpus

Source	%
Online newspapers and periodicals	22.7
Primary school textbooks	15
Texts from websites of organizations	10.4
Texts from government websites	8.6
Miscellany	16.5
Blog	15
Texts from website of IRCAM	12.8

The Table 3 provides source statistics of our corpus, which includes 6714 sentences (approximately 75,340 words).

5   Results and Discussion

5.1   Results

In the majority of the part of speech tagging approaches, the sample is often subdivided into "training" and "test" sets. The training set is generally used for learning, i.e. fitting the parameters of the tagger. The test set is for assessing the performance of the tagger. In our experiments, we repeated the experiments five times and each time we used a random sample of sentences, 20% from the gold corpus, as the test set and used the rest

Table 4. Number of tokens in training and test sets

Run	Training tokens/Percent	Test tokens/Percent	Total
1	60,140/79.82	15,200/20.18	75,340
2	59,540/79.02	15,800/20.98	75,340
3	60,040/79.69	15,300/20.31	75,340
4	60,480/80.27	14,860/19.73	75,340
5	59,900/79.50	15,440/20.50	75,340
Avg.	60,020/79.66	15,320/20.34	

of the files for the training. Table 4 shows the number of tokens and their percentages in the training and test sets respectively.

5-fold cross validation was used to calculate the accuracy of a tagger during all five rounds of evaluation processes. We divided the gold standard data into five equal folds using stratified sampling by the sentence length. Then we used with four folds of the data for training. In the training process, the tagger "learned" the language model from the training data set based on statistical possibility. The remaining one fold was for testing. During the testing process, the tagger assigned tags to the testing data set (a version of data without tags) with the learned language model. After this, we yielded a tagged version of the testing data set. We evaluated the tagged version of the testing data with its "gold standard" version, and get accuracy for one fold of the data set. After five times of training and testing, the whole data set was tested. We then calculated the average of five accuracies as the final accuracy of the tagger. The tagging accuracy, therefore describes how well the tagger performs.

Considering the tagging accuracy as the percentage of correctly assigned tags, we have evaluated the performance of the TreeTagger from two different aspects: (1) the overall accuracy (taking into account all tokens in the test corpus) and (2) the accuracy for known and unknown words, respectively. The latter is interesting since after training the tagger, it could be used for other text than the training text. It is interesting to know how it would cope with words that did not appear in its training. Tables 5, 6 and 7 depict the results of the experiments. For each run, Table 5 shows the percentage of seen words (words that exist in the training set), number of tokens in the test set, number of tokens correctly tagged and the percentage of accuracy for that run. Similarly, Table 6 shows the same for words that are new for the tagger. Table 7 shows the overall result for each run and its average in general:

1. The overall part-of-speech tagging accuracy is around 93.15%.
2. The accuracy for known tokens is significantly higher than that for unknown tokens (93.78% vs. 65.10%). It shows 28.68% points accuracy difference between the words seen before and those not seen before.

5.2   Discussion

In our work, we used a data set of 75,000 tokens and 28 tags, we have studied also the resulting tagged corpora and we concluded that Most of the errors could be categorized as follows:

Table 5. Known tokens results

Run	Tokens	Correct	Accuracy
1	14,870	13,921	93.62
2	15,300	14,380	93.98
3	15,100	14,190	93.97
4	14,562	13,665	93.84
5	15,120	14,125	93.41
Avg.	15,292	14,339	93.78

Table 6. Unknown tokens results

Run	Tokens	Correct	Accuracy
1	330	220	66.67
2	500	312	62.28
3	200	134	67.00
4	298	203	68.12
5	320	204	63.73
Avg.	329.6	214.6	65.10

Table 7. Overall results

Run	Tokens	Correct	Accuracy
1	15,200	14,141	93.03
2	15,800	14,692	92.98
3	15,300	14,324	93.62
4	14,860	13,868	93.32
5	15,440	14,329	92.80
Avg.	15,320	14,270.8	93.15

- Errors in the case of the word are the highest. Those are partially due to the fact that some of the tags do not reflect the case of the word, and hence it is hard for the learner to conclude the reason of the next word being given its tag, examples of that are proper nouns, common noun and pronouns.
- Unknown proper nouns (of people and places) cannot be guessed. Only few rules may lead to realizing a proper noun. Having a large corpus would reduce this problem by inserting many names in the lexicon.
- A distinction between adverb and compounds is not easily guessed by our model.

The results obtained in this paper are better than those obtained in [23]; the size of corpus is increased and the features used in the training step are improved. Another point is the representativeness of training corpus; the texts are collected from various sources and that concerned diverse areas (economics, politics, sport, art,…).

Finally, taking in consideration the tag set used we worked with, and the unavailability of a standard truth corpus, we think the results obtained here are very promising, and can be enhanced by many actions like: enlarging the training corpus, and enhancing the lexical analysis program.

6   Conclusion

In this work we have presented and evaluated TreeTagger as a machine-learning based algorithm for obtaining statistical language models oriented to Amazigh POS tagging. We have directly applied the acquired models in a simple and fast tree-based tagger obtaining fairly good results. As future work, there are some improvements to be considered to enhance the performance of the system.

A corpus of different types of articles may be considered to train the model such as social media content, stories, and sport reports and so on in order to increase the accuracy of the system for these types. The variety and the size of the training data is an important factor to enhance the accuracy of the Amazigh POS tagger for assigning POS tags to unknown words correctly.

References

1. Manning, C., Schütze, H.: Foundations of Statistical Natural Language Processing. The MIT Press (1999)
2. Brill, E.: Transformation-based error-driven learning and natural language processing: a case study in part-of-speech tagging. pp. 543–565, In ACL Cambridge (1995)
3. Ratnaparkhi, A.: A maximum entropy model for part-of-speech tagging. In: Proceedings of EMNLP, Philadelphia, USA, (1996)
4. Toutanova, K., Manning, C.: Enriching the knowledge sources used in a maximum entropy part-of speech tagger. pp. 63–71, In EMNLP/VLC (1999)
5. Toutanova, K. Manning, C.D, Yoram, S.: Feature-rich part-of-speech tagging with a cyclic dependency network. In: Proceedings of HLT-NAACL. pp. 252–259 (2003)
6. Giménez, J., Màrquez, L..: SVMTool: a general POS tagger generator based on support vector machines. In: Proceedings of the 4th International Conference on Language Resources and Evaluation (LREC). pp. 43–61, Lisbon, Portugal, (2004)
7. Kudo, T., Matsumoto, Y.: Use of Support Vector Learning for Chunk Identification (2000)
8. Lafferty, J., McCallum, A., Pereira, F.: Conditional random fields: probabilistic models for segmenting and labeling sequence data. In: Proceedings of ICML. pp. 282–289 (2001)
9. Tsuruoka, Y., Tsujii, J., Ananiadou, S.: Fast full parsing by linear-chain conditional random fields. In: Proceedings of the 12th Conference of the European Chapter of the Association for Computational Linguistics (EACL). pp. 790–798 (2009)
10. Brants, T.: Tnt—a statistical part-of-speech tagger. In: ANLP. pp 224–231, Seattle (2000)
11. Black, E., Jelinek, F., Lafferty, J.,. Mercer, R., Roukos, S.: Decision tree models applied to the labeling of text with parts-of-speech. In: Proceedings of the DARPA workshop on Speech and Natural Language, Harriman, New York (1992)
12. Màrquez, L., Rodríguez, H.: Part of speech tagging using decision trees. In: Lecture Note in AI 1398 Nédellec, C., Rouveirol, C. (eds.) Proceedings of the 10th European Conference on Machine Learning, ECML'98. Chemnitz, Germany (1998)

13. Outahajala, M., Benajiba, Y., Rosso, P., Zenkouar, L.: POS tagging in amazigh using support vector machines and conditional random fields, In: Natural Language to Information Systems LNCS (6716). pp. 238–241, Springer Verlag, (2011). https://doi.org/10.1007/978-3-642-22327-3_28

14. Schmid, H.: Probabilistic part-of-speech tagging using decision trees. In: International Conference on New Methods in Language Processing. pp. 44–49 (1994)

15. Schmid, H.: Improvements in part-of-speech tagging with an application to German (1995)

16. Bishop, C.: Pattern Recognition and Machine Learning. Springer-Verlag, New York Inc, Secaucus, NJ, USA (2006)

17. Chafiq, M.: Forty four lessons in Amazigh. éd. Arabo-africaines (1991)

18. Aston, G., Burnard, L.: The British National Corpus. p. 256, Edinburgh University Press (1998)

19. Ide, N., Macleod, C., Grishman, R.: The american national corpus: a standardized resource of Americanenglish. In: Proceedings of Corpus Linguistics vol. 3 (2001)

20. Outahajala, M., Rosso, P., Zenkouar, L.: Building an annotated corpus for Amazigh. In: Proceedings of 4th International Conference on Amazigh and ICT, Rabat, Morocco (2011)

21. Outahajala, M., Zenkouar, L., Rosso, P.: Construction d'un grand corpus annoté pour la langue Amazigh. La revue Etudes et Documents Berbères, pp. 57–74, n°33 (2014)

22. Amri, S., Zenkouar, L., Outahajala, M.: Amazigh part-of-speech tagging using markov models and decision trees. Int. J. Comput. Sci. Inf. Technol. 8(5), 61–71 (2016)

Designing CBR-BDI Agent for Implementing Reverse Logistics System

Fatima Lhafiane[(✉)], Abdeltif Elbyed, and Mouhcine Adam

Mathematics and Computer Science Department, Faculty of Sciences Ain Chock,
Hassan II University, Casablanca, Morocco
{lhafianefatima, mouhcineadaml}@gmail.com,
a.elbyed@fsac.ac.ma

Abstract. Over a few last decades, the enterprises make a great effort to avoid the risk of losing competition and strive to respond precisely to the customer return demands by improving their flexibility and agility, while maintaining productivity and quality. Reverse logistical (RL) activities including all operations that seize products from their final destination and bring them back to their origin in the purpose of recapturing value, recycling or disposing the return can be quite complex to manage due to dynamicity and uncertainty in demand. Thus, to deal with these issues we propose a Belief-Desire-intention (BDI) agent modeling which performs the reverse logistics decision process. Nevertheless, the use of intentional or (BDI) agent is uncomplicated and its decision process is easy to understand, its inability of learning from the environment remains the main problem faced in the development of this kind of intelligent agent. To solve this problem our (BDI) agents utilize the features of case-based reasoning (CBR) in order to improve the agent capabilities of learning from environment and to take the best decision about returned product based on the previous cases. The agent system design was implemented in Jason open source agent programming platform and the CBR system was designed using jCOLIBRI design tools.

Keywords: Reverse logistics · Intelligent agent · BDI agent · Case-based reasoning · CBR-BDI agent

1 Introduction

One of the most commonly encountered definition in the literature is that given in 1998 by Rogers and Tibben-Lembke [1], it is based on the definition of logistics made by the Council of Logistics Management (CLM) and describes reverse logistics as: "The process of planning, implementing, and controlling the efficient, cost effective flow of raw materials, in-process inventory, finished goods and related information from the point of consumption to the point of origin for the purpose of recapturing value or proper disposal". More precisely, the purpose of reverse logistics is to make benefits from the value of materials, or to find the proper way to dispose the returned product. Otherwise, many researchers have categorized reverse logistics process in different ways. [1–3] have separated a reverse logistics into four main processes: Gate keeping

© Springer Nature Switzerland AG 2019
M. Ezziyyani (Ed.): AI2SD 2018, AISC 915, pp. 633–646, 2019.
https://doi.org/10.1007/978-3-030-11928-7_57

(entry), collection, sorting and disposal. The first process is the recognition of produc‑
return, this is very critical to succeed in managing the system. Reference [1] defines i‑
as deciding which products are allowed to enter the system. The second process is the‑
collection permits the retrieval of products from internal or external customers; here the‑
collection may be made in several ways. Detailed sorting (or the third process) decide‑
the fate of each returned item. At that moment, the company may decide what to d‑
with the product, be it subject to inspection, tests, or other manipulations. The last ste‑
involves the choice of disposal, the destination of the product. These activities nee‑
two other important elements to be integrated as is mentioned by [2], an integrate‑
information system to keep track of what's happening and to deal with the uncertaint‑
and coordinating system which is responsible of the overall performance and decision
making management in the RL system.

The reverse logistics structure presented above, generates the main components an‑
activities that define a reverse logistics system. In this system, the decision about the‑
collected products is not as simple as we can imagine. Very often, the condition of the‑
returned material is not known and requires an inspection to know the destination i‑
must take. Otherwise the Complications in the reverse flow allocation problem will b‑
added because only parts or components of the so-called value product have to b‑
transported to the reprocessing site. What makes the task more difficult is that there i‑
not yet a model designed specifically to manage the flow of decision making durin‑
these activities and to interconnect the different components of reverse logistics. I‑
order to improve the results, it is important to optimize decision-making during it‑
activities.

Over the last decades, the BDI model had a significant impact on the developmen‑
of decision support systems and it's being used for designing the enterprise applica‑
tions, as it implies a periodical review of the agent's goals in order to amply tak‑
advantage of the changes in the environment and be able to consider the resource‑
bounded nature of the agent reasoning mechanism [4]. However, Rao and Georgeff [5‑
underline two problems about BDI architecture: (1) the powerful logicality of BD‑
architecture may not achieve full implementation; (2) this kind of agent has som‑
difficulties to have the functionality of learning.

To solve this issue, we present in this work an agent-based application for revers‑
logistics decision making that combines the Beliefs-Desires-Intentions approach wit‑
learning capabilities of Case Base Reasoning techniques. The CBR approach helps the‑
intentional agent to learn and adapt instantaneously and to imitate well the revers‑
logistics entities when the environment changes.

The structure of this paper is as follows: Section II stated some related work o‑
reverse logistics elements and the CBR-BDI model will be described in the sam‑
section. Section III illustrate the architecture based BDI-agent for reverse logistics. the‑
design of BDI agent, followed by implementation of CBR BDI agent for RL decisio‑
making respectively in section IV and V. Finally, we conclude the paper with som‑
remarks and perspectives.

2 Background

We discuss some of interesting properties of RL system and stated some RL approaches. Followed by a description of the CBR-BDI model.

2.1 Reverse Logistics Literature Review

In the literature, many researchers have shown a deep interest in the problems of designing and optimizing reverse logistics. Most of them use operational research and mathematical modeling. These works are grouped into three categories according to the model used: Deterministic, Stochastic and agent-based models. Some of this work is briefly explained as follows:

Reference [6] deal with the problem of photocopiers return, they proposed a mixed linear programming which is used to model the following processes: Return of machines, repair, preparation, storage, transport, the dismantling. This formulation considers production and disposition. Reference [7] cope with the problem of returns of electronic devices in Taiwan, they developed a mixed linear mathematical model programming (MILP) to identify the collection and recycling centers.

To optimize the return network, [8] proposed a complex inverse logistics system modeling with a large number of installations. The purpose of this work is to optimize the transport costs between the original facilities and the destination facilities: from the origin centers (wholesalers), to the collection and to the destination centers. The model also considers inauguration costs. However, these deterministic approaches deal with problems that are far removed from the real problems faced by industries.

To this end and in order to get closer to reality, the study of the design problem and the management of the reverse logistics process under uncertainty is very interesting. In the following paragraph we will discuss a series of stochastic research studies that seem quite consistent and that help researchers to obtain realistic solutions. Reference [9] have shown how uncertainty is an important feature of product recovery. Uncertainty in demand, as well as the quality and quantity of returned products. Reference [10] have a fairly rich work in the construction of logistics networks. They have developed a model at all levels, stochastic, multi-product, multi-level, direct and reverse logistics, with consideration of site capacities. Also, we distinguish the work of [11] by their interests in the design of a global chain, with the consideration of the problem of recovering a product or a component, then its integration back into the chain, using a mathematical model formulated as a nonlinear mixed integer.

Moreover, the problem of quality forecasting, we find the uncertainty of the demand is treated differently with the help of the agents of which two main works have been found: [12] developed a multi-agent system for predict the return flow. Reference [13] proposed a distributed architecture for knowledge management in the context of reverse logistics. The idea behind this architecture is based on the concepts of product sustainability. Finally, and according to the approaches mentioned above, it is deduced that the use of mathematical modeling and the exploitation of intelligent distributed methods improves the management of both decision and information flow related to the reverse logistics System. Hence the aim of our approach is to deal with dynamicity and uncertainty related to RL in distributed way to achieve collaborative goal deliberation based on CBR-BDI agent.

2.2   CBR-BDI Agent Model

Since the Reverse logistics processes are quite complexes and dynamic, in this subsection we introduce the CBR-BDI agent architecture that extends the BDI model to perform case-based reasoning. The combination of these artificial intelligence technologies allows our BDI-agent to cope with uncertainty related to returned products. Also, implementing agents in the form of CBR system yield them able to learn from the previous cases.

The BDI agent has been widely used in relatively complex and dynamically changing environments. BDI agents are based on the following core data structures: beliefs, desires, intentions, and plans [5]. These data structures represent respectively: Beliefs: What I know or don't know about the world. In other words, beliefs are informational mental states that express the word's state. Desires: What I want to do. Also known as goals, correspond to the tasks allocated to the agent. Intentions: How I plan to do what I want to do. They are plans of action an agent has committed to carry out to achieve its objectives(goals).

Beside this, the Case-based reasoning has become one of the most successful method applied in artificial intelligence. this method combines between problem-solving and learning and it's based on the reuse of previous problem solutions which is stored as cases to solve new ones.

Accordingly, the CBR-BDI agent remembers the action carried out in the past, when it was in a specified state, and the subsequent result. A desire will be any of the final states reached in the past (if the agent has to deal with a situation, which is similar to a past one, it will try to achieve a similar result to the previously obtained one.

In this context, many researchers have applied this reasoning technique in different fields. stating [14] they discuss the development of this kind of agent in a real application of a wireless tourist guide system to illustrate that CBR has been successfully applied in Multi-Agent Systems as deliberative mechanism for agents. Then, in 2009 [15] presents a guide to temporally bound the CBR to adapt it to be used as deliberative mechanism for Real-Time Agents.

Otherwise in [16] they developed a domain-independent system development tool. JCBRDT. By using JCBRDT, the system developers could use CBR to develop a BDI agent, create a CBR system easily, and save the time on designing and maintaining the CBR system.

Thereby and according to [17] the case is defined into three major parts: The problem description part: means the problem of case is happening at the time and needed to solve. The solution part: is the stated or derived solution to use for the problem. The outcome part: is the result after the case occurred. In Table 1. We summarize the relationships between CBR model and BDI architecture.

Table 1. Content of major parts of CBR and BDI Agent Model

CBR part			BDI model		
Problem description	Solution	Outcome	Belief	Desire	Intention
– Goals to be achieved – Initial state	– Solutions – Reasoning steps – Sequence of actions	– Results – Final state	– Percept – State	– Set of final state	– Sequence of actions

Thereupon, once the beliefs, desires and intentions of an agent are identified, they can be mapped into a CBR system. our contribution consists of designing BDI-agent for reverse logistics and its implementation, in the form of a CBR system.

3 Architecture Based BDI-Agent of Reverse Logistics System

To carry out an efficient reverse logistics process, returned goods must follow five key steps: Controlling, Collecting, Sorting, Processing and Disposing. Our main idea consists of decomposing the system into four layers as described in [18]: Data Source layer contains different type of data source systems (e.g. PLM, PDM, ERP and WMS). Ontology layer is used to combine data from multiple heterogeneous sources and coordinate with the multi-agent system by providing information about returned goods, all of that gathered in Service Agent's functionalities. Coordinating layer, it's a multi-agent system composed of four agents: Collection Agent, Sorting Agent, Processing Agent and Disposal Agent, each one of them implements one of the five steps of reverse logistics process described above and finally, the Decision-Making layer where the Gatekeeping Agent guarantees a better decision for the returned goods in term of costs, time for either discarding, recycling or reselling and other uncertain variables. It is important to highlight that in order to keep control of variables under uncertainty the system's agents are given the capability of calculating probabilistic relationships among a set of variables or so-called Bayesian Network.

The proposed Contribution contains four BDI-agent Collection Agent, Sorting Agent, Processing Agent and Disposal Agent that collaborate to fulfill the customer's order. First the system loads the gatekeeping program after its decision; it sends the authorization to both the customer and the collection agent. Just after the Collection agent start its behavior with initial beliefs and intentions, these beliefs are shared with the other agents after deliberation process a plan is selected and executed any data obtained just after the execution of a plan is added to the case base.

Figure 1. Showed how the agents of our system fit into our environment. Considering the architecture and definition of CBR-BDI agents stated in section above, the development of an agent-based system can follow the process defined by any agent-oriented methodology that considers the identification of deliberative agents, their responsibilities and goals, their roles in the organization, and the specification of interactions and protocols.

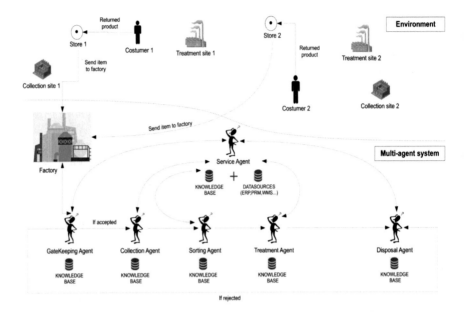

Fig. 1. Overall architecture based-agent for reverse logistics

In fact, to design these BDI agents we have chosen Prometheus as agent-oriented modeling method. We would like to stress that Prometheus methodology is intended to be able to support the design of BDI system.

4   Designing Reverse Logistics System Through CBR-BDI Agent

In this subsection we introduce the coordinating BDI agent design for reverse logistics system modeling. the Prometheus methodology it consists of three main phases: (1) system specification; (2) architecture design; (3) detailed design [19].

4.1   The System Specification Phase

In the first phase (system specification) a raw description of the system is created; a suite of use cases is formulated to depict the main functionality of the system and the goals and sub-goals are stated. The system roles are formed by grouping the similar goals. For example, the goals such as identify treatment option, optimize treatment Process, update treatment strategy, inventory management can be grouped in the return product treatment role. Consequently, Fig. 2 Groups the most important roles of the system are described below:

R1: The User Interactor Role encompass one action notify user and one agent percept related to the request of returned product and it gathers the goals that ensure the coordination and interaction between users. R2: The Return product verification Role

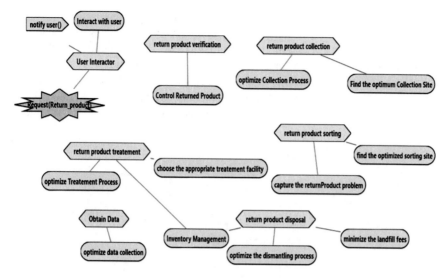

Fig. 2. System role overview

gathers the goals that ensure the return product controlling and it consists on assigning the return product authorization. R3: The Returned Product Collection Role main responsibility is to collect the returned product. In order to do this, it should handle the goals that consist in optimizing collection cost and time choosing the best site of collection and the appropriate transportation mode R04: Return product sorting Role gathers the goals of identifying the problem of return then define the sort-test optimal option. R5: Return product treatment Role should be able to optimize the treatment option by minimizing cost and decide if the return product would be processed at the producer's own facility, or secondary facility processing, in addition to finish this role is responsible of inventory management. R6: Obtain data Role gathers the goals that ensure the optimization of data collection process from ontology used by the system using SPARQL queries. R7: Return product Disposal Role gathers the goals of optimizing the dismantling process and minimizing the landfill fees.

With the system specification finalized, we have captured the basic functionalities that the system should provide. This is described through the system roles overview with their associated goals, and their relations to the percepts and actions of the system.

4.2   The Architecture Design Phase

The second phase, the architectural design, is focused respectively on deciding the agents' types in the system, describing the interactions between them using protocol diagrams and designing the overall system architecture. In the subsection above we've described the roles and tasks of these agents, and the overall interaction between them. We will now take a closer look at the interaction, defining the necessary messages and protocols.

Figure 3 illustrate how the agents of our system fit into our environment. We have already described the roles and tasks of these agents, and the overall interaction between them. The specification of functionality that we developed for the agents previously are combined to form capabilities and plans. Each agent is given a set of plans to achieve its required function, and some of the plans are grouped into capabilities. A plan is triggered either by an external message, a percept or an internal event. An internal event is usually a message sent by another plan within the same agent.

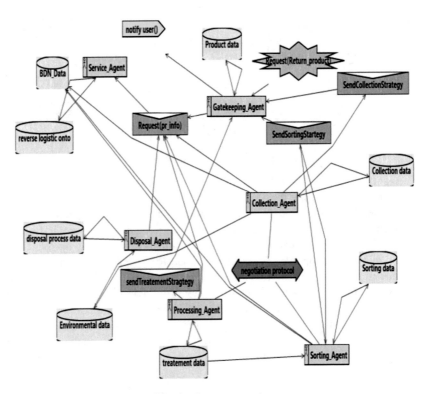

Fig. 3. System overview

4.3   The Detailed Design Phase

The following phase provides a BDI-agent overview diagrams for the internals of each agent in our system (e.g. Fig. 4 shows the internal collection agent overview). It also provides a detailed description on how the agents perform their tasks through actuating their plans and sending and receiving the messages. Each agent is given a set of plans to achieve its required function, and some of the plans are grouped into capabilities. A plan is triggered either by an external message, a percept or an internal event. An internal event is usually a message sent by another plan within the same agent. An agent contains its own data set representing its beliefs about the environment, the events that it can handle, the goals that it may assume and the plans to achieve each goal. As a new agent is built, it will wait inside the multi-agent system until it receives a goal or perceives an event that it must respond to. Then, it identifies the capability which is a set of applicable plans and selects an appropriate one after a deliberation process. If the execution of the chosen plan fails, the agent will try the next applicable.

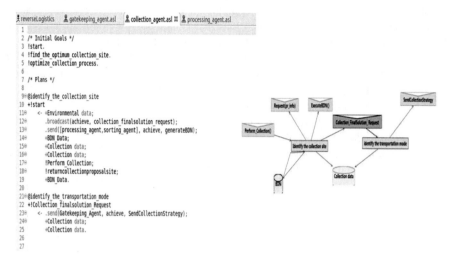

Fig. 4. Snapshot of collection agent capability implementation based on the internal design of collection agent

The capability C1: The Collection_Optimization's tasks are to identify the optimal collection site, identify the transportation mode and notify gatekeeping agent. These tasks are fulfilled through the following plans: P1 and P2.

The Plan P1 is initiated when the external Message M1 is received from the gatekeeping, first of all the Bayesian inference is executed by plan P1 to determine the most appropriate collection site to handle the Execute-BDN Messages the collection agent sends-request-Inform messages to Service-Agent for more information about Returned Product. When collection site option has been gathered initiate the plan P2 by sending the collection-site-information and the collection-final-solution-Request. The figure shows also that the plan P1 uses two data sources: BDN data with write and read access and Collection Data with only write access. Whereas the plan P2 has both write and read access for collection data.

A snapshot of the collection agent plans implementation is illustrated in Fig. 4. the agent system is developed using AgentSpeak's interpreter JASON that fully implements the BDI architecture [20].

4.4   System Development

Descriptors and diagrams of Prometheus methodology depict all necessary information like agents, goals, capabilities, functionalities, plan, percepts, data, actions, protocols, messages and scenarios. However, not all these design entities have to be implemented.

For instance, also functionalities are utilized to determine the agent types but they do not correspond to any runtime entity. otherwise, those entities are produced in the detailed design phase namely, agents, plans, capabilities, beliefs and messages, and also goals, actions and percepts.

In this subsection, we briefly observe how we endure the detailed design transition to implementation, and how particular agent platform provide a direct outlining of these concepts. as it was mentioned just before, The Prometheus methodology consists of three basic steps, the first three steps of this methodology in designing of any agent-oriented software is common but the last and the fourth step namely implementation step is different. The high heterogeneity and the vast amount of the available agent platforms for implementing proposed MAS is a fact. Hence, choosing the right or most suitable platform for a given problem is still a challenge for the developers.

Implementing the conceptual model detailed above we have opted for using the Jason platform. One strength of Jason is that it is tightly integrated with Java with the following immediate consequences as stated in [21]: the behavior of the Jason interpreter can be tailored using Java; Jason can be used to build situated agents by providing a Java API for integration with an environment model that is developed with Java; in addition, Jason has been integrated with some existing agent frameworks, including JADE [22]. The figure below shows the communication flow between the Gatekeeping agent, Collection agent and Service agent to achieve their goals (Fig. 5):

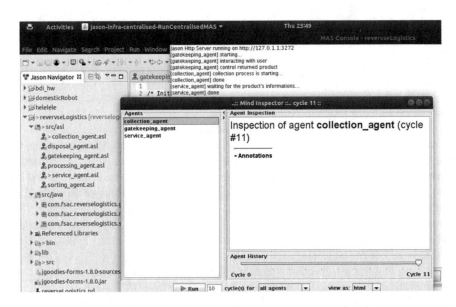

Fig. 5. Example of collaboration between agents on Jason

In order to meet the whole design objectives, agents must be cognitive enough, capable of learning and making good decisions even if it's a matter of uncertainty, for this purpose, we choose to Implement agents in the form of CBR systems because it facilitates learning and adaptation, hence a greater degree of autonomy. And There are multiple tools that can be used to use the case-based reasoning approach in the intelligent agent-based application in this work we will use jCOLIBRI tools [23], it facilitates the programmers to follow the whole CBR cycle.

5   Implementing CBR System for Processing Agent

The proposed MAS based reverse logistics system is being designed for running the reverse logistics activities with the purpose of tackling returned products properly. The decision making among the reverse logistics steps are being controlled by predefined strategies. These strategies are being designed with the help of the case-based reasoning approach executed by the intelligent agent. The CBR-BDI intelligent agents are capable of learning from the working environment.

At the first stage the intelligent agent manipulates its plan regarding the initial stage of the problem called as the beliefs. For example, the processing CBR-BDI agent has the responsibility of generating the more accurate return product treatment option. With the help of the case-based reasoning approach, the individual CBR-BDI agent generates its plan regarding to encounter the problem. This plan is based on the CBR query. The CBR query specified the all attributes of the problem faced by the intelligent agent. The resulted plan of the CBR-BDI intelligent agent helps in deriving the actions taken during the problem-solving process. Reasoning and generating its plans.

To define the case structure is the first task of the process of creating CBR-BDI intelligent agent with jColibri tools. Let's take the example of creating the Processing CBR-BDI agent.

The case designer component helps in defining the attribute names along with its type. The case structure is being stored in caseStructure.xml file. Figure 6 illustrates the process of defining the case structure of the Processing CBR-BDI agent as shown above.

The processing agent has three roles:

- To identify those believes and intentions that can be used to generate the treatment plan.
- To provide adequate plans to the other agent (collection, sorting and disposal) given a number of conditions.
- To update the believes and intentions, which are stored in the form of cases. These roles are carried out sequentially and correspond with the retrieval, reuse, and retain stages of a CBR system.

In case of remembering of how to solve the similar problem in the past, it helps processing agent finding the solution easily before executing its Bayesian network and environmental rules or sending a request to other agents. This can save the time of solving the problem. Figure 7 illustrates the existing case problem solving in the processing agent's knowledge base.

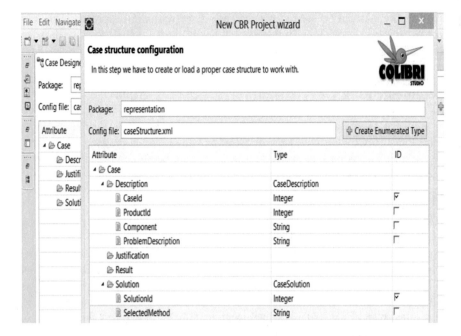

Fig. 6. Case structure of processing agent with jCOLIBRI

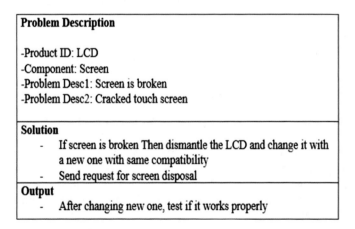

Fig. 7. Example of previous case in the processing agent's knowledge base

6   Conclusion

Recently, many industries have practiced reverse logistics primarily because of government regulation or pressure from environmental agencies. moreover, the RL has become the key strategic area that has great impact over the success of any enterprise in today's highly competitive business environment.

We have presented the design of our multi-agent system for reverse logistics which are based on BDI representation, they perform case-based reasoning (CBR) to act, instead of practical reasoning. CBR is a learning method directed towards action, which makes it very attractive for learning agents, nevertheless much more work is needed to implement the CBR for the overall architecture in combination with other supplementary reasoning method such as rule base and probabilistic reasoning.

References

1. Rogers, D.S., Tibben-Lembke, R.S.: Going backwards: reverse logistics trends and practices. Reverse logistics executive council, Reno, NV, USA (1998)
2. Lambert, S., Riopel, D., Abdulkader, W.: A reverse logistics decisions conceptual framework. Comput. Ind. Eng. **61**, 561–581 (2011)
3. Lambert, S., Riopel, D.: Logistique inverse : review of literature. Les Cahiers du GERAD, Quebec (2003)
4. Pănescu, D., Pascal, C.: HAPBA: a Holonic adaptive plan-based architecture. In: Borangiu, T., Thomas, A., Trentesaux, D. (eds.) Service Orientation in Holonic and Multi-agent Manufacturing Control. Studies in Computational Intelligence, 402, pp. 63–76. Springer, Berlin (2012)
5. Rao, A.S., Georgeff, M.P.: BDI agents: from theory to practice. In: First International Conference on Multi-Agent Systems, pp. 312–319. San Franciso, USA (1995)
6. Krikke, H.R., van Harten, A., Schuur, P.C.: A business case OCE: reverse logistics network re-design for copier's. OR Spektrum **21**(3), 381–40 (1999)
7. Shih, L.: Reverse logistics system planning for recycling electrical appliances and computers in Taiwan. Resour. Conserv. Recycl. **32**, 55–72 (2001)
8. Jarayaman, V., Patterson, R.A., Rolland, E.: The design of reverse distribution networks: models and solution procedures. Eur. J. Oper. Res. **150**, 128–149 (2003)
9. Fleischmann, M., Krikke, H., Dekker, R., Flapper, S.: A characterization of logistics networks for product recovery. Omega **28**(6), 653–666 (2000)
10. El-Sayed, M., Afia, N., Al-Kharbotly, A.: A stochastic model for forward-revere logistics network design under risk. Comput. Ind. Eng. (2008)
11. Demeril, N.O., Gökçen, H.: A mixed integer programming model for remanufacturing in reverse logistics environment. Int. J. Manufact. Technol. **3**, 1197–1206 (2008)
12. Yang, H.L., Wang, C.S.: Integrated framework for reverse logistics. In: New Trends in Applied Artificial Intelligence, pp. 501–510. Springer, Berlin, Heidelberg (2007)
13. Manakitsirisuthi, T., Ouzrout, Y., Bouras, A.: A multi-agent system for managing the product lifecycle sustainability. In: International Conference on Software, Knowledge and Application, SKIMA'09 Fes, Morocco (2009)
14. Corchado, J.M., Pavon J., Corchado E, Castillo L.F.: Development of CBR-BDI agents: a tourist guide application. In: 7th European Conference on Case based Reasoning, pp. 547–559 (2004)
15. Navarro, M., Heras, S.: Guidelines to apply CBR in real-time multi-agent systems. J. Phys. Agents **3**(3), 39–43 (2009)
16. Cheng, K.Y.R, Lee, C.H.L., Liu, A.: Applying a case-based reasoning system development tool in the design of BDI agents. J. Internet Technol. **9**(4) (2008)
17. Kolodner, J.L.: An introduction to case-based reasoning. Artif. Intell. Rev. **6**(3), 3–34 (1992)

18. Lhafiane, F., Elbyed, A., Bouchoum, M.: Reverse logistics information management using ontological approach, world academy of science, engineering and technology, international science Index 98. Int. J. Comput. Contr. Quant. Inf. Eng. **9**(2), 396–401 (2015)
19. Padgham, L., Winikoff, M.: Prometheus: A Methodology for Developing Intelligent Agents (2004)
20. Bordini, R.H., Hbner, J.F., Wooldridge, M.: Programming Multi-Agent Systems in AgentSpeak using Jason, Oct 2007
21. Bădică, C.: Software agents: languages, tools, platforms. ComSIS **8**(2), 256–295 (2011) (Special Issue)
22. Bellifemine, F., Caire, G., Greenwood, D.: Developing Multi-Agent Systems with JADE. Wiley (2007)
23. Garcia, J.A.R., Sanchez, A., Diaz-Agudo, B., Gonzalez-Calero, P.A.: jCOLIBRI 1.0 in a nutshell. A software tool for designing CBR systems. In: Proceedings of the 10th UK Workshop on Case Based Reasoning, pp. 20–28. (2005)

An Effective Parallel Approach to Solve Multiple Traveling Salesmen Problem

Abdoun Othman[1]([✉]), El khatir Haimoudi[1], Rhafal Mouhssine[1], and Mostafa Ezziyyani[2]

[1] Computer Science Department, Laboratory of Advanced Science and Technologies Polydisciplinary Faculty, University UAE, Larache, Morocco
{abdoun.otman,helkhatir,muhsiine}@gmail.com
[2] Mathematics and Application Laboratory Faculty of Science and Technics, University UAE, Tanger, Morocco
ezziyyani@gmail.com

Abstract. The evolution of computing and the appearance of the parallel architecture pushed the world to reconsider all the existing algorithm and enhance their performance given the impact that parallel programing could do to improve the performance. And it's worth to be tried on NP-Complete problems such as TSP and its variants. The traveling salesman problem (TSP) is a famous combinatorial optimization problem where a salesman must find the shortest route to n cities and return to a home base city. While the TSP restricts itself to one salesman, the mTSP generalizes the problem to account for more than one salesman. A natural approach for solving this kind of problems is to group the cities in clusters where each cluster represent a set of adjacent cities then to use one of the well know optimization, approaches for finding the optimal path route for each cluster we have. In this paper, we introduce the Ant colony optimization algorithm, and also Ag method to solve the mTSP problem using sequential and parallel programming. and then we combine the two approaches and construct a robust hybrid algorithm. and multithreading has an important role on its performance.

Keywords: TSP · MTSP · Ant colony · Genetic algorithm · Parallel · Multithread · Multiprocessor

1 Introduction

An NP-complete decision problem is one belonging to the NP complexity class. Although any given solution to an NP-complete problem can be verified quickly (in polynomial time), there is no known efficient way to locate a solution in the first place. In spite the complexity of this kind of problems, academics are trying to solve them because there is a large amount of problems that can be categorized as NP-Complete such as Graph coloring, Knapsack problem, Integer programming, Traveling salesman problem and its variations (MTSP, VRP).

The most notable characteristic of NP-complete problems is that no fast solution to them is known. That is, the time required to solve the problem using any currently

© Springer Nature Switzerland AG 2019
M. Ezziyyani (Ed.): AI2SD 2018, AISC 915, pp. 647–664, 2019.
https://doi.org/10.1007/978-3-030-11928-7_58

known algorithm increases very quickly as the size of the problem grows. Therefore, determining whether it is possible to solve these problems quickly. There is two ways to solve an NP-Complete problem:

- Exact algorithms.
- Heuristic and approximation algorithms.

In most cases you can use an exact method to solve an NP-complete problem, but you should consider the consequences, as mentioned above the time required to solve the problem using any currently known algorithm increases very quickly as the size of the problem grows, given an example close to the problem in hand (tsp).

To solve tsp using an exact algorithm you have several choices: The most direct solution would be to try all permutations (ordered combinations) and see which one is cheapest (using brute force search). The running time for this approach lies within a polynomial factor of $O(n!)$, the factorial of the number of cities, so this solution becomes impractical even for only 20 cities, you can also use branch and bound, linear programming. and still you cannot exceed 200 cities.

Various heuristics and approximation algorithms, which quickly yield good solutions have been devised. Modern methods can find solutions for extremely large problems (millions of cities) within a reasonable time which are with a high probability just 2–3% away from the optimal solution, Algorithm genetic, Ant colony optimization, and Particle Swarm Optimization. are the most known examples of this category. Although those methods have proved their effectiveness and are used to solve large set of problems, but in some cases such MTSP you still can find a gap where you can improve the result by modifying an existing approach, combine them, or improve their timing.

Since most of heuristics can be enhanced, we chose the goal of our work to be how to make this enhancement, so to improve the performance we combined the two famous approaches Genetic Algorithm and ACO, and to reduce timing we used parallel programming.

Parallel programming comes with different paradigms that suits a large number of use cases, such us multithreading that could be used on any modern computer, multiprocessing used either on multicore computer or even in clusters level. Finally GPU parallelism, which can be used on any problem that has a large input. to see a clear impact of effect of parallel programming on reducing CPU time. Figure 1 shows the huge difference between parallel and serial approach after executing a TSPLIB instance.

The rest of the paper is organized as follows. Sect. 1 describes the problem in hand. Sect. 2 solves the problem using genetic algorithm, improving performance using immigration operator, and reducing timing using multiprocessing parallelism. Sect. 3 solves the problem using ACS and how to reduce its time using multi-Threading. Sect. 4 combines the good in both worlds and construct a hybrid AG-ACO algorithm. Sect. 5 Results and comparisons, and finally we left Sect. 6 for conclusion.

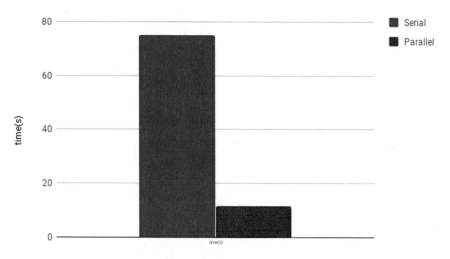

Fig. 1. ACOAG HYBRID: Serial versus Parallel

2 Studied Problem

The Traveling Salesman Problem (TSP) is a well-known and important combinatorial optimization problem. The solution of this problem is to find the shortest path that visits each city in a given list exactly once and then returns to the starting city. The multiple traveling salesman problem expands the traditional TSP to allow for multiple salesmen. Thus, each city must be visited exactly once by any salesman. Where as in mTSP, cities are clustered together and assigned to different salesman, thus converting the Multiple TSP problem into n simple TSP problem. Multiple TSP has many application areas such as the routing problems, the Pickup, Delivery Problem (Christ of ides [1], Savelsbergh [2]), print press scheduling [3] and crew scheduling [4].

Therefore, finding an efficient algorithm for the mTSP problem is important and induces to improve the solution of any other complex routing problems. Also, the mTSP can be used to solve the problem of multiple traveling robots [5, 6]. In mTSP problem we have an undirected connected graph including E nodes connecting between V vertices. every salesman will visit a subset of nodes and returns to depot vertex which will produce a tour like the simple form of TSP problem.

The total cost for visiting the nodes by each salesman man must be minimized. For each salesman we have to assign the optimal ordering of the nodes that represents the salesman's tour. The TSP belongs to the class of NP-hard problems [7] and MTSP is more difficult than TSP because it involves finding a set of Hamilton circuits without sub-tours for m (m > 1) salesmen who serve a set of n (n > m) cities so that each one will be visited by exactly one salesman.

2.1 Equation

$$\min \sum_{i=2}^{n} \sum_{j=2}^{n} c_{ij} x_{ij}$$
$$s.t \sum_{j=2}^{n} x_{1j} = m \tag{1}$$

$$\sum_{i=2}^{n} x_{i1} = m \tag{2}$$

$$\sum_{i=1}^{n} x_{ij} = 1, \quad j = 2, \ldots, n \tag{3}$$

$$\sum_{j=1}^{n} x_{ij} = 1, \quad i = 2, \ldots, n \tag{4}$$

Condition (1) ensures that m routes start at the depot node (i = 1). Condition (2) ensures that m routes also end there. Conditions (3) and (4) together ensure that all other nodes are visited exactly once (Fig. 2).

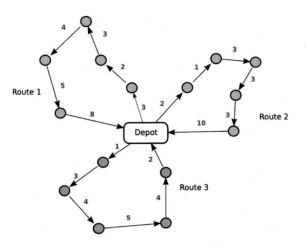

Fig. 2. Multiple traveling salesman problems

2.2 Related Work

In last few decades, many approaches have proposed to solve the mTSP problem. Like the solution in [8] is based on branch and bound algorithm. However, because of the combinatorial complexity of mTSP problem there is a need to apply a heuristic method especially for large scale instances of mTSP. In [9] the first heuristic approach was applied. Another neural network-based approach was presented in [10]. In [11] also a Taboo Search (TS) algorithm which is a metaheuristic approach used for solving nTSP. Later, genetic algorithms were also used for solving the mTSP problem [12, 13] Majd Latahs article [14] proposes an algorithm that combines the advantages of k-means clustering and the ACO algorithm to solve the mTSP problem. Its first step does n cluster using the k-means algorithm where m equals the number of vendors in the nTSP problem and for each cluster solves it independently using the modified ACO. According to its experimental results presented in without article, he demonstrated that he modified algorithm gives better results than the basic algorithm ACO and also give competitive results compared by the genetic algorithm.

3   Solving MTSP Using Genetic Algorithm

3.1   Genetic Algorithm

Genetic algorithms form a very interesting family of algorithms of optimization, initiated by Charles Darwin in the nineteenth century. The principle of genetic algorithms is directly inspired by the laws of selection natural. It is used in solving complex problems requiring high computing time Genetic algorithms are optimization algorithms based on techniques derived from genetics and mechanisms of evolution of nature: crosses, mutations, selections, etc. They belong to the class of evolutionary algorithms. The idea of a genetic algorithm is derived from Darwin's theory of evolution. Each group of individuals (animals, plant species...), also called population, gives rise to a next generation through sexual reproduction. This generation consists of crossing individuals to give offspring with the characters of both parents. In addition to this crossover, mutations of characters occur randomly in the next generation of the population. Then, this new population undergoes a selection, a metaphor for natural selection only the individuals best adapted to the environment survive. Finally, in turn, this population will give rise by the same process to a new population, which will be even more efficient in its environment. For develop a genetic algorithm, individuals are solutions, selection is thanks to their quality (evaluated through the objective function), the crossings between two solutions are made using crossover operators.

3.2   MTSP and Genetic Algorithm

There are several ways to represent the multiple traveling salesmen problem (MTSP) in a form of a genetic algorithm solution, in this paper We adopt the two-part chromosome representation technique which has been proven to minimize the size of the problem search space. Nevertheless, the existing crossover method for the two-part chromosome representation has two limitations. Firstly, it has extremely limited diversity in the second part of the chromosome, which greatly restricts the search ability of the GA.

Secondly, the existing crossover approach tends to break useful building blocks in the first part of the chromosome, which reduces the GA's effectiveness and solution quality. Therefore, to improve the GA search performance with the two-part

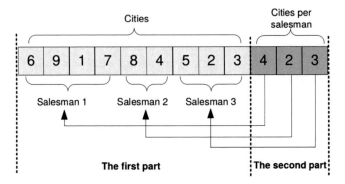

Fig. 3. Example of the two-part chromosome encoding

chromosome representation, we chose to use TCX crossover to overcome these two limitations and improve solution quality. and we used the swap approach to mutate individuals (Fig. 3).

Algorithm 1: Genetic Algorithm

1 Choose the initial random population of individuals.
2 Evaluate the fitness of individuals.
3 sort population according to fitness
4 $bestSolution \leftarrow bestIndividual$
5 **while** $i < stopCondition$ **do**
6   select individuals for use by using a Selection method
7   Generate new population using crossover and
    mutation
8   Evaluate the fitness of new individuals
9   sort population according to fitness
10   **if** $bestSolution < newBestIndividual$ **then**
11 | $bestSolution \leftarrow newBestIndividual$
12   **end**
13     $i = i + 1$
14 **end**

Using the two-part chromosome for solution representation, there are $n!$ possible permutations for the first part of the chromosome. The second part of the chromosome represents a positive vector of integers $(x_1, x_2, \ldots, x_m)$. Satisfying $x_1 + x_2 + \cdots + x_m = n$ where $xi > 0, i = 1, 2, \ldots, m$. There are $\binom{n-1}{m-1}$ distinct positive integer-valued m vectors that satisfy this requirement. Hence, the solution space for the two-part chromosome is of size $n!\binom{n-1}{m-1}$ [15].

3.3 Immigration

Given the above discussion and the usual concepts of genetic algorithms, we build our version of the genetic algorithm and it has given acceptable results. but then we noticed that it took too much time to converge, so we drew some graphs to see the problem and found that the solution stuck in some places as shown in Fig. 4.

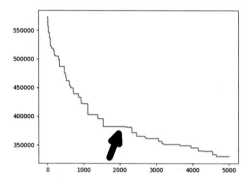

Fig. 4. Stagnation problem

Therefore, we have thought to solve this problem by using the immigration operator, which is based on the concept of exchanging some solutions of current populations with others that are already stored in memory (solutions that are not chosen in the crossover stage) every 5, 10 or 20 iterations, and the result was promising as showed in Fig. 5.

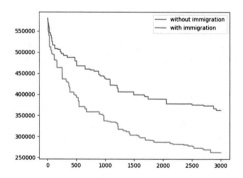

Fig. 5. Impact of immigration

3.4 Numerical Results

After constructing the application and running the programme multiple times using TSPLIB instances, we compared the results between the two version of the application (with and without immigration) and also, we compared the immigration version with the genetic algorithm in Majd's Paper.

The tables below will show the impact of immigration and also the compare The obtained results with Genetic algorithm of Majd's paper [14] (Tables 1 and 2).

Table 1. Impact of Immigration

TSPLIB	MTSP_AGS			MTSP_AGI		
	2	3	4	2	3	4
att48	34,250	36,666	44,670	35,481	**36,459**	**37,415**
berlin52	7956	8639	8880	8272	**8293**	**8775**
pr76	111,488	141,881	175,263	132,851	143,903	**158,767**
rat99	1572	2016	2016	1654	**1789**	**2087**
Bier127	149,677	181,257	218,508	**148,890**	**171,002**	**181,082**

Table 2. Comparing results

TSPLIB	AG_ar1			MTSP_AGI		
	2	3	4	2	3	4
att48	47,083	49,709	50,725	35,481	**36,459**	**37,415**
berlin52	11,736	10,898	11,066	8272	**8293**	**8775**
pr76	168,717	170,857	184,176	132,851	143,903	**158,767**
rat99	1945	1970	2487	1654	**1789**	**2087**
Bier127	233,708	257,228	282,343	**148,890**	**171,002**	**181,082**

3.5   Multiprocessing and Genetic Algorithm

Since the genetic algorithm is not so precise, and we must do the test several times to get an idea of the given results, we exploit this point, and we do these tests at the same time using multiprocessing. And we also used this point to our advantage when we wanted to know the best parameters like the mutation rate, crossover rate..., and we run the tests with different parameters in parallel, and this helped us to easily recognize the better settings for our implementation.

Table 3 shows the time difference between the classical method and the current method (Fig. 6).

Table 3. Elapsed time

No.	Sequential	Parallel
1	90.53	94.36
2	195.01	100.76
3	277.25	110.24
4	361.86	122.30

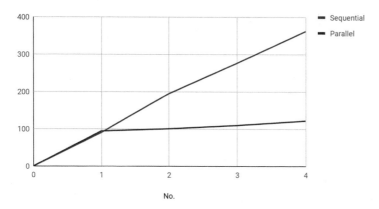

Fig. 6. Sequential versus Parallel

4   Solving MTSP Using Ant Colony Optimization

4.1   Ant Colony Optimization

ACO algorithm models the behavior of real ant colonies in establishing the shortest path between food sources and nests. Ants can communicate with one another through chemicals called pheromones in their immediate environment. The ants release pheromone on the ground while walking from their nest to food and then go back to the nest. The ants move according to the number of pheromones, the richer the pheromone trail on a path is, the more likely it would be followed by other ants. So, a shorter path has a higher amount of pheromone and in probability, ants will tend to choose a shorter path. Through this mechanism, ants will eventually find the shortest path. The main objective of the Ants Colony Optimization algorithm is to find the ideal solution through the mutual cooperation and through the exchange of information between the individual variables called ants in the algorithm (Liu and He 2014). The main advantage of ACO is that there is no priority in the information, robustness, and sensors organization requirement. ACO is also used in internet problems, assignment problems etc. related to Wireless Sensor Networks (Owen 1988; Hu et al. 2010; Gong et al. 2011) [16] (Fig. 7).

Ants are initially randomly distributed on cities. Each ant generates a complete tour by choosing the cities according to a probabilistic state transition rule: Ants prefer to move to cities which are connected by short edges with a high amount of pheromone. Once all ants have completed their tours a global pheromone updating rule (global updating rule, for short) is applied: A fraction of the pheromone evaporates on all edges (edges that are not refreshed become less desirable), and then each ant deposits an amount of pheromone on edges which belong to its tour in proportion to how short its tour was (in other words, edges which belong to many short tours are the edges which receive the greater amount of pheromone).

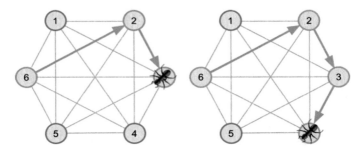

Fig. 7. Ant Colony Optimization

4.2   MTSP and Ant Colony Optimization

In this part, we will present the artificial method we used to solve the problem of the Multiple traveling salesman problems (MTSP) using k-means and ant colony optimization (ACO) and we will compare the results obtained by sequential application with article [14]. Finally, we will pass to parallel programming to reduce time of execution.

First to make use of ACO to run the problem in hand (mTSP) first we must find a way to divide the given map to m group of adjacent cities. to solve this problem, we chose to use the k-mean since it's the most famous algorithm for clustering. after getting the clusters from k-means, we run ACO on each one of them (clusters) in parallel using multi-threading this time.

4.3   k-Means

One of the most popular clustering methods is k-means clustering algorithm. In k-means n observations will be partitioned into k clusters in a way that each observation belongs to the cluster with the nearest mean. First k initialized based on the desired number of clusters. Each data point is assigned to nearest centroid and the set of points assigned to the centroid is called a cluster (Fig. 8).

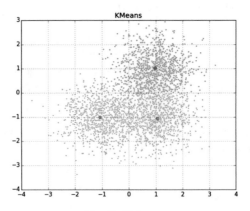

Fig. 8. K-means

Each data point is assigned to nearest centroid and the set of points assigned to the centroid is called a cluster. Each cluster centroid is updated based on the points assigned to the cluster. The process will be repeated until the centroids remain the same or no point changes clusters. In this algorithm mostly, Euclidean distance is used to find distance between data points and centroids. The main drawback of k-means algorithm is the quality of the clustering results highly depends on random selection of the initial centroids. For different runs it gives different clusters for the same input data.

4.4 Pseudo Codes

Algorithm 2: Ant Colony Optimization

---

1 Initialize parameters.
2 Initialize pheromone trails.
3 Place the ants in the source.
4 **while** *!stopCondition* **do**
5   construct a path
6   **foreach** *Ant* **do**
7   Local Update.
8   **end**
9   Global Update with the best Ant.
10 **end**

Algorithm 3: Mtsp using ACO

---

1 Run k-means clustering algorithm
2 **foreach** *cluster* **do**
3   run Aco at the same time
4   gather the solution
5   calculate total cost
6 **end**

The flow chart on Fig. 9 shows the work flow of k-means algorithm.

4.5 Numerical Results

Parameters: In our work we used a Machine with the following characteristics Table 4.

Table 5 represent the ACO Parameters used in simulation

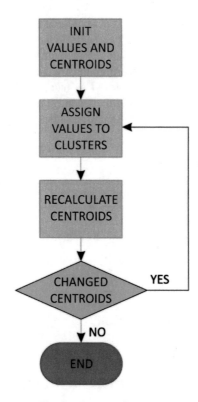

Fig. 9. K-means flowchart

Table 4. Caracteristics CPU

Characteristic	Values
Name of product	Asus N751J
Microprocessor	Intel(R) Core(TM)i7-4710HQ CPU @ 2.50 GHz UP to 3.50 GHz
Microprocessor Cache	6 MB SmartCache
Memory	8 GB RAM

Table 5. ACO Parameters

Name of Parameters	Values
Number of iterations	1000
Number of Ants	10
ρ	0.15
α	0.9
β	4

Table 6. MTSP: comparison of ACO with ACO AR1

TSPLIB	Number of vehicles	ACO_ar1	MTSP_ACO
att48	2	42,169	**39,371**
	3	51,032	**45,232**
	4	71,152	**52,157**
berlin52	2	8820	**8657**
	3	11,726	**10,145**
	4	16,354	**10,904**
ratt99	2	2814	**1430**
	3	3328	**1598**
	4	3980	**1867**
bier127	2	294,273	**140,767**
	3	349,770	**148,107**
	4	425,016	**149,336**

Table 7. MTSP: ACO Sequential versus ACO Parallele

TSPLIB	Method	K = 2	k = 3	K = 4
att48	Sequential	3000	2210	2000
	Parallel	2687	1893	1670
eil76	Sequential	6296	4297	3227
	Parallel	3769	2431	1313
ratt99	Sequential	10,937	7327	5402
	Parallel	6121	3926	1978
lin318	Sequential	221,750	148,310	71,840
	Parallel	198,000	120,430	34,000

Comparing cost: As presented in Table 6 we made a comparison between the sequential part of our program and the ACO part of article [14] made using the same instances.

Comparing time: we used multithreading to reduce execution time of our application and the result is shown in Table 7 and Fig. 10 (Fig. 11).

5 Hybrid Algorithm

5.1 The Proposed Approach

At this stage, we tried to overcome the limitation of the two above algorithms by combining the good of both of them. The idea is too simple, we construct a normal AG (the one mentioned above), and a normal ACS without any modification or complexity. The only modification worth to be mentioned is the one in k-means Algorithm, we randomized the starting points to give us different solutions each time we run the ACS.

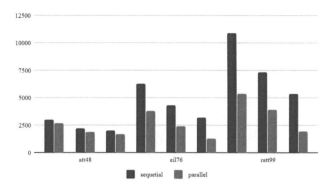

Fig. 10. MTSP: ACO sequential versus ACO parallel

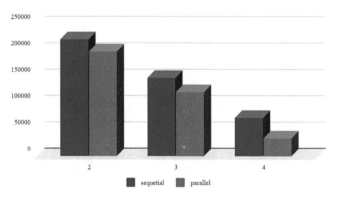

Fig. 11. MTSP: ACO sequential versus ACO parallel (Big) Instance

we used the AG as the base algorithm and after each N iteration we inject M good solution given by ACS instances and re-run them again.

And to overcome the time complexity overhead we run the ACS instances asynchronously, using the available threads, and at the same time the AG tries to enhance its solutions. To achieve performance without increasing execution time.

Algorithm 4: The proposed approach

1 Initialize parameters.
2 **while** $i < stopCondition$ **do**
3 | select.
4 | crossover.
5 | mutate.
6 | **if** $i \mod N == 0$ **then**
7 | | inject ACS solutions.
8 | | re-run ACS asynchronously.
9 | **end**
10 **end**

5.2 Numerical Results

Comparing with MTSP AGI and MTSP ACO: As presented in Table 8 we made a comparison between the ACO and AG and the proposed approach mentioned as MTSP HYB.

Table 8. MTSP: comparison of ACO and AG with proposed approach

TSPLIB	Number of vehicles	MTSP_AGI	MTSP_ACO	MTSP HYB
att48	2	35,481	39,371	**34,142**
	3	36,459	45,232	**35,570**
	4	37,415	52,157	**36,815**
berlin52	2	8272	8657	**7715**
	3	8293	10,145	**7929**
	4	8775	10,904	**8028**
ratt99	2	1654	1430	**1321**
	3	1789	1598	**1370**
	4	2087	1867	**1443**
bier127	2	148,890	140,767	**126,327**
	3	171,002	148,107	**129,577**
	4	181,082	149,336	**131,967**

Table 9. MTSP: comparison of AG methods with proposed approach

TSPLIB	Number of vehicles	2P_TCX	MP_PR	MTSP_HYB
MTSP51	3	466	465	**458**
	5	499	499	**494**
	10	**602**	662	638
MTSP100	3	28,943	**22,536**	23,560
	5	30,941	**24,292**	25,507
	10	32,802	33,416	**31,902**
MTSP150	3	51,126	**39,656**	41,144
	5	51,627	45,007	**43,448**
	10	54,473	51,962	**51,891**

Comparing with AG that exist in literature: As presented in Table 9 Comparison between the most effective ways to solve mtsp using AG and the proposed approach [17].

- 2P_TCX: two part presentation with tcx crossover.
- MP_PR: multi-part presentation [17].

Comparing with ACO benchmark
Table 10 compares ACS implementations [18] with the proposed approach.

Table 10. MTSP: comparison of ACO methods with proposed approach

TSPLIB	Number of vehicles	Optimum	KM-ACS	G-ACS	MTSP_HYB
berlin52	2	**7732**	8836	8043	**7715**
	3	**8106**	9009	8653	**7929**
	5	**[8894, 9126]**	10,335	10,164	**8479**
	7	**[9415, 9870]**	11,966	11,993	**9271**
eil76	2	**558**	594	580	**563**
	3	**579**	642	622	**594**
	5	**[623, 680]**	740	747	**634**
	7	**[675, 759]**	820	873	**677**
rat99	2	**[1296, 1350]**	1485	1398	**1321**
	3	**[1357, 1519]**	1672	1691	**1370**
	5	**[1523, 1855]**	1 996	2260	**1536**
	7	**[1712, 2291]**	2361	2859	**1763**

6 Conclusion

On this paper, we have used the most common methods that solves MTSP, and we discussed their limitations and how to improve them, and most importantly we decreased their execution time using two flavors of parallel programming multi-processing and multi-threading without affecting the quality of their solutions. And even more we combined the two methods and achieved better performance and again without increasing CPU time.

References

1. Christofides, N., Eilon, S.: An algorithm for the vehicle dispatching problem. Oper. Res. Q. **20**, 309–318 (1969)
2. Savelsbergh, M.W.P.: The general pickup and delivery problem. Trans. Sci. **29**, 17–29 (1995)
3. Gorenstein, S.: Printing press scheduling for multi-edition periodicals. Manage. Sci. **16**, 373–383 (1970)
4. Svestka, J.A., Huckfeldt, V.E.: Computational experience with an m salesman traveling salesman algorithm. Manage. Sci. **19**, 790–798 (1973)
5. Talay, S.S., Erdogan, D.R., Dept, N.: Multiple traveling robot problem: a solution based on dynamic task selection and robust execution. IEEE/ASME Trans. Mechatron. **14**, 198–206 (2009)
6. Qu, H., Yang, S.X., Willms, A.R., et al.: Real time robot path planning based on a modified pulse-coupled neural network model. IEEE Trans. Neural Networks **20**, 1724–1739 (2009)
7. Russell, R.A.: An effective heuristic for the m-tour traveling salesman problem with some side conditions. Oper. Res. **25**(3), 517–524 (1977)
8. Ali, A.I., Kennington, J.L.: The asymmetric m-traveling salesmen problem: a duality based branch-and-bound algorithm. Discrete Appl. Math. **13**, 259–276 (1986)
9. Russell, R.A.: An effective heuristic for the m-tour traveling salesman problem with some side conditions. Oper. Res. Figure 7 mTSP: ACO Sequential versus ACO **25**(3), 517–524 (1977)
10. Hsu, C.Y., Tsai, M.H., Chen, W.M.: A study of feature-mapped approach to the multiple travelling salesmen problem. IEEE Int. Symp. Circ. Syst. **3**, 1589–1592 (1991)
11. Ryan, J.L., Bailey, T.G., Moore, J.T., William, B.: Carlton Reactive Tabu Search in unmanned aerial reconnaissance simulations
12. Zhang, T., Gruver, W., Smith, M.: Team scheduling by genetic search. Proceedings of the second international conference on intelligent processing and manufacturing of materials Figure 8 mTSP: ACO Sequential versus ACO **2**, 839–844 (1999)
13. Singh, S., Lodhi, E.A.: Comparison Study of Multiple Traveling Salesmen Problem using Genetic Algorithm
14. Majd Latah Solving multiple tsp problem by k-means and, crossover based modified ACO algorithm (2016)
15. Carter, A.E., Ragsdale, C.T.: A new approach to solving the multiple traveling salesperson problem using genetic algorithms. Eur. J. Oper. Res. **175**, 246–257 (2006)
16. Ullah, A., Ashraf, M.: Wireless sensor network optimization using ACO algorithm. Sindh Univ. Res. J. (Sci. Ser.) **49**(2), 387–392 (2017)

17. Singh, D.R., Singh, M.K., Singh, T.: Multiple traveling salesman problem using novel Crossover and group theory (2017)
18. Necula, R., Breaban, M., Raschip, M.: Performance evaluation of ant colony systems for the single-depot multiple traveling salesman problem (2015)

Quadrotor Flight Simulator Modeling

Yasmina Benmoussa[1]($\boxtimes$), Anass Mansouri[2], and Ali Ahaitouf[1]

[1] Renewable Energy and Smart Systems Laboratory, Faculty of Science and Technology, Sidi Mohammed Ben Abdellah University, Fez, Morocco
yasmina.benmoussal@gmail.com
[2] Renewable Energy and Smart Systems Laboratory National, School of Applied Sciences, Sidi Mohammed Ben Abdellah University, Fez, Morocco

Abstract. It could be argued that flight simulation is the most pervasive and successful area within the simulation arena. Within simulators it is possible to deal with emergency situations and gain familiarity with new aircraft types, especially the quadrotor, which is one of the most active research topics in rotary wing unmanned aerial vehicles due to its mechanical design simplicity and human interaction safe characteristic. Visual simulation techniques have been developed to provide effective simulated real-world visual environment for flight simulators. The purpose of this work is to build a software flight simulator for quadrotor system and to display all the trajectory tracking details. The simulator was built by modeling the dynamic model of quadrotor on a software platform. The paper presents several simulation results of the quadrotor dynamics in three flight directions. The simulator results show the stable performance of the PID (Proportional-Integral-derivative) controller being used.

Keywords: Drone · Quadrotor · PID controller · Flight simulator

1 Introduction

Drones have gained widespread popularity over the last several years thanks to the recent growth of civil and military interest in Unmanned Aerial Vehicles. The quadrotor is the particular case characterized by a rotary wing platform with four rotors. Its Vertical Take-Off and Landing (VTOL) ability and excellent maneuverability make it potentially indispensable in various fields. Quadrotor dynamics can be represented using Euler-Newton equations [1] or Lagrange-Euler formalism [2].

As it is well known from the literature, due to unstable nature of quadrotor dynamics, stabilization of the quadrotor requires controller module. The suitable controller choice depends on quadrotor application. Many control algorithms were introduced to improve quadrotor stability, such as E. Abbasi, who presented a PID controller tuned using a fuzzy system in hovering mode [1], and D. C. Tosun who provided the Linear Quadratic Regulator (LQR) control [3].

This study deals with quadrotor motion 3D visualization. It proposes a flight simulator as one of the tools used for designing and validating quadrotor systems. The quadrotor dynamic model being used is based on Lagrange-Euler formalism [4]. The system is controlled using PID controller [5] and the simulation was done in MATLAB/Simulink using the Simscape Library for 3D visualization. The flight

© Springer Nature Switzerland AG 2019
M. Ezziyyani (Ed.): AI2SD 2018, AISC 915, pp. 665–674, 2019.
https://doi.org/10.1007/978-3-030-11928-7_59

simulator can provide real-time display of all flight data, including plotting, logging and modifying flight data.

The next part of this paper is organized as follows. Section 2 introduces the quadrotor dynamics using Lagrange-Euler formalism. Section 3 presents the quadrotor flight simulator being modeled in Matlab/Simulink and provides simulation results as far as results discussion. Finally, Sect. 4 provides a conclusion of this study and some research tracks.

2   Quadrotor Dynamics

The quadrotor consists of a rigid cross frame equipped with four motors. The front and the rear propeller rotate in clockwise while the right and the left rotate in counter-clockwise in order to cancel the angular momentum of the copters. The quadrotor dynamics are obtained using the coordinate system given in Fig. 1. The inertial frame [X, Y, Z] is defined with respect to the ground, with gravity pointing in the negative Z-axis. The body frame [x, y, z] is defined by the orientation of the quadrotor, with the rotor pointing in the positive z-axis and the arm-extensions pointing in the positive/negative x and y axes. The space motion of the rigid body aircraft can be divided into two parts: the center of mass movement and movement around the center of mass.

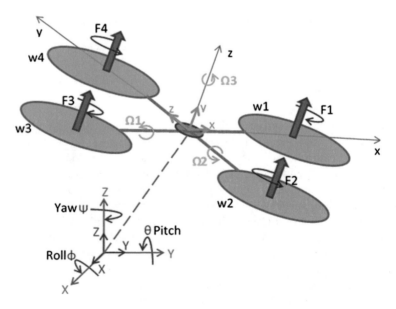

Fig. 1. Quadrotor coordinate system

2.1   Quadrotor Movement

Six degrees of freedom are required in describing any time space motion. The control for six degrees of freedom motions can be implemented by adjusting the rotational speeds of different motors, thereby changing the thrust produced. Basic motions include forward and backward movements, lateral movement, vertical motion, roll motion, and pitch and yaw motions. In order to hover, the lift force must be exactly opposite to the force of gravity. Moreover, the lift force created by each rotor must be equal to prevent the vehicle from overturning. Therefore, the thrust produced by each rotor must be identical. The upward and downward movements are achieved by increasing or decreasing total thrust of the quadrotor respectively while maintaining an equal individual thrust. The quadrotor inclines towards the slower rotor direction and then takes into account the translation along the relative axis. Therefore, as in a conventional helicopter, the quadrotor motion is characterized by translation-rotation coupling. Pitch movement is obtained by increasing (or decreasing) the front propeller speed w1 and by decreasing (or increasing) the rear speed w3. It leads to the torque which makes the quadrotor turn in the y-axis. This motion is coupled with an x-axis translation. This movement is accomplished by increasing (or decreasing) the left propeller speed w2 and by decreasing (or increasing) the right speed w4. It leads to the torque which makes the quadrotor turn in the x-axis. This motion is coupled with a y-axis translation. Yaw movement is obtained by increasing (or decreasing) the front and the rear propeller speed w1, w3 and by decreasing (or increasing) the left and the right propeller speeds w2, w4. It leads to the torque which makes the quadrotor turn in the z-axis. The total vertical thrust has to be the same with trust in hovering, such that this command only leads to acceleration of yaw angle [5]. The total vertical thrust has to be identical to trust in hovering, such that this command only leads to roll angle acceleration and makes the quadrotor move right or left.

2.2   Model Assumptions

Because of four inputs and six state outputs in a quadrotor, the quadrotor is considered an underactuated complex system. In order to control it, some assumptions are made in the process of quadrotor modeling as follows:

- The structure of the quadrotor is supposed rigid and symmetrical, which induces that the inertia matrix will be assumed diagonal.
- The structure is perfectly symmetrical.
- The propellers are supposed to be rigid to be able to neglect the effect of their deformation during the rotation.
- The center of gravity and the body fixed frame origin are assumed to coincide.
- The lift and drag forces are proportional to the squares of the rotation speed of the rotors, which is an approximation very close to the aerodynamic behavior.
- The speed of rotation of the rotors relative to the ground is not taken into account.

The rotation dynamics of the test-bench are modeled using Euler-Lagrange Formalism [6].

2.3   Euler-Lagrange Model Kinematics

For any point of the airframe expressed in the earth fixed frame, the rotational equation is given below. The demonstration is described in [7]:

$$
\begin{cases}
\underset{x}{r} = (c\psi c\theta)x + (c\psi s\theta s\phi - s\psi c\phi)y + (c\psi s\phi c\phi + s\psi s\phi)z \\
\underset{y}{r} = (s\psi c\theta)x + (s\psi s\theta s\phi + c\psi c\phi)y + (s\psi s\phi c\phi - s\psi c\phi)z \\
\underset{z}{r} = (-s\theta)x + (c\theta s\phi)y + (c\theta c\phi)z
\end{cases}
\tag{1}
$$

(c means cos, s means sin)

2.4   Control Using PID

The measurements were done on three angles (pitch, roll, yaw) and the altitude. Thus, four different PID regulators are used. This algorithm takes as input the error between the desired magnitude and the measured one, for example when the ground remote control sends nothing this error corresponds to the lack of parallelism with the ground. Mathematical operations described in Fig. 2 are used to determine the speeds to be sent to the four motors in order to minimize these errors.

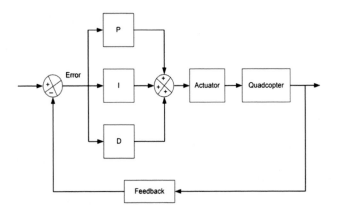

Fig. 2. Closed loop PID control system

P effect
The proportional term is obtained by multiplying the error by a constant called "proportional gain". The higher the gain, the faster the response speed and the risk of being unstable. The lower the gain, the lower the response speed and the risk of being ineffective. The aim is to find a good intermediate value between these two extremes.

I effect

Unlike a simple proportional control system, the PID controller takes into account the history of errors. Thus, the integral term is introduced, it represents the sum of all the accumulated errors in time multiplied by a constant named "integral gain".

The integral gain directly affects the height (and hence the number) of the target value being exceeded. Too little gain is problematic in some situations such as when the wind is too strong [8]. On the other hand, a gain that is too large causes an oscillation around the desired angle.

D effect

The derivative term is sometimes called "the accelerator" since it allows to compress the response in time. It is obtained by subtracting the current error and the previous error multiplied by the derived gain. However, this term is to be taken with caution, as it is very sensitive to data noise.

The effect of each gain is summarized in Table 1.

Table 1. P, I and D gains effect on the quadrotor

	Accuracy	Stability	Fastness
P	↗	↘	↗
I	↗	↘	↘
D	↘	↗	↗

Once the code of the PID regulator implemented it is necessary to determine the three gains of each regulator. As each quadcopter has particular characteristics, there are no universal PID constants. However, the determination of these values is not random. First of all, it should be noted that a method of rapid determination, called Ziegler and Nichols method [9] exists and allows to obtain correct Ki and Kd from the only value of Kp. The gains can then be adjusted according to the parameters seen above. Moreover, a quadcopter (unlike a tricopter or hexacopter) is symmetrical, constants PID pitch and roll are similar, which saves time.

3 System Modeling

A Simulink model of the system is proposed (Fig. 3) based on the relation between the thrusts of the various motors and angular accelerations.

The aim is to determine the type of correctors to put in place to ensure good stabilization of the drone on three axes yaw, pitch and roll as well as altitude [10]. Figure 3 shows the overall system Simulink model which consists of several blocks:

The "Inputs" block is used for entering instructions of the system command. These instructions are sent to the "GetErrors" block which calculates the errors between the reference signals and the real ones.

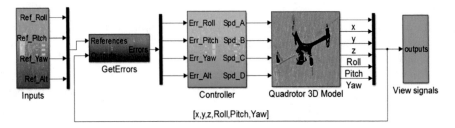

Fig. 3. Overall system Simulink model

The 3rd block "controller" contains the implementation of the model cited previously as well as the corresponding PID controller.

The "Quadrotor 3D model" block is the most significant block of this model. It was built using the Simscape library [11] by importing data from a 3D CAD [12] program into Simulink to show the quadcopter in a three-dimensional environment, it uses Simulink 3D Animation.

The "View signals" block is used for outputs plot (speeds, angles, accelerations…).

3.1   Simulation Results and Discussion

Model Inputs

The drone is controlled through four reference signals: altitude, roll, pitch and yaw as illustrated in Fig. 4. For each desired trajectory, a set of command signals shall be generated. The roll variation (segments 1, 3 of Fig. 4) produces translational motion in one direction while pitch variation (segments 2, 4 of Fig. 4) produces translational motion in the perpendicular direction. The yaw variation produces a quadrotor rotation around itself.

This trajectory plot is included in the flight simulator to ensure that the real trajectory corresponds to the reference one basing on PID factors choice. The command signals calculated according to these parameters are then sent to different motors.

Model Outputs

The model response to the reference signals previously mentioned is visualized in Fig. 5. These results correspond to the following PID gains:

- $P_Z = 100 \; I_{Yaw} = 10 \; D_Z = 20$
- $P_{Roll} = 6 \; D_{Roll} = 0.4$
- $P_{Pitch} = 6 \; D_{Pitch} = 0.4$
- $P_{Yaw} = 3 \; I_{Yaw} = 0.001 \; D_{Yaw} = 0.04$

The pitch and roll gains are identical since the system is supposed symmetrical. PD controller is sufficient for pitch and roll so integral term for them is not necessary in this case.

The output signals shown in Fig. 5 present a good trajectory tracking with the PID gains previously mentioned. The error between reference signals and output signals is

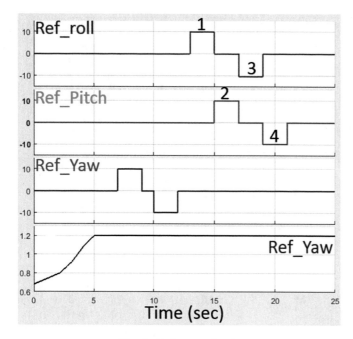

Fig. 4. Reference signals

rapidly corrected by the controller so that the quadrotor maintains its stable behaviour in the space.

Trajectory

The resulting trajectory of simulation signals is a horizontal square based on reference signals as shown in Fig. 6. The square side 1 trajectory corresponds to the first variation of roll reference signal (side 1 of Fig. 4). The square side 2 trajectory corresponds to the first variation of pitch reference signal (side 2 of Fig. 4) and so on for other sides. Any trajectory can be generated from combination of the reference signals previously mentioned. The aim of the simulation is that the quadrotor smoothly follows this trajectory.

An artificial horizon (Fig. 7) is included in the plot to provide of inclination relative to the horizontal. It indicates pitch (fore and aft tilt) and bank (side to side tilt)

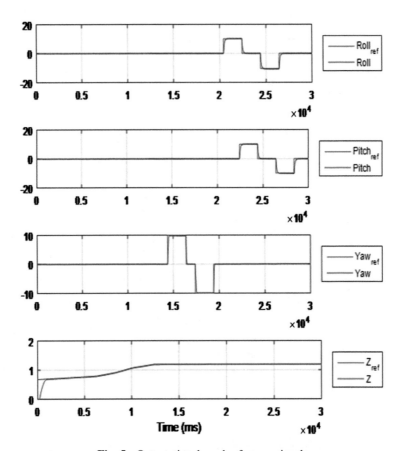

Fig. 5. Output signals and reference signals

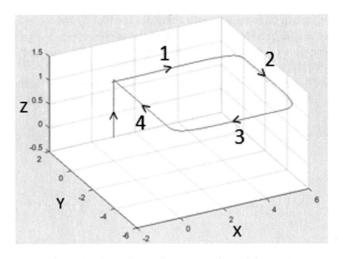

Fig. 6. Simulation trajectory (Horizontal Square)

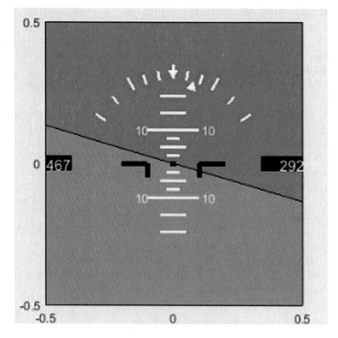

Fig. 7. Artificial horizon

4   Conclusion and Future Work

This work presented a methodology for developing a real-time flight simulator for quadrotor system. The simulator enables engineers and pilots to predict behavior of model without conducting practical test. It is very beneficial to reduce cost and time in design process. By evaluating the quadrotor dynamics in three flight directions, it can be seen that the PID controller makes the closed system stable. The PID controller was chosen due to its versatility and facile implementation, while also providing a consistent response to the model dynamics attitudes. For future work, other control algorithms will be implemented in this simulator so that a comparison between PID and other controller performance could be provided as well as optimization algorithms for trajectory generation which will be included in this research to generate paths for quadcopter in real time.

References

1. Abbasi, E., Mahjoob, M., Yazdanpanah, R.: Controlling of quadrotor uav using a fuzzy system for tuning the pid gains in hovering mode. In: 10th International Conference Advance Computer Entertainment Technology, pp. 1–6 (2013)
2. Vepa, R.: Nonlinear Control of Robots and Unmanned Aerial Vehicles: An Integrated Approach. CRC Press (2016)

3. Tosun, D.C., Isik, Y., Korul, H.: Comparison of PID and LQR controllers on a quadrotor helicopter. Int. J Syst. Appl. Eng. Dev **9**, 2074-1308 (2015)
4. Carrillo, L.R.G., López, A.E.D., Lozano, R., Pégard, C.: Quad Rotorcraft Control: Vision-Based Hovering and Navigation. Springer Science & Business Media (2012)
5. Bouabdallah, S., Noth, A., Siegwart, R.: PID vs LQ control techniques applied to an indoor micro quadrotor. In: Proceedings of the IEEE International Conference on Intelligent Robots and Systems (IROS), pp. 2451–2456. IEEE (2004)
6. Sydney, N., Smyth, B., Paley, D.A.: Dynamic control of autonomous quadrotor flight in an estimated wind field. In: 2013 IEEE 52nd Annual Conference on Decision and Control (CDC), pp. 3609–3616. IEEE (2013)
7. Bouabdallah, S., Siegwart, R.Y.: Full control of a quadrotor. In: IEEE/RSJ International Conference on Intelligent Robots and Systems, 2007: IROS 2007; 29 Oct 2007–2 Nov 2007, San Diego, CA, pp. 153–158. IEEE (2007)
8. Vachtsevanos, K.P., Valavanis, G.J.: Handbook of Unmanned Aerial Vehicles. Springer, Dordrecht, Heidelberg, New York, London (2015)
9. Frenot, A., Gossmann, A., Guillerm, R.: Stabilisation D'un Quadrirotor (2005)
10. Sanahuja, G.: Drone quadrirotor suivant une ligne par vision
11. Khebbache, H.: Tolérance aux défauts via la méthode backstepping des systèmes non linéaires: application système UAV de type quadrirotor (Doctoral dissertation) (2018)
12. Café, J.: Flight Control and Attitude Estimation of a Quadrotor

The Immigration Genetic Approach to Improve the Optimization of Constrained Assignment Problem of Human Resources

Said Tkatek[1]([✉]), Otman Abdoun[2], Jaafar Abouchabaka[1], and Najat Rafalia[1]

[1] LaRIT, Faculty of Sciences, Ibn Tofail University Kenitra, Kenitra, Morocco
`saidtkinfo@yahoo.fr`, {`abouchabaka.depinf,abouchabaka.depinf`}`@gmail.com`
[2] Polydisciplinary Faculty, Abdelmalk Essaadi University, Larache, Morocco
`otman.fpl@gmail.com`

Abstract. In this work, we are interested to propose a new genetic approach to improve the optimal solution of a constrained assignment problem of human resources within the multi sites enterprise. By taking into consideration various constraints, this problem can be defined as a NP-hard combinatorial problem as we have showed [2]. In this work, we have developed the mathematical formulation of this problem and proposed a genetic approach to the search for an optimal solution, but we have noticed that the phenomenon of stagnation of this proposed genetic algorithm persists although increases in the number of iterations lead to a significant consumption of computing time and memory space. To remedy this problem, we propose in this paper to integrate new genetic methods, such as Standard Immigration Genetic (SIG) [2], able of improving the convergence towards the optimum. This process is based on the insertion of a percentage of best individuals from previous generations in the genetic population to improve the diversity of the population and to bias the search direction for obtaining the best solution. The results are being evaluated and compared with other results obtained using the last proposed genetic approach.

Keywords: Assignment · Human resources · Optimization · Hard problem · Stagnation · Improvement · Genetic algorithm · Immigration

1 Introduction

The evolution of organizational structures, the search for productivity, performance, and rationalization of costs and flexibility of work are a strategic challenge that pushes leaders to invest in a perpetual search for new solutions. To meet this challenge, organizations are moving towards qualitative investment in human capital, which is a source of activity and productivity. This orientation drives organizations to optimize their human resources by valuing their skills, qualifications and experiences.

This orientation leads the enterprises to optimize their human resources by enhancing their skills, qualifications and experiences. In this perspective, the proposed strategy requires a human resources allocation policy based on a spatial-organizational

© Springer Nature Switzerland AG 2019
M. Ezziyyani (Ed.): AI2SD 2018, AISC 915, pp. 675–685, 2019.
https://doi.org/10.1007/978-3-030-11928-7_60

restructuring to transfer their profiles, increase their activities. This restructuring is to set up a human resources reassignment plan.

In this perspective, the proposed strategy requires a human resources assignment strategy based on a spatial-organizational restructuring to transfer their profiles and competency. Additionally, the assignment problem human resources optimization has been the subject of numerous studies [2], since it affects several fields like production management [3], maintenance management [4, 5], management projects [6], management hospital systems [7]. For this raison, it is therefore important to ask this question: How to optimize an assignment of human resources for attaining the objectives fixed?

In answering this question, we have initially focused on formulation of the human resources assignment problem under many constraints. This problem is a constrained combinatorial optimization problem, which usually provides solutions to maximize the profit while satisfying some operational constraints. For solving it, we used the uniform genetic approach and to propose the approaches to improve the optimal solution of this problem in order to optimize a best repartition of staff for achieving the prefixed objectives. In the work [1], we considered that an employee is identified by an individual weight calculated using the evaluation criteria regrouping the competency, the profitability, the individual performance, etc.).

By taking into consideration various constraints, this problem can be defined as a NP-hard combinatorial problem [1]. In this work, we have developed the mathematical formulation of this problem and proposed a genetic approach to the search for an optimal solution with a best choose of genetic parameters such as: size of the population N, and L is the length of the coding of each individual, Probability of crossing Pc and Probability of mutation Pm. initial population, a matrix crossover and a matrix mutation operators and elitism selection.

The optimal solution obtained using the proposed genetic approach (GA) after a number of iteration, but, we have noticed that the phenomenon of stagnation of this proposed genetic algorithm persists although increases in the number of iterations lead to a significant consumption of computing time and memory space.

For this, we are going in this paper which is an extension of our previous works, to propose a genetic immigration approach based on the insertion of a percentage of best individuals from previous generations in the genetic population to improve this optimal solution have been obtained using the last genetic approach. This processes called by Standard Immigration Genetic Algorithm (SIG). In this work, to optimize a constrained assignment problem of human resources (CAPHR) by the last proposed genetic algorithm, we will present each individual of population by the most adapted method of data representation which is the path representation method. A crossover and mutation operator adapted to the (CAPHR) is used in addition to structured immigration operator in order to bring dynamism and then diversity to the current population to perform the algorithm and obtain a best optimal solution in a reduced number of iterations.

This rest of this paper is organized as follows: Firstly we will present a global formalism of our constrained assignment problem that it have been solved by using the proposed genetic approach detailed in work 2. Secondly, we will present the random immigration SIG approach will be used [8] to improve the solution. In Sect. 3, computational experiments were performed through the same instance of problem exploited n work 2. The comparison with the results obtained the numerical result with last proposed genetic approach and with SIG random immigration genetic shows the performance to introducing of SIG for assignment problem of human resources for improving the solution and therefore can make an important contribution to improving the average productivity within the sites.

2 Formulation of the Problem and Last Optimal Solution

2.1 Global Formulation of the Problem

The developed formulation of this problem is written as follows [02]:

$$Max(F^a) = Max \sum_{k=1}^{NS} Trace\left(\beta_k^{\alpha_k} X_k\right) \tag{1}$$

Under theses constraints:

$$
\begin{cases}
\overline{W}_k \geq \alpha_k \, \overline{W}_k^0 \ \forall k \in [1, NS] \\
X_{jk}^i \left(\sum_{i=1}^{l} X_{jk}^i - l \right) = 0 \forall l \in \left[1, \tilde{N}_{jk}\right] \\
\sum_{\substack{j=1 \\ j \neq k}}^{NS} \sum_{i=1}^{\tilde{N}_{jk}} X_{ij}^k \leq C_k \forall k \in [1, NS] \\
\sum_{k=1}^{NS} X_{jk}^i \leq 1 \forall i \in \left[1, \tilde{N}_{jk}\right], \forall j \in [1, NS]
\end{cases}
\tag{2-5}
$$

With:

- (1) is the optimized objective function $F(x)$ related to productivity weight;
- (2) is the objective constraint can be also written as: $Trace\left(\beta_k^{\alpha_k} X_k\right) \geq 0 \forall k \in [1, NS]$;
- (3) is the priority constraint [1];
- (4) is the capacity constraint;
- (5) is the uniqueness constraint [1];
- E is symbol of an multi-sites enterprise;
- NS is the number of sites;
- E_j is the original site of the enterprise E;
- E_k is the destination site of the enterprise E;
- $E_{jk} = \left\{ E_{jk}^1, E_{jk}^2, E_{jk}^3, \ldots, E_{jk}^{\tilde{N}_{jk}} \right\}$ is the set of sites;
- $\tilde{N}_j = \sum_{k=1}^{NS} \tilde{N}_{jk}$ is the number of the employees wanting to reassign from E_j to E_k;
- X_{jk}^i is the decision variables explain that the employee can be reassigned from the site E_j to the site E_k where $X_{jk}^i = 1$ and 0 otherwise;
- W_{jk}^i is the weighted of employee;

- $\beta_{jk}^{i\alpha_k} = (W_{jk}^i - \alpha_k \bar{W}_k^0)$ is an element of sub matrix β_{jk}^α that represent the reduced weighted of an employee i can be reassigned from Ej to Ek;
- α_k is the tolerance coefficient the constraint (2);
- $\bar{W}_k^0$ is the average weight of employee worked in the site E_k before their assignments.

The assignment problem of HR under multi constraint is a NP hard problem [1, 9 10]. A standard genetic algorithm problem described in the work [1] has been implemented to solve because the AG is efficiency algorithm for solving NP-hard problems [8]. The optimal solution obtained must be ensured the improvement the average productivity for each site of production.

2.2   Last Solving Approach and Stagnation of Fitness Function

- *Last Solving Approach*

The last solving approach uses a genetic algorithm that is a one of the family of evolutionary algorithms. The genetic algorithm is a one of the family of evolutionary algorithms. The population of a genetic algorithm evolves by using genetic operators inspired by the evolutionary in biology [11]. In Genetic Algorithm, a population of potential solutions termed as chromosomes are evolved over successive generations using a set of genetic operators selection, crossover and mutation. First of all, based on some criteria, every chromosome is assigned a fitness value and then the selection operator is applied to choose relatively fit chromosomes to be part of the reproduction process. In reproduction process new individuals are created through application of operators. Large number of operators has been developed for improving the performance of GA, because the performance of algorithm depends on the ability of these operators [1]. The mutation and crossover operator is used to maintain adequate diversity in the population of chromosomes and avoid premature convergence In the last genetic approach applied in our work 2, we have used as a binary encoding method to represent the solution, each solution is formed by a the sub matrixes and each sub matrix is composed by lines vectors encoded by *0* or *1*. Also, the other applied genetic methods can be given as follow:

- Random generation of the initial population;
- Uniform Selection (US);
- Matrix Crossover (MOX);
- Matrix Mutation (MMP);
- Insertion Method (inserting elitism).

Generally, the resolution of our problem integrating these methods is carried out by this global algorithm composed of the following steps:

- *Stagnation* the using the proposed approach genetic

In the first phase of experimentation, we have constructed a randomly generated instances using an algorithm coded in c++ language in a computer CPU Pentium i5 2.5 GHz with 4 GB of RAM. This instance generated is constituted of try sites

$(NS = 3)$ and $\check{N} = \sum_{k=1}^{NS} \check{N}_k = \sum_{k=1}^{NS} \sum_{j=1}^{\check{N}_{jk}} \check{N}_{jk} = 29$ as number employees desiring to reassign from site E_j to site E_k, the evaluated weight W_{jk}^i of an employee i (competence, productivity, profitability) with $W_{\min} \leq W_{jk}^i \leq W_{\max}$.

We have run the last proposed GA algorithm to solve the problem proposed in work 2 with a size population equal at 40 individuals.

The optimal weight β^α obtained using the approach proposed 2 is illustrated in this figure:

The fitness Function F^α is showed in Fig. 2, it is corresponds to assigning 16 qualified employees from 29 employees:

So, we noticed from the figured results in Fig. 1 that the fitness function remains stagnant even though the number of iterations was increased, causing the important consumption of computation time and space memory. To remedy this problem, we propose in this paper to integrate new genetic methods, such as Standard Immigration Genetic (SIG).

STEP 1   Generating Instances

   Define α, NS, Construct $E_k, C_k, \tilde{N}_{jk}, W_{jk}^i,$

   Calculate $\beta_{jk}^{i,\alpha} = W_{jk}^i - \alpha \bar{W}_k^0$

   Construct the weighted matrix $\beta^\alpha = \{\beta_k^{\alpha} / 1 \leq k \leq NS\}$

STEP 2

   Generate the initial population of N sub matrix: $X = \{X_k / 1 \leq k \leq NU\}$

STEP 3

   Calculate $F^\alpha(X) = \sum_{k=1}^{NS} Trace(\beta_k^\alpha X_k)$ and check constraints,
   Arranging the solutions in the list N of population

STEP 4

   Itt=1   // Start iteration

   Repeat
   Select two solutions X1 and X2 from the list N
   If $Max(F^\alpha(XC1), F^\alpha(XC2)) > Max(F^\alpha(X1), F^\alpha(X2))$ and check constraints
      Then   Cross (X1 ,X2)   // Crossover Matrix of XC1 and XC2
                           X1 $\longrightarrow$ XC1
                           X2 $\longrightarrow$ XC2
      If $F^\alpha(XC1) > F^\alpha(XC2)$ then
                  Mutate (XC1) : XC1 $\longrightarrow$ XM   // Mutation Matrix of XC1
      Else
                  Mutate (XC2 : : XC2 $\longrightarrow$ XM)   // Mutation Matrix of XC2
      End if

      If   F(XM) > Max(F(XC1),F(XC2)) and XM check Constraints then
                        Insert the solution in the list N
      Itt = Itt +1   //Next iteration
      Else   Reject XM   // Reject solution
      End if
                  Until $(F^\alpha(XM) - F^\alpha(X0))/F^\alpha(X0) < Precision$

Fig. 1. Last proposed genetic approach to solve the constrained assignment problem

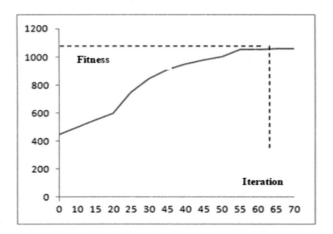

Fig. 2. Variation of fitness function depending on number of iterations

3   Genetic Immigration Algorithm to Improve the Solution

The immigration is based on structured immigration which consists in benefiting individuals not inserted during the previous generations (resulting from the crossover and mutation operators of the selected individuals). Thus, a percentage of the most powerful individuals will immigrate after an interval of time instead of the same number of the lowest individuals in the last generation. The complexity of immigration is decreased by executing it only every several generations [8].

The pseudo-code for the standard GA with random immigrants investigated in this paper, denoted SIG, is also shown in Fig. 2, where random immigrants replace worst individuals in the population, p_c is the crossover probability, and p_m is the mutation probability. Random Immigration" where the randomly created individuals are inserted into the population every generation by replacing the worst individuals or some individuals randomly selected (Figs. 3, 4 and 5).

$$X = \begin{pmatrix} X1 \\ X2 \\ X3 \end{pmatrix}$$

$$X1 = \begin{pmatrix} 1\ 1\ 1\ 1\ 0\ 0\ 0\ 0\ 0 \\ 1\ 1\ 0\ 0\ 0\ 0\ 0\ 0\ 0 \end{pmatrix},$$

$$X2 = \begin{pmatrix} 1\ 1\ 1\ 1\ 0\ 0\ 0 \\ 1\ 1\ 0\ 0\ 0\ 0\ 0 \end{pmatrix}$$

$$X3 = \begin{pmatrix} 1\ 1\ 0 \\ 1\ 1\ 0 \end{pmatrix}$$

Fig. 3. The optimal matrix assignment (**16 employees**) of HR using last Genetic Approach

```
Begin
  Initialize population P randomly with constraints validation
  evaluate population P
  for (iitr=1; iitr<=iter; iitr++)
      Sel := Select For Reproduction(P)        // N individuals
      CX := Crossover(Sel, Px)                 // Px is the crossover probability
      Mut := Mutate(CX, Pm)                     //Pm is the mutation probability
      Evaluate new individuals                 // Evalute Mut and sort in descendant
          P' = Elitisme(Mut(1; N/2))           // Perform elitism
      if mod(iitr, ItInser) == 0 then          // Execution of RIG
          Generate n random immigrants
          Evaluate these random immigrants
          Replace the worst individuals in P
      endIf
  endfor
End
```

Fig. 4. Random Standard Immigration Genetic (SIG)

4 Results and Discussion

To evaluate the performance of the new proposed genetic approach to improve the solution of the Optimization of Constrained Assignment Problem of Human Resources, we consider the same instance (of try sites (NS = 3) and) in order to compare the results of this approach with that in Sect. 3 and in work 2.

Experimentally we encoded the SIG algorithm by the C++ on Pentium i5 2.5 GHz with 4 GB of RAM. The population size chosen is 40 individuals. We have run this proposed GA algorithm including the SIG method. Ten runs of the algorithm were launched for this problem. The parameters of the GA are the crossover probability and the mutation probability Pm varying inversely proportional respectively with the number of rows and number of column in the matrix of solution X.

The optimal weight β^{α} obtained using the approach proposed in the work 2 is illustrated in this figure:

Figure 6 illustrates the results for $\alpha = \frac{1}{4}$ of fitness function using the SIG approach (LGA). The optimal solution obtained using this approach is Wop = 1260.70 during 40 iterations. If we compare these results with those of last genetic approach, which has been applied in the section illustrated in Fig. 3 (Wop = 1061.61 during 65 iterations).

In the same figure, we can also say that the fitness function remain in stagnation even thought we increase the number of iteration. This is can be explained that the last algorithm does not progress by finding any better solutions called by saturation of genetic population. For this, we have applied the SIG algorithm. These results show that we could improve the fitness function by 18% and we were able to reduce the number of iterations and the computational time by 35% using the SIG approach.

STEP 1   Define α, NU, E_j, Precision

Construct the weighted matrix $\beta^\alpha = \{\beta_k{}^\alpha \ /1 \leq k \leq NS\}$

STEP 2   Generate the initial population of N Sub matrix: $X = \{X_k \ /1 \leq k \leq NU\}$

STEP 3   Calculate $F^\alpha(X) = \sum_{k=1}^{NS} Trace(\beta_k^\alpha X_k)$ and check constraints,

Arranging the solutions in the list N of population

STEP 4   Itt=1   // Start iteration

Repeat

Select two solutions X1 and X2 from the list N

If   Max($F^\alpha(XC1), F^\alpha(XC2)) > Max(F^\alpha(X1), F^\alpha(X2))$, check constraints

Then   Cross (X1 ,X2)   // Crossover of XC1 and XC2

X1 ⟶ XC1 and   X2 ⟶ XC2

If $F^\alpha(XC1) > F^\alpha(XC2)$ then

Then   Mutate (XC1) : XC1 ⟶ XM   // Mutation of XC1

Else   Mutate (XC2 :: XC2 ⟶ XM)   // Mutation of XC2

End if

If   F(XM) > Max(F(XC1),F(XC2)) and XM check Constraints

Then   Insert the solution in the list N

Itt = Itt +1   //Next iteration

Else   Reject XM and   // Reject solution

// Introducing the pseudo code of sig algorithm

If iter= Itt /10   // iteration processes of SIG

itInser= iter

Evaluate population P   // (STEP3) ;

For (iitr=1; iitr<=iter; iitr++)

Sel:=Select For Reproduction (P)   // N individuals

XC := Crossover (Sel, P_x)   // P_x is the crossover probability

XM := Mutate (XC, P_m)   //P_m is the mutation probability

Evaluate new individuals Mutate   // EvaluteMut and sort in descendant

P' = Elitisme(Mutate(1; N/2))   // Perform elitism

ImPop = (Mutate(N/2; N))

If mod(iitr, _Itinsert_) == 0 then   // Execution of SMIGA

Evaluate immigrant's subpopulation ImPop

Replace the n worst individuals in P

Endif

Endfor

End if

Until $(F^\alpha(XM) - F^\alpha(X0))/F^\alpha(X0) < Precision$

END

Fig. 5. New approach genetic integrating the SIG to improve the solution the constrained assignment problem

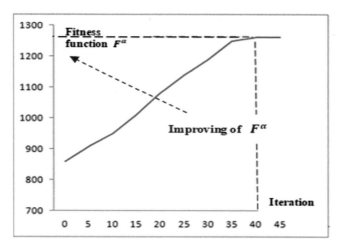

Fig. 6. Improvement of fitness function using the SIG approach

In other hand, The optimal solution X corresponds to the stagnation of fitness function F^α is showed in Fig. 2, it is corresponds to assigning 17 qualified employees from 29 employees These results show that we could increase the number of qualified employees to 17 using the SIG method for inducing the Wop (Fig. 7).

$$X = \begin{pmatrix} X1 \\ X2 \\ X3 \end{pmatrix}$$

$$X1 = \begin{pmatrix} 1\ 1\ 1\ 1\ 0\ 0\ 0\ 0\ 0 \\ 1\ 1\ 1\ 0\ 0\ 0\ 0\ 0\ 0 \end{pmatrix},$$

$$X2 = \begin{pmatrix} 1\ 1\ 1\ 1\ 0\ 0\ 0 \\ 1\ 1\ 0\ 0\ 0\ 0\ 0 \end{pmatrix}$$

$$X3 = \begin{pmatrix} 1\ 1\ 0 \\ 1\ 1\ 0 \end{pmatrix}$$

Fig. 7. The improvement of matrix assignment (**17 employees**) using the SIG

Also, in order to justify the integration the SIG to improve the optimization of our problem, we have tackled the same instance to search the different number of employees to be reassigned or displaced from a site to other according the tolerance factor, using the last proposed genetic approach and the SIG approach. The results obtained by two types of resolution approach are presented in Tables 1 and 2.

Tables 1 and 2 presents the numerical values retrieved after the implementation of standard immigration (SIG) and the similar values by last genetic approach generated. We note that the application of the proposed approach allows us to improve the weight and the number of employees assigned for different values of α (Table 1).

Table 1. Induced weight and number of possible displacement using the last proposed approach

Tolerance coefficient	Number of possible displacements	$Trace\left(\beta^{k,\alpha}X^k\right)$
$\alpha = 0$	18	1435
$\alpha = 1/4$	**16**	1061.7
$\alpha = 1/3$	14	948.91

Table 2. Induced weight and number of possible displacement using the SIG approach

Tolerance coefficient	Number of possible displacements	$Trace\left(\beta^{k,\alpha}X^k\right)$
$\alpha = 0$	19	1536
$\alpha = 1/4$	17	1261.7
$\alpha = 1/3$	15	1048.91

5 Conclusion

In this paper, we have proposed a new genetic approach to improve the solution and to remedy the stagnation of fitness for a constrained assignment problem of human resources which is a NP-hard problem. This new genetic approach is based on immigration genetic method which is consist to insert of a percentage of best individuals from previous generations in the genetic population to improve the diversity of the population and to bias the search direction for obtaining the best solution. The results obtained show the effectiveness and robustness of the new proposed immigration procedure to produce dynamism and diversity to the population and provides better optimal solution with reduction the number of iteration and computation time. Compared to the last proposed genetic applied in the our work 2. It is also observed that the new proposed genetic approach serves to improve an optimal matrix of assignment in order to get a best repartition of staff contributing to increase the average productivity in enterprise.

References

1. Tkatek, S., Abdoun, O., Abouchabaka, J., Rafalia, N.: An optimizing approach for multi constraints reassignment problem of human resources. Int. J. Electr. Comput. Eng. (IJECE) **6** (4), ISSN: 2088-8708@2016
2. Tan, S., Weng, W.: Scheduling of worker allocation in the manual labor environment with genetic algorithm. In: Proceedings of the International Multi Conference of Engineers and Computer Scientists, vol. 1 (2009)
3. Hegazy, Z., Sabry, A., Mohamed, W., Khorshi, M.: An alternative differential evolution algorithm for global optimization. J. Adv. Res. **3**, 149–165 (2012)
4. Bennour, M., Addouch, S., El Mhamedi, A.: RCPSP sous contraintes de compétences dans un service de maintenance. Comput. Oper. Res. **32**, 491–507 (2005)
5. Dakkak, B., Chater, Y., Talbi, A.: Modélisation d'un problème d'allocation des agents de maintenance. In: CIGIMS '2012, pp. 1–14 (2012)

6. Selaru, C.: Resource allocation in project management. Int. J. Econ. Pract. Theor. **2**(4), 274–282 (2012)
7. Lanzarone, E., Matt, A.: Robust nurse-to-patient assignment in home care services to minimize overtimes under continuity of care. Operations Research for Health Care (2014)
8. Tkatek, S., Abdoun, O., Abouchabaka, J.: A hybrid heuristic method to solve an assignment problem of human resource. Int. Rev. Comput. Softw. (I.RE.CO.S.) **10**(9) (2015)
9. Tkatek, S., Abdoun, O., Abouchabaka, J., Rafalia, N.: A Meta-heuristically approach of the spatial assignment problem of human resources in multi-sites enterprise. Int. J. Comput. Appl. **77**(7) (2013)
10. Afilal, M., Yalaoui, F.: The human resources assignment with multiple sites problem. Conference paper in International Journal of Modeling and Optimization, Feb 2015
11. Abdoun, O., Abouchabaka, J., Tajani, C.: Analyzing the performance of mutation operators to solve the traveling salesman problem. Int. J. Emerg. Sci. (IJES) **2**(1) (2012)
12. Abdoun, O., Tajani, C.: Genetic algorithm adopting immigration operator to solve the asymmetric traveling salesman problem. Int. J. Pure Appl. Math. **115**(4), 801–812 ISSN: 1311-8080 (printed version); ISSN: 1314-3395 (2017)
13. Yang, Q., Guozhu, H., Li, L.: Application of genetic algorithm on human resources optimization. In: ICCTAE International Conference on Computer and Communication Technologies in Agriculture Engineering (2010)
14. Lampinen, J., Zelinka, I.: On stagnation of the differential evolution algorithm. In: Proceedings of 6th International Mendel Conference on Soft Computing, pp. 76–83 (2000)
15. Liu, J., Lampinen, J.: On setting the control parameter of the differential evolution algorithm. In: Proceedings of the 8th International Mendel Conference on Soft Computing, pp. 11–18 (2002)
16. Das, S., Abraham, A., Chakraborty, U.: Differential evolution using a neighborhood-based mutation operator. IEEE Trans. Evol. Comput. **13**(3), 526–553 (2009)
17. Bouajaja, S., Dridi, N.: Survey on human resource allocation problem and its applications. Oper. Res. Int. J. **17**, 339–369. (2017). https://doi.org/10.1007/s12351-016-0247-8

Analysis of Real Transient Multiexponential Signals Using Matrix Pencil Method in Labview Environment

Lina El Alaoui El Abidi[1]([⊠]), Mounir Hanine[2], and Brahim Aksasse[1]

[1] Department of Computer Science, FST Errachidia,
Moulay Ismail University, Errachidia, Morocco
`elalaouielabidilina@gmail.com`,
`b.akssasse@fste.umi.ac.ma`
[2] ASIA Team, M2I Laboratory, Department of Science, FP Errachidia,
Moulay Ismail University, Errachidia, Morocco
`mounir.hanine@gmail.com`

Abstract. It has been a challenge for us to determine the most powerful and exact method for estimating parameters of a sum of real multi-exponentials signals. Indeed, in this study, we present and analyze two powerful methods for estimating these parameters. The first one is Matrix Pencil (MP) method, which is a linear technique for estimating the parameters. The second one is Pony method. In this work, we opted to reprogram the Matrix Pencil method and the Prony method in the Labview environment to automate signal processing and parameters estimation. The comparison between these methods shows that the Matrix Pencil method is more efficient in computation and faster. Simulation and experimental results indicate that Matrix Pencil method is less sensitive to noise than Prony method.

Keywords: Matrix pencil · Prony method · Multiexponential signals

1 Introduction

Many experiments in science and engineering generate data that can be accurately modelled by a sum of real exponentials signals (1, 2). Some of the areas they arise include electromagnetic field analysis, nuclear magnetic resonance, etc. This makes the estimation of the parameters very important. The signals are of the form

$$y(t) = \sum_{i=1}^{M} a_i e^{-\lambda_i t} + b(t) \tag{1}$$

where M represents the number of components, a_i and λ_i denote respectively the amplitudes and the relaxation times.

$b(t)$ represents the noise part that contaminates the multi-exponential signal.

Relaxation times are very close to one another. Hence the need to compare the different methods to find the one that has a higher resolving power. In this study we

© Springer Nature Switzerland AG 2019
M. Ezziyyani (Ed.): AI2SD 2018, AISC 915, pp. 686–696, 2019.
https://doi.org/10.1007/978-3-030-11928-7_62

will compare two high resolution methods, Matrix Pencil (MP) represented in (5), (7), and (8) developed in (3), (4), (6) and Prony method (9), (10).

The term « high resolution » can be applied to any digital analysis method able to treat multi-exponential signals and to extract the amplitudes and time constants from each exponential component more accurately than traditional methods. This explains our particular interest in these methods allowing treating information with enhanced quantity and quality.

The rest of the paper is organized as follows: in Sect. 2, we give the notations used in MP method. Section 3 recalls the Prony method. In Sect. 4, we deal with some simulations results and finally Sect. 5 concludes the paper.

2 Notion of Matrix Pencil

The term "pencil" originated with Gantmacher [11], in 1960. The historical context behind the word pencil in matrix pencils. The pencil in Greek represents a group bound by a property. In the projective geometry the term a pencil of lines, means lines passing through a common point. It is the definition of the pencil forms that some sort of bundling or parameterization is involved. However, the definition itself of the word pencil does not introduce the context.

After sampling, the time variable, t, is replaced by kT, where T, is the sampling period. The sequence can be rewritten as (1):

With $k = 0, 1, \ldots, N - 1$, and $t = kT$,

We note

$$x_i = e^{-\lambda_i T} \tag{2}$$

The poles x_i, are found as the solution of a generalized eigenvalue problem. For noiseless data, we can obtain the parameters from two $(N - L) \times L$ matrices Y_1 and Y_2 formed from data with N samples uniformly selected as follows:

$$Y_1 = \begin{pmatrix} A(0) & A(1) & \cdot & \cdot & \cdot & A(L-1) \\ A(1) & A(2) & & & & A(L) \\ A(2) & A(3) & & \cdot & \cdot & A(L+1) \\ \cdot & \cdot & \cdot & & & \cdot \\ \cdot & \cdot & & \cdot & & \cdot \\ \cdot & \cdot & & & \cdot & \cdot \\ A(N-L-1) & A(N-L) & \cdot & \cdot & \cdot & A(N-2) \end{pmatrix} \tag{3}$$

$$Y_2 = \begin{pmatrix} A(1) & A(2) & \cdot & \cdot & \cdot & A(L) \\ A(2) & A(3) & & & & A(L+1) \\ A(3) & A(4) & & \cdot & \cdot & A(L+2) \\ \cdot & \cdot & \cdot & & & \cdot \\ \cdot & \cdot & & \cdot & & \cdot \\ \cdot & \cdot & & & \cdot & \cdot \\ A(N-L) & A(N-L+1) & \cdot & \cdot & \cdot & A(N-1) \end{pmatrix} \tag{4}$$

where L is referred to the pencil parameter.

One can write:

$$Y_1 = X_1 R X_2 \tag{5}$$

$$Y_2 = X_1 R X_0 X_2 \tag{6}$$

where X_0, X_1, X_2 and R are given by:

$$X_1 = \begin{pmatrix} 1 & 1 & . & . & . & 1 \\ x_1 & x_2 & . & . & . & x_M \\ . & . & . & & & . \\ . & . & & . & & \\ x_1^{N-L-1} & x_2^{N-L-1} & & & . & x_M^{N-L-1} \end{pmatrix} \tag{7}$$

$$X_2 = \begin{pmatrix} 1 & x_1 & . & . & . & x_1^{L-1} \\ x_1 & x_2 & . & . & . & x_2^{L-1} \\ . & . & . & & & . \\ . & . & & . & & \\ 1 & x_M & . & . & . & x_M^{L-1} \end{pmatrix} \tag{8}$$

$$X_0 = \begin{pmatrix} x_1 & 0 & . & . & . & 0 \\ 0 & x_2 & . & . & . & 0 \\ . & . & . & & & . \\ . & . & & . & & . \\ . & . & & & . & . \\ 0 & 0 & . & . & . & x_M \end{pmatrix} \tag{9}$$

$$R = \begin{pmatrix} r_1 & 0 & . & . & . & 0 \\ 0 & r_2 & . & . & . & 0 \\ . & . & . & & & . \\ . & . & & . & & . \\ . & . & & & . & . \\ 0 & 0 & . & . & . & r_M \end{pmatrix} \tag{10}$$

with this method the multi-exponential signals is supposed to be multi-exponential such that:

We can write the Matrix Pencil in the following form:

$$Y_2 - \lambda Y_1 = X_1 R (Z_0 - \lambda I) X_2 \tag{11}$$

where I is the $M \times M$ identity matrix. The mathematical entity named Matrix Pencil means any linear combination of two matrices, such that $Y_2 - \lambda Y_1$ for the matrices (Y_1, Y_2), where λ is a scalar parameter.

Moreover, it is easy to demonstrate that the matrix product $Y_1^+ Y_2$ (the symbol + represents the Moore-Penrose pseudo inverse) has M non-null eigenvalues equal to the z_i parameters searched for and L-M non-null eigenvalues. Note that the $Y_1^+ Y_2$ matrix product has M non-null eigenvalues equal to the x_i^{-1} parameters and L-M null eigenvalues. This result is easy to yield when decompositions (6) and (7) of Y_1 and Y_2 are introduced in the product. The eigenvalues of $Y_2 - \lambda Y_1$, which are also those of $Y_1^+ Y_2$: may be computed according to the following steps

Step 1: The pseudo inverse Y_1^+ is computed through a Singular Value Decomposition (SVD) of Y_1

$$Y_1 = \sum_{i=1}^{M} s_i u_i v_i^H \tag{12}$$

Such that

$$Y_1 = USV^H \tag{13}$$

where the symbol H denotes the transpose-conjugate. $U = [u_1, u_2, \ldots, u_M]$ and $V = [v_1, v_2, \ldots, v_M]$, u_i and v_i being respectively the ith eigenvectors on the left and on the right of Y_1.

$$S = \begin{pmatrix} s_1 & 0 & . & . & . & 0 \\ 0 & s_2 & . & . & . & 0 \\ . & . & . & & & . \\ . & . & & . & & . \\ . & . & & & . & . \\ 0 & 0 & & & & s_M \end{pmatrix} \tag{14}$$

s_i are the singular values of Y_1. Note that for a (noiseless) ideal signal, the M number of damped signals can be estimated on the base of the singular values to the extent that

$$s_1 \geq s_2 \geq \cdots \geq s_M \geq \cdots \geq s_{\min(N-L,L)} \tag{15}$$

and that

$$s_{M+1} = \cdots = \cdots s_{\min(N-L,L)} = 0 \tag{16}$$

For noisy samples, Y_1 tends to reach a maximum rank. Then we select $s_1, \ldots, s_M$ as the M dominant singular values of Y_1 A jump into the singular values allows determining the preponderant singular values. The best approximation of Y_1, in the sense of the least squares, can be obtained by reducing the other L-M singular values to zero. Thus, the Y_1 matrix data is replaced by a M-rank matrix Y_{1T} computed through a singular value decomposition of Y_1. The Moore-Penrose pseudo inverse Y_{1T}^+ becomes indeed:

$$Y_{1T}^+ = \sum_{i=1}^{M} \frac{1}{\hat{s}_i} \hat{v}_i \hat{u}_i^H \tag{17}$$

Such that

$$Y_{1T}^+ = VS^{-1}U^H \tag{18}$$

where $\hat{s}_i$ denotes the largest singular values of Y_1; $\hat{u}_i$ and $\hat{v}_i$ are respectively the n left and right eigenvectors

Step 2: The computation of the largest M eigenvalues of the $(L \times L)$ matrix is stated as:

$$Y_{1T}^+ Y_2 \tag{19}$$

These M eigenvalues represent approximations of the emission rates of the damped signals, since $x_i = e^{-\lambda_i . T}$. Moreover, note that the multiplication of Y_{1T}^+ times Y_2 boils down to filtering the matrix of Y_2 data thanks to the SVD used. Should it also be applied to Y_1, such a decomposition would not be very helpful since the noise in Y_2 is strongly correlated with that in Y_1.

3   The Prony Method

The objective of the Prony method is to identify a sample of N values of a signal represented by a finite linear combination of M complex exponentials. In this section we will work with the real exponentials.

These exponentials identified by amplitudes, phases, damping factor and frequencies obviously characterized the signal.

We have more data than exponential parameters to be determined. He is more question to calculate a_i and x_i by resolution of

$$Y(t) = \sum_{i=1}^{M} a_i e^{-\lambda_i t} \tag{20}$$

with $t = kT$ and, $k = 0, 1, \ldots, N - 1$.

The system is on—determined and only an estimate by lesser squares of 2 M parameters a_i and x_i suits. By taking estimate:

$$y(t) = \sum_{i=1}^{M} a_i e^{-\lambda_i t} \tag{21}$$

with $t = kT$ and $k = 0, 1, \ldots, N - 1$.

We tried to minimize the mean squared error:

$$\xi = \sum_{k=1}^{N} |||Y(k) - y(k)||^2 \tag{22}$$

By taking as parameters of minimization a_i and x_i. This problem is in itself delicate because the problem to minimize ξ in comparison with a_i and x_i is a nonlinear problem which is very unstable, that is to say very sensitive to errors of roundness on stocks X (n) (to see HILDEBRANDT [7], pp. 380–381).

Let us introduce the error of approximation of linear prediction defined by:

$$e(k) = \sum_{n=0}^{p} f(n)Y(k - n) \tag{23}$$

with, p + 1 < k < N and f(0) = 1.

We should minimize the quantity:

$$\xi = \sum_{k=p+1}^{N} ||e(k)||^2 \tag{24}$$

In comparison with the parameters of $f(n)$, n = 1, 2, ..., p

After calculus, we can say that the acknowledgement of f(n) can lead us to find the a_i and x_i.

4   Simulation Results

- Case 1:

Using (2) we test the program with two exponentials and we choose very close values of the damping factors λ_i. In this case, we work without noise:

In Table 1. We mentioned the values used in case 1 for testing if Matrix Pencil method and Prony Method can estimate the parameters. In all cases the number of samples used is 512.

Table 1. Values of amplitudes and damping factors

i	1	2
ai	10	12
λi	0.001	0.0011

In Fig. 1, we display the result obtained by Matrix Pencil. We can find the results obtained by Matrix Pencil method when it estimate the parameters of amplitudes, damping factors and the noise.

We can say that Matrix Pencil can estimate and calculate correctly the parameters.

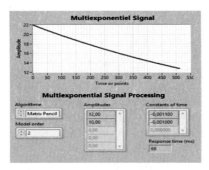

Fig. 1. Results of Matrix Pencil method

Now let tray to estimate the model parameters by using the Prony Method. Figure 2, display the obtained result.

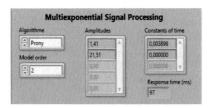

Fig. 2. Results of Prony method

As shown by Fig. 2, the values for parameters giving by the Prony method are wrong. And time response is bigger than the time response of Matrix Pensil method.

Now in Table 2, we will add a White Gaussian Noise with a very low standard deviation:

Table 2. Values of amplitudes, damping factors and the noise

i	1	2
ai	10	12
λi	0.001	0.0011
Standard deviation	1E-5	1E-5

The result obtained by the Matrix Pencil method are shown in Fig. 3. In this case, Matrix Pencil is unable to calculate correctly the values of parameters.

Now, let tray to estimate the model parameters in the noisy case by using the Prony Method. The result are given in Fig. 6.

As we can see in Fig. 4, like Matrix Pencil, the Prony method in this case is unable to calculate the correct values of the parameters of the signal.

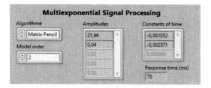

Fig. 3. Results of Matrix Pencil method

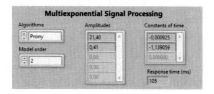

Fig. 4. Results of Prony method

• Case 2:

In this case, we choose very close amplitudes values for the two exponentials. The parameters chosen are illustrated in Table 3.

Table 3. Values of amplitudes and damping factors

i	1	2
ai	10.01	10.02
λi	0.1	0.2

The result obtained by the Matrix Pencil method are shown in Fig. 5. As we can see, the Matrix Pencil method can estimate correctly the parameters and faster.

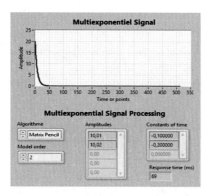

Fig. 5. Results of Matrix Pencil method

The result obtained by the Prony Method are displayed in Fig. 9. According to Fig. 6, we can conclude that in this case Prony method can also estimate correctly the parameters, but the time response is bigger than Matrix Pencil method.

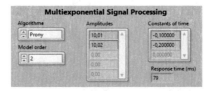

Fig. 6. Results of Prony method

Now in Table 4. We add the white Gaussian noise with a standard deviation equal to 0.001:

Table 4. Values of amplitudes, damping factors and the noise

i	1	2
ai	10.01	10.02
λi	0.1	0.2
Standard deviation	0.001	0.001

Result obtained by Matrix Pencil are displayed in Fig. 7.

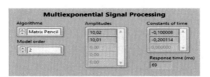

Fig. 7. Results of Matrix Pencil method

We can conclude according to Fig. 7, that Matrix Pencil method with the presence of noise can estimate the parameters of the signal.

The result obtained by Prony Method are displayed in Fig. 8.

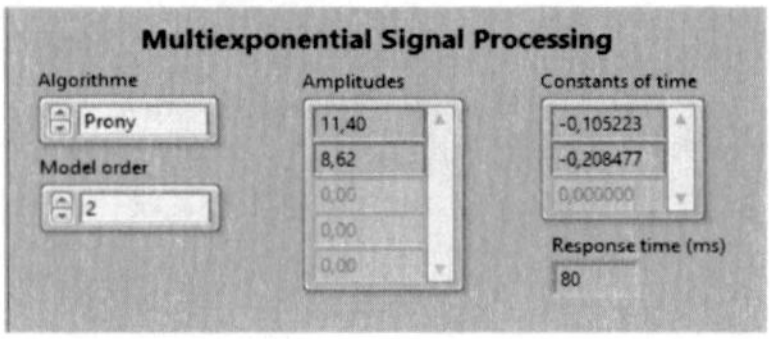

Fig. 8. Results of Prony method

As we can see in the Fig. 8, we can conclude in this case that Prony method is unable to calculate the parameters of the signal.

- Case 3:

In case 3 we will apply more noise to the signal and the values of amplitudes and damping factors we will choose them far from each other.

Table 5. Illustrate the parameters chosen in this case.

Table 5. Values of amplitudes, damping factors and the noise

i	1	2
ai	10	50
λi	1	5
Standard deviation	0.01	0.01

According to simulation results, we can conclude from this test that both of Prony method and of Matrix Pencil method can gives us results very near from the true values. Therefore, they can estimate the parameters of the signal given. However, Matrix Pencil method is faster than Prony method.

5 Discussion and Conclusions

For all tests presented in this paper, the other ones not treated, and writing in the paper, we can say that both of the high resolution methods Matrix Pencil and Prony method can estimate the parameters of the signal if the noise is very low. However, Matrix Pencil method is more efficient in computation and faster. Simulation and experimental results indicate that Matrix Pencil method is less sensitive to noise than Prony method. Prony method is iterative so when we do a huge signal processing the Prony method does not give any results. However, when the noise is high, Matrix Pencil does not give a good performance. It is for that we will revisit the methods of smoothing which does not modify the signal and will apply it to the method in order to improve the yield of Matrix Pencil method.

References

1. Shubair, R.M., Chow, Y.L.: Efficient computation of the periodic Green's function in Layered Dielectric Media. In: IEEE Transactions 011 Microwave Theory & Techniques, MTT-41, pp. 498–502, March 1993
2. Miller, E.K., Burke, G.J.: Using model based parameter estimation to increase the physical interpretability and numerical efficiency of computational electromagnetics. Comput. Phys. Commun. **68**, 43–75 (1991)

3. Evans, A.G.: Least squares systems parameter identification and time domain approximation, Ph.D. thesis, Drexel University, 1972. 20. Stieglitz, K.: On simultaneous estimation of
   poles and zeros in speech analysis. In: IEEE Transactions Acoustics, Speech and Signal
   Processing, ASSP-25, pp. 229–234, June 1977
4. Goodman, D.M., Dudley, D.G.: An output error model and algorithm for electromagnetic
   system identification. Circ. Syst. Signal Process. 6(4), 471–505 (1987)
5. Gantmacher, F.R.: Theory of Matrices, vol. I. Chelsea, New York (1960)
6. Ouibrahim, H., Weiner, D.D., Sarkar, T.K.: A generalized approach to direction finding.
   IEEE Trans. Acoust. Speech. Signal Process. **ASSP-36**, 610–612 (1988)
7. Ouibrahim, H.: A generalized approach to direction finding, Ph.D. dissertation, Syracuse
   Univ., Syracuse, NY, Dec 1986
8. Hua, Y., Sarkar, T.K.: Further analysis of three modern techniques for pole retrieval from
   data sequence. In: Proceedings of the 30th Midwesr Sytnp. Circuirs Sysr. Syracuse. NY,
   Aug 1987
9. Ouibrdhim, H., Weiner, D.D., Wei, Z.Y.: Angle of arrival estimation using a forward-back
   moving window. In: Proceedings of the 30th Midwesf Symnp. Circuirs Syst. Syracuse, NY,
   pp. 563–566, Aug 1987
10. Hua, Y., Sarkar, T.K.: Matrix Pencil method and its performance. In: Proceedings of the
    ICASSP-88, Apr 1988
11. Hua, Y., Sarkar, T.K.: A variation of ESPRIT for harmonic retrieval from a finite noisy data
    sequence. IEEE Trans. Acoust. Speech Signal Process. (submitted for publication)

Automated Checking of Conformance to SBVR Structured English Notation

Abdellatif Haj[(⊠)], Youssef Balouki, and Taoufiq Gadi

LAVETE Laboratory, Faculty of Sciences and Technics,
Hassan 1st University, Settat, Morocco
Haj.abdel@gmail.com

Abstract. Business rules are generally captured in a natural language. The inherit ambiguity of the latter is often seen as a cause for project failure, which makes it necessary to translate natural language business rules statements to another language sufficiently formal. However, business experts are generally not familiar with formal languages, which can complicate the communication between stakeholders. For this reason, Object Management Group (OMG) had proposed SBVR Standard (2008) for modeling complex organizations in a natural language but in a formal and detailed way. As a result, several studies have succeeded to increase the accuracy of their approaches by transforming their models from/to SBVR standard. Clearly then, the success of these approaches depends on the quality of the SBVR based statements used or generated. This paper presents an approach for checking conformance of both lexicon and syntax of Business Rules (BR) expressed with Semantic of Business Vocabulary and Rules (SBVR), to SBVR Structured English notation (SBVR-SE) using Natural Language Processing (NLP).

Keywords: Business rules · Semantic of business vocabulary and rules · Natural language processing · NLP · BR · SBVR · SBVR structured english

1 Introduction

Traditionally, the software modeling starts initially with the identification of the business needs before analyzing and abstracting the application, to conclude with the production of the source code us final step. Consequently, the reliability of each step is related to the level of reliability of its previous step, which explains the fact that the inception step is the most important phase. That is to say, the success of any project is related to the level of consistency, correctness and clarity of its gathered business needs. With this in mind, business needs are generally captured in a natural language, which not only suffers from ambiguity due to its informal nature, but also extremely difficult to automate due to its complexity. In the other hand, transforming natural language specifications directly to another language sufficiently formal (such as UML), conflict with the fact that business experts are generally not familiar with formal languages, which can make the communication between stakeholders a complex tasks, to say nothing of erroneous comprehension. For this reason, Object Management Group (OMG) [1] presented in 2008 a new standard called "Semantic Business

© Springer Nature Switzerland AG 2019
M. Ezziyani (Ed.): AI2SD 2018, AISC 915, pp. 697–706, 2019.
https://doi.org/10.1007/978-3-030-11928-7_63

Vocabulary and Rules" (SBVR) [2], providing a way to capture specifications in Natural Language (NL) understandable to all business people, and represent them in formal logic understandable to machines, so they can be automatically processed. Such a solution can help simplifying communication and bridging the gap between business experts and engineers. As a result, several studies have succeeded to increase the accuracy of their approaches by using SBVR standard as a pivot in their transformations between models, such as generating UML diagram from SBVR based business (SBVR to Use Case [3], SBVR to Class Diagram [4, 5], SBVR to Activity Diagram [6]), or vice versa, by extracting SBVR element from models (Use Case to SBVR [7], UML/OCL to SBVR [8], BPMN to SBVR [9]). Other approaches deal with checking consistency of SBVR based business rules by its translation to formal representation such as Alloy [10], SMT-LIBv2 [11], or OWL ontologies [12].

This large number of approaches dealing with SBVR standard confirms the efficiency of using SBVR standard as both input and output in models transformations. Although this may be true, the success of these approaches depends on the conformance level of the SBVR based statements (used or generated) to the SBVR standard, which will reflect the level of their reliability. Despite this interest, no one as far as we know has proposed an approach to check the conformance of the business statement to the SBVR standard.

Using Natural Language Processing (NLP), this paper presents an approach for checking lexical and syntactical conformance of SBVR based Business statements to SBVR Structured English (SBVR-SE) [2] as one of possibly notation that can map to the SBVR Meta-model. SBVR-SE was chosen due to its popularity; otherwise, there are other SBVR notations such as Rule-Speak.

In the first step, syntactical analyse will be done to make sure of the existence of SBVR elements in each statement (Modality, Quantifiers, Roles of Atomic/instantiation formulation and Fact type). Figure 2 shows an overview of SBVR main elements. Then, a lexical analyze will be performed by verifying the vocabulary conformance to that specified in SBVR-SE.

As illustrated in Fig. 1, our approach proceeds following the steps outlined below:

1. The input document: an English file text including business rules written in a natural language.
2. Parse the file text and extract statements supposed separated by full stop "." mark.
3. Store statements separately in a list.
4. Part-Of-Speech (POS) tagging: statement will be POS tagged to identify the basic POS tags for each statement.
5. Generate the dependency grammar for each statement.
6. Extract SBVR elements: modality, Roles, fact types, quantifiers.
7. Flagg statements suffering from missing elements.
8. Compare the vocabulary used with the SBVR-SE wordlist.
9. Flagg not conform words.
10. A list of statements not conform to the SBVR-SE will be shown to the user with an explication of the source of problem.

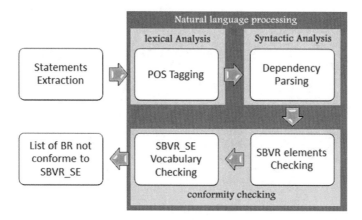

Fig. 1. General architecture of the methodology

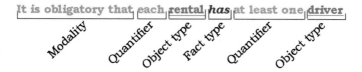

Fig. 2. Overview of SBVR main elements

The next chapter looks at technologies used in our approach (SBVR, and Stanford CoreNLP), Section 3 describes our approach. Section 4 presents a case study for our approach, and our conclusions are drawn in the final section.

2 Background

2.1 SBVR (Semantic Business Vocabulary and Rules)

Founded on the basic mantra of SBVR "Rules are constructed of fact types, and fact types are constructed of terms" (Fig. 3), Semantic Business Vocabulary and Rules (SBVR) [2] is an Object Management Group (OMG) standard to capture specifications in natural language understandable to all business people, and represent them in formal logic understandable to machines, which can help bridging the gap between business experts and engineers, thus, simplifying communication between them. Its compatibility with MDA increases its adoption by several organizations.

An overview of SBVR main elements is presented in Fig. 2:

(1) **Business Vocabulary (BV):**

Business Vocabulary is the concepts used by the organization to define the business domain. Two major types of concepts are used:

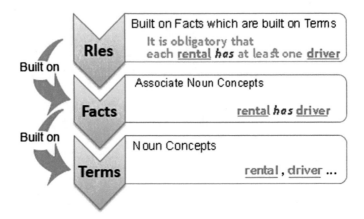

Fig. 3. SBVR realizes the 'Business Rules Mantra'

Noun Concept:

'Concept that is the meaning of a noun or noun phrase', and has as sub-types:

- Object type: 'noun concept that classifies things on the basis of their common properties'.
- Role: 'noun concept that corresponds to things based on their playing a part, assuming a function or being used in some situation'.
- Individual concept: 'a (noun) concept that corresponds to only one object [thing]'.

Verb Concepts (Fact Type):

'A concept that is the meaning of a verb phrase that involves one or more noun concepts and whose instances are all actualities.' (e.g. renter achieves rental).

(2) Business Rules (BR):

There are 2 types of SBVR Rules:

Structural (Definitional) Business Rules:

Also called alethic constraints, that cannot be violated by the business and can take one of the following forms: necessity, impossibility, restricted possibility.

e.g. '**It is necessary that each** rental_car *has* **exactly one** car_model'.

Behavioral (Operative) Business Rules:

Also called deontic constraints that can be broken by people, and can take one of the following forms: obligation, prohibitive and restricted permissive statement.

e.g. '**A** rental **must** *be refused* **if a** driver **of the** rental *is* **in** renter blacklist'.

(3) **Semantic Formulation:**

SBVR rules are semantically formulated using logical formulations. Here are the main categories of semantic structure of SBVR Semantic Formulations:

Atomic Formulation:

Based exactly on one fact type which in turn involves noun concepts. (e.g. <u>renter</u> *achieves* <u>rental</u>).

Instantiation Formulation:

When a Noun Concept is an instance of another Noun Concept. (e.g. "<u>Luxury car</u> *is* **an instance** **of a** <u>Car</u>").

Logical Operation:

Used to create more complex logical expression:

- Negation: "it is NOT p"
- Conjunctions/Disjunctions: "p AND/OR q"
- Implication: "IF p THEN q", "q IF p"
- Quantification: Introduces Concepts to quantify them.
- Universal: a, an, each, all...
- Existential: At least/most n | more/less than n
- Numeric range: between n and m
- Exactly n.
- Modality: different modality are provided
- Structural:
     It is necessary that | Always
     It is impossible that | Never
     It is possible that | Sometimes.
- Behavioral:
     It is obligatory that | Must
     It is prohibited that | Must not
     It is permitted that | May.

SBVR Structured English notation [2] will be used in this paper to describe our vocabularies and formalize the syntax of rules. There are four font styles with formal meaning:

Term:	Noun concepts. e.g. "<u>person</u>";
Name:	Individual concepts. e.g. "<u>USA</u>"
Verb:	Verb concepts e.g. "<u>*Insert*</u>" (italicized).
Keywords:	e.g. **each**, **obligatory** (bolded).

2.2 Stanford CoreNLP

As defined in [13]: "Stanford CoreNLP provides a set of human language technology tools. It can give the base forms of words, their parts of speech, whether they are names of companies, people, etc., normalize dates, times, and numeric quantities, mark up the structure of sentences in terms of phrases and syntactic dependencies, indicate which noun phrases refer to the same entities, indicate sentiment, extract particular or open-class relations between entity mentions, get the quotes people said, etc."

2.3   Natural Language Processing (NLP)

As a discipline of computer science, Natural language processing (NLP) [14] is used to make human language understandable by machines. Generally it involves tasks such as: Lemmatization, Morphological segmentation, Part-of-speech tagging, Parsing, Sentence breaking, Stemming, Word segmentation, Terminology extraction, in order to solve diver problems, in particular: Lexical semantics, Machine translation & Automatic summarization.

3   Our Approach

Our goal is to verify the lexicon and syntax of SBVR-SE based business rules using NLP techniques.

- Looking for the SBVR semantic formulations in each statement: Modality, Quantifiers, Roles of Atomic/instantiation formulation, Fact types.
- Verifying the vocabulary conformance to that specified in SBVR Structured English.

Verifying lexicon and syntax of BR can help to obtain a well formed BR statement and reveal weak ones. We choose "Stanford CorNLP" [13] to perform Natural Language Processing, according to the following steps.

3.1   Lexical Analyzing

The Part-Of-Speech (POS) tagging is performed to identify the basic POS each word.

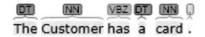

3.2   Syntactic Analysis

Dependency parse is performed to generate the parse tree for further semantic analysis.

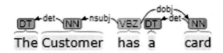

3.3 Analyze of SBVR Semantic Formulation

Statement without Verb will be flagged as "Fact type missing".

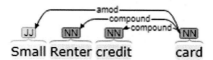

Verb without subject (or agent in passive voice) or predicate will be flagged as "Role missing".

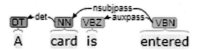

Subject/object (or agent in passive voice) without determinant, or numeric modifier is flagged as "quantifier missing".

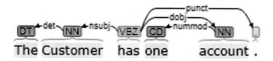

Sentence witch not begin with "it is <modality> that" statement and don't have a modal auxiliary verb is flagged as "missing modality".

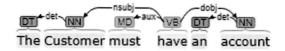

3.4 Verifying the Vocabulary Conformance to that Specified in SBVR Structured English

Determinants:

Each determinant will be compared with a list of determinants in a dictionary. If the detected determinant doesn't exist in the dictionary, the statement will be flagged as "determinant error".

Cardinality:

If a noun has no determinant, so we look for cardinality which may have only a noun modifier in form of Adjective superlative "least" or "most".

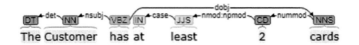

The Customer has at   least   2   cards

Or may have only an adverb modifier in form of Adjective comparative "more" or "less".

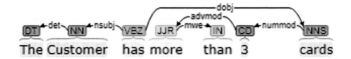

The Customer has more   than 3   cards

Else the statements will be flagger as "Cardinality error".

Implication:

A statement contains the "if" word but no adverbial clause found, so the statement is flagged as "Missing Consequence".

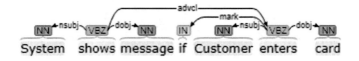

System shows message if Customer enters   card

In the other hand, if a statement contains an adverbial clause, but no "if" word found, so the statement is flagged as "error keyword (if)".

4   Case Study

Our approach will be illustrated using few rules extracted from EU-Rent Car Rental case-study.

- R1: **Each** car rental **must** *be insured.*
- R2: **Each** luxury car rental *is* **a** car rental.
- R3: **Each** luxury car rental **must** *be insured* **by** credit cards.
- R4: car rental credit card validating **a** credit card.

Figures 4 and 5 clearly show that:

- R1 has no agent which means that the rule misses the role 1 of the statement.
- R2 has no auxiliary verb in form of modality (MD) which means that the rule misses a modality.
- R3 has no determinant for the noun "credit card" which means that it misses a cardinality.
- R4 has no verb which means it misses a fact type.

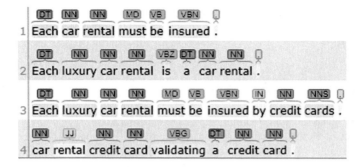

Fig. 4. The generated POS tagging

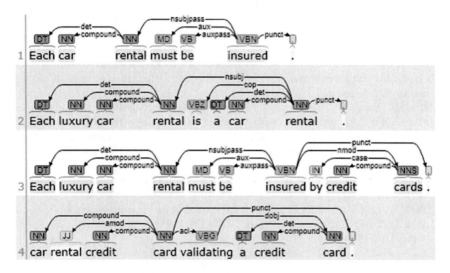

Fig. 5. The generated dependency parse

5 Conclusion and Future Works

We have not followed the trend and translate models from/to SBVR standard, but rather presented an approach for checking lexical and syntactical conformance of SBVR based Business statements to SBVR-SE using Natural Language Processing (NLP), to increase the level of BR reliability.

Our work clearly has some limitations related in particular to the accuracy of results obtained from the parser used. Nevertheless, we believe our work not only can help to obtain a well formed BR statement and reveal weak ones, but also could be a starting point for detecting and resolving more BR problems such as inconsistencies, ambiguity and duplication.

However, the approach should be validated by implementing a solution for a larger sample size including complex ones. Further improvements are also needed to remove irrelevant results.

References

1. OMG: Object Management Group. http://www.omg.org/
2. Semantics of Business Vocabulary and Rules (SBVR), Version 1.4. Version 1.4, Object Management Group (2017). www.omg.org/spec/SBVR/
3. Thakore, D., Upadhyay, A.R.: Development of use case model from software requirement using in-between SBVR format at analysis phase. Int. J. Adv. Comput. Theory Eng. (IJACTE) **2**, 86–92 (2013)
4. Awasthi, S., Nayak, A.: Transformation of SBVR business rules to UML class model. In: Pfeiffer, H.D., Ignatov, D.I., Poelmans J., Gadiraju, N. (eds.) Conceptual Structures for STEM Research and Education. ICCS-Conceptual Structures 2013. Lecture Notes in Computer Science, vol. 7735. Springer, Berlin, Heidelberg (2013)
5. Bajwa, I.S., Naeem, M.A., Ali, A., Ali, S.: A controlled natural language interface to class models. In: 13th International Conference on Enterprise Information Systems, ICEIS 2011, Beijing, China, pp. 102–110 (2011)
6. Iqbal, U., Bajwa, I.S.: Generating UML activity diagram from SBVR rules. In: The Sixth International Conference on Innovative Computing Technology (INTECH 2016)
7. Skersys, T., Danenas, P., Butleris, R.: Extracting SBVR business vocabularies and business rules from UML use case diagrams. J. Syst. Softw. (2018). https://doi.org/10.1016/j.jss.2018.03.061
8. Cabot, J., Pau, R., Raventós, R.: From UML/OCL to SBVR specifications: A challenging transformation. Inf. Syst. **35**(4), 417–440 (2010)
9. Malik, S., Bajwa, I.S.: Back to origin: transformation of business process models to business rules. In: La Rosa, M., Soffer, P. (eds.) BPM 2012 Workshops, pp. 611–622. Springer, Berlin, Heidelberg (2012)
10. dos Santos Guimarães D., et al.: A method for verifying the consistency of business rules using alloy. In: Proceedings of the Twenty-Sixth International Conference on Software Engineering & Knowledge Engineering, pp. 381–386 (2014)
11. Chittimalli, P.K., Anand, K.: Domain independent method of detecting inconsistencies in SBVR-based business rules. In: Proceedings of the International Workshop on Formal Methods for Analysis of Business Systems, pp. 9–16. ACM (2016)
12. Karpovic, J., et al.: Requirements for semantic business vocabularies and rules for transforming them into consistent owl2 ontologies. In: International Conference on Information and Software Technologies, pp. 420–435. Springer (2012)
13. Stanford NLP [Online]. Available: nlp.stanford.edu/
14. Kurdi, M.Z.: Natural Language Processing and Computational Linguistics: Semantics, Discourse, and Applications, vol. 2. ISTE-Wiley. ISBN 978–1848219212 (2017)

Image Analysis by Hahn Moments
and a Digital Filter

Hicham Karmouni[1(✉)], Tarik Jahid[1], Mhamed Sayyouri[2],
Abdeslam Hmimid[1], Anass El-Affar[1], and Hassan Qjidaa[1]

[1] CED-STIC, LESSI, Faculty of Sciences Dhar El-Mehraz,
Sidi Mohamed Ben Abdellah University, Fez, Morocco
hicham.karmouni@usmba.ac.ma
[2] LabSIPE, National School of Applied Sciences,
Chouaib Doukkali University, El Jadida, Morocco

Abstract. In this paper, we propose a new method of the fast and stable computation of the discrete orthogonal moments of Hahn. In this method, we have combined two main concepts. The first concept is the digital filters based on the Z-transform to accelerate the calculation process and their inverses of the Hahn moments. The second concept is the partitioning of the image into a set of blocks of fixed sizes where each block is processed independently. The first concept to accelerate the computation time and the second to improve the quality of images reconstruction. Experimental results show that both the proposed algorithms to compute Hahn moments and inverse perform better than existing methods in term of computation speed and the quality of images reconstruction.

Keywords: Hahn moments · Image reconstruction · Lapped block-based method

1 Introduction

Function moments of various types have been extensively used in pattern recognition and image analysis tasks [1–5]. Geometric moments and their translation, scaling and rotation invariants were firstly introduced by Hu [6]. Moment based image reconstruction was pioneered by Teague who noted that image can be reconstructed from a set of orthogonal moments [7]. The computation of continuous orthogonal moments requires a suitable transformation of the coordinates of the image in the space, and an appropriate approximation of the integral. This increases the computational complexity and error of the discretization [8–11]. To eliminate this error, a set of discrete orthogonal moments such as Tchebichef, Krawtchouk, Meixner, Charlier, and Hahn [12–19] have been recently introduced in the field of image analysis. The use of discrete orthogonal polynomials as basic functions for the computation of the image moments eliminates the need for numerical approximation and satisfies exactly the property of orthogonality in the discrete domain of the image space coordinates [12]. This property makes the discrete orthogonal moments superior to the continuous orthogonal moments in the sense of the capacity of the image's representation [12–15]. But, the use of these discrete

© Springer Nature Switzerland AG 2019
M. Ezziyani (Ed.): AI2SD 2018, AISC 915, pp. 707–718, 2019.
https://doi.org/10.1007/978-3-030-11928-7_64

orthogonal moments generates two major problems which are high computational cost and the propagation of numerical errors in the computation of discrete orthogonal polynomials [12, 13]. This field of research was confronted to cost of calculation and quality of reconstruction. So, many algorithms were implemented for fast computation of moments and its inverses. Spiliotis [20] proposed an algorithm based on blocks representation of binary image which reduces considerably the numerical fluctuation caused by computation of high order and high dimensions. Papakostas [21] introduced a new method based to use on gray-scale image; he proposed a partial image block representation PIBR, to compute moments rapidly and efficiently, which was proven for orthogonal moments by Hmimid et al. [13]. Wang and Wang [22] used a Clenshaw recursion formula to accelerate the calculation of Tchebichef moments. Honarvar [23–25] introduced the 1D and 2D all-polar digital filter using the properties of the Z transformation in terms of Tchebichef and Krawtchouk polynomials. Previous works using the digital filter have been introduced by Hatamian [26] and then by Wong and Siu [27], both are focused on geometric moments.

In this paper, we propose a new method to accelerate the computation time of Hahn's discrete orthogonal moment based on two notions. The first one is the digital filters based on the Z-transform allowed the acceleration of the moments calculation processes and their inverses. The second one is the block image representation, which represents the image as a set of fixed size blocks. This method is purely local, where each block is processed independently. Thus, the reduction of the image space allows the use of low order discrete orthogonal moments during the calculation process [28–30]. The computation of discrete orthogonal moments of image blocks provides better image representation. In order to demonstrate the effectiveness of the proposed approach in comparison to existing method in terms of numerical stability, computation time and the quality of reconstruction and noise robustness, some simulations have been carried out.

The paper is organized as follows. In Sect. 2, we introduce the polynomes and the moments of Hahn. In Sect. 3, we define the calculation of Hahn moments and its inverse using the digital filters based on the Z-transform. In Sect. 4, the reconstruction method based on Lapped blocks (LBBRM) is presented. In Sect. 5, provides some experimental results concerning the reduction of the time calculation of Hahn moments and the image reconstruction for binary and gray-scale images. Section 6 concludes this work.

2 Discrete Orthogonal Polynomials and Moments of Hahn

2.1 Hahn Polynomials

The nth Hahn polynomials of one variable x, with the order n, defined in the region of $[0, N-1]$, are represented by using hypergeometric function as [15]:

$$h_n^{(a,b)}(x) = \frac{(-1)^n (b+1)_n (N-n)_n}{n!} \sum_{k=0}^{n} \frac{(-n)_k (n+a+b+1)_k (-x)_k}{(b+1)_k (1-N)_k k!} \tag{1}$$

where $x, n = 0, 1, 2, \ldots, N - 1$, N is a natural number representing the degree of the Hahn polynomial, $a \succ -1$ and $b \succ -1$.

We show a relationship between the Hahn polynomials and monomials. First, by expanding the Pochhammer symbol in terms of binomial coefficients, we obtain:

$$(-x)_k = (-1)^k k! \binom{x}{k} \tag{2}$$

More explicit form is defined in:

$$h_n^{(a,b)}(x) = \frac{(-1)^n (b+1)_n (N-n)_n}{n!} \sum_{k=0}^{n} \frac{(-1)_k (-n)_k (n+a+b+1)_k (-x)_k}{(b+1)_k (1-N)_k} \binom{x}{k} \tag{3}$$

Equation (3) can be expressed in terms of binomial $\binom{x}{k}$ as:

$$h_n^{(a,b)}(x) = \sum_{k=0}^{n} \Gamma_k(n, a, b) \binom{x}{k} \tag{4}$$

where $\Gamma_k(n, a, b)$ is a lower triangle matrix:

$$\Gamma_k(n, a, b) = \frac{(-1)^n (b+1)_n (N-n)_n}{n!} \times \frac{(-1)_k (-n)_k (n+a+b+1)_k}{(b+1)_k (1-N)_k} \tag{5}$$

To avoid fluctuation in numerical computation, we use the normalized form of Hahn polynomials defined by:

$$\tilde{h}_n^{(a,b)}(x) = h_n^{(a,b)}(x) \sqrt{\frac{w(x)}{\rho(n)}} \tag{6}$$

With $w(x)$ is the weight function of Hahn discrete orthogonal polynomials and $\rho(n)$ is the squared norm of Hahn discrete orthogonal polynomials defined as:

$$w(x) = \frac{(N-x+a-1)!(x+b)!}{(N-x-1)!x!} \quad \text{and} \quad \rho(n) = \frac{(a+n)!(b+n)!(a+b+n+1)_N}{(a+b+2n+1)(N-n-1)!n!}$$

2.2   Hahn Moments

For a digital image $f(x, y)$ with size $N \times M$, that is $x \in [0, N-1]$ and $y \in [0, M-1]$, the $(n+m)$th order Hahn moments is defined as follows

$$HM_{nm} = \sum_{x=0}^{N-1} \sum_{y=0}^{M-1} \tilde{h}_n^{(a,b)}(x) \tilde{h}_m^{(a,b)}(y) f(x, y) \tag{7}$$

which we can express as follow:

$$HM_{nm} = \frac{1}{\sqrt{\rho(n,m)}} \sum_{x=0}^{N-1} \sum_{y=0}^{M-1} h_n^{(a,b)}(x) h_m^{(a,b)}(y) \sqrt{w(x,y)} f(x,y) \tag{8}$$

We can replace it by for later purpose:

$$HM_{nm} = A_{nm} \sum_{x=0}^{N-1} \sum_{y=0}^{M-1} h_n^{(a,b)}(x) h_m^{(a,b)}(y) \tilde{f}(x,y) \tag{9}$$

where:

$$A_{nm} = \frac{1}{\sqrt{\rho(n,m)}} = \frac{1}{\sqrt{\rho(n)\rho(m)}} \quad \text{and}$$

$$\tilde{f}(x,y) = \sqrt{w(x)w(y)} f(x,y) = \sqrt{w(x,y)} f(x,y)$$

3   Fast Computation of Hahn Moments Based on Digital Filters

In this section, it is shown that a cascaded feed-back digital filter outputs can be sampled at the earlier time intervals. The second subsection is meant to show how the Hahn moments can be computed efficiently in terms of the cascaded digital filter outputs. Finally, a matrix representation of 2D Hahn moments expresses the direct calculation of these moments based on the filter outputs.

3.1   Digital Filter Outputs

The transfer function of a cascaded filter $H_n(z) = \frac{1}{(1-z^{-1})^{n+1}}$ can be created by a series of n cascaded accumulators. Such a filter as shown in Fig. 1a, given an input the image $f(x)$, produces a sampled output at earlier points of $N - n - 1$ as:

$$y_n(N - n - 1) = \sum_{x=0}^{N-1} f(x) \binom{x}{n} \tag{10}$$

This formulation shows that the digital filter outputs are sampled at earlier points, $N - 1, N - 2, N - 3 \ldots N - n - 1$. Meanwhile, this set of output values starts to decrease after $n/2$ moments orders. The 2D accumulator grid is shown in Fig. 1b and consists of one row and $n + 1$ columns based on single-pole single-zero filters. The filter output for an input scaled image $\tilde{f}(x,y)$ with size $N \times M$ is given by the following expression:

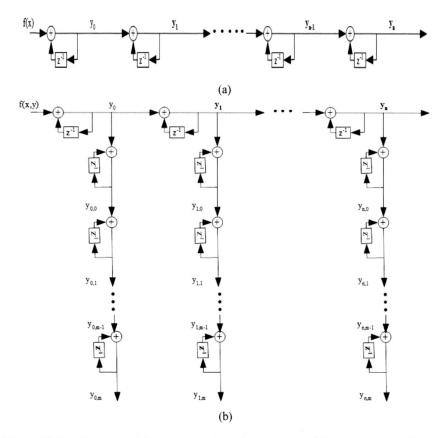

(a)

(b)

Fig. 1. Digital filter structure for generating desired outputs. **a** y_n of *1D* up to (n) order. **b** $y_{n,m}$ of *2D* up to $(n + m)$ order

$$y_{nm}(N - n - 1, M - m - 1) = \sum_{x=0}^{N-1}\sum_{y=0}^{M-1}\tilde{f}(x,y)\binom{x}{n}\binom{y}{m} \qquad (11)$$

3.2   Computation of Hahn Moments Using a Digital Filter

In this subsection, a direct relationship between Hahn moments and digital filter outputs is derived. Then, by using the *2D* Hahn moments definition in Eq. (12), the binomials form of Hahn polynomials in Eq. (4) we have

$$HM_{nm} = A_{nm} \sum_{x=0}^{N-1} \sum_{y=0}^{M-1} h_n^{(a,b)}(x) h_m^{(a,b)}(y) \tilde{f}(x,y)$$

$$= A_{nm} \sum_{x=0}^{N-1} \sum_{y=0}^{M-1} \sum_{k=0}^{n} \Gamma_k(n,a,b) \binom{x}{k} \sum_{l=0}^{m} \Gamma_l(m,a,b) \binom{y}{l} \tilde{f}(x,y)$$

$$= A_{nm} \sum_{k=0}^{n} \sum_{l=0}^{m} \Gamma_k(n,a,b) \Gamma_l(m,a,b) \sum_{x=0}^{N-1} \sum_{y=0}^{M-1} \binom{x}{k} \binom{y}{l} \tilde{f}(x,y) \qquad (12)$$

$$= A_{nm} \sum_{k=0}^{n} \sum_{l=0}^{m} \Gamma_k(n,a,b) \Gamma_l(m,a,b) y_{kl}$$

with y_{kl} is the filter output for the input scaled image $\tilde{f}(x,y)$

$$y_{kl} = \sum_{x=0}^{N-1} \sum_{y=0}^{M-1} \tilde{f}(x,y) \binom{x}{k} \binom{y}{l} \qquad (13)$$

3.3 Image Reconstruction Using Hahn Moments

The original image function can be approximated by a truncated series:

$$\hat{f}(x,y) = \sum_{n=0}^{max} \sum_{m=0}^{n} HM_{nm} \tilde{h}_n^{(a,b)}(x) \tilde{h}_m^{(a,b)}(y) \qquad (14)$$

If 'max' tends to infinity, the difference between the original image and the reconstructed image tends to zero.

The difference between the original image $f(x,y)$ and the reconstructed images $\hat{f}(x,y)$ is measured using the mean squared error *(MSE)* defined as follows [24]:

$$MSE = \frac{1}{MN} \sum_{i=1}^{M} \sum_{j=1}^{N} \left(f(x_i, y_j) - \hat{f}(x_i, y_j) \right)^2 \qquad (15)$$

4 Lapped Block-Based Reconstruction Method for Hahn Moments

In this section, we present the Lapped Block Image Analysis [28] method to compute the Hahn moments of each block and to reconstruct the image from these blocks instead of the global reconstruction.

Then, let the image function be associated to each f^{p_1,p_2}, thus, each subset will be defined as follows:

$$f^{p_1,p_2}(x,y) = \{f(i,j)/i,j \in f^{p_1,p_2}\} \tag{16}$$

From that, we can get a reconstructed image:

$$\hat{f}(x,y) = \bigcup_{p_1=0}^{(s_1-1)} \bigcup_{p_2=0}^{(s_2-1)} \hat{f}^{p_1,p_2}(x,y) \tag{17}$$

According to these definitions, we introduce the Hahn moments using a digital filter related to each image block, we obtain:

$$HM_{nm}^{p_1,p_2} = A_{nm} \sum_{r=0}^{n} \sum_{s=0}^{m} \Gamma_k(n,a,b)\Gamma_l(m,a,b)y_{rs}^{p_1,p_2} \tag{18}$$

where

$$y_{rs}^{p_1,p_2} = \sum_{x=p_2k}^{(p_2+1)k} \sum_{y=p_1l}^{(p_1+1)l} \tilde{f}^{p_1,p_2}(x,y)\binom{x}{r}\binom{y}{s} \tag{19}$$

Figure 2 summarises the block diagram of Hahn via digital filters based on the transformation Z. The significant reduction of the image space during partitioning makes it possible to represent the minute details of the image with only low orders of Hah discrete orthogonal moments, which ensures the digital stability during the processing of the image.

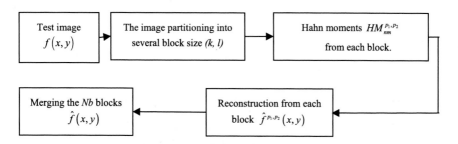

Fig. 2. Image reconstruction process diagram

5   Results and Simulations

In this section, we give experimental results to validate the theoretical results developed in the previous sections. This section is divided into two sub-sections. In the first sub-section, we will compare the time computation of Hahn moments by the recursive methods respect to x and the proposed methods. In the second part, we will test the ability of Hahn moments using the proposed method for the reconstruction of binary and gray-scale images.

5.1   The Computational Time of Hahn Moments

In order to validate the theoretical results developed in the previous sections and to test the yield of the proposed method in terms of computation time, our algorithm is tested by a set of the three binary images and the three gray-scale images of size 256×256, extracted from the MPEG-7 image database CE-shape-1 Part B [MPEG-7, 2014] [31] (Figs. 3 and 4). Each of the six images contains 4096 size $[4 \times 4]$ and 1024 size $[8 \times 8]$.

Fig. 3. a Binary images: chicken, guitar and pocket. **b** Gray-scale images: lena, cameraman, and pirate

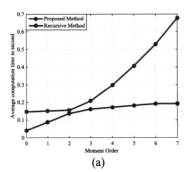 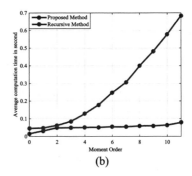

(a)   (b)

Fig. 4. Average computation time of Hahn moments of three binary images, using two differents method, image as blocks of siz **a** $[4 \times 4]$ and **b** $[8 \times 8]$

The Hahn discrete orthogonal moments are computed for orders ranging from 0 to 7 for blocks of size $[4 \times 4]$ and from 0 to 11 for blocks of size $[8 \times 8]$. The two figures in Figs. 4 and 5 represent the average time of calculation of the Hahn discrete orthogonal moments for the three binary images and the three gray-scale images respectively. The average time of the calculation of the discrete orthogonal moments of Hahn by the proposed method is compared by the recursive method respect to x [32].

The two figures show that the proposed methods are faster than the direct one because the computation of Hahn moments by two proposed methods depends only on the number of blocks instead of the image's size. For both types of images as blocks of size $[4 \times 4]$, the computation time of Hahn moments has accelerated considerably, and the gain of time arrives until 80% for binary images and 82% for images in gray-scale.

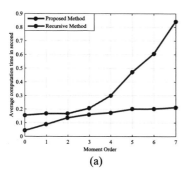 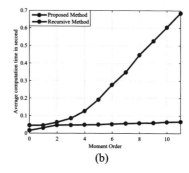

(a)   (b)

Fig. 5. Average computation time of Hahn moments of three gray-scale images using two differents methods, image as blocks of size **a** [4 × 4] and **b** [8 × 8]

5.2 Image Reconstruction via Hahn Moments

In this sub-section, we will discuss the ability of Hahn moments in terms of reconstruction quality our algorithm is tested on two types of images of size 256×256 pixels (Fig. 3). The image reconstruction test by blocks of sizes [4 × 4] and [8 × 8] is performed using the discrete orthogonal moments of Hahn by the two methods:

- The recursive method [32].
- The proposed method based on LBBRM on Eq. (29).

The two figures in Figs. 6 and 7 represent the mean square errors between the reconstructed images and the original images as a function of the orders. The order varies between 0 and 7 for blocks of size [4 × 4], and between 0 and 11 for blocks [8 × 8].

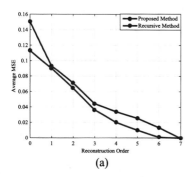 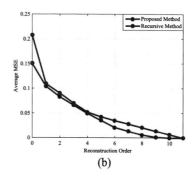

(a)   (b)

Fig. 6. Average MSE of three binary images, using two differents method, image as blocks of size **a** [4 × 4] and **b** [8 × 8] using Hahn moments

The two Figs. 6 and 7 show that the reconstruction errors by the proposed method are smaller using the Hahn moments. This shows that the proposed approach is effective in terms of reconstruction quality for binary and gray-scale images as block of size [4 × 4] and [8 × 8].

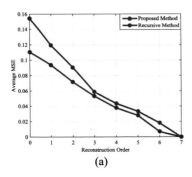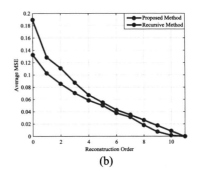

Fig. 7. Average MSE of three gray-scale images using two differents methods **a** image as blocks of size [4 × 4] **b** image as blocks of size [8 × 8] using Hahn moments

In this experience, we will test the robustness of Hahn's moments in relation to different types of noise. For this, two numerical experiments are performed using two types of noise. The first type of noise is the "salt and pepper" noise while the second is the sound of the strong "white Gaussian noise", for gray-scale images are shown in Fig. 8.

The images contaminated by the two types of noise are presented in Fig. 8 for gray-scale image are reconstructed using Hahn discrete orthogonal moments. Figure 9 shows the mean squared error (MSE) of the reconstructed images for gray-scale images.

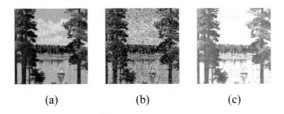

Fig. 8. **a** Zawaka binary image, **b** noisy image by salt and pepper, and **c** noisy image by white Gaussian

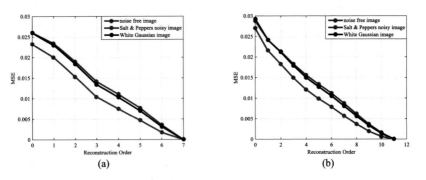

Fig. 9. MSE of noisy image "Lake", image as blocks of size **a** [4 × 4] and **b** [8 × 8] using Hahn moments

It can be seen that the three errors decrease with the increase of Hahn moments until a stable minimum value is obtained, which proves the robustness of the proposed approach to Gaussian and salt & Pepper noise for gray-scale images.

6   Conclusion

In this paper, we have presented a fast and stable method for the computation of Hahn's moments for binary and gray-scale images. This method is performed using the digital filters based on the Z-transform to accelerate the calculation process Hahn moments and we have adopted a method of partitioning the image into a set of fixed size blocks (LBBRM), where each block is processed independently. When we have worked on the image with only Hahn moments of low orders, to solve this numerical instability. The experiment was carried out with a comparison of the performance speed of the proposed method in presence of the existing method and image reconstruction using Hahn moments has been used as an example to illustrate the stability of the results of images with and without noise.

References

1. Khotanzad, A., Hong, Y.: Invariant image recognition by Zernike moments. IEEE Trans. Pattern Anal. Mach. Intell. **12**(5), 489–497 (1990)
2. Hsu, H.S.: Moment preserving edge detection and its application to image data compression. Optim. Eng. **32**, 1596–1608 (1993)
3. Heywood, M., Noakes, P.: Fractional central moment method for movement invariant object classification. IEE Proc. Vis. Image Signal Process. **142**(4), 213–219 (1995)
4. Belkasim, S., Shridhar, M., Ahmadi, M.: Pattern recognition with moment invariants: a comparative study and new results. Pattern Recogn. **24**(12), 1117–1138 (1991)
5. Flusser, J., Suk, T.: Pattern recognition by affine moment invariants. Pattern Recogn. **26**(1), 167–174 (1993)
6. Hu, M.K.: Visual pattern recognition by moment invariants. IRE Trans. Inform. Theory **8**(2), 179–187 (1962)
7. Teague, M.R.: Image analysis via the general theory of moments. J. Opt. Soc. Amer. **70**(8), 920–930 (1980)
8. Liao, S.X., Pawlak, M.: On image analysis by moments. IEEE Trans. Pattern Anal. Mach. Intell. **18**, 254–266 (1996)
9. Chong, C.W., Paramesran, R., Mukundan, R.: Translation and scale invariants of Legendre moments. Pattern Recogn. **37**, 119–129 (2004)
10. Lin, H., Si, J., Abousleman, G.P.: Orthogonal rotation invariant moments for digital image pr cessing. IEEE Trans. Image Process. **17**, 272–282 (2008)
11. Yang, B., Li, G., Zhang, H., Dai, M.: Rotation and translation invariants of Gaussian-Hermite moments. Pattern Recogn. Lett. **32**, 1283–1298 (2011)
12. Mukundan, R., Ong, S.H., Lee, P.A.: Image analysis by Tchebichef moments. IEEE Trans. Image Process. **10**(9), 1357–1364 (2001)
13. Hmimid, A., Sayyouri, M., Qjidaa, H.: Image classification using a new set of separable two-dimensional discrete orthogonal invariant moments. J. Electron. Imag. **23**(1), 013026 (2014)

14. Sayyouri, M., Hmimid, A., Qjidaa, H.: A fast computation of novel set of Meixner invariant moments for image analysis. Circuits Syst. Signal Process. 1–26 (2014). Springer 2014. https://doi.org/10.1007/s00034-014-9881-7

15. Sayyouri, M., Hmimid, A., Qjidaa, H.: Image analysis using separable discrete moments of Charlier-Hahn. Multimedia Tools Appl. **75**(1), 547–571 (2014)

16. Karmouni, H., Jahid, T., El Affar, I., Sayyouri, M., Hmimid, A., Qjidaa, H., Rezzouk, A.: Image analysis using separable Krawtchouk-Tchebichef's moments. In: International Conference on Advanced Technologies for Signal and Image Processing (Atsip'2017). Fez, Morocco, 22–24 May 2017

17. Karmouni, H., Jahid, T., Lakhili, Z., Hmimid, A., Sayyouri, M., Qjidaa, H., Rezzouk, A.: Image reconstruction by Krawtchouk moments via digital filter. In: International Conference on Intelligent Systems and Computer Vision, ISCV'2017. Fez, Morocco, 17–20 Apr 2017

18. Sayyouri, M., Hmimid, A., Karmouni, H., Qjidaa, H., Rezzouk, A.: Image classification using separable invariant moments of Krawtchouk-Tchebichef. In: 12th International Conference of Computer Systems and Applications (AICCSA). Marrakech, Morocco, 17–20 Nov 2015

19. Jahid, T., Karmouni, H., Hmimid, A., Sayyouri, M., Qjidaa, H.: Image moments and reconstruction by Krawtchouk via Clenshaw's recurrence formula. In: 3rd International Conference on Electrical and Information Technologies (ICEIT), Rabat, Morocco, 15–18 Nov 2017

20. Spiliotis, I.M., Mertzios, B.G.: Real-time computation of two-dimensional moments on binary images using image block representation. IEEE Trans. Image Process. **7**(11), 1609–1615 (1998)

21. Papakostas, G.A., Karakasis, E.G., Koulouriotis, D.E.: Accurate and speedy computation of image Legendre moments for computer vision applications. Image Vis. Comput. **28**(3), 414–423 (2010)

22. Wang, G., Wang, S.: Recursive computation of Tchebichef moment and its inverse transform. Pattern Recognit. **39**(1), 47–56 (2006)

23. Honarvar, B., Paramesran, R.: A new formulation of geometric moments from lower output values of digital filters. J. Circ. Syst. Comput. 1450055 (2014)

24. Honarvar, B., Paramesran, R., Lim, C.-L.: The fast recursive computation of Tchebichef moment and its inverse transform based on Z-transform. Digital Signal Process. **23**(5), 1738–1746 (2013)

25. Honarvar, B., Flusser, J.: Fast computation of Krawtchouk moments. Inf. Sci. **288**(20), 73–86 (2014)

26. Hatamian, M.: A real-time two-dimensional moment generating algorithm and its single chip implementation. IEEE Trans. Acoust. Speech Signal Process. **34**(3), 546–553 (1986)

27. Wong, W.-H., Siu, W.-C.: Improved digital filter structure for fast moments computation. IEE Proc. Vis. Imag. Signal Process. **146**(2), 73–79 (1999)

28. El Fadili, H., Zenkouar, K., Qjidaa, H.: Lapped block image analysis via the method of Legendre moments. EURASIP J. Appl. Signal Process. **2003**(9), 902–913 (2003)

29. Karmouni, H., Hmimid, A., Jahid, T., Sayyouri, M., Qjidaa, H., Rezzouk, A.: Fast and stable computation of the Charlier moments and their inverses using digital filters and image block representation. Circuits Syst. Signal Process. (2018)

30. Jahid, T., Hmimid, A., Karmouni, H., Sayyouri, M., Qjidaa, H., Rezzouk, A.: Image analysis by Meixner moments and a digital filter. Multimed. Tools Appl. (2017)

31. http://www.dabi.temple.edu/~shape/MPEG7/dataset.html

32. Hmimid, A., Sayyouri, M., Qjidaa, H.: Fast computation of separable two-dimensional discrete invariant moments for image classification. Pattern Recogn. **48**, 509–521 (2015)

A New Web Service Architecture for Enhancing the Interoperability of LMS and Mobile Applications Using the Next Generation of SCORM

Abdellah Bakhouyi[1][(✉)], Rachid Dehbi[2], and Mohamed Talea[1]

[1] LTI Laboratory, Faculty of Science Ben M'Sik, Hassan II University
Casablanca, Casablanca, Morocco
abdellah.bakhouyi@gmail.com, taleamohamed@yahoo.fr
[2] LR2I Laboratory, Faculty of Science Aïn Chock, Hassan II University
Casablanca, Casablanca, Morocco
dehbirac@yahoo.fr

Abstract. The evolution of mobile learning has changed the way of learning. With the growing popularity of using mobile devices, mobile learning has become important in teaching and learning in education. Most m-learning services are provided by the Learning Management Systems. This article aims to design a software architecture with LMS and focuses on integrating mobile applications to improve interoperability. This architecture is being implemented for the famous open source LMS Moodle.

Keywords: Interoperability · SOA · LMS · Moodle · M-learning · E-learning · SCORM · LRS

1 Introduction

In recent years, the rapid evolution of information technology has supplied new learning modalities and innovative ways to address the limitations of traditional learning [1]. In brief, mobile learning is characterized by the ability to enhance strong interaction between learners, teachers and tutors, supporting greater motivation, convenience and resilience in the learning process. By virtue of mobile devices [2], teachers, tutors and learners can use the power of ubiquitous computing to contribute, participate and access to learning materials anytime, anywhere [3]. This is possible because of the interconnectivity between web technology and the portability and integration of these devices, offering a high degree of communication and cooperation between their users [4]. Adapting the e-learning systems and stretching for the mobile applications permit users to access learning content and functions using mobile devices [5]. The main objective of this article is to propose a software architecture that aims to adapt the features of the learning management system and its extension to the mobile scenario. For this study, we first tried to analyze the evolution of certain learning standards and enumerate the contributions related to the interoperability of LMS with mobile applications based on the SOA architecture and define the limits of these

© Springer Nature Switzerland AG 2019
M. Ezziyani (Ed.): AI2SD 2018, AISC 915, pp. 719–726, 2019.
https://doi.org/10.1007/978-3-030-11928-7_65

initiatives in Sect. 1 after, presenting in Sect. 2, an overview of the interoperability architecture that we proposed. This architecture is being implemented for the most used open source LMS software Moodle.

2 The Learning Standards for Interoperability and SOA Works

The standards of content and online learning structure are established to ensure the interoperability of e-learning systems so that access to sources of information such as reuse of content or discrimination of subjects from different sources at different times is possible [6]. Standards such ADL SCORM [7] have been widely implemented and adopted, so that standards have been implemented to provide data models and communication protocols conforming to have an interoperable content between e-learning systems [8]. One of the great challenges of e-learning systems is the exchange of data between different systems. In addition, learning interoperability is not just about content thus, the interoperability goals we are looking for are not only related to the interoperability of the content, but to a wider range of features and services that learning applications can provide. For the above reasons, the service orientation approach is used to address the problem of interoperability between different e-learning systems.

2.1 The E-learning Standards for Interoperability

The need for standardization to achieve better interoperability between e-learning systems is widely discussed [9, 10]. Different standards have been proposed to put the learning content in a machine-readable form, as well as creating a unified way for e-learning systems to communicate with each other.

a. SCORM Standard

In its development, the SCORM standard [7] is characterized by the use of XML technology, to define the structure of the course in its first versions as well as the use of metadata to determine the details of the content, while the SCORM specification 2004 and in particular, brought two more important aspects to avoid any ambiguity in later versions; Navigation and sequencing to verify compliance and interoperability in learning environments [10]. The evolution of SCORM has been extremely positive and does not end in the 2004 version [10], but it lacks good practices in terms of the means and mechanisms for exploiting tracing data and tracking learning experiences and does not support the features and services that learners can take their courses in mobile applications. All of these issues discussed above are not available in this interoperability standard. The requirements listed above are presented as new features and capabilities in a new specification that has been co-developed by two organizations ADL and AICC, while defining the components necessary for the interoperability of the system, such as packaging, launching, accreditations and the information model.

b. New Generation of SCORM: xAPI and CMI5

In 2013, the third version of Tin Can API formalized under the name Experience API or xAPI is part of the Training Learning Architecture (TLA) [10, 11]. This is a Representational State Transfer (REST) Web service based on JavaScript Object Notation (JSON) for its data format. xAPI is a specification that has produced an application program interface (API), that captures learning data in the stream and stores it in a repository as "instruction" objects using the following structure (Fig. 1).

xAPI is selected from the reviewed and compared specifications xAPI, ActivityStrea.ms [12], IMS[1] Caliper [13], CAM[2] (which is an early approach to capturing and storing attention metadata for single users), NSDL paradata[3] (defined to capture aggregated usage data about a resource which is designated by audience, subject or education level) and Organic.Edunet format [14] (to store social data provision activities and designed in an extendable way, so other user activities) for communication between heterogeneous learning environments in a major contribution that was published [15].

CMI-5 (Computer-Managed Instruction) [10] is a set of rules with the use of xAPI protocol (or profile xapi) which is intended for scenarios launch contained within a learning management system. It is indispensable to know that xAPI as it is does not replace SCORM, because it is only responsible to match the learning experience with an LRS to LMS. In addition, the set of rules includes some verbs: Launched, Initialized, Completed, Passed, failed, Abandoned, and Terminated. They are used to match the learning content (AU) with an LMS, and correlate its data with the LRS, which is considered as a communication path between LMS and the AU[4] (Fig. 2).

The use of xAPI by CMI-5 permit the development of interoperability capabilities far than this the traditional and non-traditional LMS paradigm [16]. Table 1 shows a general comparison of SCORM and CMI-5 characteristics [17].

Some E-learning application suppliers have already incorporated CMI-5 support into their products: Trivantis,[5] Zavango Corp.,[6] iSpring Solutions,[7] Rustici Software [8] and other brands more and less known and one of our main challenges is to integrate xAPI and CMI-5 learning standards features for interoperability in order to adapt the content of an LMS like Moodle to the specific characteristics of the mobile device.

2.2 The SOA Works for Interoperability

Learning standards [18] have been implemented to create, share and use educational content, with the exploitation of technological progress in learning has led to advanced

---

[1] IMS Global Learning Consortium.
[2] Contextualized Attention Metadata.
[3] National Science Digital Library Paradata.
[4] Assignable Unit (Data).
[5] https://www.trivantis.com/.
[6] https://www.zavango.com/.
[7] https://www.ispringsolutions.com/.
[8] https://rusticisoftware.com/.

```
{
  "actor": {
    "name": "Sally",
    "mbox": "mailto:sally@example.com"
  },
  "verb": {
    "id": "http://adlnet.gov/expapi/verbs/completed",
    "display": { "en-US": "completed" }
  },
  "object": {
    "id": "http://example.com/activities/solo-hang-gliding",
    "definition": {
      "type": "http://adlnet.gov/expapi/activities/assessment",
      "name": { "en-US": "Solo Hang Gliding" },
      "extensions": {
        "http://example.com/gliderClubId": "test-435"
      }
    }
  },
  "result": {
    "completion": true,
    "success": true,
    "extensions": {
      "http://example.com/flight/averagePitch": 0.05
    }
  },
  "context": {
    "extensions": {
      "http://example.com/weatherConditions": "rainy"
    }
  }
}
```

Fig. 1. Representation JSON of a xAPI statement

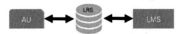

Fig. 2. CMI-5 communication paths

Table 1. Comparative table

Characteristics	E-learning standards		
	SCORM	Tin Can (xAPI)	CMI-5
LMS-to-AU-communication	+	−	+
Operation based on rules	+	−	+
Easy implementation	−	±	+
Course sequencing	+	+	+
Enhanced tracking options	−	+	+
Multi-score report	−	+	+
Online and offline availability	−	+	+
Distributed content and full interoperability	−	±	+
Compatibility of mobile devices	−	+	+

growth in this area through e-learning applications over the last decade and currently by the appearance of a new concept called Mobile Learning. For the above reasons, new technologies that do not focus only on learning content such as Service Oriented Architecture SOA, which is a software architecture, defines the use of services to support the needs of software users [19]. A service is defined as a software component that performs a specific function, which is exposed by a service provider and available to users or the system for consumption in order to achieve the desired results [20, 21].

There have been several contributions that could be considered for the integration of SOA services for LMS and their extension to mobile applications, such as:

- A study on the use of LMS with a mobile application [22].
- Designing a new MRLA Application Architecture optimized for M-learning [23].
- Integrating mobile educational apps with a LMS Moodle via web services [24].
- A Service-Oriented Reference Architecture for Mobile Learning Environments [25].

In all cases, these scientific contributions are limited by the following problems:

- A field of application defined: All the services of online learning systems are not supplied, only those that are useful in a field of application defined.
- Single-way interoperability: Architectures only work in one direction, that is, provide information from the e-learning system or integrate it with other tools. But it is not possible to supply this information and to integrate the tools into the e-learning system in a transparent way for the users.
- Specifications of Interoperability Standard: Designate a service structure that does not use the specifications for interoperability. Especially which does not include the specification that support the features and services related to using mobile apps.

In any case, what is planned with this approach is to solve these problems by defining a responsive and flexible architecture, open and bidirectional.

3 A Web Service Architecture for Interoperability of LMS and Mobile Applications

This approach consists of four parts:

- **Smart Mobile Device**: a mobile device (learner) that has access to the Internet to be able to consume web services.
- **Middleware**: A Web application that contains the RESTful API Web Services.
- **LMS**: it represents the learning management system with their modules, plugins, software components and database.
- **LRS**: it represents the data warehouse experience and learning activities between customers and suppliers of activities.
- **CDN**: Content delivery network in which learning resources and assignable units (learning content) reside.

In this article, we have proposed a software architecture that focuses on integrating external educational applications (mobile or not) with existing LMSs and taking advantage of LMS resources and activities through their extensions to mobile client devices (Fig. 3-A). As shown (Fig. 3-B), a web service layer (ws) is implemented and used by external applications and is represented by the LRS system which acts as a Restful services middleware between the external applications and the functionalities of the xAPI standard. Data and learning activities are delivered to external applications via LRS.

On the one hand, the proposed architecture takes advantage of web technologies and integrates learning standards functionality for interoperability such as xAPI and

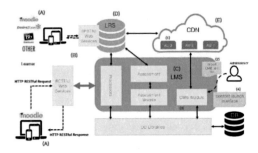

Fig. 3. SOA architecture for interoperability of LMS and mobile applications

CMI5. They are used as basic standard communication mechanisms, in order to adapt the content of the LMS to the specific characteristics of the mobile device. The course content must conform to CMI-5 in the form of one or more assignable units AU (Fig. 3-1) that can be stored anywhere in the Distributed Content Network CDN that is, these AUs do not need to reside all the content in the LMS; only the course structure which has to be imported and saved as an XML file named "cmi5.xml" (Fig. 3-2). The CMI-5 module (Fig. 3-3) is responsible for writing the appropriate data to the LRS and launching (launching mechanism) the AUs by the administrator (LMS) via a launch interface (Fig. 3-4) with the necessary parameters based on the import file "cmi5.xml". Moreover, this set of web services is used to extend the LMS system to develop an advanced mobile application (offline mobile client) that accesses LMS resources and activities, to overcome the limitations of traditional mobile browsers.

The proposed structure is characterized by significant advantages such as:

- LMS personalization would be kept to a minimum so a web service software layer was defined by a set of necessary service to provide easy access to the contents and activities of all LMS.
- The learning content would not need to be located in the e-learning system, each unit of this content could have its own launching mechanism through an interface.
- The LRS, which is an element also for storing special data, which represents to query the results of the data when its consumption is required by another assignable unit or an e-learning system.
- The ability to work offline on the mobile client application via any type of mobile device (tablet, smartphone …).
- The interoperability of learning content compatible with the CMI-5 standard and its integration into the LMS which must comply with CMI-5, would guarantee compared to only use the protocol xAPI or a custom content solution devoid of any rules as well as to solve the problem of interoperability with mobile devices.

4 Conclusion

According to this article, content standards are established to ensure the interoperability of learning systems and in particular, most standards have an important perspective such as xAPI and CMI5 to improve the level of interoperability and reuse of online learning content thus to deal with the problem of interoperability between different e-learning systems, we have analyzed contributions that have considered for the integration of SOA services for LMS and their extension to mobile applications. For the reasons mentioned previously, this article aimed at designing a software architecture with LMS that focuses on integrating mobile applications to improve interoperability with open source systems like Moodle. We have seen that this architecture will always be in development and in perspective. In the future, more research is needed on the implementation of this architecture for open source environments by integrating other new technologies (Big Data and BI) which help teachers and administrators to perform statistics and reports from non-SQL data and also integrate objects smaller than the mobile (Internet of Things IoT).

References

1. Basaeed, E., Berri, J., Zemerly, J., Benlamri, R.: Webbased context-aware m-learning architecture. Int. J. Interact. Mob. Technol. (iJIM) **1**(1), 5–10 (2007)
2. Martin, S., Peire, J., Castro, M.: M2Learn: towards a homogeneous vision of advanced mobile learning development. In: Education Engineering (EDUCON), pp. 569–574, IEEE (2010)
3. Jones, A.C., Scanlon, E., Clough, G.: Mobile learning: two case studies of supporting inquiry learning in informal and semiformal settings. Comput. Educ. **61**, 21–32 (2013)
4. Ozdamli, F., Cavus, N.: Basic elements and characteristics of mobile learning. Proc. Soc. Behav. Sci. **28**, 937–942 (2011)
5. García-Peñalvo, F.J., Conde, M.Á.: The impact of a mobile personal learning environment in different educational contexts. Univ. Access Inf. Soc. **14**, 375–387 (2015)
6. Fallon, C., Brown, S.: E-learning Standards: A Guide to Purchasing, Developing, and Deploying Standards-Conformant E-learning. CRC Press (2016)
7. Advanced Distributed Learning (ADL) Initiative, http://www.adlnet.gov/, last accessed 08 June 2018
8. Del Blanco, Á., Serrano, Á., Freire, M., Martínez-Ortiz, I., Fernández-Manjón, B.: E-learning standards and learning analytics. Can data collection be improved by using standard data models? In: Global Engineering Education Conference (EDUCON), pp. 1255–1261, IEEE (2013)
9. Karavirta, V., Ihantola, P., Koskinen, T.: Service-oriented approach to improve interoperability of e-learning systems. In: IEEE 13th International Conference on Advanced Learning Technologies (ICALT), pp. 341–345 (2013)
10. Bakhouyi, A., Dehbi, R., Lti, M.T., Hajoui, O.: Evolution of standardization and interoperability on E-learning systems: an overview. In: 16th International Conference on Information Technology Based Higher Education and Training (ITHET), pp. 1–8 (2017)
11. Total Learning Architecture—ADL Net, https://www.adlnet.gov/tla/, last accessed 21 May 2018

12. Vozniuk, A., Govaerts, S., Gillet, D.: Towards portable learning analytics dashboards. In: IEEE 13th International Conference on Advanced Learning Technologies (ICALT), pp. 412–416 (2013)
13. Sakurai, Y.: The value improvement in education service by grasping the value acceptance state with ICT utilized education environment. In: International Conference on Human Interface and the Management of Information, pp. 90–98, Springer, Cham (2014)
14. Niemann, K., Wolpers, M., Stoitsis, G., Chinis, G., Manouselis, N.: Aggregating social and usage datasets for learning analytics: data-oriented challenges. In: Proceedings of the Third International Conference on Learning Analytics and Knowledge, pp. 245–249 (2013)
15. Santos, J.L., Verbert, K., Klerkx, J., Duval, E., Charleer, S., Ternier, S.: Tracking data in open learning environments. J. Univ. Comput. Sci. **21**(7), 976–996 (2015)
16. The CMI5 Project Homepage, https://aicc.github.io/CMI-5_Spec_Current/, last accessed 02 Mar 2018
17. cmi5 vs SCORM Comparison Document AICC/CMI-5_Spec_Current Wiki GitHub, https://github.com/AICC/CMI-5_Spec_Current/, last accessed 01 Feb 2018
18. Bakhouyi, A., Dehbi, R., Talea, M.: Multiple criteria comparative evaluation on the interoperability of LMS by applying COPRAS method. In: Future Technologies Conference (FTC) pp. 361–366, IEEE (2016)
19. Rosen, M., Lublinsky, B., Smith, K.T., Balcer, M.J.: Applied SOA: service-oriented architecture and design strategies. Wiley (2012)
20. Vasista, T.G.K., AlSudairi, M.A.: Service-oriented architecture (SOA) and semantic web services for web portal integration. In: Advances in Computing and Information Technology, pp. 253–261, Springer, Berlin, Heidelberg (2013)
21. Garriga, M., Rozas, K., Anabalon, D., Flores, A., Cechich, A.: RESTful mobile architecture for social security services: a case study. In: Computing Conference (CLEI) on XLII Latin American, pp. 1–11, IEEE (2016)
22. Hung, P., Lam, J., Wong, C., Chan, T.: A study on using learning management system with mobile app. In: International Symposium on Educational Technology (ISET) , pp. 168–172, IEEE (2015)
23. Wang, N., Chen, X., Song, G., Lan, Q., Parsaei, H.R.: Design of a New Mobile-Optimized Remote Laboratory Application Architecture for M-Learning. In IEEE Trans. Ind. Electron. **64**(3), 2382–2391. IEEE (2017)
24. Casany Guerrero, M. J., Alier Forment, M., Mayol Sarroca, E., Piguillem Poch, J., Galanis, N., García Peñalvo, F.J., Conde González, M.Á.: Extending Moodle services to mobile devices: the Moodbile project. In: UBICOMM 2012: The Sixth International Conference on Mobile Ubiquitous Computing, Systems, Services and Technologies pp. 24–28 (2012)
25. Duarte Filho, N.F., Barbosa, E.F.: A service-oriented reference architecture for mobile learning environments. In: Frontiers in Education Conference (FIE), pp. 1–8, IEEE (2014)

Porosity Estimation in Carbonate Rock Based on Voronoi Diagram and 2D Histogram Segmentation in HSV Color Space

Safa Jida[✉], Brahim Aksasse, and Mohammed Ouanan

M2I Laboratory, ASIA Team, Department of Computer Science,
Faculty of Sciences and Techniques, Moulay Ismail University,
Errachidia, Morocco
s.jida@edu.umi.ac.ma,
{b.aksasse,m.ouanan}@fste.umi.ac.ma

Abstract. In this work, we propose a new segmentation method for color image in HSV color space as it was demonstrated to be a perceptual color space closely associated with the way human eyes perceived colors. Voronoi diagram (VD) are widely used in image processing but it costs an important execution task if applied directly on the image. In this paper, we propose to apply Voronoi diagram on some selected points extracted from an improved 2D histogram in HSV color space. The results are then exploited in porosity estimation in carbonate rocks using thin section image.

Keywords: Segmentation · Color image · HSV color space · 2D histogram · Voronoi diagram · Delaunay triangulation · Convex hull · Knn classification · Porosity · Carbonate rock · Borsotti evaluation · Thin section image

1 Introduction

In image processing, segmentation is a crucial step that can be considered as a factor of success or failure for further treatment. The major challenge in image segmentation is the choice of its criterion that can be either color, texture or shape. The choice is basically based on the nature of the processed image and also on the segmentation's objectives. Color space plays a vital role in image segmentation as it differentiates the color information from space to another. All the set of colors are specified using a 3D coordinate system and a subspace which has all buildable colors with specific models. Commonly, an image is characterized using three components: red, green and blue. But small color differences are quite difficult to comprehend. Different application uses different color space. The most used in color segmentation are RGB, HSV and YIQ [1–3] but it was demonstrated that the HSV is more close to the way human eyes perceive colors [4].

Voronoi diagram is a powerful tool that has, unfortunately, gained less attention especially in image segmentation due to the fact of the high computational time and its complexity. Among the work founded on VD, we can cite [5–10] for face segmentation and detection. To overcome this situation, we proposed to work on improved 2D histograms in HSV color space instead of the image itself to a better vision and

© Springer Nature Switzerland AG 2019
M. Ezziyani (Ed.): AI2SD 2018, AISC 915, pp. 727–735, 2019.
https://doi.org/10.1007/978-3-030-11928-7_66

understanding of the image. Next issue we overcame using this new approach is the high correlation between the R, G and B components [11] due to the fact that the measurement of a color in RGB space does not represent color differences in a uniform scale; Therefore, it is impossible to evaluate the similarity of two colors from their distance in RGB space. However, the color and intensity information are separated in the HSV space which leads to a successful segmentation.

The structure of the paper is as follow: first, we present the improved 2D histogram in HSV space. Next, we give the details about the segmentation method using VD. Finally, the experimental results and discussion.

2 Two-Dimensional Histogram

Despite the construction complexity of two dimensional histograms, the provided informations are priceless and reliable and its presentation is nothing more than a grey level image, thus a whole package of classic image processing techniques can be exploited.

2D histograms are the extension of the concept of image histogram to two channel images. Speaking of image processing, a 2D histogram shows the relationship of intensities at the exact position between two images. For a RGB color image I, a 2D-histogram p_n maps the number of pixels in I image presenting the colorimetric components (x_1, x_2). it can be represented by a J image whose spatial resolution is equal to 256×256. The value $p_n(x_1, x_2)$ of the pixel of coordinates (x_1, x_2) in J is obtained by a linear dynamic contraction of the histogram between 1 and M [12].

$$p_n(x_1, x_2) = round \left[\frac{(M-1)p(x_1, x_2) - Mp_{min} + p_{max}}{p_{max} - p_{min}} \right] \qquad (1)$$

where p_{min} and p_{max} are respectively the minimum and the maximum values of p and $M = min(p_{max}, 255)$.

The HSV is widely different from RGB space because it separates the intensity from the color. Sural et al. [13] proved the existence of a liaison between the three component: hue, saturation and value of HSV space. For a given intensity and hue, if the saturation is altered from 0 to 1, the observed color changes from a shade of grey to the purest form of the color represented by its hue. Thus, any color in HSV space can be immigrated to a shade of grey by decreasing the saturation. To choose the suited saturation threshold, we should take in consideration the intensity since the saturation depends on it. This hypothesis is illustrated by Sural et al. [13] where they confirmed that for a higher saturation values a saturation of 0.2 distinguish between hue and intensity dominance. For a maximum intensity value of 255, the thresholding function to decide if the pixel should be presented either by its intensity or its hue as the assertive attribute is as follow:

$$Ths\,(V) = 1 - \frac{0.8\,V}{255} \qquad (2)$$

By applying the equation, we obtain a feature vector composed of two parts: the hue value between 0 and 2p quantified after a transformation and a quantized set of intensity values. Based on the Eq. (2), we define an intermediate image (Fig. 1a): for lower values of saturation, a color can be approximated by a grey value specified by the intensity level, whereas for higher saturation; the color can be approximated by its hue value.

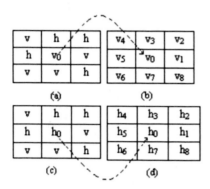

Fig. 1. 3 × 3 block: **a** and **c** intermediate image; **b** and **d** their component in the original image

Afterward, the 2D color histogram for the intermediate image is constructed as follow: for each block of 3x3 pixels of the intermediate image, we consider the central pixel which can be either an intensity or a hue component (Fig. 1a, c) according to the Eq. (2). Then, we calculate the maximum (Max) and the minimum (Min) in its corresponding component (H or V) in the original image (Fig. 1b, d) [14]. Where the Max is the maximum hue or intensity in the 3 × 3 neighbour excluding pixels of the four-neighbour and Min is the minimum hue or intensity in the four-neighbour.

We note that Max = maximum [(v4, v2, v6, v8) or (h4, h2, h6, h8)] and Min = minimum [(v0, v1, v3, v5, v7) or (h0, h1, h3, h5, h7)]. Next, we construct the 2D-histogram by mapping the number of pixels presenting the minimum and the maximum (Min, Max) in all 3 × 3 block of the image according to P_h (Min; Max) and P_v (Min; Max) for central pixel represented by H or V component respectively (Fig. 2).

Once the histogram is built, we proceed to the next step of our segmentation method. As shown in Fig. 3, the obtained histogram is made of dotted points that can form connected blobs. We calculate the convex hull to extract the feature points from which we will build Voronoi diagram.

The convex hull is widely used in computer graphics [15] and image processing [10, 16, 17] and he is one of the first sophisticated geometry algorithms and there are many variations of it. The most common form of this algorithm involves determining the smallest convex set containing a discrete set of points.

Convex hull of a planar point set S is defined as the intersection of all the half-planes containing S. The shape of convex hull is a convex polygon whose vertices belong to S. For an edge pq, all other points lie on one side of the line running through p and q. The most popular hull algorithms are the "Graham scan" algorithm [18] and

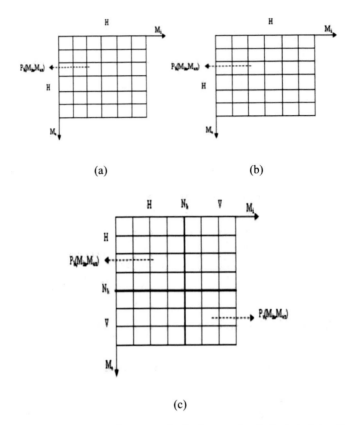

Fig. 2. a, b Histograms representing respectively the associated pixels to intensity values and hue. c 2D histogram

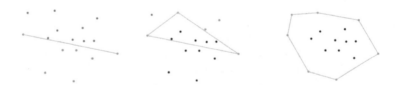

Fig. 3. Quickhull steps illustration (Wikipedia)

the "divide-and-conquer" algorithm [19]. In this work, we have used the *Quickhull* [20], it uses the divide and conquer approach. The algorithm selects the two points x1 and x2 with the smallest and largest x coordinate. These points will be in the convex hull. A line is drawn between x1 and x2 that divides the set into two subsets of points. The algorithms now find the point x3 that is furthest away from the line. A triangle is drawn between x1, x2 and x3 while eliminating points inside the triangle. This procedure is done in each subset recursively until there are no points left.

For its application on the two dimensional histogram mentioned before, we obtain a polygon of point which contains the original image pixel's representation by their hue or value in HSV space. To locate the closest convex hull set, we are going to apply knn classification using the Euclidian distance.

Knn classification is a non-parametric learning algorithm that classifies data sets based on their similarity with neighbours. "K" stands for number of data set items that are considered for the classification. In this paper, we are going to locate the closest convex hull set in HSV color space using the Euclidian distance.

3 Experimental Results

Below, we give the results of the segmentation method mentioned before and compared with other the same method using only 2D histogram in RGB color space [10] (Fig. 4).

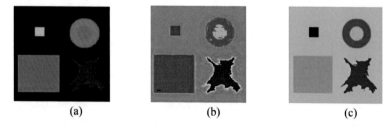

(a)   (b)   (c)

Fig. 4. Segmentation results **a** original image **b** segmented image using 2D histogram in RGB **c** segmented image with the proposed method

We considered this image due to its importance in term of color and shape. The image consists of four pattern with different shape and colors and the circular pattern contains two shapes that alter only by the variation of saturation component which make it more difficult to separate them. Thus, by adding the background, we have six class in total.

It can be seen from experimentation results that the new approach gives better results. The two circular pattern are well separated using the new method, the boundaries are more sharpen and clear while in RGB space, the edge of the non-geometric and the circular pattern are merged with the background giving birth to a new region.

Visually talking, it is difficult to estimate the quality of any segmentation method in the absence of a reference segmentation. But, there ere a few quantitative criteria for comparing segmentation results [21], we propose to use Borsotti, noted Q ([22, 23] [Eq. (3)]), which is especially entrusted for evaluating the quality of color image segmentation [24]. The lower Q it is, the better the segmentation method it is

$$Q(I) = \frac{1}{10,000 \times N} \sqrt{R} \times \sum_{i=1}^{R} \left(\frac{e_i^2}{1 + \log N_i} + \frac{R(N_i)^2}{N_i^2} \right) \qquad (3)$$

where I is the segmented image, N is the image size, N_i is the area of the region R_i in term of pixels, R is the number of the obtained region, $R(N_i)$ is the number of regions having an area equal to N_i and e_i is the average color error of the region. Table 1 summarize the results obtained by applying the Q value on RGB segmentation versus HSV segmentation.

Table 1. Values of evaluation function 'Q' for various images

Method	Pattern image	Rock 1	Rock 2
2D-histogram using RGB space	6728	2873	2198
2D-histogram using HSV space	867	1092	993

4 Application in Porosity Estimation in Carbonate Rock

One of various characteristics to describe rocks in a qualitative manner is porosity measurement as it is considered one of properties with "kill or cure" effectiveness. Diverse porosity estimation methods are known in chemistry field. In this work, we propose an alternative method for estimation 2D porosity from thin section images for carbonate rocks basis of core samples picked out from carbonate reservoir rocks of Tournasian age [25, 26]. Porosity is determined by the ratio of pore area to the total area of the image, i.e. the ratio of the number of pixels corresponding to pores to the total number of pixels after obtaining pore region by applying the proposed VD segmentation technique.

Here after, we present the segmentation results along with the pore region (Fig. 5).

After obtaining the pore regions which correspond to the black pixels [25, 26], we then proceed to estimate the porosity as explained before. Table 2 summarize the results and compare our calculus with the obtained with chemical experiments.

Based on the results shown in the table and the liquid injection's results [27], we can notice a close and satisfying estimation to the experimental results using the new method applied in HSV color space compared to method in RGB color space [10] which can be explained to the high correlation between color components that doesn't allow to treat separately each component.

Regarding the results, porosity depends on many factors such as the type of rocks, porous space and methodical differences. Liquid injection method gives insufficient results in case of connected porosity. While in thin section, the total of 2D porosity is measured in the cavernous and fractured sample. Consequently, a significant excess of 2D evaluation of porosity is expected.

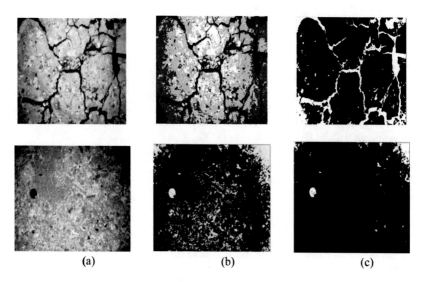

Fig. 5. Segmentation results **a** original image **b** segmented image **c** pore region

Table 2. Values of estimated porosity

Image	Method	
	Segmentation in HSV (%)	Segmentation in RGB (%)
Rock 1	12.97	14.25
Rock 2	6.37	7.86

5 Conclusion

In this paper, we have developed a new approach for color image segmentation based on analyzing two dimensional histograms in HSV space. We applied this technique on synthetic image with different challenges starting from shape to intensity variation. We obtained a satisfying results backed by evaluation using Borsotti value compared with those obtained in RGB space. The method is successfully applied too in porosity estimation for carbonate rock using thins section image and showed a closer and logic results.

References

1. Wang, H., Suter, D.: Color image segmentation using global information and local homogeneity. In: Proceeding of 7th Conference of Digital Image Computing: Techniques and Applications, pp. 10–12 (2003)
2. Mythili, C., Kavitha, V.: Color image segmentation using ERKFCM. Int. J. Comput. Appl. **41**(20), 21–28 (2012)

3. Rathore, V.S., Kumar, M.S., Verma, A.: Colour based image segmentation using L*A*B* colour space based on genetic algorithm. Int. J. Emerg. Technol. Adv. Eng. **2**(6), 156–162 (2012)

4. Cheng, H.D., Jiang, V., Sun, Y., Wang, J.: Color image segmentation: advances and prospects. Pattern Recogn. **34**, 2259–2281 (2001)

5. Dan, D.: Image segmentation using Voronoi diagram. In: Eighth International Conference on Digital Image Processing, International Society for Optics and Photonics, 100331P (2016)

6. Hettiarachchi, R., Peters, J.F.: Voronoi region-based adaptive unsupervised color image segmentation. Pattern Recogn. **65**, 119–135 (2016)

7. Tuceryan, M., Jain, K.: Texture segmentation using Voronoï polygons. IEEE Trans. Pattern Anal. Mach. Intell. **12**(2), 211–216 (1990)

8. Cheddad, A., Dzulkifli, M., Abd Manaf, A.: Exploiting Voronoi diagram properties in face segmentation and feature extraction. Pattern Recogn. **41**(12), 3842–3859 (2008)

9. Jida, S., Aksasse B., Ouanan, M.: Face segmentation and detection using Voronoi diagram and 2D histogram. In: Intelligent System and Computer Vision, pp. 1–5. Fez (2017)

10. Jida, S., Ouanan, M., Aksasse, B.: Color image segmentation using voronoi diagram and 2D histogram. Int. J. Tomogr. Simul. **30**(3), 14–20 (2017)

11. Uchiyama, T., Arbib, M.: Color image segmentation using competitive learning. IEEE Trans. Pattern Anal. Mach. Intell. **16**, 1197–1206 (1994)

12. Clément, A., Vigouroux, B.: Unsupervised segmentation of scenes containing vegetation (Forsythia) and soil by hierarchical analysis bi-dimensional histograms. Pattern Recogn. Lett. **24**, 1951–1957 (2003)

13. Sural, S., Qian, G., Pramanik, S.: Segmentation and histogram generation using the HSV color space for image retrieval. In: Proceeding of International Conference on Image Processing. IEEE, vol. 2, II589–II592 (2002)

14. Zennouhi, R., Masmoudi, L.H.: A new 2D histogram scheme for color image segmentation. Imag. Sci. J. **57**(5), 260–265 (2009)

15. Bhaniramka, P., Wenger, R., Crawfis, R.: Isosurface construction in any dimension using convex hulls. IEEE Trans. Vis. Comput. Graph. **10**(2), 130–141 (2004)

16. Yuan, B., Tan, C.L.: Convex hull based skew estimation. Pattern Recogn. **40**(2), 456–475 (2007)

17. Sirakov, N.M., et al.: Search space partitioning using convex hull and concavity features for fast medical image retrieval. In: Proceeding of the IEEE International Symposium on Biomedical Imaging: Nano to Macro, pp. 796–799 (2004)

18. Graham, R.L.: An efficient algorithm for determine the convex hull of a finite linear set. Inf. Prec. Lett. **1**(1), 132–133 (1972)

19. Preparata, F.P., Hong, S.J.: Convex hulls of finite sets of points in two and three dimensions. CACM **20**(2), 87–93 (1977)

20. Barber, C.B., Dobkin, D.P., Huhdanpaa, H.: The quickhull algorithm for convex hulls. ACM Trans. Math. Softw. **22**(4), 469–483 (1996)

21. Philipp-Foliguet, S.: Evaluation de méthodes de segmentation d'images couleur. In: Actes de l'école de printemps du GDR ISIS Opération Imagerie Couleur (2001)

22. Zhang, H., Fritts, J.E., Goldman, S.A.: Image segmentation evaluation: a survey of unsupervised methods. Comput. Vis. Image Underst. **110**, 260–280 (2008)

23. Borsotti, M., Campadelli, P., Schettini, R.: Quantitative evaluation of color image segmentation results. Pattern Recogn. Lett. **19**, 741–747 (1998)

24. Macaire, L., Vandenbroucke, N., Postaire, J.G.: Color image segmentation by analysis of subset connectedness and color homogeneity properties. Comput. Vis. Image Underst. **102**, 105–116 (2006)

25. Nurgalieva, N.D., Nurgalieva, N.G.: New digital methods of estimation of porosity of carbonate rocks. Indian J. Sci. Technol. **9**(20) (2016)
26. Nurgalieva, N.D., Nurgalieva, N.G.: Cluster image processing technique for porosity estimation of carbonate rocks. ARPN JEAS **10**(4), 1668–1671 (2015)
27. Nurgalieva, N.G.: Microfacies, petrophysics and sequence-stratigraphic frame of carbonate reservoir rocks of Kizelovskian formation. J. Oil Ind. **3**, 38–40 (2015)

An Extended Data as a Service Description Model for Ensuring Cloud Platform Portability

Abdelhak Merizig[1](✉), Hamza Saouli[1], Maite Lopez Sanchez[2],
Okba Kazar[1], and Aïcha-Nabila Benharkat[3]

[1] LINFI Laboratory, Computer Science Department, University of Biskra,
Biskra, Algeria
merizig.abdelhak@gmail.com, {Hamza_saouli,okbakazar}
@yahoo.fr
[2] Mathematics and Computer Science Department, University of Barcelona,
Barcelona, Spain
maite_lopez@ub.edu
[3] LIRIS Laboratory, INSA Lyon, University of Lyon, Lyon, France
nabila.benharkat@insa-lyon.fr

Abstract. Nowadays there is a myriad of different Cloud services deployed in datacenters around the world. These services are presented by means of models offered as services on demand (SaaS, PaaS and IaaS). At a different level, the companies aim at finding some services that manage their data in order to enhance their process and increase their benefits. The massive quantity of data and the heterogeneous types of data deployed in the Cloud made the discovery task much important. In addition, one big problem in discovery task is the absence of a description model to represent data services (Data as a service; DaaS). Moreover, the location of services made the selection and composition process much very hard, especially for functional and non-functional parameters. In this paper, we plan to solve these problems by introducing an extended description model for data services, in order to reduce the number of services during the selection and composition process. The implementation shows the effectiveness of the proposed model.

Keywords: Data as a service · Service model · Service discovery · Extensible language · Cloud computing · QoS · XML

1 Introduction

Recently Cloud computing emerged as a new paradigm that offers solutions presented across the virtualization [1], also, it represents the fifth commodity after water, electricity, gas, and phone bills [2]. In addition, it emerged as a service on demand presented in different service delivery models [3]. These models represented now in everything as a service (XaaS) [4], which gives to different end user any type of services on demand under the basis of payment pay as you go [5]. The growing number of societies and companies right now present a challenge to these companies in terms

© Springer Nature Switzerland AG 2019
M. Ezziyyani (Ed.): AI2SD 2018, AISC 915, pp. 736–744, 2019.
https://doi.org/10.1007/978-3-030-11928-7_67

of offers and services. Cloud service discovery selection and composition are the most important tasks that allow us to manipulate and control Internet services [6]. These issues depend on the massive number of services deployed in the Cloud and the absence of a standard description model to represent services [7]. Moreover, it is a difficult task for a user to rank the best cloud services from thousands of selected services [8]. Since the emergence of the Internet, data represent the kernel of any operation. These last year cloud service providers' interest on providing data on demand under the model titled data as a service (DaaS). Moreover, data services are involved in many services especially in the big companies. Since the service data was founded, it has many characteristics. In addition, the way of describing data in the cloud by service providers without using the predefined model to present their services lead to a problem when selecting services. To select a data service it is a hard task due to the data's nature. In addition, companies look for a manner to compose data services together to enhance their results. As we know the data are presented as heterogeneous entities, to handle all majority of existing information in different types (relational, social networks, live analysis, CRM systems, HR & ERP) [9]. To satisfy the client's demands we need a description model for data service. To solve all these mentioned problems this paper present an extended model to describe data service.

The reminder of this paper is structured as follows: Sect. 2 surveys some related works. Section 3 presents our extended data service description model. Section 4 gives an implementation of the proposed model. Section 5 provides the conclusion of this paper with some perspectives.

2 Related Works

There are several works created to resolve the problem of data services discovery and composition using different approaches. In this section, we present some works corresponding to this issue.

The works of Tbahriti et al. presented in [10, 11] the authors present a privacy model based in order to introduce data services description. The proposed model is given as a formalism which gives us the possibility to determine a new and efficient privacy policy. In addition, the privacy model is indented to match privacy constraints with DaaS description. However, this work focus is limited to privacy characteristics.

Rajesh et al. [12] present the importance of data in cloud computing. In addition, this work gives a study on the concept of data as a service, which represents the challenges and the benefits. However, this work does not give any details about the data services description.

In [13] the authors proposed a framework that allows data from different sources to be integrated with the semantic data. Moreover, this work tries to solve interoperability issues and proposes an access control system in order to define an explicit privacy constraint. However, the authors do not present a full description of data services.

In [14] the authors extend semantically the WSDL description files in order to facilitate annotation and selection. In [15] the authors extended the QoS representation in order to integrate it in ERP selection combined with a multi-criteria decision making system [16]. However, industrial and data cloud sides are completely ignored with these methods.

In both [17, 18] the authors deployed a new P2P method for cloud service selection. Although, [17] ignored the non-functional side of cloud services, and [18] did not provide any implementation or testing.

3   Data Service Description Model

This section introduces the proposed description model for data services. The DaaS services have common characteristics as in SaaS services. In addition, DaaS services extended from the basic cloud computing models (SaaS, PaaS, and IaaS). Therefore, these services proposed under the payment basis pay as you go [5]. This model is proposed specially to big society that needs different data services. The provided description model presented in this paper is collected from the literature based on the SaaS description presented in [19]. Thus the characteristics collected from [20–23]. The next table gives a description of this model (DaaS).

Table 1. Summary of data part characteristics

Category	Characteristic	Description/value
Numerical values	Clients' number	Integer
	Brand value of vendor	Float
	Versioning	Converted to integer
	Experience	Integer
	Engineers' Skill levels	Integer
Textual values	Contributor	The name of the organization that contributes to the development of new versions of the target DaaS
	Creator	The name of the organization that creates the target DaaS
	Owner	The name of the organization that possess the target DaaS
	Publisher	The target DaaS organization name
	Location	The country name where DaaS is deployed
	Identifier	The unique identifier of DaaS
	Language support	It's the list of the languages supported by the target DaaS
	Standard adhered	Underlying technologies used to creat DaaS (e.g. WSDL, OVF, TOSCA… etc.)
	Certification	The name(s) of the certificate(s) earned by the target DaaS, to proove the required skills levels

(continued)

Table 1. (*continued*)

Category	Characteristic	Description/value
Pre-determined values	Payment system	(i) Free (ii) dynamic (iii) pay per use
	Cloud deployment	(i) Private (ii) public (iii) hybrid (iv) community
	Cloud openness	(i) Unknown_Limited (ii) basic (iii) moderate (iv) complete
	Standardization	(i) No (ii) public API (iii) part (standard, organization)
	Formal Agreement	(i) No SLA (ii) SLA (service level agreement)
	Licence type	(i) Open source (ii) propriety
	Integration	(i) Yes (ii) no
	Support for mobile devices	(i) Yes (ii) no
	Offline support	(i) Yes (ii) no
	External security	(i) None (ii) SSL (iii) PKI (iv) VPNs
	Accessibility to data	(i) Read only (ii) CRUD
	Type of data	(i) Structured (ii) unstructured (iii) semi-structured
	Pricing model	(i) Quantity based pricing (ii) pay per call (iii) data type based model
	Supported semantic model	(i) OWL-S (ii) WSMO (iii) SAWSDL (iv) RDF
	Representation model	(i) Relational (ii) XML (iii) object (iv) parallel (v) network (vi) non structural
	Operation type	(i) Based on request (ii) Based on function

As we have seen in the previous Table 1, we used the categorization mentioned in [19], which classifies the characteristics in three main categories: the category of numerical values, the category of textual values and category of pre-determined values. In order to describe the data services, all the data services description are represented as WSDL files. Figure 1 represented an XML representation of the proposed model.

```
<?xml version="1.0" encoding="UTF-8" ?>

<Categories>
  <NumericalValues>
    <ClientsNumber Type = " Integer " > 10000 </ClientsNumber>
    <Versioning> 1.1 </Versioning >
    < Experience Type = "Integer"> 20 </ Experience >
    .......
  </NumericalValues>
  < TextualValues Type = " String " >
    < Contributor > IBM </Contributor>
    <Creator> BSA Development </Creator >
    < Location > Oran </ Location >
    < StandardAdhered Description = "WSDL"/>
    < StandardAdhered StorageFormat = "OVC"/>
    < StandardAdhered CloudService = " TOSCA"/>
    .......
  < TextualValues Type>
   </ PreDeterminedValues >
    < PaymentSystem > Dynamic</ PaymentSystem >
    <CloudDeployment> Public </CloudDeployment >
    < CloudOpenness > Basic </ CloudOpenness >
    < FormalAgreement > SLA</ FormalAgreement >
    < DataType> Semi Structured </ DataType >
    <PricingModel> Quantity pricing </PricingModel >
    .......
  </PreDeterminedValues>
</ Categories >
```

Fig. 1. Extensible Cloud data platform language

4   Implementation and Results

This section shows the used method and equations that help to implement the proposed model. First, we will introduce some tools used to implement the model. Then we will give an implementation that shows some results with a discussion.

4.1   Used Equations

In this work, we present each service by a vector each element of these vectors defined by a couple of the term value and the weights of the data services characteristics that mentioned in Table 1. To calculate the weight of each characteristic we used tf-idf formulation (term frequency –inverse document frequency) [24] given as follows in Eq. 1.

$$W(\text{term}) = \text{tf} - \text{idf}(\text{term}) = \text{tf}(\text{term}) * \log_2(N/\text{df}(\text{term})) \tag{1}$$

where W is the term weight, tf is the term frequency defined the number of occurrences of the term in the document (WSDL), N is the number of documents in the collection, and df is the document frequency which gives the number of times that the term appears in the other documents in the collection. After the client introduces his request, we will transform his request into a vector of weight using Eq. 1. Then we will use the similarity function to select the appropriate service among the rest [25]. In this work, we used the similarity function presented in Eq. 2.

$$Sim(r,d) = \frac{\vec{r} \cdot \vec{d}}{|\vec{r}| \times |\vec{d}|} = \frac{\sum_{i=1}^{N} r_i \times d_i}{\sqrt{\sum_{i=1}^{N} r_i^2} \times \sqrt{\sum_{i=1}^{N} d_i^2}} \tag{2}$$

where $|\vec{r}|$ and $|\vec{d}|$ are norms of the request and the document vectors, N number of terms in the vectors. Since $r_i \geq 0$ and $d_i \geq 0$, sim(r, d) varies from 0 to +1 and shows the degree of similarity between a request r and a document d.

4.2 Results and Discussion

In our experiment, we used CloudSim simulator to calculate the time response for a growth number of clients' requests. This simulator is composed of a user interface that allows us to introduce the necessary parameters to determine the chosen task distribution policies with a combination between the core virtual machine management system and the number of clients' requests that a data centre can process at the same time [26, 27]. Figure 2 shows the response time of the used model given for a number of clients (requests number).

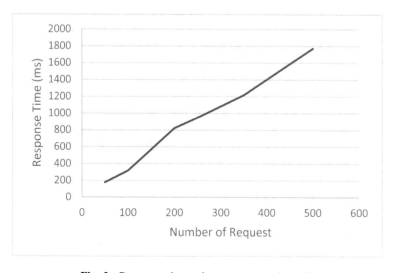

Fig. 2. Response time using our proposed model

As we see in the previous figure that shows response time to a given number of clients (depicted in the number of requests axis) using our model. From Fig. 1, we can observe the obtained data are given to clients in a reasonable time. In the present graph, we can saw there is variation in response time values at 100, 200 and 350 (number of requests). The changes in the graph it depends on a number of selected services for each request (e.g. request number 1 have a match with 10 data services, the second request have a match with five data services).

Table 2 shows a comparison between the main cloud description models and the proposed Extensible Cloud data platform language.

Table 2. Comparison study

Attributes models	Industrial parameters	Economic parameters	Data parameters	QoS parameters
Chen et al. [14]	Ignored	Uninsured	Ignored	Insured
Park and Jeong [15]	Ignored	Uninsured	Ignored	Insured
Hussain and Hussain [16]	Insured	Insured	Uninsured	Ignored
Proposed model	Insured	Insured	Insured	Insured

Finally, the comparison between the proposed description models and its previous peers shows that it is more efficient on covering all the cloud, functional and non-functional parameters with a possible implementation with an XML extensible language to ensure an effective service selection and discovery.

5   Conclusion

Service composition, selection and discovery are the most important challenges due to the massive number of services. In addition, the absence of service description makes this issue more difficult. To solve the mentioned problems we presented in this paper a description of data services in the cloud, that take into consideration, industrial, economic, and especially data sides (that can be sold as geographic or meteorological information for example, offered as a service through cloud datacenters). As we mentioned the presented model is extended from some works in the literature.

In the future, we aim to add other characteristics in order to improve the search task for the discovery/selection process of and composition. As we mentioned earlier to describe a data services we need to provide description language of cloud service cloud. Moreover, we will extend a short description for data services using WSDL. In addition, to limit the number of discovered services we also plan to focus on data quality. We plan also to use the proposed model to solve the problem of service composition in the cloud.

References

1. Androcec. D., Vrcek. N., Seva. J.: Cloud computing ontologies: a systematic review. In: Proceedings of the 3rd International Conference on Models and Ontology based Design of Protocols, Architectures and Services, Chamonix/Mont Blanc, France, pp. 9–14 (2012)
2. Wang, L., Ranjan, R., Chen, J., Benatallah, B.: Cloud Computing: Methodology, Systems, and Applications, p. 3. CRC Press, Boca Raton (2011)
3. Yorozu, Y., Hirano, M., Oka, K., Tagawa, Y.: Effective use of cloud computing in education: education as a service. Int. J. Commun. Networks Distrib. Syst. **11**(3), 297–309 (2013)
4. Xu, X.: From cloud computing to cloud manufacturing. Robot. Comput. Integr. Manuf. **28**(1), 75–86 (2012)
5. Kar, A.K., Rakshit, A.: Pricing of cloud IaaS based on feature prioritization—a value based approach. In: Recent Advances in Intelligent Informatics, pp. 321–330. Springer International Publishing, Berlin (2014)
6. Jula, A., Sundararajan, E., Othman, Z.: Cloud computing service composition: a systematic literature review. Expert Syst. Appl. **41**(8), 3809–3824 (2014)
7. Zhang, M., Ranjan, R., Hallerl, A., Georgakopoulos, D., Menzel, M., Nepal, S.: An ontology-based system for cloud infrastructure services, discovery. In: Proceedings of the 8th International Conference on Collaborative Computing: Networking, Applications and Worksharing (Collaboratecom), pp. 524–530 (2012)
8. Tahamtan, A., Beheshti, S.A., Anjomshoaa, A., Tjoa, A.M.: A cloud repository and discovery framework based on a unified business and Cloud service ontology. In: Proceedings of the Eighth World Congress on Services, pp. 203–210. IEEE (2012)
9. Glay, E., Sauceda, M.J.: Post-implementation practices of ERP systems and their relationship to financial performance. Inf. Manage. **51**(3), 310–319 (2014)
10. Tbahriti, S.E., Mrissa, M., Medjahed, B., Ghedira, C., Barhamg, M., Fayn, J.: Privacy-aware DaaS services composition. In: International Conference on Database and Expert Systems Applications, pp. 202–216. Springer, Berlin (2011)
11. Tbahriti, S.E., Ghedira, C., Medjahed, B., Mrissa, M., Benslimane, D.: How to Enhance privacy within DaaS service composition? IEEE Syst. J. **7**(3), 442–454 (2013)
12. Rajesh, S., Swapna, S., Shylender Reddy, P.: Data as a service (Daas) in cloud computing [data-as-a-service in the age of data]. Glob. J. Comput. Sci. Technol. Cloud Distrib. **12**(11), 25–29 (2012)
13. Terzo, O., Ruiu, P., Bucci, E., Xhafa, F.: Data as a service (DaaS) for sharing and processing of large data collections in the cloud. In: IEEE Seventh International Conference on Complex, Intelligent, and Software Intensive Systems, pp. 475–480 (2013)
14. Chen, F., Bai, X., Liu, B.: Efficient service discovery for Cloud computing environments. In: Proceedings of Advanced Research on Computer Science and Information Engineering, pp. 443–448 (2011)
15. Park, J., Jeong, H.-Y.: The QoS-based MCDM system for SaaS ERP applications with social network. J. Supercomput. **66**(2), 614–632 (2013)
16. Hussain, O.K., Hussain, F.K.: IaaS Cloud selection using MCDM methods. In: Proceedings of IEEE Ninth International Conference on e-Business Engineering (ICEBE), pp. 246–251 (2012)
17. Zhou, J., Abdullah, N., Shi, Z.: A hybrid P2P approach to service discovery in the Cloud. Int. J. Inf. Technol. Comput. Sci. **3**(1), 1–9 (2011)

18. Lin, W., Dou, W., Xu, Z., Chen, J.: A QoS-aware service discovery method for elastic cloud computing in an unstructured peer-to-peer network. Concurr. Comput. Practice Exp. **25**(13), 1843–1860 (2013)
19. Saouli, H., Kazar, O., Benharkat, A.N.: SaaS-DCS: software-as-a-service discovery and composition system-based existence degree. Int. J. Commun. Networks Distrib. Syst. **14**(4) (2015)
20. Vu, Q.H., Pham, T.V., Truong, H.L., Dustdar, S., Asal, R.: Demods: a description model for data-as-a-service. In: IEEE 26th International Conference on Advanced Information Networking and Applications, pp. 605–612 (2012)
21. Zehoo, E., Hong. Y.W.: Pro ODP. NET for Oracle Database 11g. Apress, p. 20 (2010)
22. Rankins, R., Bertucci, P., Gallelli, C., Silverstein, A.T., Cotter, H.: Microsoft SQL Server 2012 Unleashed. Pearson Education, London (2012)
23. Truong, H.L., Dustar, S.: On analyzing and specifying concerns for data as a service. In: Proceedings of the 2009 IEEE Asia-Pacific Services Computing Conference (APSCC) (2009)
24. Safeer, Y., Mustafa, A., Ali, A.N.: Clustering unstructured data (flat files) an implementation in text mining tool. Int. J. Comput. Sci. Inf. Secur. (IJCSIS) **8**(2) (2010)
25. Özel, S.A.: A Web page classification system based on a genetic algorithm using tagged-terms as features. Expert Syst. Appl. **38**, 3407–3415 (2011)
26. Long, W., Yuqing, L., Qingxin. X.: Using cloudsim to model and simulate cloud computing environment. In: IEEE 9th International Conference on Computational Intelligence and Security (CIS), pp. 323–328 (2013)
27. Merizig, A., Kazar, O., Lopez-Sanchez, M.: A dynamic and adaptable service composition architecture in the cloud based on a multi-agent system. Int. J. Inf. Technol. Web. Eng. **13**(1), 50–68 (2018)

Security Analysis in the Internet of Things: State of the Art, Challenges, and Future Research Topics

Karim Ennasraoui[1]([⊠]), Youssef Baddi[2],
Younes El Bouzekri El Idrissi[1], and El Mehdi Baa[1]

[1] Systems Engineering Laboratory, National School of Applied Sciences
of Kenitra (ENSAK), Ibn Tofail, Kenitra, Morocco
karim.ennasraoui@gmail.com, y.elbouzekri@gmail.com,
aba.elmehdi@gmail.com
[2] STIC Laboratory, ESTSB School, Chouaib Doukkali University,
El Jadida, Morocco
baddi.y@ucd.ac.ma

Abstract. Internet of Things is a big new technology that will make new future concepts and technologies. The work of this paper is to a brief survey security analysis in the internet of things. We provide an overview and discuss a qualitative way the recent development of the most relevant security field in the context of the internet of things (IoT). It outlines the key characteristics of the security analysis and summarizes various representative studies for IoT, including Blockchain. An important focus is the inclusion of how value is extracted from the security in the IoT. We also discusses some recent techniques for the existing activities and future opportunities related to the security in the internet of thing, outlining some of the key underlying issues that need to be tackled.

Keywords: Internet of things · Security · Blockchain · Privacy · Trust

1 Introduction

The Internet of things (IoT) was a fixture in the news last year, has recently become an important research topic because it integrates various sensors and objects to communicate directly with one another without human intervention at many level. It touches everything not just the data, but how, when, where and why you collect it. The IoT incorporates everything from a minuscule to big machines, appliances to building, body sensors to cloud computing which includes major types of networks, for instance, building, smart home, grid, healthcare, and vehicular networks. The security of the Internet of Things is a constant topic of discussion, with the focus typically on the devices it connects. However, the IoT also intersects with the worlds of law enforcement and public safety, and that connection has been growing in recent years.

Unlike much more other networking systems of what we talk about with the IoT, the Human-as-a-Sensor (HaaS) paradigm is one typically subject worth focusing on, its based on people users rather than automated sensor systems, detecting and reporting

© Springer Nature Switzerland AG 2019
M. Ezziyyani (Ed.): AI2SD 2018, AISC 915, pp. 745–752, 2019.
https://doi.org/10.1007/978-3-030-11928-7_68

events or incidents they witness through mobile apps. Law enforcement is then able to aggregate this data in order to build a better sense of the emergencies at hand, and which ones to respond to first [1].

The goal of this paper is to review the background and state-of-the art of security of the Internet of Things to provide an overview of the related work in IoT, together with the open challenges and future research directions.

2 Internet of Things Security Background and Terminologies (Fundamental Concept)

The security of the Internet of Things is a constant topic of discussion, with the focus typically on the devices it connects. However, the IoT also intersects with the worlds of law enforcement and public safety, and that connection has been growing in recent years. With the expansion of the IoT market, new issues are raised, in term of security and privacy, caused by its specific characteristics. We propose the following services [2, 3] to make sure that any IoT device is secure every developer need. These criteria are based on extensive review literature [4].

2.1 Authentication

The big challenge for IoT is to authenticate. With the new standard and self-configuring protocol authentication becoming more complex compare to traditional approach [5, 6]. Authentication ensure that the supposed sender is the real sender, For instance, when we go to unlock our connected car with our mobile phone, we want to be reassured that only we, the owners, are authorized to do so preceded by successful authentication [7].

2.2 Confidentiality

Confidentiality is about keeping data private, so that only authorized users (both humans and machines) can access that data. Cryptography is a key technology for achieving confidentiality. For example, confidentiality breaches in home monitoring systems can lead to the inadvert release of sensitive medical data. Even seemingly innocuous data, such as the internal home temperature, along with knowledge of the air conditioning system operation parameters, could be used to determine whether a house is occupied or not, as a precursor to burglary. Loss of confidentiality in things such as keys and passwords will lead to unauthorized system access threats [8].

2.3 Data Integrity

IoT security is about securing data that the information contained in the original message is kept intact. It is required that the data exchanged between IoT devices is immensely secured and the devices themselves are protected. This is because the data shared between devices is very confidential and important as it contains personal credentials, health status, financial statements and other confidential stuff. Thousands of IoT-connected devices deliver new experiences to people throughout the world and lowering costs.

2.4   Access Control

Access control known as the central element to address the security and privacy problems in computer networks. It can prevent unauthorized users from gaining access to resources, prevent legitimate users from accessing resources in an unauthorized manner, and enable legitimate users to access resources in an authorized manner [9]. Access control lets only authorized users to access a resource, such as a le, IoT device, sensor or URL. All modern operating systems limit access to the le system based on the user. For instance, the superuser has wider access to les and system resources than regular users. In the IoT context, access control is needed to make sure that only trusted parties can update device software, access sensor data or command the actuators to perform an operation.

Access control helps to solve data ownership issues and enables new business models such as Sensors As a Service, where you might for instance sell temperature sensor data to customers. Access control enables companies to share IoT device data selectively with technology vendors to allow both predictive maintenance and protection of the sensitive data [10].

3   Secure the Internet of Things (IoT) with Blockchain

With billions of connected devices filling our homes, workplaces and cities, security of data must keep pace. The billions of smart devices coming to the Internet of Things (IoT) could transform homes, cities and lives. But they also could create a serious security headache. The common enterprise security model of today is centralised, yet the IoT encourages exactly the opposite [11]. However, the biggest challenge facing IoT security is coming from the very architecture of the current IoT ecosystem; its all based on a centralized model known as the server/client model, Fig. 1.

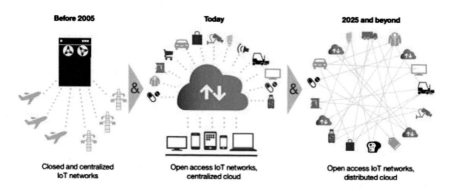

Fig. 1. The biggest challenge facing IoT security [15]

All devices are identified, authenticated and connected through cloud servers that support huge processing and storage capacities. The connection between devices will have to go through the cloud, even if they happen to be a few feet apart. While this model has connected computing devices for decades and will continue to support today IoT networks, it will not be able to respond to the growing needs of the huge IoT ecosystems of tomorrow [12]. Existing IoT solutions are very expensive caused by high infrastructure and maintenance cost associated with centralized clouds, large server farms and networking equipment [13].

A decentralized approach to IoT networking would solve many of the questions above. Adopting a standardized peer-to-peer communication model to process the hundreds of billions of transactions between devices will significantly reduce the costs associated with installing and maintaining large centralized data centers and will distribute computation and storage needs across the billions of devices that form IoT networks. However, establishing peer-to-peer communications will present its own set of challenges, chief among them the issue of security. And as we all know, IoT security is much more than just about protecting sensitive data. The proposed solution will have to maintain privacy and security in huge IoT networks and offer some form of validation and consensus for transactions to prevent spoofing and theft [14].

To perform the functions of traditional IoT solutions without a centralized control, any decentralized approach must support three fundamental functions [15], Fig. 2: Kevin Curran, IEEE Senior member and Professor of Cybersecurity at Ulster University in Northern Ireland, the next potential for securing the IoT coming from another trending technology: blockchain [16].

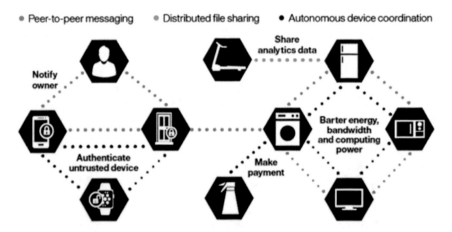

Fig. 2. The three fundamental functions: peer-to-peer messaging, distributed le sharing, autonomous device coordination [15]

- Peer-to-peer messaging
- Distributed le sharing
- Autonomous device coordination

4 Related Work

4.1 Blockchain

Blockchain the distributed technology provides everyone with a working proof of a decentralized trust. All cryptocurrencies, such as BitCoin, Ethereum, Litecoin and Dash, utilize what can best be described as a public ledger that is impossible to corrupt. Every user or node has the exact same ledger as all of the other users or nodes in the network. This ensures a complete consensus from all users or nodes in the corresponding currencies blockchain [17].

Blockchains success as a foundation for cryptocurrencies has spawned new research within the industry aimed at securing systems and technologies using the distributed ledger technology. In 2017, many business initiatives focused on creating limited prototypes and proofs-of-concepts that serve mostly to master the intricacies of this complex technology [18].

In the blockchain, a block is used to securely store information. Every block contains a hash value of the previous block header that forms a type of chain. It is then used to authenticate the data and guarantee the blocks integrity [17].

A blockchain service includes two main components:

- Transactions are the actions created by the participants in the system. A transaction records the transfer of a value (altcoin) from some input address to output addresses. Transactions are generated by the sender and distributed amongst the peers in the network. Transactions are only valid once they have been accepted into the public history of transactions, the blockchain [15, 17].
- Blocks record these transactions and make sure they are in the correct sequence and have not been tampered with. Blocks also record a time stamp when the transactions were added [15] (Table 1).

Table 1. Use cases of the IoT security and blockchain

Category	Paper	Usage of the blockchain and IoT
Agriculture	[20, 21]	Food safety, using RFID and blockchain technology in building the agri-food supply chain traceability system
		The blockchain in the agricultural world, what uses for what benefits
Energy	[22, 23]	The evolving smart energy ecosystem, support micro-transactions between individuals for new internet of energy
		Security and privacy in decentralized energy trading through multi-signatures, blockchain and anonymous messaging streams
Health	[24, 25]	Consortium explore blockchain for healthcare IoT security
		IoT and blockchain may streamline transition to digital healthcare
Environment	[26]	Blockchain technology help fight air pollution

The big advantage of Blockchain technology implementation can be public or private. For example the benefits offered by a private blockchain, are all the participants are known and trusted. This is useful when the blockchain is used between companies that belong to the same legal mother entity [12]. For public blockchain, everyone participating can see the blocks and the transactions stored in them. This doesn't mean everyone can see the actual content of your transaction, however; that's protected by your private key [19].

4.2 The Blockchain and IoT Security

Ahmed Banafa, general engineering faculty and advisor in the Davidson College of Engineering at San Jose State University, believes blockchain offers new hope for IoT security. The astounding conquest of cryptocurrency, which is built on blockchain technology, has put the technology as the flag bearer of seamless transactions, thereby reducing costs and doing away with the need to trust a centered data source, he says. Blockchain works by enhancing trustful engagements in a secured, accelerated, and transparent pattern of transactions. The real time data from an IoT channel can be utilized in such transactions while preserving the privacy of all parties involved.

Security will be the major challenge that needs to be addressed (in 2018), Banafa says. As the world becomes increasingly high-tech, devices are easily targeted by cybercriminals. Consumers not only have to worry about smartphones (but also) other devices such as baby monitors, cars with Wi-Fi, wearables, and medical devices can be breached. Security undoubtedly is a major concern, and vulnerabilities need to be addressed.

5   Perspective and Conclusion

The work of this paper gives a brief survey security analysis in the internet of things. We provided an overview and discussed a qualitative way the recent development of the most relevant security field in the context of the internet of things (IoT). It outlines the key characteristics of the Security analysis and summarizes various representative studies for IoT, including Blockchain. An important focus is the inclusion of how value is extracted from the security in the IoT. We also discussed some recent techniques for the existing activities and future opportunities related to the security in the internet of thing, outlining some of the key underlying issues that need to be tackled.

References

1. Rahman, S.S., Hearteld, R., Oli, W., Loukas, G., Filippoupolitis, A.: Assessing the cyber-trustworthiness of human-asa-sensor reports from mobile devices. In: IEEE 15th International Conference on Software Engineering Research, Management and Applications (SERA), pp. 387–394. IEEE (2017)
2. Yu, H., He, J., Zhang, T., Xiao, P., Zhang, Y.: Enabling end-to-end secure communication between wireless sensor networks and the internet. World Wide Web 16(4), 515–540 (2013)
3. Garcia-Morchon, O., Keoh, S.L., Kumar, S., Moreno-Sanchez, P., Vidal-Meca, F., Ziegeldorf, J.H.: Securing the ip-based internet of things with HIP and DTLS. In: Proceedings of the Sixth ACM conference on Security and privacy in Wireless and Mobile Networks, pp. 119–124. ACM (2013)

4. Lopez, J., Zhou, J.: Wireless Sensor Network Security, vol. 1. Ios Press (2008)
5. Ferrag, M.A., Maglaras, L.A., Janicke, H., Jiang, J., Shu, L.: Authentication protocols for internet of things: A comprehensive survey. Secur. Commun. Networks **2017** (2017)
6. Kim, H., Lee, E.A.: Authentication and authorization for the internet of things. IT Profess. **19**(5), 27–33 (2017)
7. Privacy and authentication in the internet of things (2018). http://www.information-age.com/privacy-and-authenticationinternet-things-123461082/
8. Lin, H., Bergmann, N.W.: Iot privacy and security challenges for smart home environments. Information **7**(3), 44 (2016)
9. Liu, J., Xiao, Y., Chen, C.P.: Authentication and access control in the internet of things. In: 2012 32nd International Conference on Distributed Computing Systems Workshops (ICDCSW), pp. 588–592. IEEE (2012)
10. Access control for the internet of things (2018). https://www.intopalo.com/blog/2015-05-25-access-controlfor-internet-of-things/
11. Blockchain for IoT security (2018). https://blog.nordicsemi.com/getconnected/blockchain-foriot-security
12. IoT and blockchain: challenges and risks (2017). https://www.linkedin.com/pulse/iot-blockchain-challengesrisks-ahmed-banafa/
13. How to secure the internet of things (IoT) with blockchain (2017). https://dataoq.com/read/securing-internet-of-things-iotwith-blockchain/2228
14. Decentralizing IoT networks through blockchain (2016). https://techcrunch.com/2016/06/28/decentralizing-iotnetworks-through-blockchain/
15. How to secure the internet of things (IoT) with blockchain (2018). https://dataoq.com/read/securing-internet-of-things-iotwith-blockchain/2228
16. Can blockchain secure the internet of things (2018). http://transmitter.ieee.org/can-blockchain-secure-internetthings/
17. Ouaddah, A., Elkalam, A.A., Ouahman, A.A.: Towards a novel privacy-preserving access control model based on blockchain technology in IoT. In: Europe and MENA Cooperation Advances in Information and Communication Technologies, pp. 523–533. Springer, Berlin (2017)
18. Biswas, K., Muthukkumarasamy, V.: Securing smart cities using blockchain technology. In: High Performance Computing and Communications; IEEE 14th International Conference on Smart City; IEEE 2nd International Conference on Data Science and Systems (HPCC/SmartCity/DSS), 2016 IEEE 18th International Conference, pp. 1392–1393. IEEE (2016)
19. A secure model of IoT with blockchain (2016). https://www.bbvaopenmind.com/en/a-secure-model-of-iotwith-blockchain/
20. Tian, F.: An agri-food supply chain traceability system for china based on rd & blockchain technology. In: 2016 13th International Conference on Service Systems and Service Management (ICSSSM), pp. 1–6. IEEE (2016)
21. La blockchain dans le monde agricole, quels usages pour quels bénéfices (2018). http://www.acta.asso.fr/actualites/communiquesde-presse/articles-et-communiques/detail/a/detail/lablockchain-dans-le-monde-agricole-quels-usages-pour-quelsbeneces-vers-une-agriculture.html
22. The evolving smart energy ecosystem (2018). https://www.gemalto.com/iot/inspired/smart-energy
23. Aitzhan, N.Z., Svetinovic, D.: Security and privacy in decentralized energy trading through multi-signatures, blockchain and anonymous messaging streams. IEEE Trans. Depend. Secure Comput. (2016)

24. UK and India consortium explore blockchain for healthcare IoT security (2017). https://internetofbusiness.com/consortiumblockchain-iot-security/
25. How IoT and blockchain may streamline transition to digital healthcare (2018). https://www.kaaproject.org/iot-blockchainmay-streamline-transition-digital-healthcare/
26. How can blockchain technology help fight air pollution (2016). https://media.consensys.net/how-can-blockchain-technologyhelp-ght-air-pollution-3bdcb1e1045f/

Steganographic Algorithm Based on Adapting Secret Message to the Cover Image

Youssef Taouil$^{(\boxtimes)}$ and El Bachir Ameur

Computer Sciences Department, Faculty of Sciences, Ibn Tofail University,
Kenitra, Morocco
taouilysf@gmail.com, ameurelbachir@yahoo.fr

Abstract. Steganography is the art of dissimulating secret data into digital files in an imperceptible way that does not arise the suspicion; it is one of the techniques of information security field. In this paper, a steganographic method based on the Faber-Schauder discrete wavelet transform is proposed, the embedding of the secret data is performed in the Least Significant Bits of the integer part of the high frequency coefficients. The secret message is decomposed into packets of K bits, and then each packet is transformed into another packet based on a permutation that allows obtaining the most matches possible between the message and the K-LSBs of the coefficients. To assess the performance of the proposed method, experiments were carried out on a large set of images, and a comparison to prior works is accomplished. Results show a good level of imperceptibility and a good trade-off imperceptibility-capacity compared to literature.

Keywords: Steganography · Data hiding · Faber-Schauder-DWT · Permutation · Least significant bit

1 Introduction

The main branches in the information security system are the cryptography and data hiding. Cryptography protects information through coding its content to make it unintelligible to unauthorized parties; the content cannot be interpreted without the key. Data hiding techniques consist of inserting information into digital media. Watermarking and steganography are data hiding techniques. In steganography, the information is hidden invisibly in harmless media file; the objective is that no one should suspect the existence of the information inside the host file. Various media files have been utilized in steganography as host to embed data such as audio, image, video and plain text. However, the most popular one is image; it is considered as inoffensive file, it is shared everyday on networks; and more importantly, the human visual system is insensitive to slight changes within the image intensity.

Steganography techniques can be classified into two major categories: the spatial domain and the frequency domain. In the first one, data is hidden directly in the pixels of the cover image. In the frequency domain techniques, data is hidden in the coefficients of the transform domain.

© Springer Nature Switzerland AG 2019
M. Ezziyani (Ed.): AI2SD 2018, AISC 915, pp. 753–771, 2019.
https://doi.org/10.1007/978-3-030-11928-7_69

In this paper, we propose a steganographic scheme based on the Faber Schauder DWT. This transform allows us to hide data in the integer part of the coefficients without worrying about the problem of the floating point i.e. the pixels of the stego image are guaranteed to be integers. The message is dissimulated in the LSBs of the coefficients details. The message and the coefficients LSBs are decomposed into packets of K bits $\overline{m_r}$ and $\overline{z_r}$ respectively. We search for the permutation of the packets $\overline{m_r}$ that gives the minimal error possible of the hiding by substitution. Experiments were performed on a large set of a variety of images to assess the performance of the proposed work, and comparison to prior works is accomplished. Results indicate a good amelioration in the imperceptibility and better values compared to literature.

The remaining of the paper is organized as follows: Sect. 2 presents a literature review. Section 3 details the algorithms of decomposition and reconstruction of the Faber-Schauder DWT. In Sect. 4, the proposed steganographic method is explained. In Sect. 5, experimental results of the test and comparison are discussed. Section 6 concludes the paper.

2 Literature Review

The earliest technique in the spatial domain technique is the Least Significant Bit (LSB) Substitution [1, 2]; the bit of the weakest weight is replaced by the bit of secret data. It has a good imperceptibility, but it leaves statistical traces in the histogram; the values $2j$ and $2j + 1$ tend to have a similar frequency of appearance in the stego image. This uniformity was broken later by the LSB matching [3, 4], where the embedding does not consist of replacing the LSB, but by incrementing or decrementing the coefficients. In [5, 6], authors proposed algorithms that break the uniformity of the histogram of the LSB substitution by inserting some additional bits just to have the histogram approaches its initial values. Other techniques were proposed to increase the capacity, like the interpolation based techniques [7–9]; where data is hidden in the interpolated pixels. The interpolation error provides a large space to dissimulate data; it depends essentially on the interpolation technique adopted and on the method used to calculate the interpolation error. There is also the pixel value differencing (PVD); data is hidden into each pair of consecutive pixels in such a way that it can be extracted from their difference in the stego image [10, 11]. The greater the difference between the consecutive pixels, the larger is the capacity of hiding. This feature make those techniques adapted to the image complexity.

In the frequency domain based techniques, data is hidden in the coefficients of the transform domain that contain the less part of the image energy, such as Discrete Cosine Transform (DCT) and Discrete Wavelet Transform (DWT). The DCT based steganography techniques usually are intended to the JPEG images since the JPEG compression is based on this transform. One of the first methods in this technique is the algorithm JSTEG [12]; it utilizes the LSB substitution on the DCT coefficients. The algorithm F5 [13] offers a high level of imperceptibility using the matrix embedding but to the detriment of the capacity. Its capacity was later ameliorated in the algorithm nsF5 [14] where the shrinkage was eliminated. More works were proposed on this transform, several of them are based on the idea of manipulating the quantization table to minimize the error of dissimulation [15, 16].

In the transform domain, we still can apply several techniques used in the spatial domain such as the PVD [17]. In [18], the Integer Wavelet Transform (IWT) is applied to each 8×8 block of the cover image; then the zero tree method is utilized to select the proper location where to dissimulate data. In [19], a steganographic scheme based on Haar DWT is proposed; data is hidden in the LSB of the coefficients, and the algorithm is generalized on K-LSB with the use of the Optimal Pixel Adjustment Procedure (OPAP) in [20]. The DWT is convenient for adaptive steganography. In [21], the edge coefficients of the Integer DWT are classified based on their Most Significant Bit (MSB). The size of data to be dissimulated in a single coefficient is determined based on the value of the coefficient's MSBs. In [22], the edges are determined by thresholding the DWT coefficients. Then, data is dissimulated using the XOR coding. In [23], the proposed algorithm divides the cover image into blocks of prescribed size; every block is decomposed into one-level of Haar DWT. Then, the number of wavelet coefficients of larger magnitude decides the size of the secret data that can be hidden; the embedding is based on modulus function. The optimization algorithms can be employed in steganography in both spatial and frequency domain. In [24], authors search for the optimal pixels to dissimulate data via the Particle Swarm Optimization (PSO) algorithm. In [25], the Genetic Algorithm (GA) is used for the same purpose in the Curvelet Transform Domain.

3 Faber-Schauder Discrete Wavelet Transform

Faber-Schauder transform is a Multi-scale transform; the multi-scale is a sequence $(E_j)_{j \in \mathbb{Z}}$ of nested vector spaces $E_j \subset E_{j+1}$ satisfying certain conditions that guarantee that the passage from level j to level $j + 1$ gives an approximation with a different resolution. The space E_j is generated by a family of piecewise linear functions $(\varphi_{j,n})_{n \in \mathbb{Z}}$ on the intervals $[n2^{-j}, (n+1)2^{-j}]$ with

$$\varphi(t) = \begin{cases} 1-t & if \quad 0 \leq t \leq 1 \\ 1+t & if \quad -1 \leq t \leq 0 \\ 0 & if \quad |t| \geq 1 \end{cases} \quad and \quad \varphi_{j,n}(t) = \sqrt{2^j}\varphi(2^j t - n). \quad (1)$$

We consider the space F_j supplementary of E_j in $E_{j+1}, E_{j+1} = E_j \oplus F_j$, its basis is the basis of Faber-Schauder, and it is given by the family of functions $(\psi_{j,n})_{n \in \mathbb{Z}}$, while $\psi_{j,n}(t) = \varphi_{j,2n+1}(t)$.

A signal f is a sequence of real numbers; these numbers are considered as the coefficients of the signal f in the space E_{j+1}. Afterwards, the signal is projected on E_j and on F_j. The first projection gives an approximation of f at the level j and the second one gives the details of f at the same level.

In two dimensions, the approximation of $L^2(R^2)$ is extended by the tensor product $\widetilde{E_{j+1}} = E_{j+1} \otimes E_{j+1}$. Thus,

$$\widetilde{E_{j+1}} = \left(E_j \oplus F_j\right) \otimes \left(E_j \oplus F_j\right)$$

Hence, $\widetilde{E_{j+1}} = \widetilde{E_j} \oplus \widetilde{F_j}$, while

$$\begin{cases} \widetilde{E_j} = E_j \otimes E_j \\ \widetilde{F_j} = \left(E_j \otimes F_j\right) \oplus \left(F_j \otimes E_j\right) \oplus \left(F_j \otimes F_j\right) \end{cases} \tag{2}$$

An image C is a two dimensional signal, to obtain its Faber-Schauder transform, it is projected on every one of the four subspaces of $\widetilde{E_{j+1}}$. Figure 1 illustrates an example of the Faber-Schauder 2-D DWT using the image Peppers. These projections are named respectively A, H, V and D and given by the following equations:

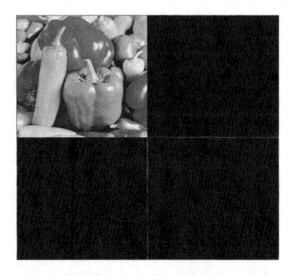

Fig. 1. Faber-Schauder DWT of the image peppers

$$\begin{cases} A_{i,j} = C_{2i,2j} \\ H_{i,j} = C_{2i+1,2j} - \dfrac{C_{2i,2j} + C_{2i+2,2j}}{2} \\ V_{i,j} = C_{2i,2j+1} - \dfrac{C_{2i,2j} + C_{2i,2j+2}}{2} \\ D_{i,j} = C_{2i+1,2j+1} - \displaystyle\sum_{k=0}^{1}\sum_{r=0}^{1} \dfrac{C_{2i+2k,2j+2r}}{4} \end{cases} \tag{3}$$

To reconstruct the projection on $\widetilde{E_{j+1}}$ from the projections on its four subspaces, we use the inverse transform given by the following equations:

$$\begin{cases} C_{2i,2j} = A_{i,j} \\ C_{2i+1,2j} = H(i,j) - \frac{A_{i,j}+A_{i+1,j}}{2} \\ C_{2i,2j+1} = V(i,j) - \frac{A_{i,j}+A_{i,j+1}}{2} \\ C_{2i+1,2j+1} = D(i,j) - \sum_{k=0}^{1}\sum_{r=0}^{1}\frac{A_{i+k,j+r}}{4} \end{cases} \tag{4}$$

4 Proposed Work

As the block A contains the low frequencies in which the human visual system is sensitive to the smallest changes, it is then mandatory to keep this bloc unchanged. Therefore, data will be hidden in the remaining three blocs H, V and D; these blocs contain the details of the image, coefficients corresponding to the high frequencies, the suitable location to hide the secret information.

4.1 Dissimulation Phase

Let m be the binary sequence of size L representing the secret data, $m = \{m_1, \ldots, m_L\}$ while $m_i \in \{0, 1\}$. Let K be the number of bits of m that we hide into one coefficient of the blocs H, V and D, and let $E_K = \{0, 1\}^K$.

If $K > 1$, we decompose the sequence m into packets of K bits, $m = \cup \overline{m_r}$ with $\overline{m_r} \in E_K$. We construct the vector $z = \cup \overline{z_r}$, while $\overline{z_r}$ contains the K least significant bits of the rth coefficient detail. The objective is to find the permutation of E_K that transforms the sequence m into another sequence m' that minimizes the error between the cover and stego images. Therefore, let us find the expression of the Mean Square Error (MSE) in term of permutation of the set E_K.

The error of the dissimulation in term of permutation

When $\overline{m_r}$ is hidden into $\overline{z_r}$, they have q different bits with $0 \leq q \leq K$, for each value of q, there is C_K^q possibilities, which makes a total of 2^K possibilities. In order to visualize all these possibilities, we introduce the matrix G whose elements denote how many times $\overline{m_r}$ encounters $\overline{z_r}$. Since both $\overline{m_r}$ and $\overline{z_r}$ are in E_K and $card(E_K) = 2^K$, then G is a matrix of 2^K rows and 2^K columns. The occurrence of $\overline{m_r}$ is between zero and $\frac{L}{K}$, hence $G \in M_{2^K}(F_K)$ with $F_K = \{0, \ldots, \frac{L}{K}\}$. The first column is associated to $(0, \ldots, 0)$, the second one to $(0, \ldots, 0, 1)$, and so on. The same thing goes for the columns. Thus, we associate to each element $\overline{m_r} = (\overline{m_{r,0}}, \ldots, \overline{m_{r,K-1}})$ of E_K an integer between 1 and 2^K that indicates the column corresponding to $\overline{m_r}$ via the following function f:

$$f : E_K \rightarrow \{1, \ldots, 2^K\}$$

$$\overline{m_r} \mapsto 1 + \sum_{q=0}^{K-1} \overline{m_{r,q}} 2^q \tag{5}$$

To construct the matrix G, we calculate the indexes $i = f(\overline{z_r})$ and $j = f(\overline{m_r})$, then the element $G_{i,j}$ is incremented, we repeat this until the end of the sequence m.

$$G_{i,j} = cardinal(\{r, f(\overline{z_r}) = i \text{ and } f(\overline{m_r}) = j\}) \tag{6}$$

On another hand, the error of the dissimulation MSE between the cover C and stego image S is expressed as follows:

$$MSE = \frac{1}{MN} \sum_{i=1}^{M} \sum_{j=1}^{N} (C_{i,j} - S_{i,j})^2 \tag{7}$$

where M and N are respectively the numbers of rows and columns of the images C and S. Let $H'_{i,j}$ be the obtained coefficient after hiding K bits of m into the K-LSB of $H_{i,j}$, and let $h_{i,j} = H'_{i,j} - H_{i,j}$ be the difference resulting from this dissimulation. We introduce the same way $v_{i,j}$ and $d_{i,j}$. Using the equations of the inverse Faber-Schauder transform, we obtain

$$MSE = \frac{1}{MN} \sum_{i=1}^{M} \sum_{j=1}^{N} h_{i,j}^2 + v_{i,j}^2 + d_{i,j}^2 \tag{8}$$

When $\overline{m_r}$ is hidden, some bits of $\overline{z_r}$ are flipped, this difference happens $G_{i,j}$ times with $i = f(\overline{z_r})$ and $j = f(\overline{m_r})$. For example, the diagonal elements G_{ii} indicate how much times data $\overline{m_r}$ can be hidden into $\overline{z_r}$ without any changes, the elements of the inverse diagonal $G_{i,2^K+1-i}$ indicate how much times data is hidden while flipping all the bits of $\overline{z_r}$. Then, we associate to the matrix G a matrix W such as each element $G_{i,j}$ is associated to a *cost* $W_{i,j}$ that denotes the difference resulting from the dissimulation of $\overline{m_r} = f^{-1}(j)$ into $\overline{z_r} = f^{-1}(i)$

$$W_{i,j} = \left| \sum_{q=0}^{K-1} (\overline{m_{r,q}} - \overline{z_{r,q}}) 2^q \right| = |j - i| \tag{9}$$

Note that the element $W_{i,j}$ can be minimized by the optimal pixel adjustment procedure when conditions are satisfied. Thus, we can reformulate the MSE as follows

$$MSE = \frac{1}{MN} \sum_{i=1}^{2^K} \sum_{j=1}^{2^K} W_{i,j}^2 G_{i,j}$$

To minimize the MSE, we propose to perform all the permutations possible of the columns of the matrix G, because such a permutation is in fact a permutation of the K-binary words $\overline{m_r}$ of the message. For each permutation, we calculate the corresponding MSE as follows

$$MSE(p) = \frac{1}{MN} \sum_{i=1}^{2^K} \sum_{j=1}^{2^K} W_{i,j}^2 G_{i,p(j)} \qquad (10)$$

At the end, we choose the permutation p^*, which gives the minimal value of MSE: $p^* = \min_{p \in S_{2^K}} (MSE)$. Based on this permutation, each $\overline{m_r}$ is transformed using p^*, thus we obtain the sequence m' which corresponds to the minimal value of MSE as follows

$$m' = \bigcup_{r=1}^{\frac{L}{K}} f^{-1} o(p^*)^{-1} of(\overline{m_r}) \qquad (11)$$

There are $(2^K)!$ permutations, so we have to calculate $(2^K)!$ value of MSE. However, $(2^K)!$ increases rapidly, so in practice, this imposes limitations to the values of K that we can use, for $K = 4$, we have $(2^K)! = 16! = 20922789888000$ permutations which the machine cannot execute, for $k = 3$, $(2^K)! = 40,320$ so we apply the proposed idea for $k \in \{1, 2, 3\}$.

First case $K = 3$

For this case, the vector z contains the three least significant bits of the coefficient details, and the sequence m is decomposed into packets of three bits. The set E is

$$E = \{(0,0,0), (0,0,1), \ldots, (1,1,1)\}.$$

The matrices G and W have 8 rows and 8 columns, W is given by

$$W = \begin{pmatrix} 0 & 1 & 2 & 3 & 4 & \alpha_{1,6} & \alpha_{1,7} & \alpha_{1,8} \\ 1 & 0 & 1 & 2 & 3 & 4 & \alpha_{2,7} & \alpha_{2,8} \\ 2 & 1 & 0 & 1 & 2 & 3 & 4 & \alpha_{3,8} \\ 3 & 2 & 1 & 0 & 1 & 2 & 3 & 4 \\ 4 & 3 & 2 & 1 & 0 & 1 & 2 & 3 \\ 3 & 4 & 3 & 2 & 1 & 0 & 1 & 2 \\ 2 & 3 & 4 & 3 & 2 & 1 & 0 & 1 \\ 1 & 2 & 3 & 4 & 3 & 2 & 1 & 0 \end{pmatrix}$$

The optimal pixel adjustment procedure (OPAP)

If $|H_{i,j}| \geq 2^{K-1}$ and $|h_{i,j}| \geq 2^{K-1}$, there exists a coefficient $H''_{i,j}$ that carries the same data hidden into $H'_{i,j}$ and verifies $|H''_{i,j} - H_{i,j}| \leq 2^{K-1}$. This coefficient is given by $H''_{i,j} = H'_{i,j} - \text{sign}(h_{i,j})$.

The bold elements in the left below are originally 5 instead of 3, 6 instead of 2 and 7 instead of 1, but they are minimized by the optimal pixel adjustment procedure because the associated coefficients satisfy the OPAP condition $|H_{i,j}| \geq 2^{K-1}$. As for the elements $\alpha_{i,j}$, they are the optimized coefficients when the conditions of the procedure are satisfied

$$\alpha_{i,j} = (j - i)(1 - p_{i,j}) + (8 - j + i)p_{i,j} \tag{12}$$

while $p_{i,j}$ is the probability that the corresponding coefficient is greater or equal to $2^{K-1} = 4$.

Second case $K = 2$

In this case, $E = \{(0,0), (0,1), (1,0), (1,1)\}$ and the matrix W is given by

$$W = \begin{pmatrix} 0 & 1 & 2 & \alpha \\ 1 & 0 & 1 & 2 \\ 2 & 1 & 0 & 1 \\ 1 & 2 & 1 & 0 \end{pmatrix}$$

The element α is obtained by the minimization of 3 (it becomes 1) by the OPAP when the condition is satisfied.

$$\alpha = p + 3(1 - p) \tag{13}$$

with p is the probability that the coefficient is greater or equal to 2.

Third case $K = 1$

This case is treated a little differently from the other two cases; the vector z contains the LSB of the coefficients details; it is decomposed into packets of two bits. The sequence m is decomposed the same way into pairs. The set E is the same as in the second case. The matrix W is given by

$$W = \begin{pmatrix} 0 & 1 & 1 & 2 \\ 1 & 0 & 2 & 1 \\ 1 & 2 & 0 & 1 \\ 2 & 1 & 1 & 0 \end{pmatrix}$$

The *MSE* in this case changes; the elements $W_{i,j}$ are not squared:

$$MSE = \frac{1}{MN} \sum_{i=1}^{4} \sum_{j=1}^{4} W_{i,j} G_{i,j} \tag{14}$$

4.2   Extraction Phase

In the extraction, two parameters are needed to be able to extract the dissimulated data successfully, the number of bits of the coefficients K used to hide data and the permutation p^*. We firstly hide K in the first two coefficients, and then we hide an identifier of p^*. In the case of $K = 1, 2$, there is 24 permutations, so the identifier of p^*

is hidden in the next five coefficients, for $K = 3$ there is 40,320 permutations, so the identifier of p^* is hidden in the next 16 coefficients. Thus, by extracting K we can retrieve the sequence m' from the K-LSB of the coefficients details, then we decompose m' into packets of size K, and we use the permutation p^* to construct the original sequence m as follows:

$$m = \bigcup_{r=1}^{\frac{L}{K}} f^{-1} op^* of \left(\overline{m'_r}\right) \tag{15}$$

4.3 Example

For example, suppose that we try to dissimulate the message $Msg = $ "*Hello!*", the binary sequence corresponding to this message is

$$m = 01001000011001010110110001101100011011110100100001$$

Third case:

In this case, we decompose the sequence m into pairs as follows:

$$m = 01|00|10|00|01|10|01|01|01|10|11|00$$
$$|01|10|11|00|01|10|11|11|00|10|00|01$$

Suppose that the LSBs of the 48 coefficients in which m is to be embedded are

$$z = 00|11|00|01|11|01|10|00|10|10|10|11$$
$$|11|10|00|10|10|10|00|00|10|00|01|11$$

We construct the matrix G:

$$G = \begin{pmatrix} 0\ 2\ 2\ 3 \\ 2\ 0\ 1\ 0 \\ 2\ 3\ 3\ 1 \\ 2\ 3\ 0\ 0 \end{pmatrix}$$

Now, the error is 30, which means there are 30 bits of the vector z among 48 that need to be flipped in order to dissimulate m. The errors are calculated by the Eq. (10) without taking M and N into consideration. Therefore, we permute the columns of G and we calculate the error for every permutation, then we choose the optimal permutation p^* associated to the lowest error. This permutation is given by:

$$p^* = \begin{pmatrix} 1\ 2\ 3\ 4 \\ 4\ 3\ 2\ 1 \end{pmatrix}$$

The error associated to p^* is 18; this means that instead of flipping 30 bits, we need to flip only 18 bits of z. We construct the sequence m' as follows:

$$(0,0) \rightarrow (1,1), (0,1) \rightarrow (1,0),$$
$$(1,0) \rightarrow (0,1), (1,1) \rightarrow (0,0).$$

Hence, we obtain the sequence m' using p^*

$$m' = 1011011110011010100100111001001110010000110111110$$

Second case:

Suppose that the two LSBs of the coefficients are

$$z = 00|11|00|01|11|01|10|00|10|10|10|11$$
$$|11|10|00|10|10|10|00|00|10|00|01|11$$

The matrix G is given by:

$$G = \begin{pmatrix} 0\ 2\ 2\ 3 \\ 2\ 0\ 1\ 0 \\ 2\ 3\ 3\ 1 \\ 2\ 3\ 0\ 0 \end{pmatrix}$$

The error is 60, by permuting the columns of G; the optimal permutation p^* reduces the error to 30 while we choose arbitrarily $\alpha = 0.25$. We find the same permutation as the third case $p^*(i) = 5 - i$. Thus, the same sequence m'.

First case:

Suppose that z contains the 3 LSBs of the coefficients. In this case, we need to decompose m and z into packets of 3 bits.

$$m = 010|010|000|110|010|101|101|100$$
$$|011|011|000|110|111|100|100|001$$

$$z = 001|100|011|101|100|010|101|011$$
$$|111|000|101|010|000|010|000|111$$

The matrix G is given by:

$$G = \begin{pmatrix} 0 & 0 & 0 & 1 & 1 & 0 & 0 & 1 \\ 0 & 0 & 1 & 0 & 0 & 0 & 0 & 0 \\ 0 & 0 & 0 & 0 & 1 & 1 & 1 & 0 \\ 1 & 0 & 0 & 0 & 1 & 0 & 0 & 0 \\ 0 & 0 & 2 & 0 & 0 & 0 & 0 & 0 \\ 1 & 0 & 0 & 0 & 0 & 1 & 1 & 0 \\ 0 & 0 & 0 & 0 & 0 & 0 & 0 & 0 \\ 0 & 1 & 0 & 1 & 0 & 0 & 0 & 0 \end{pmatrix}$$

The initial error is 140, after calculating the errors of all the permutations, the minimal error is 37 while fixing all $\alpha_{i,j}$ to 0.25, and it is associated to the permutation p^* given by:

$$p^* = \begin{pmatrix} 1 & 2 & 3 & 4 & 5 & 6 & 7 & 8 \\ 4 & 8 & 5 & 3 & 7 & 6 & 1 & 2 \end{pmatrix}$$

Using p^*, we construct the new sequence m'.

$$m' = 0110111101000111011010101000000011010000101000101011$$

To summarize, the proposed algorithm can be resumed in the following steps:

4.4 Dissimulation Algorithm

- Apply the Faber-Schauder DWT to the cover image.
- Decompose the sequence m and the vector of the coefficients details z into packets of K bits.
- Construct the matrix G.
- Calculate the error of each permutation and find the optimal permutation p^*.
- Dissimulate K and the identifier of p^* in the first coefficients.
- Transform the sequence m into a sequence m' using p^* and the function f.
- Dissimulate m' in the K-LSB of the coefficients.
- Apply the Faber-Schauder inverse DWT to obtain the stego image.

4.5 Extraction Algorithm

- Apply the Faber-Schauder DWT on the stego image.
- Extract K and the identifier of the permutation p^*.
- Extract the sequence m' from the K-LSB of the coefficients.
- Retrieve the original sequence m from the extracted m' using the permutation p^* and the function f.
- Regroup the sequence m into bytes to interpret the hidden message.

5 Experiment Results

In this section, the proposed work is tested and compared to literature in order to evaluate its performances. Tests are done on a set of 100 grayscale images of size 512×512 downloaded from the image database SIPI [26]. Some well-known which are usually used in tests are shown in Fig. 3. Comparisons are based on the same conditions utilized in the literature (images and size of hidden data).

5.1 Test of the Proposed Work

The proposed work is tested based on the imperceptibility and capacity of hiding (Fig. 2).

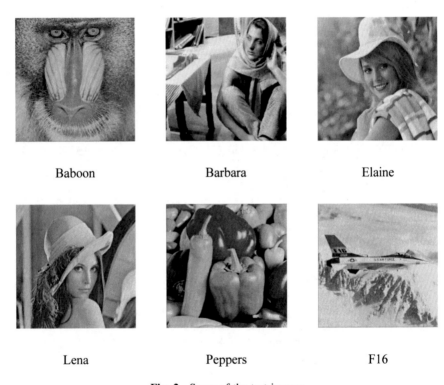

Baboon	Barbara	Elaine
Lena	Peppers	F16

Fig. 2. Some of the test images

Imperceptibility

The imperceptibility is when the human eye cannot distinguish between the cover and stego images. It is evaluated by the following metrics:

$$PSNR = 10Log_{10}\left(\frac{255}{MSE}\right)$$

$$NAE = \frac{\sum_{i=1}^{M}\sum_{j=1}^{N}|S_{i,j} - C_{i,j}|}{\sum_{i=1}^{M}\sum_{j=1}^{N}C_{i,j}}$$

$$IF = 1 - \frac{\sum_{i=1}^{M}\sum_{j=1}^{N}(S_{i,j} - C_{i,j})^2}{\sum_{i=1}^{M}\sum_{j=1}^{N}C_{i,j}^2}$$

$$NCC = \frac{\sum_{i=1}^{M}\sum_{j=1}^{N}(C_{i,j} - \mu_c)(S_{i,j} - \mu_s)}{\sqrt{\sum_{i,j}(C_{i,j} - \mu_c)^2}\sqrt{\sum_{i,j}(S_{i,j} - \mu_s)^2}}$$

The *PSNR* is the Peak Signal to Noise Ratio; the steganograhic scheme is said imperceptible when *PSNR* values are beyond 30 dB, and the greater the value of *PSNR*, the more imperceptible is the scheme.

NAE is the Normal Absolute Error; it measures the ratio of the absolute error between the cover and stego images to the cover image intensity. The scheme has a good imperceptibility when *NAE* is very close to zero.

IF is the Image Fidelity, the value $1 - IF$ measures the ratio of error energy to the cover image energy, *IF* values are between 0 and 1, it must be very close to 1.

NCC is the Normalized Correlation Coefficient, since it is a scalar product between two normalized vectors, it takes values between -1 and 1, if *NCC* is close to 1, the cover and stego images are very similar, if it is close to 0, they are uncorrelated, if it is close to -1, the images are said opposite.

Tables 1, 2 and 3 show the values of these four parameters. To exhibit the amelioration provided by the proposed work, we first hide data using the LSB substitution with the OPAP, then we use the proposed algorithm.

Table 1. Imperceptibility for K = 1

Parameter	PSNR	NAE	IF	NCC
Method	LSB Substitution + OPA			
Min	52.38	1.08e−3	0.999856	0.998287
Max	54.51	7.44e−3	0.999995	0.999996
Mean	54.20	2.05e−3	0.999984	0.999739
Method	Proposed work			
Min	53.26	8.69e−4	0.999858	0.998373
Max	55.28	7.36e−3	0.999996	0.999996
Mean	54.51	1.97e−3	0.999985	0.999742

Table 2. Imperceptibility for K = 2

Parameter	PSNR	NAE	IF	NCC
Method	*LSB Substitution + OPA*			
Min	45.32	2.81e−3	0.999148	0.990263
Max	47.41	2.48e−2	0.999980	0.999996
Mean	46.57	5.61e−3	0.999923	0.999923
Method	*Proposed work*			
Min	46.11	2.80e−3	0.999375	0.990701
Max	48.75	1.98e−2	0.999979	0.999996
Mean	47.61	5.38e−3	0.999927	0.999158

Table 3. Imperceptibility for K = 3

Parameter	PSNR	NAE	IF	NCC
Method	*LSB Substitution + OPA*			
Min	39.47	6.21e−3	0.993869	0.956163
Max	42.47	6.93e−2	0.999908	0.999995
Mean	40.65	1.29e−2	0.999601	0.996641
Method	*Proposed work*			
Min	40.54	3.94e−3	0.996811	0.959302
Max	46.58	4.61e−2	0.999950	0.999997
Mean	42.61	9.63e−3	0.999719	0.997520

We hide 16-Kilo bytes in Table 1, 40-KB in Table 2 and 60-KB in Table 3. Tables show that the proposed work has a good level of imperceptibility, the *PSNR* has high values and the other three parameters are very close to their optimal values. In comparison to the LSB substitution, the adaption of the message to the cover image via the permutation p^* improves the imperceptibility. In Table 1, the four parameters improved, even though the amelioration was slight, the *PSNR* increased by 0.3 dB, the *NAE* decreased by 10^{-4}. The coefficients *NCC* and *IF* barely changed their values. This is to be expected because the $W_{i,j}$ in this case are either 0 or 1, the error in this case is simply the distance between the LSBs of the coefficients and the bits of the message. This distance tends to the half of the message's length when the message becomes long; which means there is not a great difference between the error of the worst-case permutation and the optimal permutation.

In Table 2, the amelioration becomes important. The *PSNR* improves by 1 dB, the NAE decreases by 2.3×10^{-4}, which is more than the double of the decrease in Table 1. The effect of the permutation p^* is more profitable. The error in each coefficient $W_{i,j}$ may reach 3; when there is more error at stake, there is more to gain through the optimal permutation p^*. This can be confirmed in Table 3; when the $W_{i,j}$ can reach 7, the amelioration is more important than Tables 1 and 2, the *PSNR* improved by 2 dB and the NAE decreased by 3.27×10^{-3}. The *NCC* and *IF* do not change very much; they were already very close to 1.

The capacity of hiding

The capacity refers to the amount of data that can be dissimulated without causing visible harm to the cover image. The proposed work hides data in three blocks of the transform domain H, V and D, and each coefficient embeds K bits of data, thus the capacity is

$$capacity = \frac{3}{4}KMN.$$

The proposed work provides a large capacity of hiding as can be seen in Table 4. In general, the capacity and the imperceptibility are in conflict, improving one deteriorates the other, and here is the advantage of the proposed algorithm, we achieved a good amelioration of the imperceptibility without sacrificing a significant part of the capacity, all we need is mere 18 coefficients to hide the value of K and the identifier of the optimal permutation p^*.

Table 4. Capacity of hiding of the proposed work

K	Capacity by bits	Capacity by bit per pixel
1	195,075	0.75 bpp
2	390,150	1.50 bpp
3	585,225	3.25 pp

5.2 Comparison to Literature

In this section, the proposed work is compared to the methods developed in [18, 27].

Table 5 shows the comparison of *PSNR* to the methods of Miri et al. [27] while hiding the same amounts of data used in this article. This algorithm embeds data in the DWT domain; the genetic algorithm is used to select the proper location where to dissimulate data. For the first two lines, the work in [27] surpasses the proposed method. But, starting from 28,800 bits, the proposed offers the highest *PSNR*, with a difference of 1 dB, then as the quantity of the hidden data grows, the difference becomes larger, 1.5 dB for 51,200 bits, and as we add only 16,500 bits to 51,200, the difference in *PSNR* increases to more than 5 dB. The genetic algorithm chooses efficiently the location that minimizes the error when the size of data is small; there is too

Table 5. Capacity of hiding of the proposed work

Size of data (bits)	Method of Miri et al. [27]	Proposed work
6300	69.04	67.44
12,800	65.85	64.32
28,800	59.71	60.78
51,200	57.09	58.28
67,700	51.92	57.06

Table 6. Capacity of hiding of the proposed work

Image	Image size	Amin et al. [18]	Proposed work
Lena	128 × 128	5145	11,891
Lena	256 × 256	20,622	48,371
Lena	512 × 512	82,578	195,059
Peppers	128 × 128	5223	11,891
Peppers	256 × 256	20,694	48,371
Peppers	512 × 512	83,846	195,059

much option. However, when data becomes long, the choices become limited; hence the *PSNR* in [27] dropped rapidly at the last quantity 67,700 bits. On another hand, the quantities in the table can be hidden using only $K = 1$, the case in which the proposed algorithm does not provide strong improvement. When data size increases, the drop of *PSNR* for [27] will be remarkable, in contrast, the proposed work will pass to $K = 2$ or $K = 3$, where the amelioration will be important, hence the difference in *PSNR* will keep growing. The difference in *PSNR* in Table 5 is illustrated in Fig. 3.

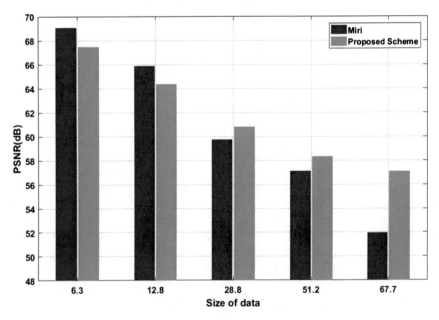

Fig. 3. Comparison of PSNR to Miri et al. [27]

As can be seen in Table 7, the proposed work provides a higher PSNR than the method in [18] with a difference of around 2.7 dB. Table 6 shows the comparison of the values of the capacity. The capacity of the proposed algorithm is larger, the authors in [18] do not use all coefficients to hide data, they hide data bloc by bloc, and each

Table 7. Capacity of hiding of the proposed work

Image	Method	100	1000	5000	10,000	15,000
Barbara	Amin et al. [18]	73.98	63.64	56.55	53.64	52.02
	Proposed	76.57	66.38	59.37	56.35	54.59
Pepper	Amin et al. [18]	74.12	63.78	56.54	53.58	51.89
	Proposed	76.61	66.42	59.34	56.34	54.57
Baboon	Amin et al. [18]	75.62	62.89	56.06	53.32	51.57
	Proposed	76.59	66.38	59.35	56.32	54.56
Lena	Amin et al. [18]	73.58	63.01	56.18	53.38	51.65
	Proposed	76.57	66.41	59.37	56.37	54.59

bloc embeds a fragment of data, the size of the bloc is greater than the size of the fragment in order to have the choice of the coefficients that will conceal data. Selecting some of the coefficients and sparing some of them diminishes the capacity of hiding, it is about 2.3 times lesser than the capacity of the proposed work. On another hand, this lack in capacity is not fully compensated in the PSNR, as illustrated in the Fig. 4; the proposed work still has higher PSNR with more than 2 dB.

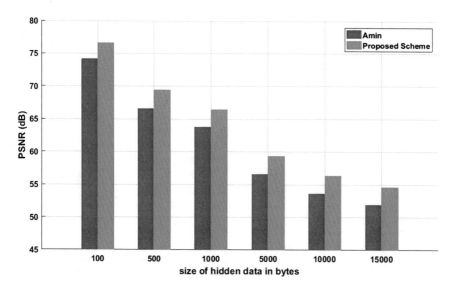

Fig. 4. Comparison of PSNR to Seyyedi and Ivanov [18]

6 Conclusion

In this paper, a steganographic method based on Faber-Schauder DWT is proposed. To minimize the distortion occurring on the cover image, secret data is transformed into another binary sequence that allows us to obtain the most matches possible to the LSBs of the coefficients details. Therefore, data is divided into packets of K bits; the same is done to the LSBs of the details in the transform domain. We construct a matrix G that calculates the number of times where each K bits combination from data encounters a K bits combination of the coefficients. Based on this matrix and the matrix of costs W, we establish the expression of the error MSE, then we permute the columns of the matrix and we calculate the error of every permutation to find the optimal permutation that corresponds to the minimal error of dissimulation. Results show satisfying amelioration of imperceptibility in comparison to LSB substitution without need to sacrifice any part of the capacity in return; we also obtained higher values compared to existing methods. In our future works, we will focus on finding a way to minimize the number of the permutations we have to test in order to extend our algorithm on $K = 4$ or $K = 5$. It will be then very efficient in adaptive schemes; in the edges where we hide more bits in one coefficient of texture zone; so the proposed algorithm will minimize significantly the error in this zone.

References

1. Chan, C.K., Cheng, L.M.: Hiding data in images by simple LSB substitution. Pattern Recogn. **37**, 469–474 (2004). https://doi.org/10.1016/j.patcog.2003.08.007
2. Bailey, K., Curtan, K.: An evaluation of image based steganography methods using visual inspection and automated detection techniques. Multimed. Tools Appl. **30**, 55–88 (2006). https://doi.org/10.1007/s11042-006-0008-4
3. Sharp, T.: An implementation of key based digital signal steganography. In: 4th International Workshop on Information hiding, vol. 2137, pp. 13–26 (2001). https://doi.org/10.1007/3-540-45496-9_2
4. Mielikainen, J.: LSB matching revisited. IEEE Signal Process. Lett. **13**, 285–287 (2006). https://doi.org/10.1109/LSP.2006.870357
5. Provos, N.: Defending against statistical steganalysis. In: SSYM'01 Proceedings of the 10th Conference on USENIX Security, vol. 10, no. 24 (2001)
6. Wu, H.T., Dugelay, J.L., Cheung, Y.M.: A data mapping method for steganography and its application to images. In: International Workshop on Information hiding, vol. 5284, pp. 236–250 (2008). https://doi.org/10.1007/978-3-540-88961-8_17
7. Hu, J., Li, T.: Reversible steganography using extended image interpolation technique. Comput. Electr. Eng. **46**, 447–455 (2015). https://doi.org/10.1016/j.compeleceng.2015.04.014
8. Benhfid, A., Ameur, E.B., Taouil, Y.: High capacity data hiding methods based on spline interpolation. In: 5th International Conference on Multimedia Computing and Systems (ICMCS), pp. 157–162 (2016). https://doi.org/10.1109/icmcs.2016.7905641
9. Tang, M., Zeng, S., Chen, X., Hu, J., Du, Y.: An adaptive image steganography using AMBTC compression and interpolation technique. Int. J. Light Electron Opt. **127**, 471–477 (2016). https://doi.org/10.1016/j.ijleo.2015.09.216
10. Wu, D.C., Tsai, W.H.: A steganographic method for images by pixel-value differencing. Pattern Recogn. Lett. **24**, 1613–1626 (2003)
11. Arya, M.S., Rani, M., Bedi, C.S.: Improved capacity image steganography algorithm using 16 pixel differencing with n-bit LSB substitution for RGB images. J. Electr. Comput. Eng. **6**, 2735–2741 (2016). http://doi.org/10.11591/ijece.v6i6
12. Upham, D.: Steganographic Algorithm JSTEG. https://zooid.org/ ~ paul/crypto/jsteg/

13. Westfeld, A.: F5-A steganographic algorithm. In: International Workshop on Information hiding, vol. 2137, pp. 289–302 (2001). https://doi.org/10.1007/3-540-45496-9_21

14. Fridrich, J., Penvy, T., Kodovsky, J.: Statistically Undetectable JPEG steganography: dead ends, challenges and opportunities. In: MM\&SEC'07 Proceedings of the 9th Workshop on Multimedia and Security, pp. 3–14 (2007). https://doi.org/10.1145/1288869.1288872

15. Chang, C.C., Chen, T.S., Chung, L.Z.: A steganographic method based upon JPEG and quantization table modification. Inf. Sci. **141**, 123–138 (2002). https://doi.org/10.1016/S0020-0255(01)00194-3

16. Wang, K., Lu, Z.M., Hu, Y.J.: A high capacity loseless data hiding scheme for JPEG images. J. Syst. Softw. **14**, 147–157 (2015). https://doi.org/10.1016/j.jss.2013.03.083

17. Gulve, A.K., Joshi, M.S.: An image steganography method hiding secret data into coefficients of integer wavelet transform using pixel value differencing approach. In: Mathematical Problems in Engineering, vol. 2015 (2014). http://dx.doi.org/10.1155/2015/684824

18. Seyyedi, S.A., Ivanov, N.: A novel secure steganographic method based on zero tree method. Int. J. Adv. Stud. Comput. Sci. Eng. **3**(3) (2014)

19. Taouil, Y., Ameur, E.B., Belghiti, M.T.: New image steganography method based on Haar discrete wavelet transform, EMENA-TSSL. Adv. Intell. Syst. Comput. **520**, 287–297 (2016). https://doi.org/10.1007/978-3-319-46568-5_30

20. Taouil, Y., Ameur, E.B., Benhfid, A., Harba, R., Jennane, R.: A data hiding scheme based on the Haar discrete wavelet transform and the K-LSB. Int. J. Imaging Robot. **17**, 41–53 (2017)

21. Miri, A., Faez, K.: An image steganography method based on integer wavelet transform. Multimed. Tools Appl. **77**, 13133–13144 (2017). https://doi.org/10.1007/s11042-017-4935-z

22. Al-Dmour, H., Al-Ani, A.: A steganography embedding method based on edge identification and XOR coding. Expert Syst. Appl. **46**, 293–306 (2016). https://doi.org/10.1016/j.eswa.2015.10.024

23. Zhiwei, K., Jing, L., Yigang, H.: Steganography based on wavelet transform and modulus function. J. Syst. Eng. Electron. **18**, 628–632 (2007). https://doi.org/10.1016/S1004-4132(07)60139-X

24. Bedi, P., Bansal, R., Sehgal, P.: Using PSO in a spatial domain based image hiding scheme with distortion tolerance. Comput. Electr. Eng. **39**, 640–654 (2013). https://doi.org/10.1016/j.compeleceng.2012.12.021

25. Mostafa, H., Fouad, A., Sami, G.: A hybrid Curvelet transform and genetic algorithm for image steganography. Int. J. Adv. Comput. Sci. Appl. **8**(8) (2017). https://doi.org/10.14569/ijacsa.2017.080843

26. Test images database. http://sipi.usc.edu/database/

27. Miri, A., Faez, K.: Adaptive image steganography based on transform domain via genetic algorithm. Optik **145**, 158–168 (2017). https://doi.org/10.1016/j.ijleo.2017.07.043

A Hybrid Machine Learning Approach to Predict Learning Styles in Adaptive E-Learning System

Ouafae El Aissaoui[1]($\boxtimes$) (ID), Yasser El Madani El Alami[2] (ID),
Lahcen Oughdir[1], and Youssouf El Allioui[3] (ID)

[1] LSI, FPT, University of Sidi Mohammed Ben Abdellah, Taza, Morocco
ouafae.elaissaoui@usmba.ac.ma
[2] ENSIAS, Mohammed V University, B.P.: 713, Agdal, Rabat, Morocco
[3] LS3M, FPK, Hassan I University, B.P.: 145, 25000 Khouribga, Morocco

Abstract. The increasing use of E-learning environments by learners makes it indispensable to implement adaptive e-learning systems (AeS). The AeS have to take into account the learners' learning styles to provide convenient contents and enhance the learning process. Learning styles refer to the preferred way in which an individual learns best. The traditional methods detecting learning styles (using questionnaires) present many limits, as: (1) the time-consuming process of filling in the questionnaire and (2) producing inaccurate results because students aren't always aware of their own learning preferences. Thus in this paper we have proposed an approach for detecting learning styles automatically, based on Felder and Silverman learning style model (FSLSM) and using machine learning algorithms. The proposed approach is composed of two parts: The first part aims to extract the learners' sequences from the log file, and then using an unsupervised algorithm (K-means) in order to group them into sixteen clusters according to the FSLSM, and the second part consists in using a supervised algorithm (Naive Bayes) to predict the learning style for a new sequence or a new learner. To perform our approach, we used a real dataset extracted from an e-learning system's log file. In order to evaluate the performance, we used the confusion matrix technique. The obtained results demonstrate that our approach yields excellent results.

Keywords: Adaptive E-Learning systems · Felder-Silverman learning style model · Unsupervised algorithm · Supervised algorithm · K-Means · Naïve bayes

1 Introduction

Adaptive E-learning refers to e-learning systems which provide customized contents for learners based on their profiles, with the final goal of enhancing their learning process. Learner profile is a representation of the learner's behavior while he/she is interacting with the system, the learner's behavior can be captured from the web logs using data mining techniques and then translated to a set of characteristics such as; skills, knowledge level, preferences, and learning style which is considered as an

© Springer Nature Switzerland AG 2019
M. Ezziyyani (Ed.): AI2SD 2018, AISC 915, pp. 772–786, 2019.
https://doi.org/10.1007/978-3-030-11928-7_70

essential factor that directly affects the student's learning process. Learning style is a vital learner's characteristic which must be taken into account in the learning personalization process, since it refers to the preferred way in which a learner perceives, treats and grasps the information. There are many learning style models where each learner is assigned to a learning style class based on the way he/she learns, a lot of LS models have been proposed such as [1–3], etc. The FSLSM is a popular learning style model which defines four dimensions (pre-processing, perception, input and understanding) and eight categories of learners (Active, reflective, sensing, intuitive, visual, verbal, Sequential and Global). In this work we have relied on the FSLSM for many reasons; firstly, because it is the most used in adaptive e-learning systems and the most appropriate to implement them [4, 5], one other reason is that the FSMSM enables the LS to be measured according to an Index of Learning Styles (ILS), The ILS consists of the four FSLSM's dimensions, each with 11 questions. Using the ILS we can link LS to appropriate learning objects.

There are many methods to detect a learning style, the traditional one consists in using questionnaires, applying this method can lead to time consuming and inaccurate results. Thus to acquire an efficient learning style, we have to detect it automatically from the log file which contains the learner's behavior using data mining techniques. In this paper we have proposed an approach which aims to detect the learners' learning styles dynamically based on Felder and Silverman [2] learning style model and using machine learning algorithms. In the first step of our approach we have extracted the learners' sequences from the log file, then we have used an unsupervised algorithm in order to group them into sixteen clusters where each cluster corresponds to a learning style, while in the second step, the clusters obtained from the first step have been considered as a training dataset which was used in order to perform a supervised algorithm on it and then predicting the learning style of a new sequence

This paper is organized as follows. Section 2 describes the learning style model and the algorithms used in our approach. Section 3 introduces a literature review of related work. Section 4 describes the methodology of our approach. The experiments and results are presented in Sect. 5; Finally, Sect. 6 presents our conclusions and future works.

2 Background

2.1 Learning Styles

Many definitions appear in the literature concerning the term learning style. Laschinger and Boss [1] defined learning style as the way in which individuals organize information and experiences, while Garity [6] defined it as the preferred way to learn and process information. Keefe [7] described learning styles as the cognitive, effective, and psychological behaviors that serve as relatively stable indicators of how learners perceive, interact with, and respond to the learning environment.

Learning style refers to the preferred way in which a learner perceives, reacts, interacts with, and responds to the learning environment. Each learner has his own preferred ways of learning; there are some students who prefer to study in a group, other prefer to study alone; some prefer to learn by reading written explanations, other by seeing visual representations, pictures, diagrams, and charts. In order to ensure an efficient learning process for learners; the e-learning system should consider the differences in learners' learning styles.

2.2 The Felder and Silverman Learning Style Model

A learning style model classifies the learners into a specific number of predefined dimensions, where each dimension pertains to the way they receive and process information. Many learning style models have been proposed in the literature, in this work we have based on the Felder and Silverman model.

According to the previous researches [4, 5], the FSLSM is the most used in adaptive e-learning systems and the most appropriate to implement them. The FSLSM presents four dimensions with two categories for each one, where each learner has a dominant preference for one category in each dimension: processing (active/reflective), perception (sensing/intuitive), input (visual/verbal), understanding (sequential/global).

Active (A) learners prefer to process information by interacting directly with the learning material, while **reflective (R)** learners prefer to think about the learning material. Active learners also tend to study in group, while the reflective learners prefer to work individually.

Sensing (Sen) learners tend to use materials that contains concrete facts and real world applications, they are realistic and like to use demonstrated procedure and physical experiments. While the **intuitive** learners prefer to use materials that contains abstract and theoretical information, they tend to understand the overall pattern from a global picture and then discovering possibilities.

The **visual (Vi)** learners prefer to see what they learn by using visual representations such as pictures, diagrams, and charts. While the **verbal (Ve)** learners like information that are explained with words; both written and spoken.

Sequential (Seq) learners prefer to focus on the details by going through the course step by step in a linear way. In the opposite, the **global (G)** learners prefer to understand the big picture by organizing information holistically.

2.3 K-Means Clustering Algorithm

The K-means is an unsupervised algorithm which aims to group similar objects into k clusters [8–10].

In machine learning, unsupervised refers to the problem of finding hidden structure within unlabeled data. Given a collection of objects each with n measurable attributes, k-means is an analytical technique that for a chosen value of k, identifies k clusters of objects based on the objects' proximity to the center of the k groups. The center is determined as the arithmetic average (mean) of each cluster's n-dimensional vector of attributes.

The following steps illustrate how to find k clusters from a collection of M objects with n attributes, where each object i is described by n attributes or property values $(P_{i1}, P_{i2}, \ldots, P_{in})$ for $i = 1, 2, \ldots, M$:

1. The first step consists in choosing the value of k and the k initial guesses for the centroids.
2. In the second step we compute the distance from each data point P_i, at $(P_{i1}, P_{i2}, ..., P_{in})$ to each centroid q located at $q_1, q_2, ...q_n$ using the following equation:

$$d(p_i - q) = \sqrt{\sum_{j=1}^{n} (p_{ij} - q_j)^2} \tag{1}$$

3. Then each point is assigned to the closest centroid. This association defines the first k clusters.
4. After determining the first k clusters, we compute the centroid, the center of mass, of each newly defined cluster from Step 3 using the following equation.

$$(q_1, q_2, ..., q_n) = \left(\frac{\sum_{i=1}^{m} p_{i1}}{m}, \frac{\sum_{i=1}^{m} p_{i2}}{m}, ..., \frac{\sum_{i=1}^{m} p_{in}}{m} \right) \tag{2}$$

5. Finally, we Repeat Steps 2, 3 and 4 until the algorithm reaches the final answer.

2.4   Naïve Bayes

The Naive Bayes is a probabilistic classification method based on Bayes' theorem with a few tweaks [11, 12]. According to the Bayes' Theorem, the conditional probability of event C occurring, given that event A has already occurred, is denoted as P(C/A), which can be found using the following formula:

$$P(c\backslash A) = \frac{P(A\backslash C) * P(C)}{P(A)} \tag{3}$$

A more general form of Bayes' theorem assigns a classified label $(C \in c_1, c_2, ..., c_n)$ to an object A with multiple attributes $(a_1, a_2, ..., a_m)$ such that the label corresponds to the largest values of $p(c_i/A)$ for $i = 1, 2, ..., n$. Mathematically, this is shown in the following equation:

$$P(C_i\backslash A) = \frac{P(a_1, a_2, a_3, ...a_m\backslash C_i) * P(C_i)}{P(a_1, a_2, a_3, ...a_m)}, \quad i = 1, 2, ..., n \tag{4}$$

With two simplifications, Bayes' theorem can be extended to become a naive Bayes classifier.

The first simplification is to use the conditional independence assumption. That is, each attribute is conditionally independent of every other attribute given a class label C_i. See the following equation:

$$P(a_1, a_2, \ldots a_m \backslash C_i) = P(a_1 \backslash C_i) P(a_2 \backslash C_i) \ldots P(a_m \backslash C_i) = \prod_{j=1}^{m} P(a_j \backslash C_i) \qquad (5)$$

The second simplification is to ignore the denominator $P(a_1, a_2, a_3, \ldots a_m)$. Because $P(a_1, a_2, a_3, \ldots a_m)$ appears in the denominator of $\boldsymbol{P}(\boldsymbol{C_i} \backslash \boldsymbol{A})$ for all values of i, removing the denominator will have no impact on the relative probability scores and will simplify calculations.

After applying the two simplifications mentioned earlier, the Eq. (4) can be extended to become a naive Bayes classifier as follow:

$$P(C_i \backslash A) \sim P(C_i) \cdot \prod_{j=1}^{m} P(a_j \backslash C_i), \quad i = 1, 2, \ldots, n \qquad (6)$$

As a result, for an object A, the naïve Bayes classifier assigns the class label C_i that maximizes the equation:

$$P(C_i) \cdot \prod_{j=1}^{m} P(a_j \backslash C_i), \quad i = 1, 2, \ldots, n \qquad (7)$$

3   Related Works

Many approaches have been proposed to automatically detect students' learning styles based on machine learning techniques. Those literature works have been relied on various classifiers. Feldman et al. [13] found that the Bayesian network classifier is one of the most widely adopted classifiers to infer the leaning style.

Garcia et al. [14] used Bayesian Networks to detect the learning style of a student in a Web-based education system. To evaluate the precision of their proposed approach, they compared the learning style detected by their approach against the learning style obtained with the index of learning style questionnaire.

Bunt and Conati [15] addressed this problem by building a BN able to detect the difficulty that learners face during the exploration process; and then providing specific assessment to guide and improve the learner's exploration of the available material.

Decision tree is a classification algorithm that is also frequently used in the field of automatic detection of learning styles. Kalhoro [16] proposed an approach to automatically detect the learners' learning styles from web logs of the students using the Data Mining technique, and the Decision Trees classifier. Kolb's learning style theory was incorporated to understand e-learners' learning styles on web. Pantho and Tiantong [17] proposed an approach to classify VARK (Visual, Aural, Read/Write, Kinesthetic) learning styles of learners by using Decision Tree C4.5 algorithm. Data concerning learning styles of learners were collected via a questionnaire responded by 1205 students. The collected data were then classified using Decision Tree C4.5 algorithm.

Neural networks are also commonly used in the automatic detection of learning styles, Hmedna et al. [18] proposed an approach that uses neural networks to identify and track learners learning styles in order to ensure efficient recommendation of resources. Their work was based on Felder-Silverman' dimensions. Hmedna et al. [18] introduced an automatic student modeling approach for identifying learning style in learning management systems according to FSLSM. They proposed the use of fuzzy cognitive maps FCMs as a tool for identifying learner's learning style. FCMs are a soft computing tool which is a combination of fuzzy logic and neural network.

Similarly to the previous algorithms; KNN is frequently used to detect the learning styles automatically, Chang et al. [19] proposed a learning style classification mechanism to classify and then identify students' learning styles. The proposed mechanism improves k-nearest neighbor (k-NN) classification and combines it with genetic algorithms (GA).

As can be noticed, all the previous works relied on a learning style model in their approaches. Most of the proposed approaches used the FSLSM's dimensions and considered that there are 8 learning styles where each one corresponds to a dimension's category. In reality, there are sixteen learning style combinations obtained by combining one category from each dimension. Similarly, to the previous work; we have also relied on the FSLSM, but by considering sixteen LSC.

4 Methodology

An adaptive E-learning system takes into account the learner's learning style and provides contents to the learners based on their preferred learning styles which are identified using the learners' sequences. To identify a learner's learning style we have to rely on a standard learning style model such as FSLSM, where the captured sequences can be labeled with a specific learning style combination using an unsupervised algorithm. In order to implement the unsupervised algorithm, the learner's sequences which have been extracted from the log file, must be transformed to the input of that algorithm.

The learning sequence of a learner is defined by the various learning objects accessed by that specific learner during a session. Each sequence contains the sequence id, session id, learner id, and the set of learning objects accessed by the learner in a session.

After detecting the learners' sequences; our first aim is to classify them according to FSLSM by assigning a specific learning style combination to each sequence, and our second aim is to use those labeled sequences as training set in order to predict the learning style of a new sequence.

In the first step we have used a clustering algorithm, while in the second step we have used a classification algorithm. In our proposed approach we have used the two following algorithms:

- K-means algorithm: in order to assign a label to each sequence based on FSLSM.
- Naïve Bayes classifier: in order to classify a new learner, or a new sequence of an existing learner according to the FSLSM.

The following schema resumes our proposed approach (Fig. 1).

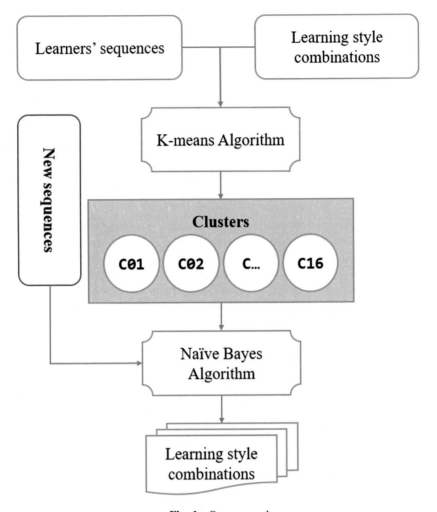

Fig. 1. Our approach

The next subsections are organized as follows: first of all, we will represent how to match each learning object with its appropriate learning style combination, then we will describe how the clustering and classification algorithms were used in our approach.

4.1 Matching LSC to Learning Objects

In order to match a LSC to a learning object, we should have relied on a LSM, in our work we have based on the FSLSM for many reasons, one important reason, is that the FSLSM considers that the student's learning style can be changed unexpectedly and in a non-deterministic way [4], therefore, our approach aims to update the student's learning style dynamically after each interaction with the adaptive e-learning systems. According to the previous researches [5], the FSLSM is the most used in adaptive e-learning systems and the most appropriate to implement them. According to FSLSM there are four dimensions, where each dimension contains two opposite categories, and each learner prefers a specific category in each dimension. Thus, to identify the learner' learning style; we have to determine a combination composed by one category from each dimension. As a result we will obtain sixteen combinations:

```
Learning  Styles  Combinations  (LSCs) = { (A,Sen,Vi,G),
(A,Sen,Vi,Seq), (R,Sen,Vi,G), (A,Sen,Ve,Seq), (A,Sen,Ve,G),
(R,Sen,Ve,Seq), (R,Sen,Ve,G), (A,I,Ve,G), (A,I,Vi,Seq), (A,
I,Vi,G), (R,I,Vi,Seq), (R,I,Vi,G), (R,S,Vi,Seq), (A,I,Ve,
Seq), (R,I,Ve,Seq), (R,I,Ve,G) }.
```

Basically, we suppose that each LSC reflects the preferred learning objects (Los) that are accessed by a learner during the learning process, so in order to identify the LSC for each learner, we first have to match the Los with its appropriate LSC. Based on the matching table presented in our previous work [20, 21]; we have obtained the following table, where the mapped learning objects are considered as feature values of the K-means clustering algorithm.

4.2 The K-Means Algorithm

The first step in our approach consists in using the K-means algorithm in order to classify the learners' sequences according to the sixteen learning style combinations where the sequences of learners are given as an input to the algorithm, and the sixteen LSCs are given as the labels to assign to the resulted clusters.

After extracting the learners' sequences from the log file using data mining techniques, we can use them as an input to the K-means by turning them into a matrix with M rows corresponding to M sequences and sixteen columns to store the attribute values where the attributes of each sequence correspond to the sixteen Los presented in the previous mapping table (Table 1). Therefore each sequence S_i is described by sixteen attributes values $(a_{i1}, a_{i2}, \ldots, a_{i16})$ for $i = 1, 2, \ldots, M$ where a_{i1} corresponds to the number of occurrences of the Lo video in a sequence S_i, a_{i2} Corresponds to the number of occurrences of the Lo PTT, and so on.

In order to perform the k-means algorithm we used the R software framework for statistical analysis and graphics, and in order to write and execute the R code easily, we used the RStudio as a graphical user interface. The dataset employed in our approach was extracted from the E-learning platform's log file[1] of Sup'Management Group.[2] This dataset records 1235 learners' sequences. The following steps describe how we used the K-means with the R language.

- Firstly, we installed the following necessary packages: plyr, ggplot2, cluster, lattice, graphics, grid, gridExtra.
- Secondly, we have imported the data file that contains 17 columns, where the first column holds a sequence identification (ID) number, and the other columns store the number of occurrences of the sixteen Los in each sequence. Because the

---

[1] http://www.supmanagement.ma/fc/login/index.php.
[2] http://www.supmanagement.ma/fc/.

Table 1. Learning objects as per FSLSM

Cluster ID	Combination	Videos	PPTs	Demo	Exercise	Assignments	PDFs	Announcements	References	Examples	Practical material	Forum	Topic list	Images	Charts	Email	Sequential
C01	(R, I, Ve, G)	3	2	0	1	1	3	2	3	0	0	1	2	0	0	1	0
C02	(A, I, Ve, G)	3	2	1	2	2	2	1	2	0	0	1	2	0	0	1	0
C03	(R, Sen, Ve, G)	3	1	0	1	1	3	2	2	1	1	0	1	0	0	1	0
C04	(A, Sen, Ve, G)	3	1	1	2	2	2	1	1	1	1	0	1	0	0	1	0
C05	(R, I, Vis, G)	3	2	0	1	1	2	1	4	0	0	1	2	1	1	0	0
C06	(A, I, Vi, G)	3	2	1	2	2	1	0	3	0	0	1	2	1	1	0	0
C07	(R, S, Vi, G)	3	1	0	1	1	2	1	3	1	1	0	1	1	1	0	0
C08	(A, S, Vi, G)	3	1	1	2	2	1	0	2	1	1	0	1	1	1	0	0
C09	(R, I, Ve, Seq)	3	2	0	1	1	3	2	3	0	0	1	1	0	0	1	1
C10	(A, I, Ve, Seq)	3	2	1	2	2	2	1	2	0	0	1	1	0	0	1	1
C11	(R, Sen, Ve, Seq)	3	1	0	1	1	3	2	2	1	1	0	0	0	0	1	1
C12	(A, Sen, Ve, Seq)	3	1	1	2	2	2	1	1	1	1	0	0	0	0	1	1
C13	(R, I, Vi, Seq)	3	2	0	1	1	2	1	4	0	0	1	1	1	1	0	1
C14	(A, I, Vi, Seq)	3	2	1	2	2	1	0	3	0	0	1	1	1	1	0	1
C15	(R, Sen, Vi, Seq)	3	1	0	1	1	2	1	3	1	1	0	0	1	1	0	1
C16	(A, Sen, Vi, Seq)	3	1	1	2	2	1	0	2	1	1	0	0	1	1	0	1

sequence id was not used in the clustering analysis, it was excluded from the K-means input matrix.

- Finally, the K-means algorithm was executed giving k = 16, the results are displayed in the two following captured pictures (Fig. 2).

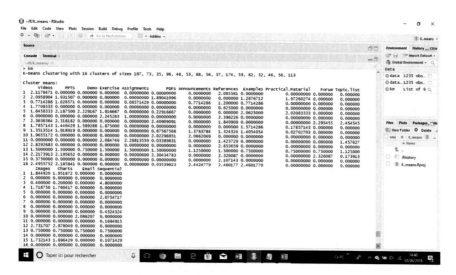

Fig. 2. The location of the cluster means

The picture above shows the number of sequences in each cluster and the coordinates of the clusters' centroid. The obtained clusters were labeled with the LSCs based on the minimum distance between the clusters' centroid and the LSCs' vectors that were presented in Table 1. The result of the clustering is shown in Table 2.

4.3 Naïve Bayes Algorithm

After applying the K-means algorithm and labeling the sequences with the LSCs, the labeled sequences were used as a training dataset to train the classification algorithm, and then use it to predict the LSC for a new sequence.

In our work we have applied the Naive Bayes classifier for many reasons. First of all, because it's one of the most efficient machine leaning algorithms, it learns fast and predicts equally so, and it doesn't require lots of storage. A very important characteristic of Naïve Bayes for our work is that it is a probabilistic classification method, therefore, in our approach we consider that the learner's LSC is not deterministic and not stationary since it can be changed during the learning process in an unexpected way, thus we can measure the LSC for a given learner after each iteration using a probabilistic method.

Given a sequence with a set of attributes $A = \{a_j/j = 1, 2..., 16\}$ where j corresponds to one of the sixteen learning objects existed in the matching table (Table 1),

Table 2. Result of k-means clustering algorithms

Cluster ID	Combination	Number of sequences in each cluster	Total
C01	(R, I, Ve, G)	58	1235
C02	(A, I, Ve, G)	73	
C03	(R, Sen, Ve, G)	174	
C04	(A, Sen, Ve, G)	48	
C05	(R, I, Vis, G)	82	
C06	(A, I, Vi, G)	56	
C07	(R, S, Vi, G)	187	
C08	(A, S, Vi, G)	59	
C09	(R, I, Ve, Seq)	35	
C10	(A, I, Ve, Seq)	32	
C11	(R, Sen, Ve, Seq)	113	
C12	(A, Sen, Ve, Seq)	56	
C13	(R, I, Vi, Seq)	46	
C14	(A, I, Vi, Seq)	96	
C15	(R, Sen, Vi, Seq)	37	
C16	(A, Sen, Vi, Seq)	53	

and a_{ij} takes one value: (yes or No), yes if the jth learning object exists in the sequence, No if the jth learning object doesn't exist in the sequence,

Given a set of classified labels $C = \{C_1, C_2, \ldots, C_{16}\}$ where C_i corresponds to one of the sixteen LSCs.

According to the Naive Bayes Classifier, for each new sequence S_i, we will assign the classifier label C_i that maximizes the following equation:

$$P(C_i) \cdot \prod_{j=1}^{16} P(a_j \backslash C_i), \quad i = 1, 2, \ldots, 16 \tag{8}$$

In order to predict the LSC for new sequences, we used the Byes naïve in R with the package e1071, and in order to be sure about the efficiency of the algorithm, we did an experiment using the confusion matrix in R with caret. The following section describes the experiment steps and the obtained results.

5 Experiment and Results

5.1 Performance Metrics for Classification Problems

In order to evaluate the performance of the classifier used in our approach, we have used the confusion matrix technique. The confusion matrix technique is a specific table layout that summarizes the number of correct and incorrect predictions in each class, and it is used to compute several validation metrics.

We suppose that we have a confusion matrix with n classes; the following Eqs. (9)–(12) show how to compute the total number of false negative (FN), false positive (FP), true negative (TN), and the true positive (TTP).

FN is the number of instances the classifier predicted as negative but they are positive.

$$FN_i = \sum_{\substack{*20cj = 1 \\ j \neq 1}}^{n} x_{ij} \tag{9}$$

(FP) is the number of instances the classifier predicted as positive but they are negative.

$$FP_i = \sum_{\substack{*20cj = 1 \\ j \neq 1}}^{n} x_{ji} \tag{10}$$

(TN) is the number of negative instances the classifier correctly identified as negative.

$$TN_i = \sum_{\substack{*20cj = 1 \\ j \neq i}}^{n} \sum_{\substack{*20cj = 1 \\ j \neq i}}^{n} x_{jk} \tag{11}$$

(TP) is the number of positive instances the classifier correctly identified as positive.

$$TTP_{all} = \sum_{j=1}^{n} x_{jj} \tag{12}$$

In order to evaluate the performance of a classifier, the following measures (Eqs. 13–17) can be computed for each class i based on the equations described above.

Precision (Positive Predictive value) is the fraction of true positive instances among the predicted positive instances.

$$P_i = \frac{TP_i}{TP_i + FP_i} \tag{13}$$

Negative Predictive Value (NPV) is the fraction of true negative instances among the predicted negative instances.

$$NPV_i = \frac{TN_i}{TN_i + FN_i} \tag{14}$$

Recall (Sensitivity) is the proportion of positive instances that are correctly classified as positive.

$$R_i = \frac{TP_i}{TP_i + FN_i} \tag{15}$$

Specificity (True negative rate) is the proportion of negative instances that are correctly classified as negative.

$$S_i = \frac{TN_i}{TN_i + FP_i} \tag{16}$$

Accuracy, defines the rate at which a model has classified the records correctly.

$$A = \frac{TTP_{all}}{total\ number\ of\ classifications} \tag{17}$$

5.2   Experiment

In order to compute a confusion matrix we need a dataset with expected outcome values, and a test dataset with predicted outcome values. In our experiment, the dataset with expected outcome value corresponds to the 128 sequences that we have taken from the training dataset obtained after performing the k-means algorithm. While the test dataset with predicted outcome values corresponds to the same 128 sequences after removing their LSCs' classes and predicting them again using the naive Bayes classifier. Therefore we have obtained a confusion matrix with sixteen LSCs' classes, where for each class we have computed the number of correct and incorrect predictions using the expected and predicted classes' values.

To compute the confusion matrix and the validation metrics described in the precedent subsection we have used the R with the package caret, the following subsection describes the obtained results.

5.3   Results and Discussion

A well performed model should have for each class a high Precision (PPV), NPV, Recall (Sensitivity) and Specificity that are perfectly 1, and it should also have a high Accuracy.

The captured picture below shows the results obtained after computing the confusion matrix using R with the package caret. As can be noticed, all the validation metrics mentioned above have high values, so we can say that the classifier used in our approach has well performed (Fig. 3).

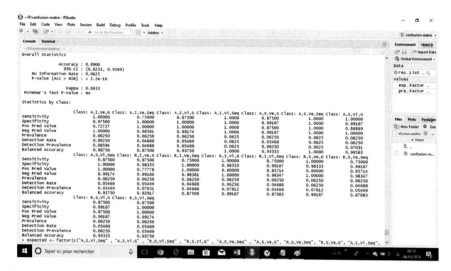

Fig. 3. The confusion matrix obtained from the expected and predicted datasets used in the experiment

6 Conclusion

In this work, we have proposed an approach which aims to predict the learners' learning style automatically, this approach consists of two steps; in the first step the learners' sequences were extracted from the log file then transformed to an input of the K means algorithm. The k means algorithm was used to group students into sixteen clusters based on FSLSM, where each cluster was labeled with a learning style combination. The second step consists in performing an unsupervised algorithm (Naive Bayes) to predict the LS for a new sequence. We evaluated the performance of our approach using the confusion matrix. The produced results show that our approach performs well. In the future work we will have compared the performance of the naive Bayes classifier with other machine learning techniques such as the neural networks and decision tree.

References

1. Laschinger, H.K., Boss, M.W.: Learning styles of nursing students and career choices. J. Adv. Nurs. **9**(4), 375–380 (1984)
2. Felder, R.M., Silverman, L.K.: Learning and teaching styles in engineering education. Eng. Educ. **78**(7), 674–681 (1988)
3. Biggs, J.: Study process questionnaire manual. Student approaches to learning and studying (1987)
4. Graf, S., Kinshuk.: Advanced adaptivity in learning management systems by considering learning styles. In: 2009 IEEE/WIC/ACM International Joint Conference on Web Intelligence and Intelligent Agent Technology, vol. 3, pp. 235–238 (2009)

5. Kuljis, J., Liu, F.: A Comparison of learning style theories on the suitability for elearning. In: IASTED International Conference on Web Technologies, Applications, and Services, pp. 191–197 (2005)
6. Garity, J.: Learning styles basis for creative teaching and learning. Nurse Educ. **10**(2), 12–16 (1985)
7. Keefe, J.W.: Learning style: an overview. Student Learn. styles Diagnosing Prescr. Programs **1**, 1–17 (1979)
8. Chandola, V., Banerjee, A., Kumar, V.: Anomaly detection: a survey. ACM Comput. Surv. **41**(3), 1–18 (2009)
9. Huang, Z.: Extensions to the k-means algorithm for clustering large data sets with categorical values. Data Min. Knowl. Discov. **2**(3), 283–304 (1998)
10. Kaufman, L., Rousseeuw, P.J.: Partitioning around medoids (Program PAM). In: Finding Groups in Data: An Introduction to Cluster Analysis, pp. 1–67 (2008)
11. EMC.: Data Science & Analytics: Discovering, Analyzing, Visualizing and Presenting Data. Willey, India (2015)
12. Richert, W., Coelho, L.P.: Building Machine Learning Systems with Python, 1st edn. Packt Publishing Ltd., Birmingham (2013)
13. Feldman, J., Monteserin, A., Amandi, A.: Automatic detection of learning styles: state of the art. Artif. Intell. Rev. **44**(2), 157–186 (2015)
14. García, P., Amandi, A., Schiaffino, S., Campo, M.: Using Bayesian networks to detect students' learning styles in a web-based education system. In: Argentine Symposium on Artificial Intelligence (ASAI'2005), vol. 11, pp. 115–126 (2005)
15. Bunt, A., Conati, C.: Probabilistic student modelling to improve exploratory behaviour. User Model. User-Adapted Interact. **13**(3), 269–309 (2003)
16. Kalhoro, A.A., Rajper, S., Mallah, G.A.: Detection of E-learners' learning styles: an automatic approach using decision tree. Int. J. Comput. Sci. Inf. Secur. **14**(8), 420–425 (2016)
17. Pantho, O., Tiantong, M.: Using decision tree C4. 5 algorithm to predict VARK learning styles. Int. J. Comput. Internet Manage. **24**(2), 58–63 (2016)
18. Hmedna, B., El Mezouary, A., Baz, O., Mammass, D.: A machine learning approach to identify and track learning styles in MOOCs. In: 2016 5th International Conference on Multimedia Computing and Systems (ICMCS), pp. 212–216 (2016)
19. Chang, Y.C., Kao, W.Y., Chu, C.P., Chiu, C.H.: A learning style classification mechanism for e-learning. Comput. Educ. **53**(2), 273–285 (2009)
20. El Allioui, Y.: Advanced prediction of learner's profile based on felder silverman learning styles using web usage mining approach and fuzzy C-means algorithm. Int. J. Comput. Aided Eng. Technol. (in press)
21. El Aissaoui, O., El Madani El Alami, Y., Oughdir, L., El Allioui, Y.: Integrating web usage mining for an automatic learner profile detection: a learning styles-based approach. In: 2018 International Conference on Intelligent Systems and Computer Vision (ISCV), pp. 1–6 (2018)

Toward Adaptive and Reusable Learning Content Using XML Dynamic Labeling Schemes and Relational Databases

Zakaria Bousalem[1(✉)], Inssaf El Guabassi[2], and Ilias Cherti[1]

[1] Faculty of Sciences and Technologies, Hassan 1st University, Settat, Morocco
zakaria.bousalem@gmail.com
[2] Faculty of Sciences, Tetuan, Morocco

Abstract. A learning object is "any digital resource that can be reused to support learning." A learning object should meet several characteristics: interoperability, reusability, self-contentedness, accessibility, durability and adaptability. In order to achieve the accessibility, reusability and interoperability and in the aim of allowing learners the freedom to choose the learning objects they wish to appear in their courses we propose an approach to build an adaptive and reusable learning content. The general idea of our paper is to automatically generate a course for each learner according to his individual preferences to ensure a better adaptation. For this aim we opted for the XML language to represent the course materiel. So as to avoid the weaknesses of XML databases and to benefit from the strengths of Relational databases, the XML document of the course materiel will be stored in Relational databases and in order to identify the relationships between nodes and accelerate the query processing, we use the XML labeling schemes.

Keywords: Learning object · Adaptive learning · XML · Relational databases · XML labeling schemes

1 Introduction

E-learning is being considered as a widely recognized option to address drawbacks of traditional learning environment [1]. Adaptive educational systems are designed for the purpose of allowing learners the freedom to choose the learning objects they wish to appear in their courses. Yet, learning objects have several characteristics such as: interoperability, reusability, self-contentedness, accessibility, durability and adaptability [2]. The accessibility, reusability and interoperability can be achieved by using XML Language [3]. The XML language is a widely recognized standard to ensure the portability of data using structural and semantic markup. Thanks to its nesting and the fact that contains both the data itself and information about their structure (self-describing structure), it provides a simple and flexible way for applications to model and exchange data in a way that is readable by humans and easily verified, transformed, and published.

There are three approaches to storing XML data. The first is a native XML repository that supports XML data models and query languages directly (Native XML

© Springer Nature Switzerland AG 2019
M. Ezziyyani (Ed.): AI2SD 2018, AISC 915, pp. 787–799, 2019.
https://doi.org/10.1007/978-3-030-11928-7_71

Databases). The second is storing the data in Relational tables via Relational databases (RDB) and finally, storing the XML data in the first approach suffers from several limitations (like access control information, returns the data only as a XML format…). To overcome these limitations many approaches [4–6] have been proposed, for taking advantages of the mature technologies that are provided by current relational DBMSs (like indexes, triggers, data integrity, security and query optimization by SQL), and also in order to exploit the full power of this technology.

In this paper we will propose an approach that aims to support learners by supplying them with course materials. There are several technologies to represent a structured course. In our approach we opted for the XML language to represent them. So as to overcome limitations of XML databases and to exploit advantages of Relational databases, the XML document of the course materiel will be stored in Relational databases and in order to identify the relationships between nodes and accelerate the query processing, we use the XML labeling schemes.

The remaining of the paper is organized as follows: Sect. 2 concentrates on background; in this section we briefly present the Adaptive educational systems and XML Labeling Schemes. In Sect. 3, we present our approach. Finally, Sect. 4 concludes our paper.

2   Background

2.1   Adaptive Educational Systems

E-learning is being considered as a widely recognized option to address drawbacks of traditional learning environment. E-learning can be defined as the use of the Internet and its technologies to deliver a broad array of solutions, that enhance knowledge of the learners through a computer interface.

Adaptive educational systems (AESs) is based on the principle that every learner is unique and has a different experiences, educational needs, background, level, learning style, etc.

The goal of AESs is being able to capture those differences, and then translate them into training processes and contents which are relevant for each individual learner.

The components of Adaptive educational systems (AESs) have the following building blocks, as show in Fig. 1:

- Educational Resources Model: Represents the set of knowledge that needs to be transmitted to learner.
- Learner model: Represents information about the interests, knowledge, skills, preferences, level, learning style, etc. of each learner.
- Learning model: Contains the intelligence that making decisions about which content elements, (examples, definitions, illustrations, exercises, materials, etc.) will be presented to the learner in order to acquire the knowledge contained within the educational resources model. The learning model bridges the gap between the knowledge and the learner.

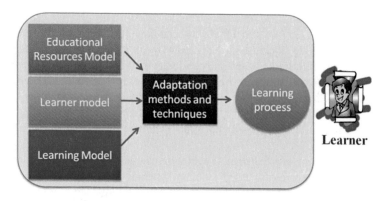

Fig. 1. Components of an adaptive learning system

2.2 XML Labeling Schemes

XML Labeling Schemes: An Overview. With the increasing popularity of XML in data exchange and in order to facilitate the queries processing, achieve efficient indexing and also preserve relationships between nodes to quickly determine the ancestor-descendant, parent-child, sibling and ordering structural relationships [7] many approaches have been proposed. These approaches can be classified into two types [8–10]: (i) static labeling schemes that can deals with static XML documents [11–14] and the most crucial type; (ii) dynamic labeling schemes which are adequate for XML documents that are frequently updated.

Labeling Schemes Taxonomy. XML labeling schemes can be divided into four categories [9, 15–17], that is, interval-based labeling schemes, Prefix-based schemes, Multiplicative labeling schemes, Hybrid labeling schemes:

(a) *Interval-Based Labeling Schemes.* (also known as Containment labeling schemes, Range-based labeling schemes, or Region Encoded labeling schemes) [9] it's the simplest category, it consist to decode the (i) startPos and endPos by using the depth first traversal of the XML Data tree or by counting the number of words or letters from the beginning of the document at the start of the element and the end of the element, respectively and (ii) level of the node in the document is the depth of the element in the XML Data tree [18] the main strength of this category is that the label of the node is usually compact however this XML labeling scheme category suffer from decline in performance in an update intensive environment [16]. According to Almelibari [19] the labeling schemes into this category can be divided into three forms; the containment labeling schemes [20], the pre-post labeling [21] and the order/size schemes [11]. The ancestor–descendant or parent–child structural information of two nodes in XML Data tree N1 and N2 can be extracted by using these two rules: (i) ancestor–descendant: N2 is descendant of N1 if and only if N1.start < N2.start and N2.end < N1.end (ii) parent–child: N2 is a child of N1 if and only if N2 is a descendant of N1 and N2.level = N1.level + 1. There are many approaches in this category like [11, 20, 22–24].

(b) *Prefix-Based Schemes.* Prefix-based labeling systems(also known as path-based labeling schemes) [16] are structured such that they directly encode the parent label as a prefix of a node label into an XML data tree by using depth-first tree traversal [13, 17]. Thus, determining the ancestor/descendant and parent/child relationships between two nodes is simply to find out if one label is a prefix to another [25, 26]. After the labeling process the final node label is composed of a set of labels separated by a delimiter ("." Or ";") each one of them represents the local order of the node among nodes of its ancestor. There are many approaches in this category like [13, 17, 27–31].

(c) *Multiplicative Labeling Schemes.* Several researchers [9, 26, 32, 33] report the weaknesses of the Interval-based labeling schemes approaches. They claim that this approaches group generates long labels which require a large storage space and affect the query processing [9, 34] also this type of approaches does not identify the Sibling relationship [33, 34]. The prefix labeling approaches are also suffering from several drawbacks. Al-Shaikh et al. [32] states that the labels and separators generated require a very large storage space in case of deep trees, which affects the space required for labels storage as well as the performance of query processing. To overcome these problems, researchers have proposed the Multiplicative labeling schemes. This labeling schemes class uses atomic numbers based on arithmetic properties to label nodes and use mathematical operations to identify the structural relationships between nodes [9, 26], usually A-D and P-C relationships. The fact that this type of labeling schemes uses atomic numbers to label nodes and mathematical operations to identify structural relationships, that's simplify query processing and minimizes label storage space [9] but they are costly in computation processes [19].

(d) *Hybrid Labeling Schemes.* This class of XML labeling schemes consists to combine two or more approaches by using their strengths and overcoming their weaknesses with the aim of speeding up the query processing and minimizing the storage space of nodes labels [9, 34].

3   Our Approach

The general idea is to automatically generate a course for each learner according to his/her individual preferences, but the problematic is how to structure, store and index the learning contents to ensure a better adaptation. For this aim we opted for the XML language to represent our course materiel. So as to avoid the weaknesses of XML databases and to benefit from the strengths of Relational databases, the XML document of the course materiel will be stored in Relational databases and in order to identify the relationships between nodes and accelerate the query processing, we use the XML labeling schemes.

As described in Fig. 2 "Data Mapper" Component maps XML document that contains the course materiel into Relational database using the "DOM Parser" that gives as result a "XML DOM Tree". The function "XMap.TreeBrowser" iterates the "XML DOM Tree" and executes the SQL insert statement to store the XML data in

RDB, The role of "Query Mapper" Component is to translate the XML Query to SQL statement and launch it in the database engine to obtain the results. "Relational to XMap Mapper" Component reconstructs XML document from RDB by transforming the SQL Result to hierarchical data format (XML) that contains the learning object adapted to learner preferences.

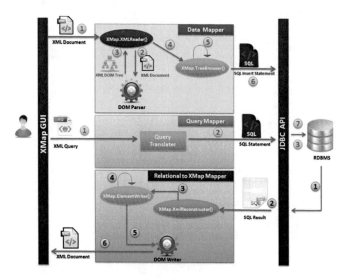

Fig. 2. The proposed model for mapping process [4]

3.1   Course Material

In this section we will introduce the course components, which is an essential element in all learning systems.

We create the structure of a personalized course, by specifying the different layers constituting a course, based on content hierarchy of Duval and Hodgins [35] as shown in Fig. 3, and by presenting the course using XML language.

- Raw Media Elements: Include a single sentence or paragraph, example, exercise, illustration, animation, etc.
- Information Objects: contain sets of raw media elements
- Learning Objects: contain information objects
- Aggregate Assemblies: This level corresponds with lessons or chapters

The structure of the course is illustrated in Fig. 4, with a focus on the "Python introduction" unit.

The course structure comprises four levels: Course, Unit, Learning object and Concept.

Modular Content Hierarchy

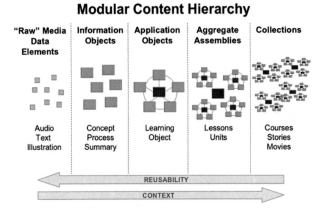

Fig. 3. Content hierarchy

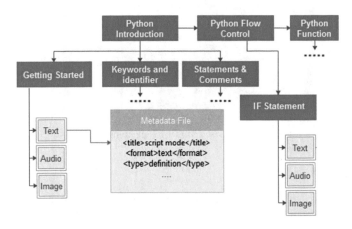

Fig. 4. Python course hierarchical organization

- Course: Describes the pedagogical resource, each resource has several units.
- Unit: Represents the parts that constitute a course, each unit contain several Learning objects.
- Concept: Describes the set of concepts for a given unit, these concepts are linked by relationships.
- Learning object: Describes the content of resources; it includes four types of content: Definition, Illustration, Example, and Exercise. These types are represented in different formats (text, image, and audio).

Figure 5 represents the XML course document for the Python course.

```xml
<?xml version="1.0" encoding="UTF-8"?>
<course>
    <about>
        <title>Python</title>
        <identifier>C1234F</identifier>
        <level>beginner</level>
        <authors>Zakaria BOUSALEM</authors>
        <keywords>Python, Python programming</keywords>
    </about>
    <unit title="Python introduction" number="1">
        <concept title="Getting starting">
                <text>Python is a cross-platform programming ...</text>
                <image>whatIsPython.png</image>
                <audio>whatIsPython.mp3</audio>
        </concept>
    </unit>
    <unit title="Python control flow " number="2">
        <concept title="The if statement">
                <text>The if statement is used to check a condition: ...</text>
                <image>ifStatement.png</image>
                <audio>ifStatement.mp3</audio>
        </concept>
    </unit>
</course>
```

Fig. 5. The XML document for the Python course

3.2 Labeling Schemes and Course Material

In this section we will give a brief presentation of some XML dynamic labeling schemes that allow update in XML document. Since our course materiel will be presented in XML language and it can be arbitrary updated, we will apply those XML dynamic labeling schemes in the XML tree (Fig. 6) of our course material in Fig. 5. After the labeling of the XML document of our course materiel, the generated XML document will be stored in Relational databases as shown in Fig. 2.

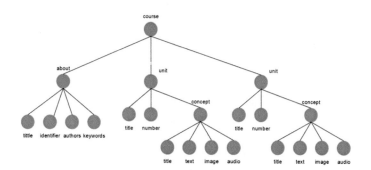

Fig. 6. Python course in tree representation

ORDPATH Labeling Scheme. ORDPATH is the first labeling system that allows overcoming the re-labeling in case of structure update. Besides its effectiveness in insertion and compression, ORDPATH [27] is conceptually similar to the Dewey technique.

ORDPATH provides the possibility of effective insertion at any position in an XML document. The changes in the structure of an XML tree can be done in several ways:

- New sub-trees can be inserted.
- Sub-trees can be removed.
- Sub-trees can be moved in the tree.

ORDPATH materializes the parent-child relationship in the ID attribute. The concept is to set the child node by concatenating the label of the parent with the local ID of the Child (e.g. 1.3 is the parent node ID of 1.3.5).

In initial load only odd, positive integers are assigned. The other integers (even-numbers and negatives) are reserved for later insertions.

For inserting a new node X between two existing nodes, we use even numbers for example, to insert a new node between two nodes: 1.3.5 and 1.3.7, the new id is 1.3.6.1.

However, this technique is less compact; due to its insertion mechanism it wastes half of the total numbers [9, 19, 34]; it's not suitable for deeper trees. Figure 7 shows the XML tree of our course materiel labeled with ORDPATH. The grey nodes with dashed edge indicating newly inserted nodes.

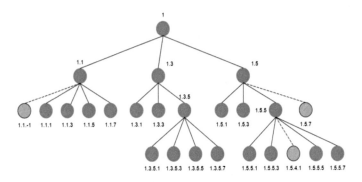

Fig. 7. ORDPATH labeling scheme

Dynamic XDAS. Dynamic XDAS [34] approach can be classified in Hybrid labeling schemes category; it uses IBSL approach [36] to avoid relabeling nodes in update processing. To label nodes, Dynamic XDAS uses IP addressing and subnetting technique commonly used in computer networks. In labeling phase Dynamic XDAS set to each node a label in the form of <Level, Number> where Level is the depth of the node in the document, it's represented only by one byte and Number is generated using IP addressing and subnetting technique, it's represented using hexadecimal numbers which minimize the space required for the storage of labels. To identify the ancestor-descendant, parent-Child and Sibling structural relationships, Dynamic XDAS uses logical operations which improve significantly the time needed to determine the relationships between nodes.

Ghaleb et al. have modified the IBSL approach to be compatible with the original XDAS. For insertion operation, there are four main cases in modified approach:

- Insert a node before the leftmost node (2 sub-cases)
- Insert a node after the rightmost node (2 sub-cases)

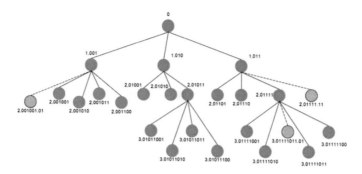

Fig. 8. Dynamic XDAS labeling scheme

- Insert a node between any two nodes at any position (3 sub-cases)
- Insert a sub-tree at any position of the tree (1 sub-case)

Figure 8 shows the XML tree of our course materiel labeled with Dynamic XDAS. The grey nodes with dashed edge indicating newly inserted nodes. There are 8 sub-cases of node insertion operation; in this figure only three are applied.

GroupBased Approach. This approach [19] is based on the parent-child grouping in order to rapidly identify the structural relationships and to ease insertion of new nodes in the XML document knowing that the dealt with small tree structure is easy than the dealt with big tree structure.

In this technique each node has two labels; global label and local label. The global label is used to identify easily the relationships between nodes by linking the small groups to the whole tree. The role of local label is to facilitate performing the identification of structural relationships and insertion operations in the same group.

The labeling process is involved in two steps:

1. First step: consists to divide the whole XML tree to simple groups which contain each node with its child nodes. Each simple group will be labeled by a global label which composed by two parts. The first part is the Dewey label. In order to maintain the document order this approach uses the second part which is the order of the child node from left to right.
2. Second step: consists to set the local label to each node.

This approach can identify the ancestor-descendant, parent-Child, Sibling, Lowest Common Ancestor and ordering structural relationships.

For insertion operation, the GroupBased approach has four main cases:

- Leftmost insertion (2 sub-cases)
- Rightmost insertion (2 sub-cases)
- Insertion between two siblings (3 sub-cases)
- Insertion below a Leaf Node (2 sub-cases)

Figure 9 shows the XML tree of our course materiel labeled with GroupBased Approach. The grey nodes with dashed edge indicating newly inserted nodes. There are 9 sub-cases of node insertion operation; in this figure only three are applied.

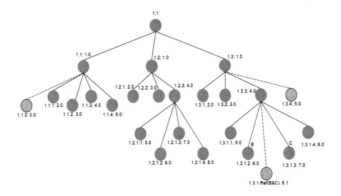

Fig. 9. GroupBased approach labeling scheme

Dynamic Prefix-based Labeling Scheme (DPLS). DPLS [17] can be categorized in Prefix-based schemes class. DPLS has a distinguishing characteristic that is, reusing the deleted node labels when frequent insertions and deletions occur. The objective of this approach is to significantly reduce the update and query processing time, to minimize the space required for the storage of node labels and to avoid relabeling nodes in dynamic context. DPLS uses Dewey labeling scheme in initial labeling phase.

For insertion operation, the DPLS approach has four main cases:

- Leftmost insertion
- Rightmost insertion:
- Insertion between two siblings:
- Insertion below a Leaf Node

Yet, to insert new node between two siblings, DPLS uses fractional part for the node self-label component as a floating-point number. Furthermore, to overcome the overflow problems related to fraction representation, DPLS adopt variable-length storage format used in ORDPATH approach.

Figure 10 shows the XML tree of our course materiel labeled with GroupBased Approach. The grey nodes with dashed edge indicating newly inserted nodes.

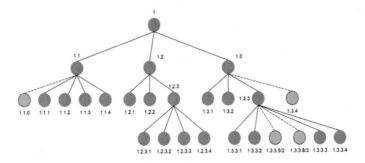

Fig. 10. DPLS labeling scheme

Moreover, in order to reduce the node labels size, DPLS approach uses the "reduction technique" when insertions between two siblings and deletions take place alternately.

4 Conclusion and Future Work

In this paper we proposed an approach to build an adaptive and reusable learning content by using the XML language to represent the course materiel. The XML document of the course materiel will be stored in Relational databases and in order to identify the relationships between nodes and accelerate the query processing, we use the XML labeling schemes. The benefit of this approach is to avoid limitations of XML databases and benefit from the strengths of the mature technologies that are provided by current relational DBMSs. To further our research we plan to implement the four XML labeling schemes presented in our paper (ORDPATH, Dynamic XDAS, GroupBased Approach and DPLS) then evaluate and compare the efficiency of these approaches in term of size of generated databases and time of query processing to choose the right one for our approach and finally compare our presented approach with others approaches.

References

1. Deborah, L.J., Baskaran, R., Kannan, A.: Learning styles assessment and theoretical origin in an E-learning scenario: a survey. Artif. Intell. Rev. **42**(4), 801–819
2. Chawla, S., Gupta, N., Singla, R.K.: LOQES: model for evaluation of learning object. Int. J. Adv. Comput. Sci. Appl. (IJACSA) **3**(7) (2012)
3. Bray, T., Paoli, J., Sperberg-McQueen, Michael, C., et al.: Extensible markup language (XML). World Wide Web J. **2**(4), 27–66 (1997)
4. Bousalem, Z., Cherti, I.: XMap: a novel approach to store and retrieve XML document in relational databases. JSW **10**(12), 1389–1401 (2015)
5. Qtaish, A., Ahmad, K.: XAncestor: an efficient mapping approach for storing and querying XML documents in relational database using path-based technique. Knowl. Based Syst. **114**, 167–192 (2016)
6. Zhu, H., Yu, H., Fan, G., et al.: Mini-XML: An efficient mapping approach between XML and relational database. In: 16th International Conference on. IEEE Computer and Information Science (ICIS). IEEE/ACIS, pp. 839–843 (2017)
7. Gabillon, A., Fansi, M.: A new persistent labelling scheme for XML. J. Digital Inform. Manage. **4**(2), 5 (2006)
8. Lu, J.: XML Labeling scheme. In: An Introduction to XML Query Processing and Keyword Search, pp. 9–32. Springer, Berlin (2013)
9. Al Zadjali, H.: Compressing labels of dynamic XML data using base-9 scheme and Fibonacci encoding. Thèse de doctorat. University of Sheffield (2017)
10. Thonangi, R.: A concise labeling scheme for XML data, pp. 4–14. In: COMAD (2006)
11. Li, Q., Moon, B., et al.: Indexing and querying XML data for regular path expressions. In: VLDB, pp. 361–370 (2001)

12. Bruno, N., Koudas, N., Srivastava, D.: Holistic twig joins: optimal XML pattern matching. In: Proceedings of the 2002 ACM SIGMOD International Conference on Management of Data, pp. 310–321. ACM (2002)
13. Tatarinov, I., Viglas, S.D., Beyer, K., et al.: Storing and querying ordered XML using a relational database system. In: Proceedings of the 2002 ACM SIGMOD International Conference on Management of Data, pp. 204–2015. ACM (2002)
14. Lu, J., Ling, T.W., Chan, C.-Y., et al.: From region encoding to extended dewey: on efficient processing of XML twig pattern matching. In: Proceedings of the 31st International Conference on Very Large Data Bases, pp. 193–204. VLDB Endowment (2005)
15. Nguyen, X.-T., Haw, S.-C., Subramaniam, S., et al.: Dynamic node labeling schemes for XML updates
16. Haw, S.-C., Lee, C.-S.: Data storage practices and query processing in XML databases: a survey. Knowl. Based Syst. **24**(8), 1317–1340 (2011)
17. Liu, J., Zhang, X.: Dynamic labeling scheme for XML updates. Knowl. Based Syst. **106**, 135–149 (2016)
18. Al-Khalifa, S., Jagadish, H.V., Koudas, N., et al.: Structural joins: a primitive for efficient XML query pattern matching. In: 18th International Conference on Data Engineering, pp. 141–152. IEEE (2002)
19. Almelibari, A.: Labelling Dynamic XML Documents: A GroupBased Approach. University of Sheffield, Sheffield (2015)
20. Zhang, C., Naughton, J., Dewitt, D., et al.: On supporting containment queries in relational database management systems. In: ACM Sigmod Record, pp. 425–436. ACM (2001)
21. Dietz, P.F.: Maintaining order in a linked list. In: Proceedings of the Fourteenth Annual ACM Symposium on Theory of Computing, pp. 122–127. ACM (1982)
22. Amagasa, T., Yoshikawa, M., Uemura, S.: QRS: a robust numbering scheme for XML documents. In: 19th International Conference on Data Engineering, pp. 705–707. IEEE (2003)
23. Min, J.-K., Lee, J., Chung, C.-W.: An efficient XML encoding and labeling method for query processing and updating on dynamic XML data. J. Syst. Software **82**(3), 503–515 (2009)
24. Subramaniam, S., Haw, S.-C., Soon, L.-K.: Relab: a subtree based labeling scheme for efficient XML query processing. In: 2014 IEEE 2nd International Symposium on Telecommunication Technologies (ISTT), pp. 121–125. IEEE (2014)
25. Assefa, B.G., Ergenc, B.: Order based labeling scheme for dynamic XML query processing. In: International Conference on Availability, Reliability, and Security, pp. 287–301. Springer, Berlin, Heidelberg (2012)
26. Al-Khazraji, S.H.A.: A labelling technique comparison for indexing large XML database. Dissertation, University of Sheffield (2017)
27. O'neil, P., O'neil, E., Pal, S., et al.: ORDPATHs: insert-friendly XML node labels. In: Proceedings of the 2004 ACM SIGMOD International Conference on Management of Data, pp. 903–908. ACM (2004)
28. Duong, M., Zhang, Y.: LSDX: a new labelling scheme for dynamically updating XML data. In: Proceedings of the 16th Australasian Database Conference, vol. 39, pp. 185–193. Australian Computer Society, Inc. (2005)
29. Cohen, E., Kaplan, H., Milo, T.: Labeling dynamic XML trees. SIAM J. Comput. **39**(5), 2048–2074 (2010)
30. Liu, J., Ma, Z.M., Yan, L.: Efficient labeling scheme for dynamic XML trees. Inform. Sci. **221**, 338–354 (2013)

31. Xu, L., Ling, T.W., Wu, H., et al.: DDE: from dewey to a fully dynamic XML labeling scheme. In: Proceedings of the 2009 ACM SIGMOD International Conference on Management of Data, pp. 719–730. ACM (2009)
32. Al-Shaikh, R., Hashim, G., Binhuraib, A.R., et al.: A modulo-based labeling scheme for dynamically ordered XML trees. In: 2010 Fifth International Conference on Digital Information Management (ICDIM), pp. 213–221. IEEE (2010)
33. Fu, L., Meng, X.: Triple code: an efficient labeling scheme for query answering in XML data. In: 10th IEEE Web Information System and Application Conference (WISA), pp. 42–47 (2013)
34. Ghaleb, T.A., Mohammed, S.: A dynamic labeling scheme based on logical operators: a support for order-sensitive XML updates. Proc. Comput. Sci. 57, 1211–1218 (2015)
35. Duval, E., Hodgins, W.: A LOM research agenda. In: WWW (Alternate Paper Tracks) (2003)
36. Ko, H.-K., Lee, S.K.: A binary string approach for updates in dynamic ordered XML data. IEEE Trans. Knowl. Data Eng. 22(4), 602–607 (2010)
37. Zniber, N., Cauvet, C.: Systèmes pédagogiques adaptatifs: état de l'art et perspectives. In: MajecSTIC 2005: Manifestation des Jeunes Chercheurs francophones dans les domaines des STIC, pp. 300–315 (2005)

A Honey Net, Big Data and RNN Architecture for Automatic Security Monitoring of Information System

Alaeddine Boukhalfa$^{(\boxtimes)}$, Nabil Hmina, and Habiba Chaoui

Ibn Tofail University, Kenitra, Morocco
{alaeddine.boukhalfa, mejhed90}@gmail.com,
hmina@univ-ibntofail.ac.ma

Abstract. The security monitoring of the information system represents a major concern for organizations. Attackers can use multiple and different ways to harm or abuse system resources, this variety of attacks raises issues related to how to treat it. In addition, these attacks can evolve and be undetectable by the existing methods of security. To solve these problems, we propose, in this paper, the implementation of an automatic security monitoring system of the information system, based on exposing Honeypots and collecting data of attacks from them, storing the variety of attacks using Big Data techniques, and processing and analyzing them by Recurrent Neural Network (RNN) which is a Deep Leaning method, in order to extract knowledge from these threats and face the others unknown similar.

Keywords: NIDS · Security monitoring · Big data · Deep learning · RNN · Honeypot · Honey net

1 Introduction

Currently, with the rapid evolution of information technology and its large application in all life domains, the detection and prevention of intrusions constitute a major security challenges. The role of Network Intrusion Detection Systems (NIDS) is to inspect and analyze data traffic passing through network in order to detect anomalies, and raise an alert or block communication between the communicating entities. This analyze is based on predefined algorithms and rules that rely on signatures or suspected traffic behavior.

Moreover, attackers and intruders are always trying with impatience to find new means and possibilities to destroy the security obstacles and attack the system. While current methods of analysis and detection of the NIDS are inefficient, they do not evolve to automatically detect and reveal this unidentified new manner of attacks. What makes thinking about smart new methods of analysis and recognition which can adapt to changing aspects of menaces.

In addition, attacks can be of different shapes like SQL Injection or probing attacks, this issue of variety of attacks pushes us to find solution to treat them all in a unique way.

© Springer Nature Switzerland AG 2019
M. Ezziyyani (Ed.): AI2SD 2018, AISC 915, pp. 800–808, 2019.
https://doi.org/10.1007/978-3-030-11928-7_72

To solve these problems, we have proposed, in this paper, architecture of a local organization network which evolves to detect automatically intrusions. This new approach relies on attracting attackers and gathering there attacks using Honeypots, storing the variety of attacks with a Big Data storage system, and applying the Recurrent Neural Network (RNN) which is a Deep Learning method in order to recognize attacks and exploit it to stop new threats.

The paper has the following structure. We provide an overview of related work in Sect. 2. In Sect. 3 we present our proposed architecture. Sect. 4 is reserved for conclusion and future work.

2 Related Work

The idea of a NIDS based on Deep Learning was discussed in [1], the authors applied Self-Taught Learning (STL) which is a Deep Learning approach on a set of traffic data of network called NSL KDD [2], which contains normal records and attack records. They compared the attack recognition performance with an old classification method Soft-Max Regression (SMR) and proved with experimentations that the STL recognizes attacks better. This solution presents a good approach to distinguish normal traffic from suspected traffic, but no illustration of the implementation of NIDS in the real world is described.

Almost the same work was done in [3], KDD CUP 99 [4] which is an old version of NSL KDD and which also gathers the traffic data, was used to perform a precision benchmarking of traffic detection, between Support Vector Machine method based on Restricted Boltzmann Machine (SVM-RBMs) [5], and classic classification methods. The researchers do not showed any proof of choice of the employed Deep Learning method. The study concluded clearly that SVM-RBMs can better identify the origin of threats and it takes evidently less time processing big amount of data.

In the paper [6], a new approach to detect code injection attacks have been established. A new hybrid of Deep Learning called Hybrid Deep Learning Network (HDLN) was built. The injection attacks are attached to JavaScript code. They used the Abstract Syntax Tree (AST) to identify more features and employed three methods to distinguish key features. HDLN has been evaluated, firstly, relatively to the number of hidden layer, the number of filters and number of neurons, the results showed that the accuracy is higher as the number of filters increases. Secondly, it was evaluated against the other traditional classifiers using IG feature vectors, the accuracy was greater than all the other classifiers. Finally, they compared the precision of the model to a work of a machine learning already done by the team, they showed that this modern model is more efficient than the previous. The submitted effort is prestigious, except that they only focused on injection attacks related to JavaScript code and not all kinds of attacks. Thanks to this solution.

Paper [7] proposes also a hybrid of Deep Learning which combines Auto-Encoder and DBN. The Auto-Encoder was employed in order to decrease the dimensionality of data and identify the principal features of data, whereas the DBN had the role of discovering the malicious code. The new Deep Learning was applied on KDD CUP 99 [4], and assessed against the DBN alone, the results indicated effectively that the new

Deep Learning is the best in term of accuracy, and it consumes less time than the DNB. The authors have not specified the motivation to use this combination of DBN and Auto-Encoder to form the presented Deep Learning model.

A distributed way to detect attacks in the space of Internet of Things (IoT) was adopted in [8], the authors applied Deep Learning on each node of fog-to-things networks, the purpose was to obtain independence of identifying locally attacks and sharing parameters with neighbors, in order to accelerate the identification and optimize the update of parameters. The safety of system was verified by NSL KDD [2], and Big Data management system Spark to concretize the design of fog nodes. The results were demonstrated that the scattered concept is better effective then centralized conception and Shallow Learning which is a machine learning method. The proposal is very interesting, it is an advanced and significant enhancement of detection, except that the researchers have not shown exactly which method of the Deep Learning family have been adopted.

In an environment where Big Data transits, network security monitoring was discussed, the manuscript [9] cited, in the first, the raisons of need of network security monitoring which are prediction issues, security devices and mechanisms are not suitable for amount data environments, abnormal alarm must be detected quickly and equitable diagnostics of alert information must be done, the correlation algorithms are employed only for anomaly identification and not for the full devises and tools for network security. Secondly the authors illustrate a network security monitoring system based on accumulation of Big Data, its integration which consists of purification and classification, and analyzing to extract information to expose it in order to make decisions. Finally, they give an overview on some correlation algorithms used for analyzing data. The paper proposed a schema of a security monitoring system but it did not think about improving correlation methods to effectively accompany the evolution of attacks.

Another approach for security monitoring of Internet of Things (IoT) networks was debated in [10], a big and variety of security logs was gathered from consumer electronic devices, then it was stored in a parallel way in the nodes of Big Data management system Hadoop, the operation of normalization was applied to get a unique format of data, the analysis was performed by applying methods of aggregation and correlation adopting Complex Event Processing (CEP) which aims to detect and analyze information contained in the events then take action in real time, the results was visualized using advanced tools of visualization. The principle of the article is founded solely on displaying and reporting data without taking action against attacks.

Our work will be different by comparing it with the existing works, it is a concrete representation of a system of security monitoring of the organization network, it treats any type of attack and will be evolutionary to take decisions against the new threats.

3 System Architecture

3.1 Components

The proposed architecture of monitoring security of information system is described in Fig. 1, it is based on the establishment of the mechanisms of the collection and analysis of attacks, to infer knowledge from them and to cope with others which have some points of resemblance. It is composed of an organization network separated by two firewalls. We depict the components one by one:

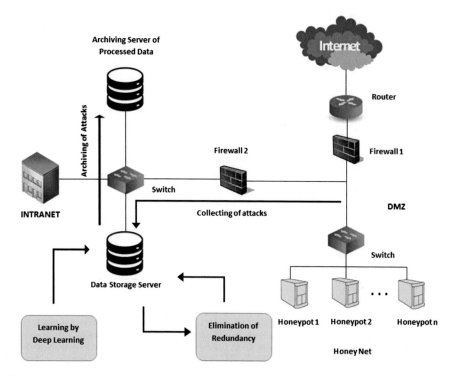

Fig. 1. Architecture of automatic security monitoring of the information system based on Honey Net, Big Data and RNN

Demilitarized Zone

The Demilitarized Zone (DMZ) is an isolated subnet of the local network and the internet. It contains:

Honey Net

Honeypots are devices dedicated to attract attackers and record information about their attacks. So, any attempt to interact with a Honeypot server is a proof of an unwanted activity.

The interaction level of a Honeypot defines at which point the intruder can attack the system. Low interaction Honeypots minimize the level of interaction of the provided services, however, attackers can easily reveal their natures. Medium interaction Honeypots have a reduced set of services with some ability to hide from the attackers. With a high interaction level, Honeypots expose themselves as attractive real machines with complete operating systems.

Research Honeypots are intended for scientific research, they are used only to memorize intrusion attempts, contrary to production Honeypots which protect the system and take action when it is about menace [11].

We opt for a collection of a high interaction research Honeypots which constitutes a Honey Net to gather as much data as possible, the non-use of production Honeypots lies in the fact that an action produced against threats may make the hackers believing that the machine is monitored, however, we want them to keep attacking and using more means, it will help us to gather more data. Therefore, our Honeypots will play the role of a network machines with security flaws intended to be attacked from the internet.

Firewall 1

Honeypots are attractive, we have to think about the prevention of our network. The Firewall 1 is configured to block traffic coming from the internet to the local network to ensure its security, and allow only traffic from the internet to the DMZ. Thus, we offer permission to intruders to attack Honeypots from the internet.

Firewall 2

Firewall 2 will stop all traffic to prevent intruders from infiltrating via Honeypots, and allow only traffic coming from a specific ports dedicated for loading data from Honeypots to our production machines.

In order to obtain more security, we try to get the two firewalls from two different builders because they will have different security bugs, this will enhance the security of our local network [12].

Thus, in case of compromise of our local network, two obstacles must be overcome.

Intranet

It is our network of organizations which groups production machines, in addition to:

Data storage server.

Given the variety and mass of data that can be collected from our Honeypots, we thought about setting up a Big Data management system for storing and analyzing this data, two of the most famous open source Big Data frameworks are:

- Hadoop is a dedicated framework for storage and processing of Big Data in a distributed way, it is based mainly on two parts, one part for storage called Hadoop Distributed File System (HDFS), and one part for the processing called MapReduce. To managing cluster, Hadoop use master/slave architecture [13].

- Spark is a framework also designed for Big Data management, it does not have its own distributed storage file, it relies on storage systems such as that of Hadoop (HDFS) or others, but it is considered faster than Hadoop regarding iterative treatments [14].

We will try to test them both during our futures experiments and choose the most efficient and suitable for our architecture.

Archiving server of processed data

Because of the amount of data which can be processed over time, this server is a Big Data management system, it is dedicated for the archiving of the data of the attacks after the treatment by the RNN.

3.2   Treatments

After exposing the set of Honeypots, the treatment operations are as follows:

Collecting of attacks

In this phase, we use an Extract Transform Load (ETL) tool to load the data of attacks recorded by Honeypots to the Big Data storage server, we attempt to choose the most efficient and adequate during our researches.

We describe in detail the loading algorithm in Table 1 and following program:

```
LoadData (StartDate)
{
EndDate = Null;
If (StartDate == null)
{
StartDate = SysDate;
}
 While (DataDate >= StartDate)
{
LoadDataToServer;
}
EndDate = SysDate;
Return EndDate;
}
```

With this algorithm, the data that can be recorded by the Honeypot during the current loading will be loaded during the next loading.

Elimination of redundancy

After loading the data into the Big Data storage server, the step of elimination of redundancy is necessary, we will try to delete duplicate data with a NoSQL request to provide more performance to the next processing.

Table 1. The description of the variables of the loading algorithm

Variable	Description
StartDate	Is the start date of loading data to the Big Data storage server. During the first load, it is initialized with the current date of the operating system where it is installed the ETL which will perform the loading
SysDate	Is the current date of the operating system of machine where the ETL which will perform the loading is installed
DataDate	Is the date of the recording of the attack noted by the Honeypot
LoadDataToServer	Is the operation which consists of loading data from the Honeypot to the Big Data storage sever
EndDate	Is the end date of loading data, noted by the operating system where it is installed the ETL which will perform the loading. It is returned and kept at the end of loading in order to be the start date of the next data loading

Learning by Deep Learning

Although Big Data constitutes a processing challenge related to volume, variety, velocity, and veracity, Deep Learning appears to extract knowledge and perform predictive analytics from it, it is a promising research field [15]. It is a set of machine learning techniques inspired from the deep structure of the human brain [3]. Several models of Deep Learning have appeared recently, those who are original and typically used are: Stacked Auto-Encoder (SAE), Deep Belief Network (DBN), Convolutional Neural Network (CNN) and Recurrent Neural Network (RNN), the others are hybrids based on these [16].

Unlike other Deep Learning models, the RNN is characterized by its memory, as depicted in Fig. 2, it includes Input Layer, Hidden Layer and Output Layer, to make decision at the time step t, it takes into his input in addition to the current input, the information about decision at time step t − 1 stored in the Hidden Layer. Moreover, it is designed to draw knowledge from sequences of data like sentences, word sequence and speech [6]. Which justifies our choice of model, in order to have a memory on the old attacks.

So the RNN will be applied to all the data loaded to learn about the different attacks.

Archiving of processed attacks

At the end of each analyze by the RNN, We will archive all processed data in another Big Data storage server so as not to lose our data, and we will empty the server which is dedicated for processing to prepare a blank server for future operations of loading of the new data and treatment by the RNN.

With this native and particular design of the system, we have illustrated a new manner of monitoring security, which can progress automatically, by learning, to discover new menaces.

Reccurent Neural Network

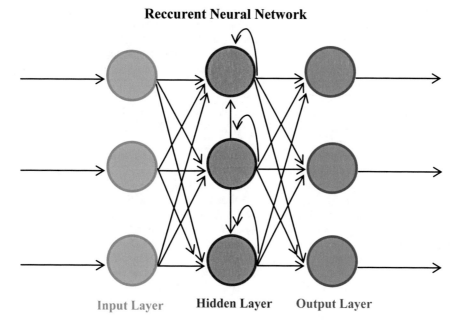

Input Layer   **Hidden Layer**   **Output Layer**

Fig. 2. Design of layers of RNN

4 Conclusion and Future Work

We have presented in this paper, an automatic security monitoring system of the information system in order to recognize old attacks and cope with new others which look like them, our architecture is based on collection of Honeypots to collect threats, Big Data storage server to store the amount and the variety of data of attacks, and the applying of the RNN method to learn about menaces.

In the future, we will implement our work in a real-life environment and, at the same time, try to exploit our RNN in a NIDS with keeping our architecture running to allow it to know more about attacks. Moreover, we will try to schedule loading, processing and archiving of data in order to have automatic real time monitoring of security.

References

1. Niyaz, Q., Sun, W., Javaid, A., Alam, M.: A deep learning approach for network intrusion detection system. In: Proceedings of the 9th EAI International Conference on Bio-inspired Information and Communications Technologies (BICT'15). pp. 21–26. ACM, United States (2015). https://doi.org/10.4108/eai.3-12-2015.2262516
2. NSL KDD. https://github.com/defcom17/NSL_KDD

3. Dong, B., Wang, X.: Comparison Deep learning method to traditional methods using for network intrusion detection. In: 2016 8th IEEE International Conference on Communication Software and Networks, pp 581. https://doi.org/10.1109/iccsn.2016.7586590

4. KDD Cup 99. http://kdd.ics.uci.edu/databases/kddcup99/kddcup99.html

5. Yang, J., Deng, J., Li, S., Hao, Y.: Improved traffic detection with support vector machine based on restricted Boltzmann machine. Soft Comput. **21**(11), 3101–3112 (2017). https://doi.org/10.1007/s00500-015-1994-9

6. Yan, R., Xiao, X., Hu, G., Peng, S., Jiang, Y.: New deep learning method to detect code injection attacks on hybrid applications. J. Syst. Softw. **137**, 1–27 (2018). https://doi.org/10.1016/j.jss.2017.11.001

7. Li, Y., Ma, R., Jiao, R.: A hybrid malicious code detection method based en deep learning. Int. J. Secur. Appl. (IJSIA) **9**(5), 205–216 (2015). https://doi.org/10.14257/ijsia.2015.9.5.21

8. Abeshu Diro, A., Chilamkurti, N.: Distributed attack detection scheme using deep learning approach for Internet of Things. Int. J. Future Gener. Comput. Syst. (FGCS) **82**, 761–768 (2018). https://doi.org/10.1016/j.future.2017.08.043

9. Lan, L., Jun, L.: Some special issues of network security monitoring on big data environments. In: 2013 IEEE 11th International Conference on Dependable, Autonomic and Secure Computing, pp. 10–15. (2013) https://doi.org/10.1109/dasc.2013.30

10. Saenko, I., Kotenko, I., Kushnerevich, A.: Parallel processing of big hterogeneous data for security monitoring of IoT networks. In: 2017 25th Euromicro International Conference on Parallel, Distributed and Networks-Based Processing, pp 329–336 (2017). https://doi.org/10.1109/pdp.2017.45

11. Campbell, M.R., Padayachee, K., Masombuka, T.: A survey of Honeypot research: trends and opportunities. In: The 10th International Conference for Internet Technology and Secured Transactions (ICITST-2015), pp. 208–210 (2015). https://doi.org/10.1109/icitst.2015.7412090

12. Designing a DMZ.: SANS Institute 2003. https://www.sans.org/reading-room/whitepapers/firewalls/designing-dmz-950

13. Saraladevi, B., Pazhaniraja, N., Victer Paul, P., Saleem Basha, M.S., Dhavachelvan, P.: Big data and Hadoop—a study in security perspective. In: 2nd International Symposium on Big Data and Cloud Computing (ISBCC'15), p. 598 (2015). https://doi.org/10.1016/j.procs.2015.04.091

14. Gu, L., Li, H.: Memory or time: performance evaluation for iterative operation on hadoop and spark. In: 2013 IEEE International Conference on High Performance Computing and Communications & 2013 IEEE International Conference on Embedded and Ubiquitous Computing, pp. 721–722 (2013). https://doi.org/10.1109/hpcc.and.euc.2013.106

15. Chen, X., Lin, X.: Big data deep learning challenges and perspectives. IEEE Access **2**, 514 (2014). https://doi.org/10.1109/access.2014.2325029

16. Zhang, Q., Yang, L.T., Chen, Z., Li, P.: A survey on deep learning for big data. Inform. Fusion **42**, 147 (2017). https://doi.org/10.1016/j.inffus.2017.10.006

A New Langage for Adaptatif System Structured Decision Network Language (SDNL)

Soumaya El Mamoune[✉], Mostafa Ezziyyani,
and Maroi Tsouli Fathi

Faculty of Science and Technology/Computer Science, Tangier, Morocco
{soumayamgi,ezziyyani,maroi.tsouli}@gmail.com

Abstract. Based on adaptatif system and decision theory, this paper introduces a new language to manage Decision Network for proposing services to a dynamic event after an adaptation. The new approach presents several solutions to critiques situations but the most problem was how we can manage and structure the decisions in the database. To solve this problem, we propose a Structured Decision Network Language (SDNL) to define all the operations that can be used like add a decision, update, delete and link the decisions. The new language is some instructions to execute for having some operations. The main objective of this article is to present the new language and the instruction of this language. We also propose a case study on which we apply the instructions of the language. For that, we suggest a network for the managements of accidents during pilgrimage and we take part of the network to show how to construct a network decision by the language SDNL.

Keywords: SDNL · Decision network · Adaptation · Network management · Structured language · Network evolution

1 Introduction

A major challenge of adaptive systems is to present a comprehensive approach to adaptation to the environment for the construction of an optimal and effective action plan [1]. The organization of data in the adaptatif system was also a big problem of research [2, 3]. In this context, the Decision Network is a new approach that allows the system to adapt and offer services according to environmental data and the user profile [4]. The approach has been proposed as a graphical model used to structure the services offered according to rules and well-defined constraints. The components of this model must to allow an easy and effective use. The proper implementation of this model will facilitate communication and collaboration to meet the users with quality services.

This paper is structured as follows. In Sect. 1, we present a system for disaster and the basic information of Decision Network that is used in Disaster emergency system. In the Sect. 2, we propose the new language for managing the network decision and the syntax of this language. Finally, to clear up the instructions of this new language, we apply on a real case.

© Springer Nature Switzerland AG 2019
M. Ezziyyani (Ed.): AI2SD 2018, AISC 915, pp. 809–820, 2019.
https://doi.org/10.1007/978-3-030-11928-7_73

2 Disaster Emergency System

Human security means protecting fundamental freedoms that are the essences of life. It also means protecting the individual against serious threats or generalized. It's necessary to build on the strengths and aspirations of each individual, but it also signifies creating systems that give people environmental elements essential to their survival, their lives and their dignity. In this context, we present a new concept to create an adaptive system to save lives and help the individual in danger, the system called Disaster Emergency system "D.E.S".

The mine objective of our research is to propose a conception of an intelligent emergency system in disaster. The system proposes an optical plan to save the user if he is in danger. In this perspective, the system must adapt to user's context to offer an adequate plan. Our interests are the trust and the quality of our support which will guarantee an efficient operation depending on the services offered by the system that occurs spontaneously known as the best rescue system that gives individuals the essential elements of survival and several partial objectives which are:

- Reduce the probability of accidents: After studying the context information and analyzing the existence of an accident, the system can prevent the probability of the accident and notify the user.
- Inform the public about preventive behavior to be a disaster or an emergency: If the system receives information concerning a disaster, it shall inform any person who can be exposed to this disaster and propose an emergency plan to save him.
- Reduce the severity, if disasters occurred despite the taken precautions: the severity of a disaster can be judged by the amount of damage and the latter to limit the severity. Our system improves the efficiency and quality of aid by implementation rules such as call emergency rescue, fire …

To achieve these goals, we propose in Fig. 1 architecture of system that allows adapting to context user and environment and offering an adequate service. The user

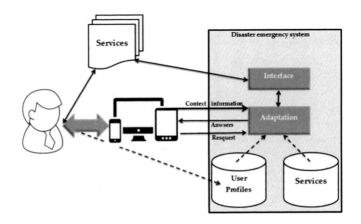

Fig. 1. Architecture of disaster emergency system

must fulfil his profile and be in interaction with system by using his phone, pc or tablet. The system picks up the environment change by analyzing the environment data and decides which service can be suitable after an adaptation process that select the best service and tend at any moment towards the adequate function.

In the related literature, we find several adaptive systems [2, 5, 6]. But, the problem is that each researcher proposes its own concept or his/her own proposal and we do not find an approach of common adaptation. The concept of adaptation is different for each case as each one defines the concept of the context according to its proposed system. So, the idea of our work is to present a process of adaptation and decision-making aid standard which could be used for any adaptive system. In this article, we present the description of user profile and how the system offers the services to each profile.

The suggested solution is a novel method to model the behavior of the adaptive system of decision-making aid, which makes the system to pertinently act in its medium according to its perceptions of the environment by using the sensors and its knowledge.

In the critical situation like Dynamic Medical [3], Flood Forecasting [7], autonomy for time-critical takeoff decisions [8], lot of suggestions and lot of architectures can be cited but it's useful just in the situation where it's cited. So, we propose an architecture that can be used in every critical situation based to the environmental data.

3 Decision Network

3.1 Definitions

The decision network is a new approach and adaptive decision support that can be used by adapting systems to provide an adaptive solution to the situation [4]. The idea is to structure the solutions offered by the system as a network. This includes services that are represented by elementary decisions interlinked by rules and constraints that we have defined for the operation of the system.

For the definition of our approach, we proposed several terms as "final decision" which is the set of services to be rendered in a given situation. Each service is called elementary decision and they are connected with each other via connectors used to specify the sequence of use of elementary decisions. Graphically depicts our approach as dependency graph structure where the decision network from the system knowledge base to model the dynamic behavior of the system.

3.2 Why a New Approach

The new approach improves the system's ability to be scalable, adaptive and intelligent. The proposal provides very important features such as the assessment, improvement, and evolution. The degree of adaptability and using a decision used to verify the effectiveness of the decision for a given situation. This level is used to evaluate the efficiency of a decision for an improvement that can be deletion or update decision. The evolution of the system is through the development of the network which is enlarged in progressively use. The network is initially empty and is in operation, gradually creating decisions for a given context. The creation of decisions by them-selves is sufficient that's why we offer other components that connect these decisions according to well defined rules.

3.3   The Representation of Decision Network

The decision network (RDD) is an evolutionary graph to model the final decision of the system according to a dependency graph. A node in the graph represents a basic decision that could also be a final decision in a simple situation.

The graph proposed by us uses the standard notion of the directed graphs besides the new notations in order to formalize the new features of the decision graph proposed for the adaptive system. The decision graph is defined by the triplet $GD = \{ <N^{in}, C, N^{out}> \}$ whose elements are N^{in} (the node of entry), N^{out} (the node of exit) and C (the connector connecting the nodes realized by an arc) and, graphically, it is presented as shown in Fig. 2.

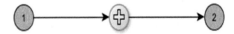

Fig. 2. triplet of the graph

After creating several triplets, we represent our decision network as a graph. Each decision graph node (GD) is a separate item (basic decision) and connected these points with connectors and bows.

4   The New Language SDNL

4.1   Why a New Language?

After the proposal of the new approach, we continue our research and development of decision network by defining a new language that will handle the data of the proposed network. We aim to provide a total manipulation RDD by ordinary operations like creating basic decisions, updating and deleting. The new language will also manage all components of the graph as connectors and arcs. This language helps everyone to create his network and apply all operations whatever his level in computer sciences.

The proposed language is called SDNL (Structured Decision Network Language). SDNL is a computer language used to manipulate and organize all the components of decision network such as the creation of the elementary decisions and making the connection between connectors.

The new language addresses two areas:

- Manipulation of decision (nodes): create, search, add, edit or delete decision making in the network.

- The manipulation of the entire network such as the creation of links between decisions by creating connectors or arcs or generally modify the organization of decision making in the network.

4.2   SDNL Syntax

SDNL instructions are written in a simple way. They resemble that of ordinary declarative sentences in English according to a precise syntax. This resemblance referred facilitates learning, reading and understanding of the new language. The latter is a declarative language, that is to say, it can describe the transaction or the desired action, without describing how to get it and in parallel we are developing a program that automatically determines the optimal way to perform these operations.

The proposed language will define the main operations performed to manage the organization of network components.

Creation of Graph

The graph is the element that collects the decision network. Before creating the components of the latter, we must create the graph that will be initially empty but filled as and creating custom other components. To create an empty graph, we use the following statement:

Create graph '*Id graph to create*'

Creation of Elementary Decision

The elementary decision is one of the main components of the graph. It represents the graph node. The elementary decision is not only the base part of the graph, but it is a member composed of a plurality of other elements which are shown below. With this, we guarantee the most important character is the evolution of the system (Table 1).

Table 1. Syntax to create elementary decision elements

Element	Syntax
Elementary decision	**Create decision** '*Id of decision to create*' **in** '*Id of graph where we add the decision*'
Action	**Create action** '*Id of action to create*' **as** '*defition of action or commande of action*' **in** '*Id of decision where we add the action*'
Condition PRE	**Create pre** '*Id of condition pre*' **as** '*the condition to verify*' **in** '*Id of decision where we add the condition*'
Condition POST	**Create post** '*Id of condition post*' **as** '*the condition to verify*' **in** '*Id of decision where we add the condition*'

Creation of Connector

Create a connector means, the birth of a relationship between two decisions to be determined later. The type of relationship is accurate according to the type of connector (Table 2).

Table 2. Syntax to create the different connectors

Type of connector	Syntax
Or	Create connector or 'Id of connector'
And	Create connector and 'Id of connector' in 'graph'
Parallel	Create connector parallel 'Id of connector' in 'graph'

Linking Components

After creating the decision network elements, it is necessary to link the components to construct the network by connecting the basic decisions with connectors and arcs. To construct this network, we suggest these instructions:

- Link decision *'Id of decision'* to connector *'Id of connector'*.

This instruction puts the link between a decision and a connector like Fig. 3.

- Link connector *'Id of connector'* to decision *'Id of decision'*.

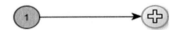

Fig. 3. Link the decision to connector

This instruction puts the link between a connector and a decision like Fig. 4.

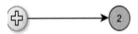

Fig. 4. Link the connector to decision

These instructions automatically create an arc between the two components but the choice of one of these instructions presented makes the difference. The first allows you to create an arc decision to the connector against the second connector creates an arc to the decision.

The arc is a single component but it plays a key role because it is impossible to connect two components without using the bow. In the language we propose, we presented above the arcing due to the relationship between the decision and the elementary connector but this relationship can also be broken following an arc suppression operation we define it according to the syntax follows:

Delete arc *'Id of arc'*

Id of arc is a combination of Id connector and Id of decision. It is created automatically after the connection between the decision and the connector.

Modification

The decision to offer network (RDD) has a very important property that is improving. This improvement can be made by changing the network elements. It shows the syntax to follow to do. The updating is a modification of one or more components of elementary decision as necessary and useful for it to be effective.

We present the syntax of the update in the following Table 3.

Table 3. Syntax to edit the elementary decision elements

Element	Syntax
Elementary decision	**Edit decision** '*Id of decision to update*' **to** '*The new of decision*' *This instruction update the name of decision*
Action	The modification of the action can be done by two things is changing the name of the action or is changing the definition of the action itself **Modification of action name:** **Edit Action name** '*Id of action to update*' **in** '*Id of decision where it is the action*' **to** '*The new name of action*' **Modification of action:** **Edit Action** '*Id of action to update*' **in** '*Id of decision where it is the action*' **as** '*the new action to execute it*'
Condition PRE	Changing the PRE condition can be done by two things is changing the name of the condition or either the change in the definition of the condition itself. **Modification of condition PRE name:** **Edit condition pre name** '*Id of condition pre to update*' **in** 'Id of decision where it is the condition pre' **to** '*the new Id of condition*' **Modification of condition:** **Edit condition pre** '*Id of condition pre to update*' **in** 'Id of decision where it is the condition pre' **as** '*the definition of condition pre*'
Condition POST	Changing the POST condition can be done by two things is also changing the name of the condition or either the change in the definition of the condition itself **Modification of condition Post name:** **Edit condition post name** '*Id of condition post to update*' **in** 'Id of decision where it is the condition post' **to** '*the new Id of condition*' **Modification of condition:** **Edit condition post** '*Id of condition post to update*' **in** 'Id of decision where it is the condition post' **as** '*the definition of condition post*'

Suppression

If necessary, the administrator can delete an elementary decision is not used or if it is incorrect. We offer several choices for this operation:

- Delete basic decision: it is total suppression that is to say after this operation all actions and all conditions constituting this decision will be deleted.

- Delete action: We can eliminate one or more shares in a decision provided it must keep at least one share in a decision. The decision will be modified but just the number of shares that will be changed following the abolition performed.
- Delete a Condition (Pre and Post): We can remove one or more conditions and this deletion just change the conditions of implementation of the decision (Table 4).

Table 4. Syntax to delete the elementary decision elements

Element	Syntax
Elementary decision	**Delete decision** '*Id of decision to delete*' This instruction deletes the decision identified by Id and all its components
Action	**Delete Action** '*Id of action to delete*' **in** '*Id of decision where the action exists*' The network administrator can remove N actions in a decision but it is forbidden to remove all the actions. The decision must have one action to execute it
Condition PRE	**Delete pre** '*Id of condition Pre*' **in** '*Id of decision where the condition exists*'
Condition POST	**Delete post** '*Id of condition Post*' **in** '*Id of decision where the condition exists*'
Connector	**Delete connector** '*Id of connector to delete*' The suppression of the connector is the suppression of the connection between the decisions.

5   Applying SDNL: Managing Pilgrimage Accidents

The year 2015 was marked by a human catastrophe during the pilgrimage. Two accidents were a cause of more than 1000 dead. This disaster has upset the stability of thousands of families around the world and even pushed us to seek solutions for a more efficient organization.

In this context, we propose a management of problems or accidents encountered during pilgrimage as path loss, loss of contact with family, looking for people in an accident … Several services can be offered but we chose some of them to present the Decision Network approach. The graph that we offer allows us to apply the instructions of the new language to better understand the utility of each instruction.

In this example, we present all steps to create a graph. For this, we will create the elements of the area surrounded with the linking of these elements (Fig. 5).

5.1   Analysis

Before creating the graph, we must list all the elements of graph: elementary decision, connectors and arc. In this case, we will take a part of graph to apply our language as shown in the following Fig. 6:

If it is necessary like in an accident, the user can look for another user to locate him to see if he is in danger.

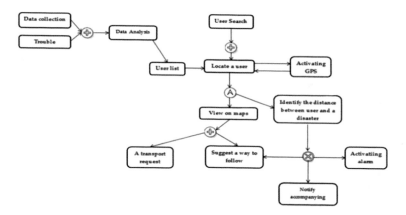

Fig. 5. Decision network to manage the pilgrimage accidents

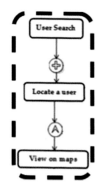

Fig. 6. The network to create

For this case, we have one graph which contains:

- Three elementary decisions
- Two connectors
- Four arcs.

5.2 The Steps of the Network Decision Creation

Creation of Graph

The creation of the graph is the first step. Create a graph is creating an empty container that will be filled by the services. This requires a graph name under which we create. In this example, we create the graph "Hajj".

Create graph "Hajj"

Creation of Elementary Decision

The elementary decision is one of the main components of the graph. It represents the graph node. The elementary decision is not only the base part of the graph, but it is an element composed of several other elements. It is composed by one or more actions that will be performed.

In this example, we have three elementary decisions: User search, Locate a user and View on maps.

First Decision: User Search

Create decision 'User Search' **in** 'Hajj'

    Create action 'information' **as** 'get information of user to search (Name, Code, Access permission)' **in** 'User Search'

    Create action 'verification' **as** 'verification of user's information' **in** 'User Search'

    Create action 'reply' **as** 'reply yes or no' **in** 'User Search'

    Create pre 'Access permission' **as** 'Verify if user A has permission to search B' in 'User Search'

    Create post 'Permission' **as** 'if the altitude is not null' **in** 'Locate a user'.

Second Decision: Locate a User

Create decision 'Locate a User' **in** 'Hajj'

    Create action 'longitude' **as** 'get longitude' **in** 'Locate a user'

    Create action 'Id user' **as** 'get Id of user to locate' **in** 'Locate a user'.

    Create action 'altitude' **as** 'get altitude' **in** 'Locate a user'

    Create action 'latitude' **as** 'get latitude' **in** 'Locate a user'

    Create pre 'gps on' **as** 'if the gps is activated' in 'Locate a user'

    Create post 'alt' **as** 'if the altitude is not null' **in** 'Locate a user'

    Create post 'long' **as** 'if the altitude is not null' **in** 'Locate a user'

    Create post 'lati' **as** 'if the latitude is not null' **in** 'Locate a user'.

Third Decision: View on Maps

Create decision 'View on maps' **in** 'Hajj'

    Create action 'gps coordinates' **as** 'get gps coordinates' **in** 'View on maps'

    Create action 'address' **as** 'get address' **in** 'View on maps'.

    Create action 'point address' **as** 'pointing the address on the map' **in** 'View on maps'

    Create pre 'gps ok' **as** 'if the gps coordinates are not null **in** 'View on maps'

    Create post 'maps ok' **as** 'if the map is correctly downloaded' **in** 'View on maps'

Creation of Connectors

To link the elementary decisions we need the connectors. In this case, we need parallel connector and or connector so we create two connectors with two different Id.

    Create connector parallel 'par1'

    Create connector or 'or1'

Linking of Components

Link decision 'User Search' **to connector** 'or1'

Link connector 'or1' **to decision** 'Locate a user'
Link decision 'Locate a user' **to connector** 'par1'
Link connector 'par1' **to decision** 'View on maps'.

The instructions are very simple to use by any user no matter his level in computer science.

6 Conclusion and Perspectives

The decisions network is the solution for modelling complex adaptive systems, which is based on the interaction with the environment or the user, the self-improvement and the evolution. The procedure suggested allows the evolution of the final decision by taking into account the limits presented in other approach.

To construct the decision network and not have just a theory, we propose this new language. It has several advantages such as evolution of network and ease of use. This advantage allows any user to build a network of decision and change it without difficulty. The instructions of this language manage the network and to apply these instructions we development also a tool of interpretation with the automatic execution of these instructions.

In future works, we will define more algorithms to manage the decisions network in order to ensure the communication with different entities from the system. Moreover. We are also planning to develop a database to store the decision graph and services in different situations because to make a good decision, multiple conditions should be met. To specify the most accurate decision, the user profile should be taken into account. So, we must propose a structuring profile to help us to choose the suitable service. It can act in a simple decision or a more or less coherent whole of dependent decisions.

References

1. George, J.-P., Gleizes, M.-P., Glize, P.: Conception de systems adaptatifs à fonctionnalité émergente : la théorie Amas (2007). Revue d'intelligence artificielle **17**/4 - 2003, 591–626. ISSN 0992-499. http://dx.doi.org/10.3166/ria.17.591-626
2. Rupert, M.: Organisation du contenu du Web selon la perspective des Systèmes Complexes Adaptatifs. In: CORIA '2006(COnférence en Recherche d'Informations et Applications), ARIA de Lyon France, pp. 283–294
3. Bouzguenda, L., Turki, M.: Designing an architectural style for dynamic medical cross-organizational workflow management system: an approach based on agents and web services. J. Med. Syst. Arch. **38**(4), pp. 1–14 (April 2014). Plenum Press, New York, NY, USA. http://dx.doi.org/10.1007/s10916-014-0032-2
4. Mamoune, S.E., Ezziyani, M., Lloret, J.: Towards a new approach for modelling interactive real time systems based on collaborative decisions network. Netw. Protoc. Algorithms (NPA) **7**(1) (April 2015). ISSN 1943-3581
5. Rattrout, A., Issa, T., Badir, H.: Intelligent web system: using intelligent web agents to achieve a self-organized system. In: IEEE Conference on SKIMA09 Fes, Morocco, pp. 93–101, 21–23 Oct 2009

6. Wang, J.: Development of a decision support system for flood forecasting and warning—a case study on the Maribyrnong River. Ph.D. thesis, Victoria University, Melbourne, Australia (Jan 2007)

7. El Mabrouk Marouane, C.L., Mostafa, E., Mohammad, E.: Conception of real-time flood forecasting system approach based on anytime techniques. In: Proceeding Engineering & Technology (PET) of the International Conference on Control, Engineering & Information Technology (CEIT'13)", vol. 1, pp. 207–211 (2013)

8. Inagaki, T.: Situation-adaptive autonomy for time-critical takeoff decisions. Int. J. Modell. Simul. **20**(2), pp. 175–180 (2000). http://dx.doi.org/10.1109/TSMCA.2009.2026428

Localization and Tracking System Using Wi-Fi Signal Strength with Wireless Sensors Network

Douae Zbakh[(✉)], Abdelouahid Lyhyaoui, and Mariam Tanana

Abdelmalek Essaâdi University, National School of Applied Sciences, LTI.
Laboratory, BP 1818, Tangier, Morocco
Douae.zbakh@gmail.com

Abstract. Indoor location and tracking systems based on Wi-Fi signals are both gainful and precise, they are able to attain certain positioning level using existing Wi-Fi infrastructure environment. The implementation within a wireless sensors network proffer an updating card that estimate true values of RSSI on the fingerprints points, and combine algorithms localization that offer accurate positions estimations. In this paper a localization algorithm will be described it offers a good accuracy using a particular filter which tracks multiple points to characterize a trajectory. Finally an evaluation of methods performance is desirable to verify that the system is more accurate and efficient on tracking.

Keywords: Wireless sensor network · Localization algorithm · Indoor location · Access point · Signal strength · Location tracking

1 Introduction

Indoor localization [1] is one of the most important problems in intelligent services. They are considered much more difficult than outdoor localization problems because GPS signal is not available within building or nearby huge structure.

The technologies of indoor location tracking are used in public building [2] like museums, transit stations or hospitals. In contrast, location errors may result in undesirable deliveries of wrong information to the wrong people at wrong place.

Location tracking and positioning systems can be classified by: Measurement attribute [3], localization Algorithms [4] and communication protocol. The classifications by the measurement techniques are employed to determine mobile device location (localization). Location tracking approach differs in terms of the specific technique used to precisely detect and measure the position of the mobile device in the target environment under observation. The Real Time Location Systems (RTLS) as a type of measurement attribute includes many basic systems able to determine positions using the following parameters:

- Cell of origin (nearest cell)
- Distance (lateration)
- Angle (angulations)
- Location patterning (pattern recognition)

© Springer Nature Switzerland AG 2019
M. Ezziyani (Ed.): AI2SD 2018, AISC 915, pp. 821–829, 2019.
https://doi.org/10.1007/978-3-030-11928-7_74

RTLS solution typically includes location sensors that are attached to various assets, using a unique ID. The system can locate the tags and report real time information about its positioning within the facility estimation, based RTLS solution enables tracking unit. This location services are preferment in finding and tracking assets (objects) and people; they deliver information for users mainly on client software.

Manufacturers of RTLS systems have combined the functionality of both systems and incorporated both technologies GPS and Wi-Fi in a device to provide the location data.

System as such utilizes the availability of GPS for outdoor location and switch to Wi-Fi when confronting obstacles.

Wi-Fi [6] based system potentially works indoor. For instance, Radar is an indoor location system based on Wi-Fi signal [7, 8]. It uses tow methods to calculate locations from signal information. The first is to use a signal propagation model, which quantifies how wireless signal fluctuates with distance. The second it estimates the distance from multiple access point from signal strengths. In this regard, there are two types of Wi-Fi based positioning technologies: time and space attributes [9] of received signal (TSARS)—based technology and received signal strength (RSS) based positioning technology. We need to update our map every in order to use a sensor network to get the value of the RSSI from each grid point; that is to say, the RSSI represents the best localization entity and a relied parameter.

Wi-Fi based location systems operate via two phases. First one is called the offline training phase, which makes a human operator able to perform a survey on those sites with signal strength indicators (RSSI), using different access points (APs) attributed to the same fixed environment sampled point. These RSSI measurements are registered in radio card, which exposes APs RSSI values of different sampled points. The second one is the online estimation. It is charged of target's location which calculated in real time by corresponding sampled points on radio card with the closest RSSI values of the target.

In this paper, the location and the tracking use the Wi-Fi strength signal. It is implemented in a wireless sensors network to estimate the positions using the fingerprinting location method. The Wi-Fi locations use the LF and sensors in two aspects: the training one, in charge of collecting different RSS values due to sensors and their databases. The second aspect is interested in position estimation using KNN Algorithm [10]. Then we employed the particular filter to track multiple points and characterize a trajectory. This solution shows many benefits as the system resulted with 3 m of location precision adapted with the indoor space.

This paper is organized as follows, in Sect. 2 we describes the design of the proposed Indoor location system based on wireless sensors networks, next presents location mythology was described. In Sect. 4, the improvement of trajectory accuracy is due to a particular filter, Sect. 5 gives a performance evaluation of location estimation. Finally the last section presents discussion of future works.

2 Localization Approach Design

The experiment was performed in the hall of the National School of Applied Sciences in Tangier; the dimension is approximately 25 × 15 m².

We use 6 AP operating on the radio channel of IEEE 802,11b at 2, 54 GHz with 3 overlapping channel. Also 300 distributed sensors as shown in Fig. 1.

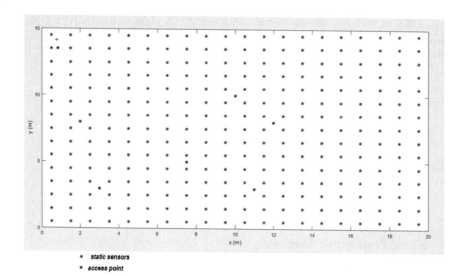

Fig. 1. The mesh description

The received signal strength is in the range of −40dBm and −90dBm, and the highly RSS value is −25dBm approximately at 1 m (APs distance).

Access points are located in the following positions (3; 3), (17; 3), (3; 13), (17; 13), (14; 10), (8; 6).

The location and the tracking system use the Wi-Fi strength signal. It is implement the wireless sensors network to estimate the positions using the fingerprinting location method.

The Wi-Fi locations algorithm use tree aspects: the training one, in charge of collecting different RSS values due to sensors and their databases. The second aspect is interested in position estimation using KNN Algorithm, finaly In order to improve the accuracy the Particular Filter is implemented

Figure 1. A figure caption is always placed below the illustration. Short captions are centered, while long ones are justified. The macro button chooses the correct format automatically.

2.1 Localization Algorithm

This section describes the algorithm used in the proposed approach: signal propagation theorem, K-nearest neighbor and a probabilistic estimation.

K-nearest neighbor is applied to specify the sensors positions after collecting the RSSi vector $F = [F_1....F_N]$ values.

With N as the number of the deployed AP in the area and Pi as an independent RSSI from a data AP.

In order to find the nearest neighbor we use KNN algorithm, which is a set of strength signal, then we also use the weighted average of geometric coordinate relative to the K nearest sensors.

$$\frac{1}{k} \cdot \sum_{i=1}^{k} \frac{P_i \cdot (x_i, y_i)}{\sum_{i=1}^{k} P_i}$$

With P_i as the mean the F_i Vector:

$$P_i = \frac{1}{N} \sum_{i}^{N} F_i$$

2.2 Signal Propagation Theorem

Wi-Fi RSS is retrieved from all grid points, the radio frequency signal obeys propagation based model.

$$r_j(d_{j,k}) = r_k(d_k) - 10\alpha \, \log_{10}(d_{j,k}) - wallLoss$$

where $r_k(d_k)$ is the initial RSS at the reference distance of d_0 of 1 m.

The variable α gives the exponent path loss, in the indoor α can be between 1 and 6 wall Loss is the sum of losses introduced by each wall on the line segment at the Euclidian distance $d_{j,k}$.

3 Probabilistic Estimation

The Wi-Fi RSS research support taking on Gaussian distribution when the size samples RSS is large. Supposing the case, the variance of Wi-Fi RSS distribution are σ_s & μ_s and the probability of getting the exact location is donate.

$$\Pr[X] = \Pr[d_i|F] = \frac{1}{\sqrt{2\pi\sigma}} \exp\left[-\frac{x - \mu_k}{2\sigma_k^2}\right]$$

With μ_k, σ_k are the distribution variance using all neighbors.

$$\mu_k = \frac{1}{k} \sum_{i=1}^{k} (f_{correct} - f_i)(f_{correct} + f_i - 2r)$$

$$\sigma_k^2 = \frac{4}{k} \sum_{i=1}^{k} (f_{correct} - f_i)^2 \sigma_s^2$$

4 Tracking Using a Particular Filter

In order to improve the accuracy the Particular Filter is implemented, so that we can estimate the state of a discrete time tracking process monitored by no linear stochastic difference equation. Then the covariance matrix is used to estimate system evolution that offers more precision than the regular tracking, which provides only the estimated location correction.

5 Performance Evaluation

This part of the work is interested in system performance, and starts by examination of errors through the mesh, then the effect of varying the number of neighbors, number of access points and also the number of sensors used, finally we evaluate the estimation of particular filter trajectory.

5.1 Error Evaluation and the Influence of Varying Several Parameters

As shown in the figure above (Fig. 2), the mesh is fully swept, where the error is calculated in meters from sensors. This figure shows also a maximal error approximately about 2.7 m and average error approximately about 1 m. So we notice that errors increase in minimum power density positions, and the received signal from various access points is a source of several errors.

In the study shown in Fig. 3, we varied the size of the mesh, also increased the distance between nodes up to 4.5 m. We notice that the more the mesh size increases, the more the error increases. And the average error attains 1 m while the distance between nodes is 1 m.

Figure 4 indicates the effect of variation neighbor numbers and shows that the location becomes more accurate. Referring to the figure, the error is minimized to 0.3 m using 8 neighbors.

5.2 Results for Adding the Location Tracking Filter

The nearest neighbor algorithm [10] uses a Map for keeping track of the status of the users in a particular location. There is a calibration process in which the tracks of all users are kept so that the location is achieved easily.

The K-Nearest Neighbor (K-NN) algorithm is used to estimate the mobile sensor location. Once the location is figured, the Particular filter is attributed to improve the

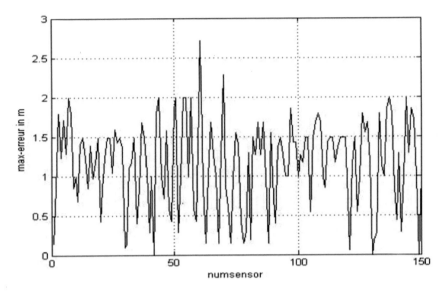

Fig. 2. MAX-ERROR in the basic mesh

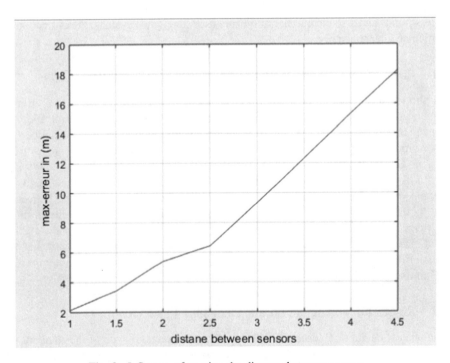

Fig. 3. Influence of varying the distance between sensors

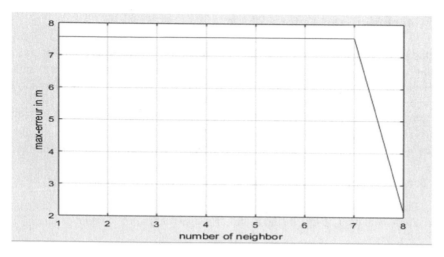

Fig. 4. Influence of varying the number of neighbor

performance. Those experiments examine the accurate trajectory when a user walks around a room with a mobile sensor.

The figure below (Fig. 5) offers the trajectory estimation using a particular filter algorithm combined with position already described. We observe that error decreases along the trajectory to an average of 1 m.

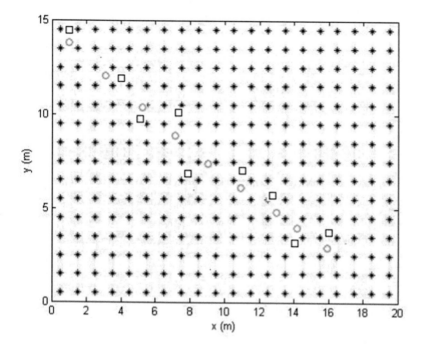

Fig. 5. Estimation of trajectory with a particular filter

6 Conclusion and Future Work

In this paper, different techniques stated for location based tracking and also concentrating on a mass usage of wireless Wi-Fi signal for location tracing. Wi-Fi signals allowing an immense field of services to track the user's location. In this scenario the distance between sensors is a major issue.

We proposed and describe a localization algorithm in this research paper that offers a good accuracy and stability using a particular filter. Many improvements could be made such as reducing the number of sensors using clustering; also using other metrics give more precision than Euclidian distance.

Some perspectives of wireless indoor positioning systems are as follows:

(1) The use of KALMAN filters to reduce error location.
(2) Implementation of this methods and also construction of 3D approach.

References

1. Ahn, H-S., Yu, W.: Indoor Localization Techniques based on Wireless Sensor Networks, Korea
2. Farid, Rosdiadee Nordin, andMahamod Ismail, Recent Advances in Wireless Indoor Localization Techniques and System
3. Al Nuaim, K., Kamel, H.: A survey of indoor positioning systems and algorithms. In: International Conference on Innovations in Information Technology (2011)
4. Zou, H., Lu, X., Jiang, H., Xie, L.: A Fast and precise indoor localization algorithm based on an online sequential extreme learning machine, Sensors (2015)
5. Huh, J.-H., Seo, K.: An Indoor Location-Based Control System Using Bluetooth Beacons for IoT Systems
6. Gosai, A., Ph.D., Raval, R.: Real time location based tracking using WIFI signals. Int. J. Comput. Appl. (0975–8887), **101**(5) (2014)
7. Xia, S., Liu, Y., Yuan, G., Zhu, M., Wang, Z.: Indoor Fingerprint Positioning Based on Wi-Fi
8. Suguna1, N., Thanushkodi, K.: An improved k-nearest neighbor classification using genetic algorithm. IJCSI Int. J. Comput. Sci. **7**(2) (2010)
9. Pan, SJ., Zheng, V.W., Yang, Q., Hu, D.H.: Transfer learning forWiFi-based indoor localization, In: Association for the Advancement of Artificial Intelligence (2008)
10. Lu-Chuan Kung Jennifer C. HouY, Chan, E.C.L., Baciu, G., Mak, S.C.: Using Wi-Fi signal strength to localize in wireless sensor networks, In: International Conference on Communications and Mobile Computing, Zero-configuration indoor localization over IEEE 802.11 wireless Infrastructure, Springer Science + Business Media, LLC (2008)
11. Chan, L.-W., Chiang, J.-R., Chen, Y.-C., Ke, C.-N., Hsu, J., Chu, H.-H.: Collaborative Localization: Enhancing WiFi-Based Position Estimation with Neighborhood Links in Clusters
12. Chen, W.-P., Hou, J.C., Sha, L.: Dynamic clustering for acoustic target tracking in wireless sensor networks, IEEE Transactions On Mobile Computing, IEEE Computer Society, pp. 258–271. (2004)
13. Baggio, A., Langendoen, K.: Monte-carlo localization for mobile wireless sensor networks, In MSN06, pp. 317–328. (2006)

14. Wang, J., Zha, H., Cipolla, R.: Coarse to-Fine vision-based localization by indexing scale-invariant features, IEEE Transactions on Systems, Man, and Cybernetics—Part B: Cybernetics, vol. 36, p. 413. (2006)
15. Ahn, H.S., Yu, W.: Indoor Localization Techniques based on Wireless Sensor Networks
16. Chen, Y.-C., Chiang, J.-R., Chu, H.-H., Huang, P., Tsui, A.W.: Sensor-Assisted Wi-Fi Indoor Location System for Adapting to Environmental Dynamics, Department of Computer Science and Information Engineering, Graduate Institute of Networking and Multimedia, Department of Electrical Engineering, National Taiwan University, Industrial Technology Research Institute
17. Lee, J., Cho, K., Lee, S., Kwon, T., Choi, Y.: Distributed and energy-efficient target localization and tracking in wireless sensor networks. School of Computer Science and Engineering, Seoul National University, San 56–1 Shilim-dong, Kwanak-gu, Seoul, Republic of Korea
18. Ropponen, A., Linnavuo, M., Sepponen, R.: LF Indoor location and identification system, Int. J. Smart Sens. Intell. Syst. 2(1) (2009)
19. Bell, S., Jung, W.R., Krishnakumar, V.: WiFi-based Enhanced Positioning Systems: Accuracy Through Mapping, Calibration, and Classification
20. Hu, L., Evans, D.: Localization for Mobile Sensor Networks, Department of Computer Science University of Virginia, Charlottesville
21. Smith, J.O., Abel, J.S.:. Closed-Form least squares source location estimation from range difference measurements. IEEE Trans. Acoust. Speech Signal Process. (ASSP) 35(12) (1987)
22. Gwon, Y., Jain, R., Kawahara, T.: Robust Indoor Location Estimation of Stationary and Mobile Users, DoCoMo Communications Laboratories USA
23. Chen, Y.-C., Chiang, J.-R., Chu, H.-H., Huang, P., Tsui, A.W.: Sensor Assisted Wi-Fi Indoor Location System for Adapting to Environment Dynamics. In: International Workshop on Modeling Analysis and Simulation of Wireless and Mobile Systems, pp. 118–125. Montreal, Canada, 10–13 Oct 2005
24. Zhou, R.: Wireless Indoor Tracking System (WITS), Communication systems/Computing Centre, University of Freiburg
25. Krishnan, P., Krishnakumar, A., Ju, W.H., Mallows, C., Gani, S.: Location estimation assisted by stationary emitters for indoor RF wireless networks. In: Proceedings of the IEEE Infocom (2014)
26. Lim, H., Kung, L.C., Hou, J.C., Luo, H.: Zero-configuration indoor localization over IEEE 802.11 wireless infrastructure. Wireless Netw. 16(2), 405–420 (2010)
27. Shu, J., Zhang, R. , Liu, L., Wu, Z., Zhou, Z.: Cluster-based three-dimensional localization, algorithm for large scale wireless sensor networks, J. Comput. (2009)
28. Pan, J.J., Yang, Q., Pan, S.J.: Online co-localization in indoor wireless networks by dimension reduction. In: Proceedings of the National Conference on Artificial Intligence (22) 1102 (2007)

A Comparative Study of Standard Part-of-Speech Taggers

Imad Zeroual[(✉)] and Abdelhak Lakhouaja

Computer Sciences Laboratory, Faculty of Sciences,
Mohammed First University, Oujda, Morocco
{mr.imadine,abdel.lakh}@gmail.com

Abstract. The Part of Speech (PoS) tagging is resolving ambiguity during text processing to assign morphosyntactic tags to each word according to the context. It is an essential task in several fields, particularly corpus linguistics and Natural Language Processing (NLP). Several PoS taggers and tools are already in service as open source or as commercialized solutions. Therefore, deeper investigation regarding their performance is required especially for under-resourced languages like Arabic. Some well-known probabilistic methods were adapted for PoS tagging such as Hidden Markov Models (HMMs), Support Vector Machines (SVM), and Decision Tree (DT). Based on these methods, language-independent PoS taggers have been developed namely TnT, SVMTool, and Treetagger. In fact, this article presents very important topic which concerns, on the one hand, an adaptation of Standard PoS taggers for the Arabic language, and in the other hand conducting very rich and comparative studies and evaluation. Basically, Arabic PoS taggers are very sensitive to the number of the tagsets used and the text form processed, therefore, four different tagsets and two text forms (i.e., Classical and Modern Standard Arabic) have been used.

Keywords: PoS tagging · TnT · SVMTool · Treetagger · Arabic

1 Introduction

For almost any language, a word can have several Part of Speech (PoS) tags. Hence, a tool that performs an automatic tagging is called a tagger and it is used to remove the ambiguity according to the context [1].

Nowadays, there are many satisfying researches on PoS tagging and the number of its available tools grew significantly over the last decade. Unfortunately, not all languages have benefited equally from this growth. An example of such languages is Arabic, which is still not very well investigated with respect in this field. There are several methods that have been proposed for automatic PoS tagging. The most known are probabilistic methods such as Hidden Markov Models (HMMs), Support Vector Machines (SVMs), and Decision Tree (DT). Later, a range of language-independent PoS taggers has been developed based on these methods namely TnT [2], SVMTool [3], and Treetagger [4].

© Springer Nature Switzerland AG 2019
M. Ezziyyani (Ed.): AI2SD 2018, AISC 915, pp. 830–840, 2019.
https://doi.org/10.1007/978-3-030-11928-7_75

PoS tagging is considered as a base stage for many Natural Language Processing (NLP) applications. For instance, PoS tagging is needed as a basic tool for spell checking and correcting, parsing system, information retrieval, and text-to-speech synthesis systems [5]. Moreover, PoS tagging is still one of the main tools required to build any language corpora [6]. Reciprocally, a corpus is still one of the main tools used to improve the performance of any PoS tagger.

Despite the progress that has been made recently in Arabic NLP and corpus linguistics [7], Arabic is relatively a resource-poor language when it comes to finding free core language processing models such as taggers, parsers and so on. In addition, conducting accurate comparative studies requires standard and common ground linguistic resources for both training and testing tasks. However, proposed Arabic PoS taggers were look only for their suitable objectives, or tend to use tagsets that are minor modifications of the Standard English tagsets (e.g., [8]).

The purpose of the described work in this paper is to create the required language models to adapt three standard taggers (TnT, SVMTool, and Treetagger) to Arabic. Then, very rich and comparative evaluation of their performances are performed using standard tagset, relevant lexical resources, and annotated corpora. After the adaptation of the three taggers, we highlight the use of them via various experiments on texts from both Modern Standard Arabic (MSA) and Classical Arabic (CA).

In addition to the introduction, the remainder of this paper is arranged in three main sections. In Sect. 2, the PoS tagging and the most relevant tagging methods are described. Further, we present the three standard PoS taggers, then, we introduce the used linguistic resources and tagset to create the language models for Arabic. In Sect. 3, various experiments of this study are presented, and the findings are discussed. Finally, we draw the conclusion and perspectives in Sect. 4.

2 Part of Speech Tagging

Basically, the average number of ambiguities for a word in MSA it reaches 19.2, while this rate reaches only 2.3 for most other languages [9]. Thus, the PoS tagging aims to automatically handle this ambiguity in the processed text to assign the appropriate PoS tags to each word according to the context. In order to begin with PoS tagging, certain requirements have to be met [10]:

- Selecting the suitable approach that will be used for the automatic tagging process.
- Preparing the required linguistic resources for training the tagger, and optional lexicon containing all possible tags for a particular word form.
- Defining the tagset, i.e., basic morphosyntactic tags that will be attached to each word.

2.1 Selecting the Tagging Method

Various methods have been designed to handle the PoS ambiguity. These methods differ from each other in the approaches they are based on it and the linguistic resources required. In this section, we present some of the most relevant methods implemented for the PoS tagging task.

The rule-based method is probably the first and the oldest method ever used for Arabic PoS tagging. In this method, the rules are hand-written by linguistics [11]. For instance, A system was designed and implemented as a rules-based expert system called Qutuf [12], it was presented as an Arabic morphological analyser and PoS tagger.

In the last decades, probabilistic methods came into existence and gained more popularity. These methods are data driven approaches based on large manually pre-tagged corpora. From those corpora, they extract probabilities where the training task consists of learning lexical probabilities and contextual probabilities. The most known statistical methods implemented for developing Arabic PoS tagger, we state: Memory based model, Maximum Entropy Model (MEM), HMMs, and SVMs. An Arabic PoS tagger were produced using the Memory based model and trained on the Arabic Penn Treebank corpus [13]. The achieved accuracy was 91.5% [14]. Further, one of the well-known taggers that integrates MEM method is the Stanford PoS tagger [15]. This tagger was trained on the training part of the Arabic Penn Treebank and the achieved accuracy was 96.42%. Regarding HMMs based method, a PoS tagger were proposed and achieved a state-of-the-art performance of 97% [16]. Finally, an SVM-based tagger is developed and called AMIRA [17]. It is reported that AMIRA performs at over 96% accuracy.

To increase the accuracy of previously proposed taggers, some hybrid systems that employ probabilistic models with rule-based methods were developed. For instance, the tagger developed by [18] performs at over 97% accuracy using only three basic tags (Noun, Verb, and Particle). Another hybrid system succeeded to reach 94% accuracy using 27 tags [19]. According to Aliwy [20], the accuracy of his statistical based model increased from 90.05 to 92.86% after involving a rule-based method. Also, Aliwy claims that the low accuracy of the statistical model is due to the small manually annotated corpus (29 k words) that was implemented in his experiments.

2.2   Standard Taggers

Various standard taggers have been developed as language-independent taggers based on different probabilistic models. Most of these taggers have not been adapted and investigated on common ground using Arabic texts. In the following, we present the investigated standard PoS taggers.

TnT. The HMMs is the most widely used method for statistical PoS tagging. As a standard HMMs tagger, Brants [2] developed the TnT tagger (short form of Tri-grams'n'Tags) which the transition probability depends on two preceding tags. TnT tagger uses the Viterbi algorithm for second-order Markov models. The states of the model represent tags while the outputs represent the words. Usually, the trigram probabilities generated from training data cannot be directly used because of data sparseness. Therefore, the TnT tagger smooths the probability with linear interpolation to handle this problem. The tags of unknown words are predicted based on the word suffix. Practically, TnT tagger provides good efficiency when the input text consists only of known words in known context. Hence, the performance of the tagger will decline while the number of unknown words increases. During its execution, the TnT tagger runs two main programs:

- "tnt-para" is a program for the training task that requires a tagged training corpus (.tt extension) to generate the parameter file (.tnt extension). By default, it generates lexical and contextual frequencies (.lex and .123 extensions) from the training corpus.
- "tnt" is the tagging program, it requires the text file to be tagged and the lexical and contextual frequencies files (.lex and .123).

In addition to these two programs, there is an auxiliary program called "tnt-diff" for counting differences between the tagged file and a correct version of it.

Treetagger. Since the HMMs based methods have difficulties in estimating transition probabilities accurately from limited amounts of training data, they require a large training corpus to avoid data sparseness. Thus, they apply different methods such as smoothing to resolve the problem of low frequencies. Consequently, by using a decision tree, a new method was developed to avoid problems that HMMs face in transition probabilities. Based on this method a language-independent PoS tagger called Treetagger has been developed [4]. Expressly, the Treetagger uses an unknown word PoS guesser similar to that of the TnT tagger. However, Treetagger estimates transition probabilities with a binary decision tree which means that the probability of a given trigram is determined by following the corresponding path through the tree until a leaf is reached. The Treetagger also runs two programs:

- "train-Treetagger" is a program for the training phase that generates the language model, i.e., a parameter file (.par), from a training corpus, a lexicon, and an open class file.
- "tree-tagging" is the tagger itself. It takes as an input the parameter file generated in the training phase and a text file to be tagged.

SVMTool. It is proposed as a standard PoS tagger by [3] based on SVMs. The SVMTool comes with the implementation of five different kinds of models for training "0 (default),1, 2, 3 and 4" with a tagging direction that can be either "left-to-right", "right-to-left", or a combination of both. Models 0, 1, and 2 differ only in the features they consider. For example, in Model 0 the unseen context remains ambiguous unlike the Model 1 that considers the unseen context already disambiguated in a previous step; while the Model 2 does not consider PoS features at all for the unseen context. Model 3 and Model 4 are just like Model 0 with respect to feature extraction. Similarly, the SVMTool runs three programs:

- "SVMTlearn" is the program responsible for the training of a set of SVM classifiers by adjusting a configuration file (config.svmt) and preparing a number of pre-tagged resources to generate the parameter files for the five training models;
- "SVMTagger" is the tagging program. It requires the path to a previously learned SVM model and a text file to be tagged;
- "SVMTeval": it is a program to evaluate the performance in terms of accuracy, it needs the tagging output and the corresponding gold-standard files.

2.3   Linguistic Resources

The Arabic is relatively a resource-poor language when it comes to finding freely available lexical resources and pre-tagged corpora. Fortunately, the Treetagger was adapted and evaluated for Arabic [21] and the used data were available and well-selected. Therefore, we adopt the same resources to adapt and evaluate the other taggers (TnT and SVMTool). To sum up, the used data to build the lexicon are extracted from:

- Morphological Analysers: AlKhalil Morpho Sys [22] and BAMA [23].
- Arabic verb conjugator: Qutrub[1];
- the Arabic Gigaword Corpus 4th Edition [24];
- Tashkeela Corpus [25];
- Named Entities extracted from the Arabic Wikipedia [26].

Regarding the data used for the training and evaluation processes, we used the following corpora:

- Al-Mus'haf corpus [27] which represents the Classical Arabic. The corpus covers the Quranic text where all the words are annotated with rich morphosyntactical information using a detailed PoS tagset. It was built using a semi-automatic method by applying "AlKhalil Morpho Sys" on the Quranic text followed by a manual treatment.
- NEMLAR corpus [28, 29]: it represents the MSA. It is an Arabic written corpus produced and annotated by RDI, Egypt for the Nemlar Consortium. It is divided into four parts: Raw diacriticized texts, PoS tagged texts, fully vowelized corpus, and lexically analysed corpus. NEMLAR contains different resources to represent various domains such as Arabic literature, politics, science, sports, etc.

Notice that, the training data and the lexicon must be in column format. Thus, we prepared the corpora and the lexicon to be in a tabular form. The column separator for the TnT and SVMTool is the blank space and a tabulation for the Treetagger. The token is expected to be in the first column of the line. The tag to predict takes the second column in the output. The rest of the line may contain additional morphological information such as the token's lemma. Table 1 presents all these resources with more details.

2.4   Tagset

A tag is a string used as a label to describe the word's morphosyntactical features (case, gender, etc.) and a tagset is a set of these tags. The Arabic language is composed of three main categories: Noun "اسم" <Asm> , Verb "فعل" <fEl> and Particle "حرف" <Hrf>. There are several projects that have been done on developing a standard Arabic PoS tagset, and they have been implemented by many taggers. These works were done by Khoja [30], Alqrainy [31], and Sawalha [32]. However, a recent study [33] was conducted to target the finest possible PoS tagset for Arabic based on an

---

[1] https://qutrub.arabeyes.org/.

Table 1. Linguistic resources

Type	Resources	Data description	Nb. Of words
Lexicon	Arabic Gigaword 4th edition	Broken plurals	2562
		High frequency words	37,716
	Arabic wikipedia	Persons names	16,000
		Places names	4587
	AlKhalil Morpho Sys	Utilities words	530
		Proper nouns	20,603
	Tashkeela	High frequency words	83,411
	Buckwalter analyzer	Obsolete words	8400
	Qutrub	Verbs	10,972
Corpora	Al-Mus'haf	CA corpus	78,121
	NEMLAR	MSA corpus	500,000

investigation involved the previously proposed tagsets. Also, this study was conducted considering the recommendations of EAGLES (Expert Advisory Group on Language Engineering Standards) and in collaboration with Arabic grammar experts. As findings of this study, a tagset was designed in form of detailed hierarchical levels of categories/subcategories. These hierarchical levels allow easier expansion when required and produce more accurate and precise results. Further, based on these hierarchical levels, four distinct collections of tagsets are generated. The aim is using a PoS tagset for the Arabic language considering both formal and functional aspects.

In the following experiments, the four distinct collections of these tagsets are involved to extend the evaluation results of the taggers. The tagsets are available for free at this site[2].

It is worth mentioning that a manual map was developed to convert the tagsets used in several linguistic resources to the newly adopted tagsets. To give an idea of the difference between the tagset collections implemented in this study, Table 2 presents the change of a tag from a simple collection to a more complicated one.

3 Experiments and Discussion

The performance of the three taggers was tested on data from the NEMLAR and Al-Mus'haf corpora. 90% words were used for training phase and the rest 10% words for testing. In this section, we highlight the use of the three taggers: TnT, Treetagger, and SVMTool via various experiments and we discuss the achieved results. Table 3 exhibits the tagging achieved accuracies of the three taggers for each collection of the proposed tagsets.

The obtained results show that the accuracy is influenced by the size and the text form of the training data as well as the tagset adopted. In addition, the experiments

---

[2] http://oujda-nlp-team.net/en/programms/standard-pos-tagset-arabic-language/.

Table 2. Illustrative examples of the implemented basic tags

Corpora	Collections	Nb. of tags	Examples
Al-Mus'haf	Col. 1	4	Noun
	Col. 2	26	Noun_Non-derivative
	Col. 3	79	Noun_Non-derivative_Verbal
	Col. 4	95	Noun_Non-derivative_Past verbal
NEMLAR	Col. 1	5	Verb
	Col. 2	12	Past verb
	Col. 3	63	Past verb_Active voice_Transitive
	Col. 4	107	Past verb_Active voice_Transitive to one object

Table 3. Tagging accuracy analysis

Corpus	Tested words	Unrecognized words	Collections	TnT (%)	Treetagger (%)	SVMTool (%)
Al-Mus'haf	7738	942	Col. 1	95.81	97.18	94.51
			Col. 2	93.87	94.02	92.32
			Col. 3	90.82	91.35	90.45
			Col. 4	90.45	91.65	90.06
Nemlar	50,000	6276	Col. 1	97.16	97.15	97.51
			Col. 2	93.94	93.86	95.32
			Col. 3	92.50	94.74	94.69
			Col. 4	90.94	97.55	93.85

have been done on a PC dual core of 1.6 GHz with 1.5 Go RAM in Perl language and the tagging speeds achieved are shown in Table 4.

Next, Table 5 summarizes the order of each tagger in terms of efficiency in performance compared to the others.

Table 4. Tagging speeds

TnT	Treetagger	SVMTool
13,700 w/s	15,000 w/s	1000 w/s

Table 5. Efficiency in performance

Criteria	Performance order		
	TnT	Treetagger	SVMTool
Training on small size of data	2	1	3
Training on medium size of data	3	1	1
Tagging unrecognized words	3	2	1
Dealing with ambiguity	2	2	1
Tagging speed	2	1	3

Generally, statistical taggers require a large training corpus to avoid data sparseness. As much as the training data is large and has high accuracy, the performance of the tagger is better. However, the tagging process achieved satisfactory results for the three taggers and for each collection of tagsets. Rather than that, using a small or medium size of training data with complex tagsets did not result in a sharp degradation of the accuracy. As can be seen from the previous tables, the following points describe the advantages of each tagger compared to the others:

- Treetagger accomplished its tagging process with high speed compared to the other taggers;
- Usually, more the used tagset is rich, more the performance decreases. However, Treetagger outperforms the TnT tagger and SVM-based tagger on tagging with extensive tagset, in fact, the accuracy starts to increase again with more complex tagset;
- Treetagger needs less training data to achieve satisfactory accuracy as binary decision trees have relatively few parameters to estimate;
- TnT performs well on known words sequences (words included in the training set) and it gives better results than SVMTool. Still, Treetagger is better in tagging these words than the other two taggers;
- TnT tagger gives relatively better results than Treetagger if they trained on medium or large data with small set of tagset, but SVMTool do better under the same conditions;
- The SVM-based tagger outperforms the TnT tagger and Treetagger on unrecognized words (words not included in training data), also achieved better results with ambiguity.

Another result assumed from Table 3 that shows the influence of a tagset complexity on tagging accuracy. In the following experiments, we demonstrate that the text form (CA or MSA) has also an influence on PoS taggers performance. In these experiments, we perform five cases of taggers implementation:

- Case 1: train and test the taggers on CA texts from Al-Mus'haf corpus.
- Case 2: train and test the taggers on MSA texts from NEMLAR corpus.
- Case 3: train the taggers on CA texts and test them on MSA texts.
- Case 4: train the taggers on MSA text and test them on CA texts.
- Case 5: train the taggers on a mixed training data that contain CA and MSA texts and test them on three different samples CA, MSA, and a combination of both forms.

The overall achieved accuracies are presented in Table 6.

The **Case 3** and **Case 4** show impressive accuracies. That is, only a 78.56% is achieved as high accuracy as possible using SVMTool. Therefore, it is not recommended at all for the Arabic language to train a tagger on MSA and use it to tag a CA text or vice versa. In **Case 5**, the mixed training data that contain text from MSA and CA achieved better accuracies of tagging process than cases **3** and **4**. However, the performance of PoS taggers is still inferior compared to the **Case 1** and **Case 2**. As a conclusion, the PoS tagger will perform better if only it is trained and tested on the same text form.

Table 6. The influence of text form on tagging performance

Cases		TnT (%)	Treetagger (%)	SVMTool (%)
Case 1		93.23	93.32	92.27
Case 2		93.94	93.56	94.88
Case 3		72.32	76.83	78.56
Case 4		65.15	69.75	63.94
Case 5	Test 1: Al-Mus'haf	81.99	82.14	82.06
	Test 2: NEMLAR	91.59	92.78	93.95
	Test 3: Test 1 + 2	87.70	88.61	89.11

The last observation in these experiments is analysing the common errors of the three PoS taggers. The rate of common errors varies from 2.21 to 3%. As all these taggers are developed using statistical methods, which means that the transition probability depends on preceding tags, we will have any impact in the case of Multi-word terms. For more illustration, Table 7 exhibits two examples of Multi-word terms and its impact on the sequence of tags in the same sentence.

This kind of problem can be resolved using rules-based methods in combination with statistical ones.

Table 7. The influence of Multi-words terms on tagging performance

Sentences	Tags order
Mohamed Ali won the final	Noun/Noun/Verb/Particle/Noun/
Mohammed Ali Clay won the final	Noun/Noun/Noun/Verb/Particle/Noun/

4   Conclusion and Perspectives

The standardization of Arabic lexicon and grammar Arabic are deeply rooted and well-established a long time ago in history. Arabic is also an international modern language and recognized as one of the six major official languages of the United Nations. On the other hand, it has not received a proportional attention when it comes to the development of open-source NLP applications and resources. The scarcity of available PoS tagger devoted to handling the complexity of Arabic morphology which leading us to adapt and study the performance of standard PoS taggers. In this paper, we highlighted probabilistic tagging methods by adapting three standard PoS taggers TnT, TreeTagger, and SVMTool. The main purpose was to evaluate these taggers and apply them to the Arabic language. Basically, these taggers are robust with respect to the size of the training corpus where they require enormous amounts of tagged data to get reasonable frequencies of PoS trigrams. However, small training data did not result in a sharp degradation of the accuracy, as it was observed in the conducted experiments.

Regarding the comparative study, many factors influenced the efficiency in performance of each tagger compared to the others such as the size of training data, the complexity of the tagset implemented, and the text forms. For instance, the TreeTagger outperforms the other taggers when the small training data and detailed tagset are used. On the other hand, the SVMTool do better with large training data and a small set of tagset. The present paper also gives an overview of most relevant PoS tagging methods and language-independent tagger. This work is another step in the direction of implementing relevant standard taggers for Arabic.

It was obvious that the accuracy could not reach its high-level using these adapted statistical taggers only. In addition, the tagging results showed that the taggers have, to a certain degree, distinct types of features. For those reasons, we highly recommend the use of a strategy that either combines the tagging results achieved by different taggers or involves other kind of tagging methods to come up with an efficient hybrid tagging system. Finally, it seems important to increase the size of the lexicon and the training corpus to decrease the number of unknown words.

References

1. Henrich, V., Reuter, T., Loftsson, H.: CombiTagger: a system for developing combined taggers. In: FLAIRS Conference (2009)
2. Brants, T.: TnT: a statistical part-of-speech tagger. In: Proceedings of the Sixth Conference on Applied Natural Language Processing, pp. 224–231. Association for Computational Linguistics (2000)
3. Giménez, J., Marquez, L.: SVMTool: a general POS tagger generator based on support vector machines (2004)
4. Schmid, H.: Probabilistic part-ofispeech tagging using decision trees. In: New Methods in Language Processing, p. 154. Routledge (2013)
5. Abumalloh, R.A., Al-Sarhan, H.M., Ibrahim, O., Abu-Ulbeh, W.: Arabic part-of-speech tagging. J. Soft Comput. Decis. Support Syst. 3, 45–52 (2016)
6. Zeroual, I., Lakhouaja, A.: Data science in light of natural language processing: an overview. Proc. Comput. Sci. 127, 82–91 (2018)
7. Zeroual, I., Lakhouaja, A.: Arabic Corpus linguistics: major progress, but still a long way to go. In: Intelligent Natural Language Processing: Trends and Applications, pp. 613–636. Springer, Cham (2018)
8. Diab, M., Hacioglu, K., Jurafsky, D.: Automatic tagging of Arabic text: from raw text to base phrase chunks. In: Proceedings of HLT-NAACL 2004: Short Papers, pp. 149–152. Association for Computational Linguistics (2004)
9. Farghaly, A., Shaalan, K.: Arabic natural language processing: challenges and solutions. ACM Trans. Asian Lang. Inf. Process. TALIP. 8, 14 (2009)
10. Utvić, M.: Annotating the corpus of contemporary Serbian. In: Proceedings of the INFOtheca '12 Conference (2011)
11. AlGahtani, S., Black, W., McNaught, J.: Arabic part-of-speech tagging using transformation-based learning. In: Proceedings of the Second International Conference on Arabic Language Resources and Tools, Cairo, Egypt (2009)
12. Altabba, M., Al-Zaraee, A., Shukairy, M.A.: An Arabic morphological analyzer and part-of-speech tagger. Thesis Present. Fac. Inform. Eng. Arab Int. Univ. Damascus Syr. (2010)
13. Maamouri, M., Bies, A., Kulick, S., Gaddeche, F., Mekki, W., Krouna, S., Bouziri, B., Zaghouani, W.: Arabic treebank: part 1 v 4.1. (2013)

14. Van den Bosch, A., Marsi, E., Soudi, A.: Memory-based morphological analysis and part-of-speech tagging of Arabic. In: Arabic Computational Morphology, pp. 201–217. Springer (2007)

15. Toutanova, K., Klein, D., Manning, C.D., Singer, Y.: Feature-rich part-of-speech tagging with a cyclic dependency network. In: Proceedings of the 2003 Conference of the North American Chapter of the Association for Computational Linguistics on Human Language Technology-Volume 1, pp. 173–180. Association for Computational Linguistics (2003)

16. Al Shamsi, F., Guessoum, A.: A hidden Markov model-based POS tagger for Arabic. In: Proceeding of the 8th International Conference on the Statistical Analysis of Textual Data, France, pp. 31–42 (2006)

17. Diab, M.: Second generation AMIRA tools for Arabic processing: fast and robust tokenization, POS tagging, and base phrase chunking. In: 2nd International Conference on Arabic Language Resources and Tools (2009)

18. Hadni, M., Ouatik, S.A., Lachkar, A., Meknassi, M.: Hybrid part-of-speech tagger for non-vocalized Arabic text. Int. J. Nat. Lang. Comput. **2**, 1–15 (2013)

19. Ababou, N., Mazroui, A.: A hybrid Arabic POS tagging for simple and compound morphosyntactic tags. Int. J. Speech Technol. **19**, 289–302 (2016)

20. Aliwy, A.H.: Arabic Morphosyntactic raw text part of speech tagging system. http://portal.mimuw.edu.pl/wiadomosci/aktualnosci/doktoraty/pliki/ahmed_hussein_aliwy/aa-dok.pdf (2013)

21. Imad, Z., Abdelhak, L.: Adapting a decision tree based tagger for Arabic. In: Presented at the 2016 International Conference on Information Technology for Organizations Development, IT4OD 2016 (2016)

22. Boudchiche, M., Mazroui, A., Bebah, M.O.A.O., Lakhouaja, A., Boudlal, A.: AlKhalil Morpho Sys 2: a robust Arabic morpho-syntactic analyzer. J. King Saud Univ.-Comput. Inf. Sci. **29**, 141–146 (2017)

23. Buckwalter, T.: Buckwalter Arabic morphological analyzer (BAMA) version 2.0. linguistic data consortium (LDC) catalogue number LDC2004L02. ISBN1-58563-324-0 (2004)

24. Parker, R.: Arabic Gigaword Fourth Edition LDC2009T30 (2009)

25. Zerrouki, T., Balla, A.: Tashkeela: novel corpus of Arabic vocalized texts, data for auto-diacritization systems. Data Brief. **11**, 147–151 (2017)

26. Attia, M.: Arabic named entities. https://sourceforge.net/projects/arabicnes/

27. Zeroual, I., Lakhouaja, A.: A new Quranic Corpus rich in morphosyntactical information. Int. J. Speech Technol., 1–8 (2016)

28. Attia, M., Yaseen, M., Choukri, K.: Specifications of the Arabic Written Corpus produced within the NEMLAR project (2005)

29. Yaseen, M., Attia, M., Maegaard, B., Choukri, K., Paulsson, N., Haamid, S., Krauwer, S., Bendahman, C., Fersøe, H., Rashwan, M., et al.: Building annotated written and spoken Arabic LR's in NEMLAR project. In: Proceedings of LREC, pp. 533–538 (2006)

30. Khoja, S.: APT: Arabic part-of-speech tagger. In: Proceedings of the Student Workshop at NAACL, pp. 20–25 (2001)

31. Alqrainy, S.: A morphological-syntactical analysis approach for Arabic textual tagging. http://ethos.bl.uk/OrderDetails.do?uin=uk.bl.ethos.505224? (2008)

32. Sawalha, M.: Arabic morphological features tag set. http://www.comp.leeds.ac.uk/sawalha/tagset_details.html (2009)

33. Zeroual, I., Lakhouaja, A., Belahbib, R.: Towards a standard Part of Speech tagset for the Arabic language. J. King Saud Univ.—Comput. Inf. Sci. **29**, 174–181 (2017)

Model-Based Security Implementation on Internet of Things

Yasmina Andaloussi[⊠] and Moulay Driss El Ouadghiri

IA Laboratory, University of Moulay Ismail, Meknes, Morocco
{andyasmina,dmelouad}@gmail.com

Abstract. The explosion in the number of smart, connected and insecure devices is changing the paradigm of security, security vulnerabilities and attacks have been increased over the last few years. Currently, myriad of nodes and smart objects are connected to each other to create smart grids and infrastructures. These environments compromise our intimate and private information about our health, our location and our business. To combat the risk to intercept our communications and compromise our privacy, research investments in security fields is steadily increasing and various security models, approaches and frameworks have been proposed. This article examines the evolution of security in the context of the Internet of Things. It proposes a secure scenario in which authentication and secure communication are granted.

Keywords: Internet of Things · Security · Privacy · Access control

1 Introduction

The Internet of Things concept aims to connect anything with anyone, anytime, and anywhere. It enables interactions between the physical and virtual worlds. With the development of this field, the range of security risks is increased and the risk of loss of critical information is increasing. Security issues, such as privacy, authorization, access control, integrity, and confidentiality, are the main challenges in an IoT environment. IoT applications simplify the user's daily life, but they generate sensitive and private data. However, security is not guaranteed. The development of IoT depends greatly on the resolution of security problems.

In IoT environments, sensitive data can be stored in a distributed manner. It is important to put in place an adequate control mechanism to control and manage the data. Confidentiality for end users is a very complex issue because it involves interactions with all the different components of the system, and affects all layers of the system structure. Obtaining and analyzing all these properties represents a significant research challenge.

Access control mechanisms focus on how people can access personal information. It is important to emphasize the need for efficient policies and mechanisms to manage different types of data and to adapt to different situations in IoT contexts. This group can include blocking approaches, lightweight protocols, and data sharing, as well as access techniques.

© Springer Nature Switzerland AG 2019
M. Ezziyani (Ed.): AI2SD 2018, AISC 915, pp. 841–846, 2019.
https://doi.org/10.1007/978-3-030-11928-7_76

To adopt IoT, this problem must be addressed in order to guarantee the user's trust in terms of confidentiality and control of personal information.

This study focuses on security threats and vulnerabilities in the context of the IoT, we present the state-of-the-art IoT security, then we propose an IoT security approach in IoT environments. We implemented the approach in a scenario composed of a Raspberry Pi and an ESP 8266.

2   Overview

Different research groups have investigated the method of securing IoT environments. In [1], the authors focused on authentication and data integrity concerns, they suggested to develop new software applications to control access to personal data.

In [2], the authors identified three key issues to be innovated: confidentiality, privacy and trust, they did not give attention to authentication, integrity and access control.

In [3, 4], the authors present analysis of existing protocols and security mechanisms of communications in IoT and presented different open research issues.

Finally, we cite [5], in which the authors divided the security aspects into three categories: security requirements (authentication, confidentiality and access control), privacy, and trust. The main limitation of this work is the lack of classification of the listed research activities according to a clear sorting logic.

3   Access Control in IoT Environments

DCapBAC has been proposed as a feasible approach for IoT scenarios even in the presence on devices with resource constraints. The concept of this approach is the concept of capability, which was originally introduced by [6] as "token, ticket, or key that gives the possessor permission to access an entity or object in a computer system".

This capability token is usually composed by privileges which are granted to the entity holding the token. Therefore, it is necessary to consider suitable cryptographic mechanisms to be used even on resource constrained devices which enable an end-to-end secure access control mechanism [6, 7].

In CapBAC [7–9], an entity, which wants to access certain information from another entity, requires to send a token together the request. Thus, the entity that receives the capability already knows the right level (i.e., permissions) that the requester has been granted when need to process the request. This simplifies the authorization mechanism and it is a relevant feature in scenarios with resources-constrained devices, since complex access control policies are not required.

4   Our Approach

An implementation was realized to demonstrate the feasibility of the approach. The elements of our architecture are: Raspberry Pi, the issuer, responsible for generating the capability token. ESP 8266, the end-device that will be read the request, verify the signature and decide to accept or not the request. The ESP 8266 is a resource-constrained device, with a 64 KiB of instruction RAM, 96 KiB of data RAM. The Raspberry PI has been implemented in Java and the ESP 8266 has been implemented in C, C++.

For this implementation, a light cryptography is used to be supported by ESP 8266 because of his limited resources. We used elliptic curve cryptography (ECC) optimizations. For that, an optimized elliptic curve digital signature algorithm (ECDSA) implementation for constrained devices was employed.

4.1 Process of Decision

1. The Raspberry PI generate the capability token: The capability token is represented by JSON [7, 10] for its suitability in constrained devices. A brief description of each field is provided following the notation of [7, 10]. This token contains the access rights that the issuer grants to the subject, and the date of validity and expiration of the token, then the Raspberry PI signs the token and sends it to the ESP 8266.
2. ESP 8266 receives the token, checks his signature, checks if the action is permitted, checks that the actions are fulfilled and checks the legitimacy of the user. Then, the ESP 8266 decides to permit access or not.

4.2 Experimental Results

For the proposed scenario, we used the token capability example shown in Fig. 1 to realize this scenario:

Raspberry Pi, the issuer, responsible for generating the capability token with the access rights for the end-device.

- The Raspberry Pi generates the capability token with the access rights.
- The Raspberry Pi signs the capability token with an elliptic curve cryptography (ECC) because of its suitability in constrained devices, for that we use elliptic curve digital signature algorithm (ECDSA) (Fig. 2).
- The Raspberry Pi hash the capability token to guarantee the integrity of the token (Fig. 3).
- The Raspberry Pi sends the capability token to the ESP 8266 (end-device).

  ESP 8266, the end-device:

- The end-device verifies the validity of the capability token, if the token is not valid, the request is refused (Fig. 4).
- The end-device verifies each one of the access rights.
- The end-device verifies the permissions of each resource.
- The end-device will recalculate the signature and compare it with the signature of the token (Fig. 5).
- If all the actions are granted, the access is permitted.

```
{
  "id": "7g3vfT_q9vTL2aQ4",
  "ii": 1415174237,
  "is": "issuer@um.es",
  "su": "zNwS5FetB4rwzSKsWwSBAxm5wDa=JgLjHU8zSnmeSFQgSG9HhdsJrE8=",
  "de": "coap://sensortemp.floor1.computersciencefaculty.um.es",
  "si": "SbUudG4zuXswFBxDeHB87N6t9hR=PBQqCN3gpu7nSkuPzDk7kaR3dq1=",
  "ar": [
    {
      "ac": "GET",
      "re": "temperature",
      "f": 1,
      "co": [
        {
          "t": 5,
          "v": 25,
          "u": "Cel",
        },
        {
          "t": 6,
          "v": 20,
          "u": "Cel",
        }
      ]
    }
  ],
  "nb": 1415174237,
  "na": 1415175381
}
```

Fig. 1. The capability token used in implementation

```
93    uECCPrivateKey privKey = new uECCPrivateKey("00038B1862B4C0FDBCDD7A035435BB20B302078399", curve
94    uECCPublicKey pubKey = privKey.computePublicKey();
95    uECCKeyPair pair2 = uECCKeyPair.from(privKey, pubKey);
96
97    signature = privKey.sign(hash);
98    System.out.println(pubKey.verify(hash, signature));
99
```

Fig. 2. The capability token signature

```
39    MessageDigest digest = MessageDigest.getInstance("SHA-256");
40    byte[] hash = digest.digest(text.getBytes(StandardCharsets.UTF_8));
41
  MessageDigest digest = MessageDigest.getInstance("SHA-256");
  byte[] hash = digest.digest((token.toString()).getBytes(StandardCharsets.UTF_8));
```

Fig. 3. The capability token hash

```
114
115    if (memcmp(secret1, secret2, 20) != 0) {
116        Serial.print("Shared secrets are not identical!\n");
117    } else {
118        Serial.print("Shared secrets are identical\n");
119    }
120
```

Fig. 4. The legitimacy of the capability token

```
121    /* Create a SHA256 hash */
122    SHA256 hasher;
123
124    /* Update the hash with your message, as many times as you like */
125    char hello[2048];
126    gen_random(hello,2048);
127    Serial.print("Message :");Serial.println(hello);
128
129
130
131    hasher.doUpdate(hello, strlen(hello));
132    /* Compute the final hash */
133    byte hash[SHA256_SIZE];
134    hasher.doFinal(hash);
135
136
137    Serial.print("Hash :");
138    /* hash now contains our 32 byte hash */
139    for (byte i=0; i < NELEMS(hash); i++){
140        if (hash[i]<0x10) { Serial.print('0'); }
141        Serial.print(hash[i], HEX);
```

Fig. 5. Signature recalculation in the end-device

5   Discussion

Due to constraints in the IoT devices, security in IoT cannot be fulfilled by traditional approaches. A distributed approach is necessary to cope with these challenges. We presented a distributed scenario based in CapBAC feasible with its implementation. In this work, an optimized ECDSA implementation for constrained devices has been realized.

6   Conclusion

The security is a challenge in IoT environments and new technologies. This implementation is considered the constraints of smart objects in term of storage, energy consumption and execution time. This paper treats the CapBAC approach that was proposed as a feasible approach for IoT environments. The light cryptography is necessary to be supported in constrained devices.

References

1. Atzori, L., Iera, A., Morabito, G.: The internet of things: a survey, Comput. Netw. **54**(15), 2787–2805 (2010). Maxwell, J.C.: A treatise on electricity and magnetism, 3rd edn., vol. 2. Clarendon, Oxford, pp. 68–73 (1892)
2. Miorandi, D., Sicari, S., de Pellegrini, F., Chlamtac, I.: Survey internet of things: vision, applications and research challenges. Ad Hoc Netw. **10**(7), 1497–1516 (2012)

3. Perera, C., Zaslavsky, A.B., Christen, P., Georgakopoulos, D.: Context aware computing for the internet of things: a survey. CoRR abs/1305.0982

4. Granjal, J., Monteiro, E., Silva, J.: Security for the internet of things: a survey of existing protocols and open research issues. IEEE Commun. Surv. Tutor. **99**, 1 (2015)

5. Sicari, S., Rizzardi, A., Grieco, L.A., Coen-Porisini, A.: Security, privacy and trust in internet of things: the road ahead. Comput. Netw. **76**, 146–164 (2015)

6. Dennis, J., Horn, E.V.: Programming semantics for multiprogrammed computations. Commun. ACM **9**(3), 143–155 (1966)

7. Andaloussi, Y., et al.: Access control in IoT environlents:Feasible scenario. Proc. Comput. Sci. 1031–1036 (2018)

8. Ellison, C., Frantz, B., Lampson, B., Rivest, R., Thomas, B., Ylonen, T.: RFC2693: SPKI Certificate theory. IETF RFC 2693 (Sep 1999). http://www.ietf.org/rfc/rfc2693.txt

9. Gusmeroli, S., Piccione, S., Rotondi, D.: A capability-based security approach to manage access control in the internet of things. Math. Comput. Model. **58**(5–6), 1189–1205 (2013)

10. Ferraiolo, D., Cugini, J., Kuhn, R.: Role-based access control (RBAC): features and motivations. In: Proceedings of 11th Annual Computer Security Application Conference, pp. 241–248 (1995)

Performance Evaluation of Multicast Routing Protocols in MANET

Safaa Laqtib[1]([✉]), Khalid El Yassini[1], and Moulay Lahcen Hasnaoui[2]

[1] Informatics and Applications Laboratory (IA),
Department of Mathematics and Computer Science, Faculty of Sciences,
Moulay Ismail University, Meknes, Morocco
{laq.safaa,khalid.elyassini}@gmail.com
[2] ISIC ESTM, L2MI Laboratory, ENSAM,
Moulay Ismail University, Meknes, Morocco
myhasnaoui@gmail.com

Abstract. A Mobile Ad hoc Network (MANET) is self-sufficient network made out of mobile devices associated by wireless links without the utilization of infrastructure. Essential issues in MANET are link failure, limited bandwidth, and restricted battery control, poses many challenging issues in accomplishing quality of service (QoS) arranged correspondence. The target of a multicast routing protocol for MANETS is to support the propagation of data from a sender to every one of the receivers of a multicast group and attempting to utilize the accessible bandwidth efficiently within the sight of successive topology changes. Multicasting can enhance the efficiency of the wireless link when sending multiple copies of messages by abusing the natural broadcast property of wireless transmission. this paper exhibits a broad investigation of multicast routing protocols MAODV, ODMRP, PUMA, AMRoute, and AMRIS for MANET under different network scenarios utilizing parameters like throughput, packet delivery ratio, and average end-to-end delay.

Keywords: Mobile ad hoc networks · Multicast routing protocols · MAODV · ODMRP · PUMA · AMroute · AMRIS

1 Introduction

Mobile ad hoc network MANET is a self-configuring and self-framing network of mobile routers connected by wireless links with no access point. Every mobile device in a network is autonomous. The mobile devices are allowed to move haphazardly and sort out themselves arbitrarily. Nodes in the MANET share the wireless medium and the topology of the network changes erratically and dynamically [1].

There are many typical applications of MANET such as: (1) military battlefield: ad hoc networking would enable the military to take advantage of commonplace network technology to keep up a data network between the soldiers, vehicles, and military data head quarter [2], (2) Personal area network and Bluetooth: A personal area network is a short range, localized network where nodes are usually associated with a given person. Short-range MANET such as Bluetooth can simplify the inter communication between

© Springer Nature Switzerland AG 2019
M. Ezziyyani (Ed.): AI2SD 2018, AISC 915, pp. 847–856, 2019.
https://doi.org/10.1007/978-3-030-11928-7_77

various mobile devices such as a laptop, and a mobile phone, and too many other applications such as Commercial Sector, Collaborative work, Local level [3].

Multicasting in MANET implies the transmission of packets from a source or a group of sources to a group of one or more nodes that are recognized by a solitary destination address. Multicasting lessens the transmission cost when sending a similar packet to multiple recipients [4].

Different multicast routing protocols proposed in the literature, as shown in Fig. 1, they classified according to two different criteria: (1) proactive and reactive and (2) tree-based or mesh-based and after that (3) Hybrid-based. Proactive conventions maintain routing state, while reactive protocols decrease the effect of frequent topological changes by rethinking routes on demand. Tree-based schemes establish a single way between any two nodes in the multicast group and they are bandwidth efficient. Be that as it may, as mobility mesh-based schemes build up a mesh of alternate paths interconnecting source and destinations. They give more solid paths and are stronger to link failures as well as to various mobility conditions of nodes and Hybrid-based which creates a bi-directional, shared tree by using only group senders and receivers as tree nodes for data distribution [5, 6].

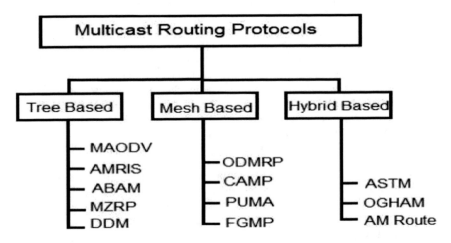

Fig. 1. Multicasting routing protocols

The criteria to group the multicast routing protocols is routing information gathering strategy, multicast initiator, multicast topology, dependence on a focal node like core, network support and disappointment administration, level of reliance on unicast routing protocol, and stateless multicast routing. A few multicasting protocols have been proposed and intended for ad hoc networks, for example, MAODV, ODMRP, AMROUTE, AMRIS, PUMA ETC. [7, 8, 9].

In this paper, we analyze the performance of some multicast routing protocols on the basis of certain performance criteria which includes throughput, delay, network lifetime using NS2 simulator. To perform the evaluation, a simulation scenario is designed to carry out the experiment [10].

The remaining paper is organized as follows: brief description of multicast routing protocols in MANET are listed in Sect. 2. The Performance evaluation and simulation scenario is described in Sect. 3 followed by conclusion in last session.

2 Brief Description of Multicast Routing Protocols in MANET

2.1 Multicast Ad Hoc on-Demand Distance Vector (MAODV)

MAODV [11] is similar to the operation of AODV [12], with AODV for unicast traffic and MAODV for multicast traffic. The MAODV is a tree-based multicast routing protocol in which every node quickly responds to breakage of links in multicast trees by correcting these periodically and consisting of only receivers and relays.

The first node to join the group in the connected component acts as a group leader for each multicast tree. It transmits a group hello packet to become aware of reconnections. Nodes can join into a group by sending a unicast route request (RREQ) if they have the address of group leader or a broadcast RREQ packet if group leader is unknown. MAODV allows each node in the network to send out multicast data packets, and the multicast data packets are broadcast when propagating along the multicast group tree. Members of the multicast group replies its distance from group leader and group sequence number by means of a route reply packet (RREP). The node demanding to join sends multicast activation (MACT) [13] message to the nearest member with an updated sequence number. After reception of MACT all the intermediate nodes become the members of the tree.

2.2 On-Demand Multicast Routing Protocol (ODMRP)

On-Demand Multicast routing protocol (ODMRP) for mobile ad hoc networks [14] is a mesh-based source-initiated protocol, mesh protocol creates a mesh of nodes which forward multicast packets via flooding, it uses forwarding group concept and multiple paths exist between sender and receiver. It applies on-demand procedures to build route and maintain multicast group membership dynamically. In ODMRP, group membership and multicast routes are established and updated by the source on demand [15].

If a multicast source has packets to send, it floods a member advertising packet called Join Query packet. On receiving the Join Query packet, every node in the network rebroadcast the packets to their neighbor nodes after storing the upstream node address into their route table. In response to these Join Query packets, the multicast receivers create and broadcast a Join Reply message to their neighbors. These Join Reply messages relayed back to the source using the known reverse path. The nodes on the reverse path become the forwarding group. Another unique property of ODMRP is its unicast capability. Not only can ODMRP coexist with any unicast routing protocol, it can also operate very efficiently as unicast routing protocol. Thus, a network equipped with ODMRP does not require a separate unicast protocol [16].

2.3   Protocol for Unified Multicasting Through Announcement (PUMA)

PUMA is distributed, receiver initiated and mesh-based protocols. Builds meshes that connect all receivers together. The main difference between a tree as constructed in MAODV and a mesh as constructed in PUMA [17] is that a mesh provides multiple paths between senders and receivers whereas a tree provides only a single path between senders and receivers. PUMA does not require any unicast routing protocol to operate. Each group has a special node called core node in the group. Every receiver connects to elected core along the shortest path, eventually forming a mesh. The first receiver acts as a rendezvous point (RP). If many receivers join the group at a time, then one with highest ID become the RP.

PUMA algorithm is used to elect one of the receivers of a group as the core of the group, and to inform each router in the network of at least one next-hop to the elected core of each group. The elected core is connected to receivers in the network through all possible shortest paths. All intermediate nodes on shortest paths collectively form the mesh structure. Data packets are sent from sender to the group via core along any possible shortest path and flooded. When the data packet reaches a mesh member, it is flooded within the mesh, and nodes maintain a packet ID cache to drop duplicate data packets. The election algorithm used in PUMA is essentially the same as the spanning tree algorithm introduced by Perlman for internetworks of transparent bridges duplicate data packets.

2.4   Ad Hoc Multicast Routing Protocol (AMRoute)

The (AMRoute) ad hoc multicast routing protocol is an endeavor to empower the utilization of IP multicast in MANETs. AMRoute make utilization of the fundamental unicast routing protocol to recognize network dynamics while it deals with the regular tree reconfigurations. The AMRoute conveyance tree expect unicast availability among part nodes and keeps on working regardless of network changes. The two key highlights that make AMRoute vigorous and proficient are [18]: (1) user-multicast trees permit group members to imitate and forward over unicast tunnels and (2) core node relocating powerfully bringing about changes to the group membership and network availability. Since non-member nodes in the tree require not be even multicast empowered, user multicast trees dispense with the need to reconfigure the tree every now and again in dynamic MANETs. In any case, the tradeoff is a decrease in bandwidth effectiveness as non-member nodes can't duplicate packets on user-multicast trees.

The AMRoute protocol comprises of a mesh creation stage following a tree creation stage. Each group member frames a 1-node mesh distinguishing itself as the core. The core node in quest for other group members periodically broadcasts join-request messages in an extended ring style. A member node, accepting join-request messages from a core node in an alternate mesh, reacts back with a join-ack setting up a bi-directional tunnel between the two nodes. Numerous cores result because of mesh mergers. All the core nodes choose a solitary core for the brought together mesh utilizing a core resolution algorithm. the core node requires not be static. It can move progressively as per group membership and network availability [18].

The core node of the unified the core node of the unified together mesh is in charge of the tree creation process. The core node intermittently sends tree-create messages along the connections episode on it in the mesh. The mesh size and node mobility in the work decides the periodicity of tree-create messages.

The core node of the brought together mesh is in charge of the tree creation process. the core node intermittently sends tree-create messages along the connections episode on it in the mesh. The mesh size and node mobility in the work decides the periodicity of tree-create messages. Gathering members that get non-duplicate tree-create messages gathering members that get non-duplicate tree-create messages forward it to every one of the links with the exception of the approaching link. In the event that the link isn't utilized as a major aspect of the tree, a tree-create-nak is transmitted through the approaching link. After accepting a tree-create-nak, the group member denotes the approaching connection as a mesh link. A member node advances information got on a tree link yet disposes of it when gotten on a mesh link and sends a tree-create-nak along that link.

Simulation studies of AMroute demonstrate that the broadcast traffic is free of group size. This thinks about the join-reqs being created at a settled rate by the core for a steady network size, the join latency increments as the group size increments. The real weakness of the convention is it shapes impermanent loops amid tree creation and non-optimal trees at high mobility.

2.5   Ad Hoc Multicast Routing Protocol Utilizing Increasing Id Numbers (AMRIS)

AMRIS is an on-demand protocol that constructs a shared multicast delivery tree to help multiple senders and recipients in a multicast session. AMRIS [18] builds up a shared tree for multicast data forwarding. Every node in the network is assigned a multicast session id number. The positioning order of id numbers is used to direct the flow of multicast data. Like ODMRP, AMRIS does not require an isolate unicast routing protocol. at first, an uncommon node called sid broadcasts a new-session packet. The new session incorporates the sid's msm-id (multicast session part id). Neighbor nodes, upon receiving the packet, compute their own msm-ids which are larger than the one. The msm id indicates the logical height of a node in the multicast delivery tree rooted at the sender that has the smallest msm id (Sid) in the tree. All other nodes in the tree have an msm id that is higher than that of its parent.

In case of a multiple sender environment, the Sid is elected among the senders. AMRIS uses the underlying MAC layer beaconing mechanism to detect the presence of neighbors. Tree Initialization Phase: During the tree-initialization phase, the Sid broadcasts a New-Session message (containing the Sid, msm id and other routing metrics) in its neighborhood. A node, receiving the New-Session message, updates the msm id in the message with a newly computed larger value that is also used to identify the node in the tree.

If a node receives more than one New-Session messages from several neighbors within a random jitter amount of time, then the message with the best routing metric is selected and updated with a newly computed msm id value. The updated New-Session message is then rebroadcast. The above strategy prevents broadcast storms. Note that the newly computed msm ids are not consecutive and the gaps can be used to locally repair the delivery tree. To join the multicast group, a downstream node X sends a unicast Join-Request message to one of a randomly chosen neighbor node that is also a potential parent node (having a lower msm id), say Y. If Y is already part of the multicast tree, then Y sends a Join-ACK message to X. Otherwise, Y forwards the Join-Request message to a set of potential parents of itself. The above process continues until the Join- Request message reaches a parent node that is part of the multicast delivery tree. The parent node responds back with a Join-ACK message to X, which can now confirm its participation in the multicast session by sending back a Join-Conf message to the parent node.

3 Performance Evaluation

3.1 Performance Metrics

Performance of multicast routing protocols in MANET can be evaluated using a number of quantitative metrics. We have used packet delivery ratio, throughput, end-to-end delay for evaluating the performance of multicast routing protocols MAODV, PUMA, ODMRP, AMRoute, and AMRIS.

Packet Delivery Ratio. It is defined as the ratio of data packets It is defined as the ratio of number of data packets delivered to all the receivers to the number of data packets supposed to be delivered to the receivers. This ratio represents the routing effectiveness of the protocol. The performance is better when the packet delivery ratio is high it can be shown as equation [19] (1):

$$PDR = \frac{\sum packets\ received\ by\ destination\ nodes}{\sum packets\ sent\ by\ source\ nodes} \tag{1}$$

Throughput. It is defined as the ratio Throughput refers to how much data can be transferred from the source to the receiver(s) in a given amount of time, Throughput include frequent topology changes, unreliable communication, limited bandwidth and limited energy. A high throughput network is desirable; it can be shown as equation It can be shown as equation [19] (2):

$$Throughput = ((Packet\ received\ size/(Simulation\ stop\ time - Simulation\ start\ time)) * (8/1000)) \tag{2}$$

Average End-to-End Delay. It is the average time taken for a data packet to move from the source to the receivers, the deadline for the end-to-end delay includes the routing and other various delays, such as the transmission delay, propagation delay and delay queue. It can be shown as equation [19] (3):

$$End\ to\ End\ delay = \frac{\sum delay}{\sum packets\ received} \tag{3}$$

3.2 Simulation Scenarios

The simulations of PUMA, ODMRP, MAODV, AMRoute, and AMRIS are implemented in NS2. Our simulation models a network of 30 mobile nodes placed randomly within a 1200 m × 1200 m area. Each simulation executes for 1000 s of simulation time. The multicast data streams are CBR streams with jitters. The size of data packet is 512 bytes as shown in Table 1. The multicast sources are selected from all 20 nodes randomly and most of them act as receivers at the same time. Receivers join one multicast group at the beginning of the simulation and never leave the group during the simulation. Nodes randomly select a destination and move with a predefined average speed.

Table 1. Simulation configuration

Parameter	Example
Channel type	Wireless
Terrain	1200 × 1200 m
Ad hoc multicast routing protocol(s)	MAODV, PUMA, ODMRP, AMRoute, AMRIS
Traffic type	CBR
Time of simulation	1000 s
Simulator	NS-2
Initial energy	10.0 J
Packet size	512 bytes
Nodes	5, 10, 15, 20

The performance metrics used for our evaluation were Packet Delivery Ratio, Throughput and End-2-End Delay. Packet delivery ratio. Throughput is defined as total packets transmitted (control packets + data packets) divided by data packets delivered. Throughput is more important metric because we are concerned about the number of packets transmitted to get a certain number of data packets to the receivers, regardless of whether those packets were data or control.

We compared the performance of PUMA, AMRoute, ODMRP, MAODV, and AMRIS multicast routing protocols for ad hoc networks [18]. PUMA and MAODV are both receiver-oriented protocols. However, PUMA is a mesh-based protocol and provides multiple routes from senders to receivers. MAODV and AMRIS on the other hand, are a tree-based protocols and provides only a single route between senders and receivers, and AMRoute is a hybrid-based protocol. ODMRP is based source-initiated protocol.

Figure 2 shown that PUMA functioning admirably contrasted with different protocols. AMRoute, ODMRP, MAODV and AMRIS demonstrated poor performance fail for a network, as they lose more CBR packets started by the source. Since every sender of ODMRP floods control messages into the whole network occasionally, the packet collision likelihood ends up higher when the quantity of senders increments. The senders in the AMRIS protocol should forward information packets to a rendezvous

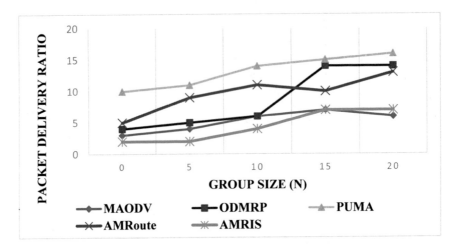

Fig. 2. Packet delivery ratio with varying group size for MAODV, ODMRP, PUMA, AMRoute, AMRIS

point, the rendezvous point is extremely bustling when numerous senders are sending data. This circumstance may likewise build the packet collision probability. The reason of poor execution of MAODV is non-formation of backup routes to go in a split second. AMRoute gives better execution due IP multicast of nodes.

PUMA is a mesh-based scheme, even if there is a link failure, the packets are transmitted using the redundant path in mesh for efficient group communication.

As shows in Fig. 3, all multicast routing protocols indicate ceaseless ascent in the throughput as the group size increments however there is contrast in the slant after the gathering size 15 the throughput of all multicast routing protocols are looked at by changing the group size of nodes. By expanding the movement stack the PUMA gives the better throughput took after by AMRoute, ODMRP, AMRIS and MAODV gives the less throughput contrasted with different protocols. So, contrasted with other. As It might be seen likewise from Fig. 3 that the throughput received in case of PUMA superior to the next multicast routing protocols.

As shown in Fig. 4, all the protocols MAODV, AMRoute and ODMRP raise with increase in the group size. This implies that slope MAODV, AMRoute and ODMRP is greater than that of PUMA and AMRIS. it is observed also that the average end to end delay is less in PUMA compared to ODMRP, MAODV, AMRoute and AMRIS. PUMA outperforms ODMRP, MAODV, AMRoute and AMRIS. With respect to average end-to-end delay. PUMA is a more suitable protocol for video streaming applications.

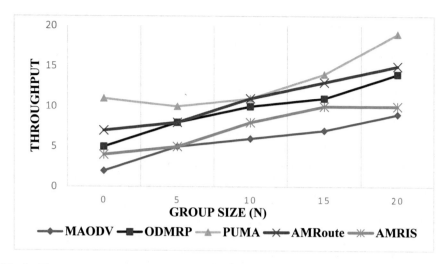

Fig. 3. Throughput with varying group size for MAODV, ODMRP, PUMA AMRoute, AMRIS

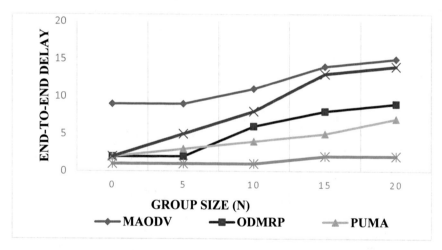

Fig. 4. End-to-end delay with varying group size for MAODV, ODMRP, PUMA AMRoute, AMRIS

4   Conclusion

In MANETs, both unicasting and multicasting can be used. But according to the performance analysis, specifically for group communications, multicast routing increases the efficiency and provides better performance.

The results obtained shows that PUMA protocol will perform better in the networks with a number of source and destination pairs relatively small for each host. In this case the number of packets send by PUMA is high then MAODV, AMRoute, AMRIS and ODMRP also in the case of throughput PUMA outperforms all the routing protocols and presents a low end to end delay, we can considerate it as the better multicast routing protocol. In future, a lot of work can be done to produce some new technologies to improve the performance of the multicast routing protocols in MANET such as ODMRP.

References

1. Chander, D., Kumar, R.: Analysis of scalable and energy aware multicast routing protocols for MANETs. Indian J. Comput. Sci. Eng. (IJCSE) **8**(3) (2017)
2. Kaur, I., Kaur, N., Tanisha, Gurmeen, Deepi, Challenges and issues in ad hoc network. Int. J. Comput. Sci. Technol. (2016)
3. Aarti, Tyagi S.S.: Study of MANET: characteristics, challenges, application and security attacks. Int. J. Adv. Res. Comput. Sci. Softw. Eng. **3**(5) (2013)
4. Adhvaryu, K.U., Kamboj, P.: Survey of various energy efficient multicast routing protocols for MANET (2013)
5. Aparna, K.: Performance comparison of MANET (mobile ad hoc network) protocols (ODMRP with AMRIS and MAODV). Int. J. Comput. Appl. (0975–8887), **1**(10) (2010)
6. Badarneh, O.S., Kadoch, M.: Multicast routing protocols in mobile ad hoc networks: a comparative survey and taxonomy. J. Wirel. Commun. Netw. (2009)
7. Kamboj, P., Sharma, A.K.: Energy efficient multicast routing protocol for MANET with minimum control overhead (EEMPMO). Int. J. Comput. Appl. (0975–8887) **8**(7), (2010)
8. Olagbegi, B.S., Meghanathan, N.: A review of the energy efficient and secure multicast routing protocols for mobile ad hoc networks. Int. J. Appl. Graph Theory Wirel. Ad Hoc Netw. Sens. Netw. (2010)
9. Jetcheva, J.G., Johnson, D.B.: A Performance Comparison of On-Demand Multicast Routing Protocols for Ad Hoc Networks. December 15, 2004
10. Jaiswal, R., Sahu, M.C., Mishra, A., Sharma, S.: Survey of energy efficient multicast routing protocols In Manet. Int. J. Adv. Res. Comput. Sci. Electr. Eng. (2012)
11. Chen, X., Wu, J.: Multicasting Techniques in Mobile Ad Hoc Networks. Computer Science Department Southwest Texas State University (2003)
12. Siva Ram Murthy, C., Manoj, B.S.: Ad Hoc Wireless Net-works Architectures and Protocols. Indian Institute of Technology (2004)
13. Harsha Chandran K.C., Jayasree P.S.: Multicast ad-hoc on-demand distance vector routing: a survey. Int. J. Sci. Eng. Technol. Res. (IJSETR) **6**(4) (2017). ISSN: 2278-7798
14. Lee, S.-J., Gerla, M., Chiang, C.-C.: On-demand multicast routing protocol. In: Proceedings of IEEE WCNC'99, pp. 1298–1304. New Orleans, LA (1999)
15. Rangarajan, J., Baskaran, K.: Performance analysis of multicast protocols: Odmrp, Puma And Obamp. Int. J. Comput. Sci. Commun. 2(2), 577–581 (2011)
16. Vaishampayan R., Zhu, Y., Kunz, T.: Efficient and robust multicast routing in mobile ad hoc networks. In: International Conference on Mobile Ad-hoc and Sensor, 2004
17. Periasamy, R., Ranjithkumar C., Panimalar, P.: A study on multicast routing protocols for MANETS: MRMP, ERAMOBILE, TSMP, LAM, PUMA. JCSNS Int. J. Comput. Sci. Netw. Secur. **13**(9) (2013)
18. Sumathy, S., Yuvaraj, B., Sri Harsha, E.: Analysis of multicast routing protocols: Puma and Odmrp. Int. J. Mod. Eng. Res. (IJMER) 2(6), 4613–4621 (2012)
19. Menchaca-Mendez, R., Garcia-Luna-Aceves, J.J.: Hydra: efficient multicast routing in MANETs using sender-initiated multicast meshes. Pervasive Mobile Comput. **6**(1), 144–157 (2010)

Analysis of Speaker's Voice in Cepstral Domain Using MFCC Based Feature Extraction and VQ Technique for Speaker Identification System

Mariame Jenhi[1(✉)], Ahmed Roukhe[2], and Laamari Hlou[1]

[1] Laboratory of Electrical Engineering and Energy System Faculty of Science,
University Ibn Tofail, Kenitra, Morocco
mariame.jenhi@uit.ac.ma
[2] Laboratory of Atomic, Mechanical, Photonics and Energy Faculty of Science,
University Moulay Ismail, Meknes, Morocco

Abstract. Automatic Speaker Recognition technology have been rapidly developed in recent years and facilely integrated with existing biometric system, which can be deployed in the identification systems to improve recognition and ensure security. An essential initial phase in Speaker Recognition (SR) system is the step of extracting accurate information from human acoustic signal that captures the unique characteristics of the speaker's voice. One popular choice for features extraction is the short-term spectral characteristics. In this paper, we proposed to investigate the performance of the Mel frequency cepstral coefficient (MFCC) to extract features in training phase for text-dependent speaker identification system. In order to evaluate the reliability of the proposed MFCCs feature sets, we use the Vector Quantization (VQ) classifier based on the best Known Linde-Buzo-Gray (LBG), and results are reported for a dataset composed of eight subject (5 male and 3 female). Moreover, we also outline the influence of changing the codebook size to find the best identification rate. The results elucidate the influence of the codebook size on the identification rate for the text-dependent speaker identification system that yield an identification accuracy of 87.5% using codebook of size 8, 16, 32 and 64.

Keywords: Automatic speaker identification · Mel-frequency cepstral coefficient (MFCC) · Vector quantization (VQ) · Codebook-size · Linde-Buzo-Gray (LBG)

1 Introduction

Human voice alongside with iris, face, signature and fingerprints recognition represent one of the major biometric tools for the identification of a person and can be used for many speech processing applications especially security, authentication and criminal investigations and does not require any sophisticated or dedicated hardware.

Speaker recognition process is the challenging task of recognizing persons from their voice. Basically this process falls into two categories: speaker verification and speaker identification. The identification task is a biometric method, which uses

© Springer Nature Switzerland AG 2019
M. Ezziyyani (Ed.): AI2SD 2018, AISC 915, pp. 857–868, 2019.
https://doi.org/10.1007/978-3-030-11928-7_78

speaker voice signal to identify a target speaker by compared with a number of prototype features obtained from speaker models [1]. On the other side, for the verification task, more specifically, consists of determining whether a voice sample was produced by a claimed speaker [2].

Speaker identification may be further categorized into text-independent and text-dependent cases. In text independent system, there is no limitation on text being spoken [3]. While text dependent recognition involves same input and target text. Speaker recognition systems employ the following two main modules: feature extraction and feature matching [4].

Feature extraction is the process of extracting unique information from the speaker's voice signal that can next be used to represent that speaker. The feature matching process aims is to identify the speaker depending on the classification techniques. Feature extraction technique is the most critical and important component that bring the important parts of the data to front [5]. Different types of feature extraction technique such as Perceptual linear prediction (PLP) [6], Linear Prediction Cepstral Coefficients (LPCC) [7], Mel-Frequency Cepstral Coefficients (MFCC) [8] have been proposed in the last years. For feature matching, different classifiers are used such as Support Vector Machine (SVM), Vector Quantization (VQ), Gaussian Mixture Model (GMM) [9], and Dynamic Time Warping (DWT).

Motivated by the great success of cepstral features in speech and speaker identification systems, this work aims to explore and evaluate the effectiveness of the Mel frequency cepstral features for text-dependent speaker identification system. The proposed system is based on three main steps: pre-processing, feature extraction, and feature matching including the Vector Quantization (VQ) based on the LBG clustering algorithm. Different codebook-sizes are used in this stage to test the performance of VQ based LBG algorithm on identification rate.

This paper is organized as follows. The process of extracting features using MFCCs is discussed in Sect. 2. VQ based LBG clustering algorithm is summarized in Sect. 3. The system implementation and results on this paper are provided in Sects. 4 and 5. Finally, conclusions and future works are discussed in Sect. 6.

2   Feature Extraction

The main objective of voice feature extraction process, is calculate parameters from the speech signal that are unique, discriminative and represent the characteristics of the input signal, in the purpose to differentiate between a wide set of distinct speakers [10]. The features extracted may be categorized into short-term spectral features, voice source features, spectro-temporal features, prosodic features etc. Short-term spectral features are extracted from speech signals by dividing them into short frames of 20–30 ms duration. Here we make use of Mel-Frequency Cepstral Coefficients (MFCC).

2.1   Computation of Mel-Frequency Cepstral Feature

The Mel-Frequency Cepstrum (MFC) is a representation of short-period power spectrum of sound wave, and the collection of coefficients of MFC is referred as MFCC, which is based on auditory characteristics of human [11]. MFCC have been used as an established and proven method to extract distinct characteristics of input speech signal [1]. Mel-frequency scale is a perceptually motivated scale that mimic the human auditory system, which is linear below 1 kHz and logarithm above, with equal numbers of samples below and above 1 kHz. The main principle of MFCC is filter-bank coefficient [3]. The overall process of MFCC analysis can be illustrated by the following block diagrams in Fig. 1.

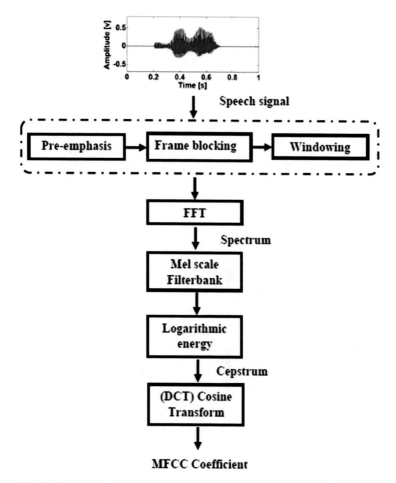

Fig. 1. Procedure for extracting Mel-frequency cepstral coefficients (MFCC)

The Pre-processing:

Acoustic signal pre-processing is the basis of the whole feature extraction system and used to increase the efficiency of the SR system, that generally including two stage: signal pre-emphasis and window framing.

Pre-emphasis: The quality of the speech signal affect strongly the signal processing applications. Although the Pre-emphasis step increases the amplitude of higher frequency band and decrease the amplitude of lower frequency band [2], in addition to that, higher frequencies are more important for signal disambiguation than lower frequencies. The most used filter is a high-pass FIR filter described in Eq. (1)

$$Y[n] = X[n] - aX[n-1] \quad \text{with } a = 0.95 \tag{1}$$

Let sound signal is $X[n]$ and $Y[n]$ the output of filter. The most typical value of is "a" is about 0.95 [12]. Various types of speech signal have their different spectral characteristics. From the spectrogram plot in Fig. 2, it can be observed that, speaker1 are distinguishable from speaker2 for their wide frequency range.

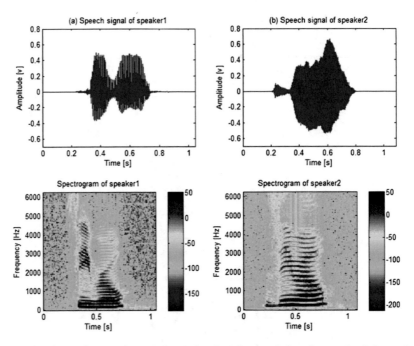

Fig. 2. Signal waveform and spectrogram showing characteristics of **a** speaker1, **b** speaker2

Window framing: windowing is carried out to reduce undesirable effects in the frequency response introduced by the discontinuities at the beginning and end of the frame. The input signal is divided into frames and each time frame is multiplied by a window function. In our study, we use Hamming window. The description of the Hamming window function is performed using Eq. (2).

$$w(n) = 0.54 - 0.46 \cos\left(\frac{2\pi n}{N-1}\right) \quad 0 \le n \le N-1 \tag{2}$$

Where N denotes the number of samples in each frame.

2.2 Fast Fourier Transform

The Fast Fourier transform is a process of converting each frame of N samples from the time domain into the frequency domain. Equation (3) represent FFT

$$X(k) = \sum_{n=0}^{N-1} x(n)e^{-\left(\frac{j2\pi k}{N}\right)}, \quad (0 \leq k \leq N) \tag{3}$$

Where $x(n)$ represents input frame, $X(k)$ represents its equivalent FFT and N correspond to the number of samples in each frame.

2.3 Mel Triangle Filter

The results of the FFT will be information about the amount of energy at each frequency band. In this step, the Mel- scale is used to plot the calculated spectrum in order to know the approximation value of the existing energy at each spot with the help of triangular filter bank. Mel-frequency scale is a perceptual scale that simulate the human auditory system which is linear below 1 kHz, and logarithm above, with equal numbers of samples below and above 1 kHz. The relationship between the frequency of speech signal and the Mel-Scale and is given in Eq. (4).

$$M_{el} = 2595 * \ln\left(1 + \frac{f_{el}}{700}\right) \tag{4}$$

Where M_{el} is the Mel frequency for the linear frequency f_{el}. The filter bank energy is obtained after Mel filtering [13]. Equation (5) represents the frequency response of the triangular filter $H_\sigma(k)$ with $\sigma = 1, 2 \ldots M$, is the number of filters,

$$H_\sigma(k) = \begin{cases} 0 & k < f_{\sigma-1} \\ \frac{2(k-f_{\sigma-1})}{(f_{\sigma+1}-f_{\sigma-1})(f_\sigma-f_{\sigma-1})} & f_{\sigma-1} \leq k \leq f_\sigma \\ \frac{2f((m+1)-k)}{(f_{\sigma+1}-f_{\sigma-1}))(f_{\sigma+1}-f_\sigma)} & f_\sigma \leq k \leq f_{\sigma+1} \\ 0 & f_{\sigma+1} < k \end{cases} \tag{5}$$

Figure 3 illustrates the MFCC filter-banks for the case of M = 20 frequency bands. The response curve of triangular window band-pass filter bank in Mel-frequency is shown in Eq. (6):

$$\sum_{\sigma-1}^{M-1} H_\sigma(k) = 1 \tag{6}$$

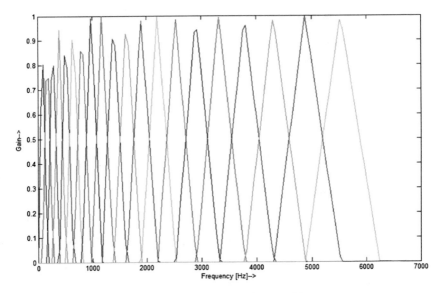

Fig. 3. The triangular filter $H_m(k)$

2.4 The Logarithmic Spectrum

Human ears smooth the spectrum and use the logarithmic scale approximately. The logarithmic spectrum of the output of each filter bank (Mel spectrum) can be computed as in Eq. (7) [1].

$$\vartheta_\sigma = \ln\left(\sum_{k=0}^{N-1} |S_f|^2 H_\sigma(k)\right) (0 \leq \sigma \leq M) \qquad (7)$$

Where ϑ_σ is the logarithmic spectrum and S_f is the disperse power spectrum.

2.5 Discrete Cosine Transform (DCT)

Finally, the discrete cosine transform (DCT) is used to converts the Mel coefficients back to time domain [2]. The DCT output is called as Mel Frequency Cepstrum Coefficients (MFCC) [14] and is performed on the log filter-bank energies ϑ_σ; the σth MFCC coefficient is represented by the Eq. (8)

$$\varsigma_\sigma = \sum_{\sigma=0}^{N-1} \vartheta_\sigma \cos\left(\frac{\pi n(\sigma - 0.5)}{M}\right), \quad (0 \leq n \leq M) \qquad (8)$$

where ς_σ is the MFCC coefficients.

3 Feature Matching

After the feature extraction stage, another important part is the feature matching [4]. In this section, the classification or clustering method known as vector quantization is discussed. This method is part of the decision making process of determining a person based on previously stored information, and it uses the features vectors extracted from speech signals as the inputs for this algorithm.

3.1 Vector Quantization

In a speaker identification system, the process of representing each speaker in a unique and efficient manner is known as vector quantization. The basic idea of this approach is to take vectors from a large feature vectors and reduce it to a finite group of feature vectors. Each vector is represented by its centroid point and is defined as a mapping function that maps "ϵ" dimensional vector space to a finite set $T = \{V_1, V_2, \ldots, V_N\}$ where T is called codebook [15] consisting of N number of code vectors and each code vector $V_i = \{v_{i1}, v_{i2}, \ldots, v_{i\epsilon}\}$ is of dimension "ϵ". This approach is popularly used to generate codebook known as Linde-Burzo-Gray (LBG) algorithm. The goal is to find the codebook that has the minimum distance measurement in order to identify the unknown word [16]. This project uses the Euclidean distance measurement for speaker similarity measure. The formula used in the function is defined as follow:

$$d(x, y) = (x - y)^{\mathrm{T}} \cdot (x - y) = \sum_{i=1}^{N} (x_i - y_i)^2 \qquad (9)$$

where x and y are multi-dimensional feature vectors

3.2 The LBG Algorithm

One of the most popular methods for the codebook training is the iterative clustering algorithm known as The Linde-Buzo-Gray (LBG) proposed by Linde, Buzo, and Gray [17]. Linde-Buzo-Gray (LBG) clustering technique was used in [18] for speaker recognition. The algorithm is applied to the set of training vectors and the resulting centroids constitute the VQ codebook.

4 Implementation and Validation

In this paper, MATLAB based program has been developed by the author for text-dependent speaker identification system. All the algorithms were executed on a desktop computer with a Core (TM) i3-350 CPU and a processing speed of 2.27 GHz. We used feature vectors composed from 20 mel-frequency cepstral coefficients (MFCC) for feature extraction technique computed using 20 mel-spaced filters.

Analysis frame was windowed by 30 ms Hamming window with 10 ms overlapping for extracting short-term features. The signal was pre-emphasized by the filter

$H(z) = 1 - 0.97 * z^{-1}$. For speaker modeling we used vector quantization (VQ) based LBG clustering algorithm. The database contains eight speakers who are five males and three females (eight speakers, labeled sp1 to sp8). Every speaker utters the same single digit, zero, once in the training session (then also in a testing session). In this paper, all speakers were modeled using a codebook-size of 1, 2, 4, 8, 16, 32 and 64.

The identification rate of any speaker identification system are computed for the correctly identified speakers out of the total number of speakers used. Identification rate is defined a follows:

$$\text{identification rate} = \frac{\text{No. of correctly identified speakers}}{\text{Total no. of speakers}} * 100\% \qquad (10)$$

5 Results and Discussion

The performance of the presented MFCC feature, applied to extract speaker's speech characteristics, is evaluated using the VQ based LBG clustering algorithm. Although, we attempt with varying the number of codebook-size from 1 up to 64 to test it influence on the identification rate of the system. Figures 4, 5 and 6 illustrates the speaker classification (clustering) process. We have shown here, just the figure of the first and second speakers (sp1 and sp2) with 4, 16 and 32 codebook-size and the plots are based on a two dimensions of the acoustic space. The raw input signal of first and second speakers (sp1 and sp2) is converting into a sequence of feature vectors extracted pevesiouly from speech signal using MFCC technique. The red cross label refer to acoustic vectors of speaker 1 while blue cross label refer to acoustic vectors of speaker 2. These feature vectors are then clustered into a set of codewords. The triangle and plus labels in black show the codewords (centroids) for feature vectors of each speaker. The distance from a vector to the nearest codeword formed the codebook is called a "VQ-distortion". We use 4, 16 and 32 codebook-size respectively.

From Figs. 4, 5 and 6 it is observed that the LBG algorithm partitions the feature vectors into centroids. As we increase the number of centroids, this means that the number of clusters will increase, so each cluster will contain less number of feature vectors and each feature vector is assigned to the nearest centroid.

The accuracy of identification rates obtained for different codebook-size is tabulated in Table 1. From Table 1, it is spotted that the accuracy of the identification rate using MFCC feature extraction technic increases from 50% (1, 2 codebook-size) and 75% (4 codebook-size) to 87.5% (8, 16, 32 and 64 codebook-size) and stays stagnant at 87.5%. The finding shows that identification rate peaks at 87.5% and gives the best results for the text-dependent speaker identification system.

Overall, codebook size determine the amount of features vectors stored for comparison and the findings show that an increase of the codebook size generally leads to a noticeable increase of the identification rate. However, increasing the codebook size beyond 8 (codebook size > 8) will not be more beneficial for the identification rate, we will only get more calculation costs.

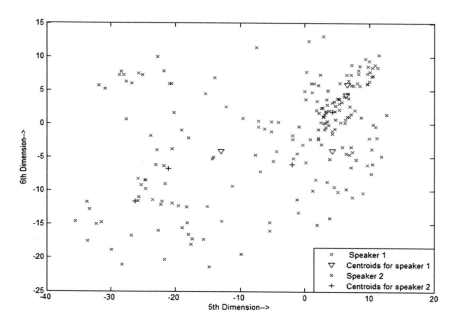

Fig. 4. 2D mixed plot of acoustic vectors with codebooks size 4 for sp1 and sp2

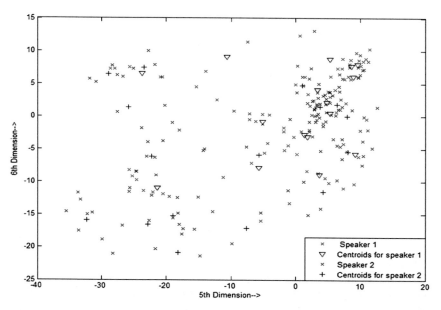

Fig. 5. 2D mixed plot of acoustic vectors with codebooks size 16 for sp1 and sp2

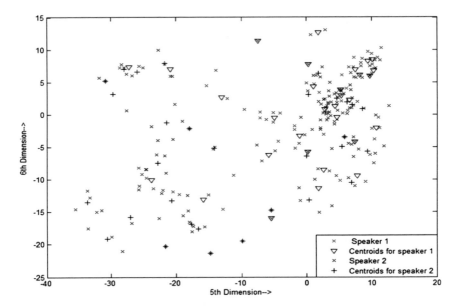

Fig. 6. 2D mixed plot of acoustic vectors with codebooks size 32 for sp1 and sp2

Table 1. Speaker identification rate of eight different speakers with seven different codebook size

Codebook size	Number of speaker	Identification rate (%)
1	8	50
2	8	50
4	8	75
8	8	87.5
16	8	87.5
32	8	87.5
64	8	87.5

6 Conclusion

Mel-cepstrum are features that simulate the characteristics of human auditory system. In this paper, we investigate the performance of the Mel frequency cepstral coefficient (MFCC) approach for a text-dependent speaker identification system. The effectiveness evaluation of the MFCCs features is done using VQ based LBG classifier algorithm for different codebook size. An interesting issue that we address in this work was that proper choice of codebook-size plays a major role in the purpose of improving the identification accuracy for text-dependent speaker identification system. In the future work we can consider using some other features to increase the robustness under a noisy environment.

References

1. Rabiner, L.R., Juang, B.-H.: Fundamentals of Speech Recognition. PTR Prentice Hall, NJ, USA (1993)
2. Sukor, A., Syafiq, A.: Speaker identification system using MFCC procedure & noise reduction method. M. Tech Thesis, Universiy Tun Hussein Onn, Malaysia (2012)
3. Kau, K., Jain, N.: Feature extraction and classification for automatic speaker recognition system. A review. Int. J. Adv. Res. Comput. Sci. Softw. Eng. 5(1), 1–6 (2015)
4. Singh, S.K.: Features and techniques for speaker recognition. M. Tech. Credit Seminar Report, Electronic Systems Group, EE Dept
5. Yanling, Z., Xiaoshi, Z., Huixian, G., Na, L.:A speaker recognition based on VQ. In: 3rd IEEE Conferences on Industrial Electronics and Applications (ICIEA), pp. 1988–1990 (2008)
6. Hermansky, H.: Perceptual linear predictive (PLP) analysis of speech. J. Acoust. Soc. Am. 87(4), 1738–1752 (1990)
7. Reynolds, D.A.: Experimental evaluation of features for robust speaker identification. IEEE Trans. Speech Audio Process. 2(4), 639–643 (1994)
8. Davis, S., Mermelstein, P.: Comparison of parametric representations for monosyllabic word recognition in continuously spoken sentences. IEEE Trans. Acoust. Speech Signal Process. 28(4), 357–366 (1980)
9. Zhang, W., Yang, Y., Wu, Z., Sang, L.: Experimental evaluation of a new speaker identification framework using PCA. In: Proceedings of the IEEE International Conference on Systems, Man and Cybernetics, pp. 4147–4152. Washington (2003)
10. Kumar, J., Prabhakar, O.P., Sahu, N.K.: Comparitive analysis of different feature extraction and classifier technique for speaker identification system: a review. Int. J. Innov. Res. Comput. Commun. Eng. 2(1), 2760–2769 (2014)
11. Reynolds, D.A.: A Gaussian mixture modeling approach to text-independent speaker identification. Ph. D. thesis, Georgia Institute of Technology (1992)
12. Verma, G.K.: Multi-feature fusion for closed set text independent speaker identification. In: International Conference on Information Intelligence, Systems, Technology and Management, Springer, 170–179 (2011)
13. Saini, P., Kaur, P., et al.: Hindi automatic speech recognition using HTK. Int. J. Eng. Trends Technol. 4 (2013)
14. Jothilakshmi, S., Ramalingam, V., Palanivel, S.: Unsupervised speaker segmentation with residual phase and MFCC features. Expert Syst. Appl. 36(6), 9799–9804 (2009)
15. Tiwari, V.: MFCC and its applications in speaker recognition. IEEE Int. J. Emerg. Technol. 1(7), 33–37 (2013)
16. Srinivasan, A.: Speaker identification and verification using vector quantization and mel frequency cepstral coefficients. Res. J. Appl. Sci. Eng. Technol. 4(1), 33–40 (2012)
17. Temko, A., Nadeu, C.: Classification of acoustic events using SVM-based clustering schemes. Pattern Recogn. 39, 684–694 (2006)
18. de Lara, J.R.C.: A method of automatic speaker recognition using cepstral features and vectorial quantization. In: Lazo, M., Sanfeliu, A. (eds.) CIARP 2005, LNCS 3773, pp. 146–153 (2005)
19. Lindasalwa, M., Begam, M., Elamvazuthi, I.: Voice recognition algorithm using Mel frequency cepstral coefficient (MFCC) and Dynamic time warping (DTW) techniques. J. Comput. 2(3), 138–143 (2010)

20. Alam, M.J., Kinnunen, T., Kenny, P., Ouellet, P., O'Shaughnessy, D.: Multitaper MFCC and PLP features for speaker verification using i-vectors. J. Speech Commun. Elsevier **55**(2), 237–251 (2013)
21. Juang, B.-H., Rabiner, L.: Fundamentals of Speech Recognition. Signal Processing Series. Prentice Hall, Englewood Cliffs, NJ (1993)
22. Tiwari, V.: MFCC and its applications in speaker recognition. Int. J. Emerg. Technol. (2010)
23. Kamale, H.E., Kawitkar, R.S: Vector quantization approach for speaker recognition. Int. J. Comput. Technol. Electron. Eng., 110–114 (2008)

A New RFID Middleware and BagTrac Application

Yassir Rouchdi[1,2]($\boxtimes$), Achraf Haibi[1], Khalid El Yassini[1]($\boxtimes$),
Mohammed Boulmalf[2], and Kenza Oufaska[2]

[1] IA Laboratory, Faculty of Sciences Meknes, Moulay Ismail University,
Meknes, Morocco
{yassir.rouchdi,Achraf.haibi,Khalid.elyassini}
@gmail.com
[2] TIC Lab, International University of Rabat, Rabat, Morocco
{Mohammed.boulmalf,Kenza.oufaska}@uir.ac.ma

Abstract. The purpose of this study is to enhance RFID application benefits as a luggage tracking system, first, by defining RFID architecture, components, functioning and middleware roles. Secondly, by discussing the implementation of Role-Based Access Control as a tool regulating access to RFID data, therefore making authentication methods more robust and flexible. To eventually presenting our UIR middleware solution and BAGTRAC application, allowing easier manipulation and real-time visualization of the luggage transportation process.

Keywords: RFID · Middleware · Role-based access control · Green logistics

1 Introduction

RFID technology has grown considerably in recent decades. The rapid advances of microelectronic transceivers have reduced the size and cost of HF and UHF RFID infrastructure, allowing longer and faster reading rates than ever before. RFID technology is now able to cope with new applications with greater mobility using a large number of components, allowing specific functionalities and general services and offering important advantages over other identification mechanisms [1].

The main objective of this study is to apply Radio Frequency Identification as a luggage tracking technology, the application have been done before, but part of this approach was to fix privacy and security issues related to RFID, by enhancing authentication protocols in existing solutions.

As to managing the tracking system, we built a middleware, but instead of building our architecture from scratch, its design is built according to already developed RFID standards, leading to a framework suitable for both RFID and WSN integration applications. Allowing adoption of RBAC model as a tool regulating access to data between 'Data and Event Management' and 'Application Abstraction' layers, leading to resolving accessibility and authorization problems occurring in anterior RFID middleware solutions.

© Springer Nature Switzerland AG 2019
M. Ezziyyani (Ed.): AI2SD 2018, AISC 915, pp. 869–884, 2019.
https://doi.org/10.1007/978-3-030-11928-7_79

The paper is presented as follows, first, an introduction to RFID technology, middleware definition, roles and existing examples. Secondly, a presentation of our middleware solution, followed by the definition of RBAC model, along with its mathematical formula and syntax. Then, we define used technologies, and present an RBAC authentication test example. Finally yet importantly, we talk about our Back-end application BagTrac, defining its architecture and capabilities, to closing the work with a general conclusion and perspectives.

2   RFID Technology

2.1   Components

RFID systems are basically composed of three elements: a tag, a reader and a middleware deployed at a host computer. The RFID tag is a data carrier part of the RFID system, which is placed on the objects to be uniquely identified. The RFID reader is a device that transmits and receives data through radio waves using the connected antennas. Its functions include powering the tag, and reading/writing data to the tag [2]. Unique identification or electronic data stored in RFID tags can be consisting of serial numbers, security codes, product codes and other specific data related to the tagged object. The available RFID tags in today's market could be classified with respect to different parameters. For example with respect to powering, tags may be passive, semi-passive, and active. In terms of access to memory, the tags may be read-only, read-write, Electrically Erasable Programmable Read-Only Memory, Static Random Access Memory, and Write-once read-many. Tags have also various sizes, shapes, and may be classified with respect to these geometrical parameters. The RFID reader is a device that transmits and receives data through radio waves using the connected antennas. RFID reader can read multiple tags simultaneously without line-of-sight requirement, even when tagged objects are embedded inside packaging, or even when the tag is embedded inside an object itself. RFID readers may be either fixed or handheld, and are now equipped with tag collision, reader collision prevention and tag-reader authentication techniques [3] (Fig. 1).

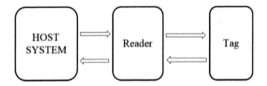

Fig. 1. RFID components

2.2   Frequency Characteristics

Frequency refers to the size of the radio waves used to communicate between RFID systems components. RFID systems throughout the world operate in low frequency (LF), high frequency (HF) and ultra-high frequency (UHF) bands. Radio waves behave differently at each of these frequencies with advantages and disadvantages associated with using each frequency band. If an RFID system operates at a lower frequency, it has a shorter read range and slower data read rate, but increased capabilities for reading near or on metal or liquid surfaces. If a system operates at a higher frequency, it generally has faster data transfer rates and longer read ranges than lower frequency systems, but more sensitivity to radio wave interference caused by liquids and metals in the environment [4].

3   RFID Middleware

Radio Frequency Identification (RFID) technology holds the promise to automatically and inexpensively track items as they move through the supply chain. The proliferation of RFID tags and readers will require dedicated middleware solutions that manage readers and process the vast amount of captured data [5]. The efficiency of an RFID application depends on the precision of its hardware components, and the reliability of its middleware which is the computer software that provides services to software applications beyond those available from the operating system [6].

Middleware makes it easier for software developers to perform communication and input/output, so they can focus on the specific purpose of their application. Middleware includes Web servers, application servers, content management systems, and similar tools that support application development and delivery. It is especially integral to information technology based on Extensible Markup Language (XML), Simple Object Access Protocol (SOAP), Web services, SOA, Web 2.0 infrastructure, and Lightweight Directory Access Protocol (LDAP) [7, 8].

3.1   Middleware's Basic Functions

The three primary functions of an RFID middleware can be broadly classified as device integration (that is, connecting to devices, communicating with them in their prescribed protocols and interpreting the data). Filtering (the elimination of duplicate or junk data, which can result from a variety of sources, for example: the same tag being read continuously or spikes or phantom reads caused by interference) and feeding applications with relevant information based on the information collected from devices after properly performing the appropriate conversions and formatting [2, 9].

Even though most RFID Middlewares share the same clear basic functions, every middleware has an architecture of its own, which is a direct result to the absence of an architecture standardization.

3.2   Security and Privacy Issues

With the adoption of RFID technology, a variety of security and privacy risks need to be addressed by both organizations and individuals. RFID tags are considered "dumb" devices, in that they can only listen and respond, no matter who sends the request signal. This brings up risks of unauthorized access and modification of tag data [10].

In other words, unprotected tags may be vulnerable to eavesdropping, traffic analysis, spoofing or denial of service attacks.

Eavesdropping (or Skimming): Radio signals transmitted from the tag, and the reader, can be detected several meters away by other radio receivers. It is possible therefore for an unauthorized user to gain access to the data contained in RFID tags if legitimate transmissions are not properly protected. Any person who has their own RFID reader may interrogate tags lacking adequate access controls, and eavesdrop on tag contents. Traffic Analysis: Even if tag data is protected, it is possible to use traffic analysis tools to track predictable tag responses over time. Correlating and analyzing the data could build a picture of movement, social interactions and financial transactions. Abuse of the traffic analysis would have a direct impact on privacy [10, 11].

Denial of Service Attack: the problems surrounding security and trust are greatly increased when large volumes of internal RFID data are shared among business partners. A denial of service attack on RFID infrastructure could happen if a large batch of tags has been corrupted. For example, an attacker can use the "kill" command, implemented in RFID tags, to make the tags permanently inoperative if they gain password access to the tags. In addition, an attacker could use an illegal high power radio frequency (RF) transmitter in an attempt to jam frequencies used by the RFID system, bringing the whole system to a halt [10, 11].

Personal Privacy as RFID is increasingly being used in the retailing and manufacturing sectors, the widespread item-level RFID tagging of products such as clothing and electronics raises public concerns regarding personal privacy. People are concerned about how their data is being used, whether they are subject to more direct marketing, or whether they can be physically tracked by RFID chips. If personal identities can be linked to a unique RFID tag, individuals could be profiled and tracked without their knowledge or consent [10, 11].

3.3   Related Work and Contribution

In the RFID domain, Savant middleware is a successful implementation of the EPC network. Currently, many of the large IT companies already offer commercial RFID software, such as SUN EPC Network and IBM WebSphere RFID Premises Server. More recently, Complex Event Processing technology was used in several RFID middleware systems, specifying that event-processing language have been adopted to define complex events. In this paper, we will be applying CEP to define unions and intersections of both RFID and WSN simple events, resulting as complex events [1, 12].

To clarify the contribution of this paper, we state that first, it proposes a new approach, instead of building our architecture from scratch, UIR middleware design is built according to already developed RFID standards, leading to a framework suitable for diverse applications. Secondly, it declares the adoption of RBAC model as a tool regulating access to data between Data & Event Management, and Application Abstraction layers, resolving accessibility and authorization problems occurring in anterior RFID middleware. Finally, the application proposed is just a basic example to test our middleware—which is still under development and improvement—and does not express the wide range of applications our middleware could handle, hence its adaptability aspect.

4 Role-Based Access Control (RBAC)

In order to resolve the security and privacy issues and prevent the RFID Tag data, we decided to use the role based access control regulation method, so that only authorized users get access to specific data.

RBAC is a method of regulating access to computer or network resources based on the roles of individual users within a network [11]. In this context, access is the ability of an individual user to perform a specific task, such as view, create, or modify a file. Roles are defined according to authority and responsibility within the Network [13]. To clarify the notions presented in the previous section, we give a simple formal description, in terms of sets and relations, of role based access control.

No particular implementation mechanism is implied.

- For each subject, the active role is the one that the subject is currently using:

  AR(s: subject) = {the active role for subject s}.

- Each subject may be authorized to perform one or more roles:

  RA(s: subject) = {authorized roles for subject s}.

- Each role may be authorized to perform one or more transactions:

  TA(r: role) = {transactions authorized for role r}.

- Subjects may execute transactions.

  The predicate exec(s,t) is true if subject 's' can execute transaction 't' at the current time, otherwise it is false:

  Exec(s: subject, t: tran) = true if subject s can execute transaction t.

4.1 RBAC Primary Rules

Role assignment: A subject can exercise a permission only if the subject has selected or been assigned a role.

- $\forall s$: subject, t : tran (, exec(s,t) $\Rightarrow$ AR(s) $\neq$ O/).

Role authorization: A subject's active role must be authorized for the subject. With rule 1 above, this rule ensures that users can take on only roles for which they are authorized.

- $\forall s$: subject(, AR(s) $\subseteq$ RA(s)).

Permission authorization: A subject can exercise a permission only if the permission is authorized for the subject's active role. With rules 1 and 2, this rule ensures that users can exercise only permissions for which they are authorized.

- $\forall s: subject, t : tran(, exec(s,t) \Rightarrow t \in TA(AR(s)))$.

4.2 RBAC Security Implementation

A properly administered RBAC system enables users to carry out a broad range of authorized operations, and provides great flexibility and breadth of application. System administrators can control access at a level of abstraction that is natural to the way that enterprises typically conduct business. This is achieved by statically and dynamically regulating users, actions through the establishment and definition of roles, role hierarchies, relationships, and constraints [13, 14].

In our case, security issues related to data access occur when backend end applications require information they are unauthorized to get. Where comes the necessity of applying RBAC. The implementation of an RBAC model in middleware security is not as simple as it seems, findings indicate that many well known middleware technologies under study fall short of supporting RBAC. Custom extensions are necessary in order for implementations compliant with each middleware to support RBAC required or optional components. Some of the limitations preventing support of RBAC are due to the middleware's architectural design decisions; however, fundamental limitations exist due to the impracticality of some aspects of the RBAC standard itself [15, 16].

4.3 RBAC Implemented Syntax

Assignment of authorizations

```
public boolean autorisation(){
if ((ReaderID ==1 && ReaderIPAddr =="192.168.1.3") || (ReaderID ==2 &&
ReaderIPAddr =="192.168.1.4"){
permission = true;
role1 = true;
role2 = true;
role3 = true;}
else{
permission = false;
role1 = false;
role2 = false;
role3 = false;}
return permission;
}
Affectation des autorisations
if (permission ==true){
```

```
if (role1 ==true){fonction 1}
if (role2 ==true){fonction 2}
if (role3 ==true){fonction 3}
else
{System.out.println("Permission denied");}
}
```

5   UIR Middleware

5.1   UIR Architecture

We propose to develop an RFID middleware called UIR, bearing in mind the design problems discussed in the second section. Our system is organized as a three-tiered architecture, with back-end applications (BagTrac), middleware (UIR) and RFID hardware.

UIR middleware offers a design that provides the application with a neutral device protocol and an independent platform interface. It integrates three hardware abstraction layer (HAL), event and data management layer (EDML) and Application Abstraction Layer (AAL).

Hardware Abstraction Layer

HAL is the lowest layer of (UIR-) and is responsible for interaction with the hardware. It allows access to devices and tags in an independent manner of their various characteristics through layers of tag abstraction and reader.

The reader abstraction provides a common interface for accessing hardware devices with different characteristics such as protocols (ISO 14443, EPC Gen2, ISO 15693), UHF (HF) and host side interface Interface (RS232, USB, Ethernet).

The abstraction of the reader exposes simple functions such as opening, closing, reading, writing, etc. To accomplish complex operations of the readers.

The abstraction of readers and tags in UIR-make it extensible to support various tags, readers and sensors.

The device management module in HAL is responsible for the dynamic loading and unloading of the reader libraries depending on the use of device hardware. This allows the system to be light because only the required libraries are loaded. This layer contains the devices for various operations, as specified by the upper layers. It is also responsible for monitoring and reporting the status of the device. Some of the functions provided by the HAL to access RFID hardware are as follows:

- The Device-opening: function is responsible for opening a connection with the device. The connection parameters are provided as an argument to this function. When a successful connection is made to the reader, a response is returned by this function. This response is then used as a reference to access the device in subsequent calls.
- The Device-reading function: reads data from the internal reader. The read parameters such as the protocol to be read by the reader, the size of the data to be

read, are specified as arguments of this function. The function responds successfully if valid data is present in the reader if not with an error code.

- The Device-Writing function writes data to the Tag. Arguments Specified with this function, the unique ID partially or totally, which triggers the data to be written to the tag. The function responds successfully if the data is written to the Tag or returns an error code (for example, when the tag is not identified only) [1, 12].

5.2   Event and Data Management Layer (EDML)

EDML handles various reader-level operations, such as reading tags and informing readers of disconnected notions such as device failure, write failure, and so on. The layer acts as a conduit between the hardware abstraction layer (HAL) and the application abstraction layer (AAL). It accepts commands from AAL, processes them and therefore issues commands to HAL. Similarly, the responses are brought from the HAL, processed and transmitted to the LAA by this layer.

The EDML is the kernel of this middleware. It filters out uninteresting data, formats the remaining useful data and builds complex events according to real-time specifications. The event specification analyzer interprets and transforms event specifications into four processes steps: filtering, grouping, aggregating, and complex construction of events. The volume of event data is very important in the NSE middleware system. The filter selects only those events in the upper layer, thus reducing the reports data dramatically. In the ratio to the upper layer, event data are separated in several groups for a clear demonstration. The aggregation provides statistical information event data. By aggregating, the volume of the declared data may be reduced again.

5.3   Application Abstraction Layer (AAL)

The Application Abstraction Layer (AAL) provides various applications with an independent interface to RFID hardware. The interface is designed as an API by which Applications use UIR-RFID services. All operations at the application level such as reading, writing, etc. Are interpreted and translated into the lower layers of UIR- by the AAL. In order to restrain unauthorized back-end application from getting acces to Data, we used Role-Based access control method of regulating access to guarantee data protection from unauthorized back-end applications.

The next figure (Fig. 2) illustrates UIR-RFID architecture.

5.4   UIR-RFID Implementation

For the UIR-RFID implementation, we propose the use of Microsoft Visual Studio.Net 2010 as Framework and development tool. The reasons for this choice are the powerful utilities for Application Development that this framework provides. The code to use to develop the Project is C Sharp (C #). We propose the use of graphical user interface features provided by the .Net Framework and Microsoft Visio 2013 to develop conceptual models and middleware architecture. For the purpose of data management and storage, we offer Microsoft SQL Server 2008, It is a cohesive set of tools, utilities and interfaces collaborating to provide excellent data management. The database schema

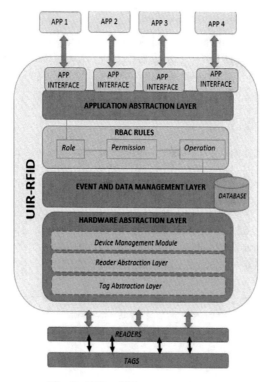

Fig. 2. UIR middleware architecture

generated by this DBMS provides a comprehensive view of the data and its relationships. To view the database, retrieve, modify, delete, and store data, we propose the use of the SQL language (Structured Query Language) [1, 14].

6   Used Technologies and Test

6.1   Eclipse

Eclipse IDE is a free, integrated development environment (the Eclipse term also refers to the corresponding IBM-initiated project) that is extensible, universal, and versatile, potentially enabling the creation of development projects that implement any programming language. Eclipse IDE is mainly written in Java (using the SWT graphical library, IBM), and this language, thanks to specific libraries, is also used to write extensions.

The specificity of Eclipse IDE comes from the fact that its architecture is developed around the notion of plug-in (in accordance with the OSGi standard): all the functionalities of this software workshop are developed as a plug-in.

Many commercial software packages are based on this free software, such as IBM Lotus Notes 8, IBM Symphony or Websphere Studio Application Developer.Units.

6.2 Supported Programming Languages

Numerous languages are already supported (most thanks to the addition of plug-ins), among which: Java, RPG for system I, C#, C++, C, Objective Caml, Python, Perl, Ruby, COBOL, Pascal, PHP, Javascript, XML, HTML, XUL, SQL, ActionScript, Coldfusion.

6.3 Abstract Application Test

TagCentric: is an open source RFID middleware that controls heterogeneous RFID devices and collects RFID-related data into a user-specified database. Its cost (free!) And its simplicity make it ideal for small businesses, RFID test centers and universities.

The goal of this project is to extend TagCentric by developing and integrating the RBAC model.

For our test, we add and activate five readers, and using the RBAC model that we added only the "authorized" readers begin to send data—For our example the readers 1 and 2 are allowed (Fig. 3).

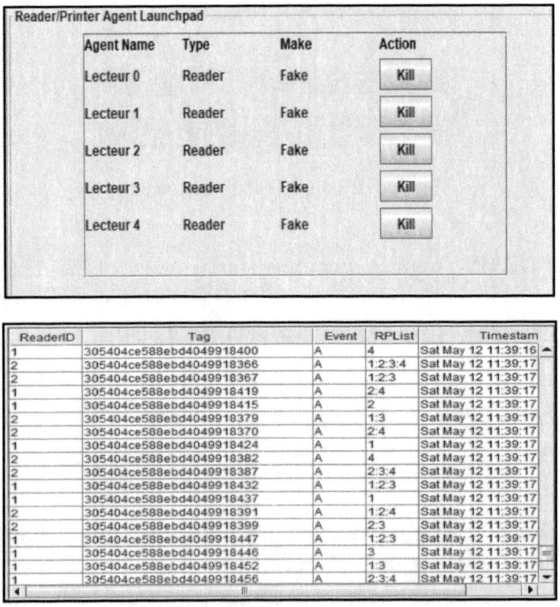

ReaderID	Tag	Event	RPList	Timestam
1	305404ce588ebd4049918400	A	4	Sat May 12 11:39:16
2	305404ce588ebd4049918366	A	1:2:3:4	Sat May 12 11:39:17
2	305404ce588ebd4049918367	A	1:2:3	Sat May 12 11:39:17
1	305404ce588ebd4049918419	A	2:4	Sat May 12 11:39:17
1	305404ce588ebd4049918415	A	2	Sat May 12 11:39:17
2	305404ce588ebd4049918379	A	1:3	Sat May 12 11:39:17
2	305404ce588ebd4049918370	A	2:4	Sat May 12 11:39:17
1	305404ce588ebd4049918424	A	1	Sat May 12 11:39:17
2	305404ce588ebd4049918382	A	4	Sat May 12 11:39:17
2	305404ce588ebd4049918387	A	2:3:4	Sat May 12 11:39:17
1	305404ce588ebd4049918432	A	1:2:3	Sat May 12 11:39:17
1	305404ce588ebd4049918437	A	1	Sat May 12 11:39:17
2	305404ce588ebd4049918391	A	1:2:4	Sat May 12 11:39:17
2	305404ce588ebd4049918399	A	2:3	Sat May 12 11:39:17
1	305404ce588ebd4049918447	A	1:2:3	Sat May 12 11:39:17
1	305404ce588ebd4049918446	A	3	Sat May 12 11:39:17
1	305404ce588ebd4049918452	A	1:3	Sat May 12 11:39:17
1	305404ce588ebd4049918456	A	2:3:4	Sat May 12 11:39:17

Fig. 3. Launch of readers and test

7 BagTrac Application

7.1 Introduction: Why BagTrac?

The purpose of this embedded application is to collect information transmitted by an RFID reader, and send them to a database in real time to process and transmit them to an application installed in a mobile terminal, working with the Android operating system, to allow a tracking of the position of luggage at airports.

7.2   BagTrac: Architecture

First, an RFID Tag is fixed on a bag or a case, by using wireless communication, the reader disposed on the path of the bag, follows its position throughout the transportation process, by sending the retrieved id of the tag to the Arduino board.

Next, it establishes a connection with the database via its USB port through a Java application, to store the location of the bag.

Finally, the mobile application communicates with the database to display to the user the location of his suitcase. The position is then collected, centralized in real time and transmitted to the corresponding user (Fig. 4).

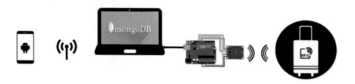

Fig. 4. Project architecture

7.3   Android Application

This application is dedicated to users to provide the location of luggage to each customer, it offers different interfaces.

Start interface
See Fig. 5.

Login space
See Fig. 6.

In case of entering an incorrect identifier or password, the identification interface generates an error message inviting the user to retype the identifiers (Figs. 7 and 8).

Client Space
After the authentication, the application makes a connection with the database to retrieve the name of the corresponding user and the location of his luggage if it was found, (Fig. 9), otherwise a message will appear to warn him that there is no checked baggage (Fig. 10).

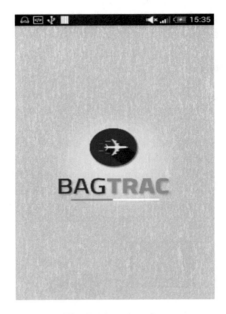

Fig. 5. Start interface

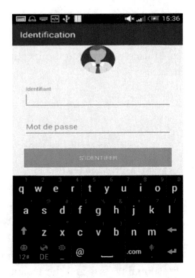

Fig. 6. Login space

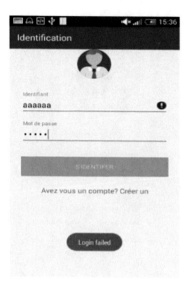

Fig. 7. Incorrect identifier

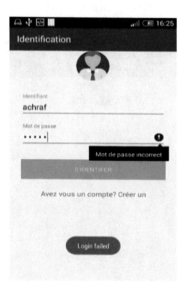

Fig. 8. Incorrect password

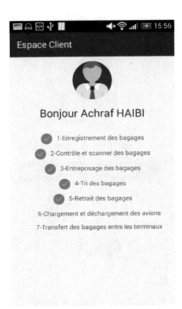

Fig. 9. Luggage location

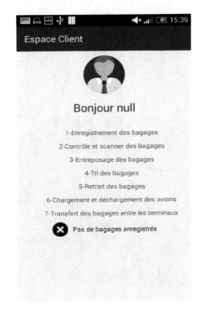

Fig. 10. No luggage

8   Conclusion

Radio Frequency Identification has shown its efficiency through its many applications in different areas such as airlines luggage tracking, Supply chain management, military use, healthcare and personal services.

Despite the technology's worldwide deployment, researches carry on the purpose of resolving many related issues cited occurring during its use in tracking networks.

In order to cover all aspects of the luggage-tracking scenario, our RFID Tracking system contains three major parts, RFID hardware, insuring the localization of bags, UIR RFID middleware, which is responsible for collecting, filtering and aggregating Data, and finally, back-end application BagTrac, that allows real-time visualization of the bag transportation process.

As for future and actual work, we intend to enhance our middleware architecture in order to offer a solution to many RFID related issues. Starting by resolving the multiple hardware support issue on the reader abstraction layer, and also, optimizing synchronization and scheduling in the middleware EDML, which manages data flow between the other layers, handling various reader level operations, servicing multiple applications and offering a device neutral interface to the applications.

References

1. Rouchdi, Y., El Yassini, K., Oufaska, K.: Complex event processing and role-based access control implementation in ESN middleware. In: Innovations in Smart Cities and Applications, pp. 966–975. LNNS 37, Springer (2018)
2. Bornhövd, M.C., Lin, T., Haller, S., Schaper, J.: Integrating automatic data acquisition with business processes—experiences with SAP's auto-ID infrastructure". In: Proceedings of the 30th International Conference on Very Large Data Bases (VLDB), Toronto, pp. 1182–1188 (2004)
3. Bell, S.: RFID Technology and Applications, pp. 6–8. Cambridge University Press, London (2011)
4. Weixin, W., Jongwoo, S., Daeyoung, K.: Complex event processing in EPC sensor network middleware for both RFID and WSN (2008)
5. Kefalakis, N., Leontiadis, N., Soldatos, J., Donsez, D.: Middleware building blocks for architecting RFID systems. Mob. Lightweight Wireless Syst. 13(9), 325–336 (2009)
6. Su, X., Chu, C., Prabhu, B.S., Gadh, R.: On the Creation of Automatic Identification and Data Capture Infrastructure via RFID and Other Technologies. Taylor & Francis Group (2007)
7. Zuluaga, M., Montanez, J., van Hoof, J.: Green Logistics—Global Practices and their Implementation in Emerging Markets, pp. 2–3, Colombia (2011)
8. Bouhouche, T., El Khaddar, M.A., Boulmalf, M., Bouya, M., Elkoutbi, M.: A new middleware architecture for the integration of RFID technology into information systems. In: International Conference on Multimedia Computing and Systems (ICMCS), pp. 1025–1030, Marrakech (2014)
9. Rouchdi, Y., El Yassini, K., Oufaska, K.: UIR-middleware. Int. J. Sci. Res. (IJSR) 7(2), 1492–1496 (2018)

10. Rouchdi, Y., El Yassini, K., Oufaska, K.: Resolving security and privacy issues in radio frequency identification middleware. Int. J. Innov. Sci. Eng. Technol. (IJISET) 5(2), 2348–7968 (2018)
11. Zhang, T., Ouyang, Y., He, Y.: Traceable Air Baggage Handling System Based on RFID tags in the airport (School of Computer Science and Engineering, Beijing University of Aeronautics and Astronautics, China). J. Theor. Appl. Electron. Commer. Res. 3(1), 106–115 (2008)
12. Sheng, Q., Li, X., Zeadally, S.: Enabling next-generation RFID applications: solutions and challenges. IEEE Comput. 41(9) (2008)
13. Weil, R., Coyne, E.: ABAC and RBAC: scalable, flexible, and auditable access management. IT Prof. 15(4), 14–16 (2013)
14. Caiyuan, J., Aodong, S., Wenxue, Y.: The RBAC system based on role risk and user trust. Int. J. Comput. Commun. Eng. (2016)
15. O'Connor, M.C.: RFID is the key to car clubs success. RFID J. (2011)
16. Russell, R.: Manufacturing execution systems: moving to the next level. Pharm. Technol., 38–50 (2004)

Portfolio Construction Using KPCA and SVM: Application to Casablanca Stock Exchange

Anass Nahil$^{(\boxtimes)}$ and Lyhyaoui Abdelouahid

Abdelmalek Essaadi University, LTI, 90000 Tangier, Morocco
anassnahil@gmail.com

Abstract. This study investigates stock market portfolio construction that is an interesting and important research in the areas of investment and applications, as it allows more profits and returns at lower risk rate with effective portfolios. To construct accurate prediction and thus good portfolio construction, various methods have been tried, among which the machine learning methods have drawn attention and been developed. This paper introduces a machine learning method of Support Vector Machine (SVM) to construct a stocks portfolio by selecting well-performing firms in Casablanca Stock Exchange (Casablanca S. E). This model can perform a nonlinear classification. However, the accuracy of SVM classification is particularly sensitive to the quality of data. To insure a better performance of the model, we bring the Kernel Principal Component Analysis (KPCA) into SVM to extract the low-dimensional and efficient feature information. As empirical results show, based on SVM, within KPCA, the stock selection model outperforms the MASI index.

Keywords: Financial market · SVM · KPCA · Portfolio

1 Introduction

Accurate prediction of prices of financial instruments is essential to take better investment decisions with minimum risk. In view of the complexity of the financial time series data, resulting from a huge number of factors which could be economic or political. Machine learning and soft computing methods have been used by several authors in the last two decades for financial time series forecasting.

Guo and Zhang [1], Kuo et al. [2] and Tsumato et al. [3] have developed many methods to forecast stock prices and maximize profitability by selecting the most profitable stocks. However, stocks selection models meet problems such as high dimension of the input and its non-linearity. Neural networks methods have made it possible to find patterns in complex and high dimensional data [4, 5].

Despite the performance of neural networks in comparison with traditional methods, this method has some weaknesses such as local minima and overfitting. Vapnik [6] has proposed a machine learning method called Support Vector Machine, SVM) that provide solutions to the neural networks model limits, especially, to the high dimension limit.

Nowadays, SVM is applied in many fields. Many researchers have used this method to predict the stock price like Yeh et al. [7] and Huang [8].

© Springer Nature Switzerland AG 2019
M. Ezziyyani (Ed.): AI2SD 2018, AISC 915, pp. 885–895, 2019.
https://doi.org/10.1007/978-3-030-11928-7_80

This article applies SVM method to the Casablanca S.E to create a portfolio that provides better performances. First, KPCA method is used to reduce the dimension of the indicators used as input. Then, The SVM model is used to select the most profitable stocks.

The reminder of this paper is organized as follows, Sects. 2 and 3 describes the KPCA and SVM methods. Section 4 describes the adopted methodology. In Sect. 5, we compare the results of the model with MASI index. Concluding remarks with suggestions for the future research are given in Sect. 6.

2   Literature Review

In recent years, there have been a growing number of studies looking at the construction of financial portfolio. Both academic researchers and practitioners have made tremendous efforts to build profitable stocks' portfolios by predicting the future movements of stock market index or its return and devise financial trading strategies to translate the forecasts into profits [9].

In the following section, we focus the review of previous studies on support vector machines (SVM) applied to stock market prediction.

Support vector machines (SVM), has been successfully applied to predict stock price index and its movements. Kim [10] used SVM to predict the direction of daily stock price change in the Korea composite stock price index (KOSPI). Experimental results proved that SVM outperform BPN and CBR and provide a promising alternative for stock market prediction. Manish and Thenmozhi [11] used SVM and random forest to predict the daily movement of direction of S&P CNX NIFTY Market Index of the National Stock Exchange and compared the results with those of the traditional discriminant and logit models and ANN. In their study, they used the same technical indicators as input variables applied by Kim [10]. The experimental results showed that SVM outperform random forest, neural network and other traditional models. Huang et al. [12], in their study, investigated the predictability of financial movement direction with SVM by predicting the weekly movement direction of NIKKEI 225 Index. To evaluate the prediction ability of SVM, they compared its performance with those of linear discriminant analysis, quadratic discriminant analysis and Elman backpropagation neural networks. The results of the experiment showed that SVM outperform the other classification methods.

Manish and Thenmozhi [13] investigated the usefulness of ARIMA, ANN, SVM, and random forest regression models in predicting and trading the S&P CNX NIFTY Index return. The performance of the three nonlinear models and the linear model are measured statistically and financially via a trading experiment. The empirical result suggested that the SVM model can outperform other models used in their study. Hsu et al. [14] developed two stage architecture by integrating self-organizing map and support vector regression for stock price prediction. They examined seven major stock market indices. The results suggested that the two-stage architecture provides a promising alternative for stock price prediction. Qiu and Song [15] utilized GA to optimize BPNN for prediction of Japanese Nikkei 225 Index and used hit ratios, which are defined as the percentage of trials when the predicted direction is correct, as criteria for predicting the direction of the stock index. They compared two basic types of input variables to predict the direction of the daily stock market index and concluded that the Type II input variables can generate a higher forecast accuracy using the proposed GA-BPNN. Qiu et al. [16] selected the input variables for BPNN for prediction of Japanese Nikkei 225 Index and employed GA and simulated annealing (SA) to improve the prediction accuracy of BPNN and overcome the local convergence performance of BPNN. Chen and Hao [17] utilized the weighted support vector machine to identify the weights and then used the feature of weighted K-nearest neighbor to effectively predict stock market indices on two well-known Chinese stock market indices: Shanghai and Shenzhen stock exchange Indices. MAPE and RMSE were employed to verify the performance of the models. Zhang et al. [18] proposed a new approach named status box method and used machine learning techniques to classify the boxes. Then they constructed a new ensemble method integrated with AdaBoost algorithm, probabilistic support vector machine (PSVM), and GA to perform the status boxes classification. They focused on Shenzhen Stock Exchange (SZSE) and National Association of Securities Dealers Automated Quotations (NASDAQ) for predicting the stock direction. The review paper of Atsalakis and Valavanis [19], which summarizes the related literature, can be useful for interested readers.

3 Kernel Principal Component Analysis

Principal component analysis (PCA) is a technique used to emphasize variation and bring out strong patterns in a dataset. It's often used to reduce the dimension. KPCA projects data in a high dimensional space before applying PCA.

Let's consider the input matrix $X = [x_1, x_2, \ldots, x_n]^T \in R^{n \times m}$ where x_i is the observation in i.

The mapping to the high dimensional space is obtained using the function $\phi(.)$:

$$R^m \overset{\phi(.)}{\longrightarrow} F^h. \tag{1}$$

The vector x_i becomes $\phi(x_i)$ in the high dimensional space. The variance covariance matrix is represented as follows:

$$S^F = \frac{1}{n} \sum_{i=1}^{n} \phi(x_i)\phi(x_i)^T, \tag{2}$$

where $\phi(x_i)$ is centered around zero. The eigenvalue decomposition in the high dimensional space [9, 10]:

$$\lambda v = S^F v = \left(\frac{1}{n} \sum_{i=1}^{n} \phi(x_i)\phi(x_i)^T \right) v = \frac{1}{n} \sum_{i=1}^{n} \langle \phi(x_i), v \rangle \phi(x_i), \tag{3}$$

where λ and v are, respectively, eigenvalues and eigen vectors in S^F. The coefficients $\alpha_{i \in \{1,2,...,n\}}$ verify [20, 21]:

$$v = \sum_{i=1}^{n} \alpha_i \phi(x_i). \tag{4}$$

Equations (3) and (4) lead to:

$$\lambda \sum_{j=1}^{n} \alpha_j \langle \phi(x_j), \phi(x_k) \rangle = \frac{1}{n} \sum_{i=1}^{n} \sum_{j=1}^{n} \alpha_j \langle \phi(x_j), \phi(x_i) \rangle \langle \phi(x_k), \phi(x_i) \rangle. \tag{5}$$

By using the kernel trick (Gaussien Kernel) and the centralization function $I_n = 1/nI_1 \in R^{n \times n}$, Eq. 5 becomes:

$$\lambda \alpha = \frac{1}{n} K \alpha, \text{ where } \alpha = [\alpha_1, \alpha_2, ... , \alpha_n]^T, \text{ Où } K - I_n K - KI_n + I_n KI_n \rightarrow K$$

The selection of the principal components is based on the value of λ. The principal components that correspond to the highest values of λ is retained. The jth principal component is calculated as follows:

$$t_j = \langle v_j, \phi(x) \rangle = \sum_{i=1}^{n} \alpha_i^j \langle \phi(x), \phi(x_i) \rangle, \quad j = 1, 2, ..., k \tag{6}$$

where k is the number of principal components taken from the principal components space.

Support Vector Machine

The SVM Linear classification lies in finding the optimal hyperplane when the data are linearly separable.

Let's consider $\{(x_1, y_1), (x_2, y_2), ..., (x_n, y_n)\}$, where x_i are the observations and $y_i \in Y = \{+1, -1\}$ (+1 for the class C_1 and -1 for the class C_2).

If the hyperplane $H_0 : \omega.x + b = 0$ divides the space into two classes, then: $y_i = +1$, $\omega x_i + b \geq +1$ and $y_i = -1$, $\omega x_i + b \leq -1$. When the distance $D = d_+ + d_-$ between the two classes is maximized, this hyperplane is an optimum.

$$d_{\pm} = min_{i,y=\pm 1} \left\{ \frac{|\omega.x_i + b|}{||\omega||} \right\} \tag{7}$$

Find the optimal hyperplane involves minimizing $||\omega||$.

To guarantee the convergence and tolerate the extreme values, the variable ζ_i is introduced. The constant C is introduced to evaluate the cost of the extreme values tolerance. The optimization problem becomes:

$$\mathbf{max} \sum_{i=1}^{n} \lambda_i - \frac{1}{2} \sum_{i=1}^{n} \sum_{j=1}^{n} \lambda_i \lambda_j y_i y_j \langle x_i, x_j \rangle$$
$$sc \quad 0 \le \lambda_i \le C, \quad i = 1, 2 \ldots n \tag{8}$$
$$\sum_{i=1}^{n} \lambda_i y_i = 0$$

The kernel function $\phi : R^n \to H : x \to \phi(x)$ is introduced to generalize to non-linear situations. H is a Hilbert space (Fig. 1):

$$\max \sum_{i=1}^{n} \lambda_i - \frac{1}{2} \sum_{i=1}^{n} \sum_{j=1}^{n} \lambda_i \lambda_j y_i y_j \langle \phi(x_i), \phi(x_j) \rangle$$
$$sc \quad 0 \le \lambda_i \le C, \quad i = 1, 2 \ldots n \tag{9}$$
$$\sum_{i=1}^{n} \lambda_i y_i = 0$$

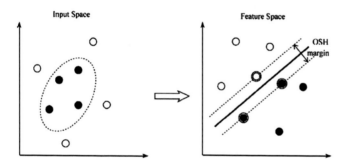

Fig. 1. Separating hyperplane in the feature space corresponding to a non-linear boundary in the input space

4   Research Data

This section describes the research data and the selection of predictor attributes. The research data used in this study is the direction of daily closing price movement in the Casablanca S.E. The entire data set covers the period from January 2012 to June 2016. The total number of cases is 1119 trading days. 70% of the observations (746) are used in the learning process. The remaining 30% are used in the test process.

The following scatter plot present the average price (MAD) of the studied stocks between January 2012 and June 2016 (Fig. 2).

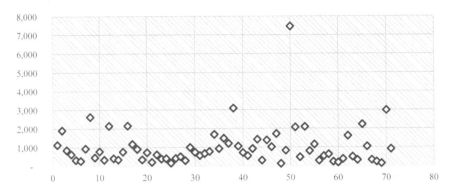

Fig. 2. Average price of the studied stocks

5 Proposed Methodology

5.1 Data Preprocessing

To increase the predictability of the model, prices are transformed to five days relative difference in prices (RDP) Thomason [22]. The transformed data are symmetrical and closer to the normal distribution.

Variables	Calculation
x_1	$DPR_5 = (P(i) - P(i - 5))/P(i - 5) * 100$
x_2	$DPR_6 = (P(i) - P(i - 6))/P(i - 6) * 100$
x_3	$DPR_7 = (P(i) - P(i - 7))/P(i - 7) * 100$
x_4	$DPR_8 = (P(i) - P(i - 8))/P(i - 8) * 100$
x_5	$DPR_9 = (P(i) - P(i - 9))/P(i - 9) * 100$
x_6	$DPR_{10} = (P(i) - P(i - 10))/P(i - 10) * 100$
x_7	$DPR_{15} = (P(i) - P(i - 15))/P(i - 15) * 100$
x_8	$DPR_{20} = (P(i) - P(i - 20))/P(i - 20) * 100$
x_9	$DPR_{25} = (P(i) - P(i - 25))/P(i - 25) * 100$
x_{10}	$DPR_{30} = (P(i) - P(i - 30))/P(i - 30) * 100$
x_{11}	$DPR_{35} = (P(i) - P(i - 35))/P(i - 35) * 100$
x_{12}	$DPR_{40} = (P(i) - P(i - 40))/P(i - 40) * 100$
x_{13}	$DPR_{45} = (P(i) - P(i - 45))/P(i - 45) * 100$
x_{14}	$DPR_{40} = (P(i) - P(i - 50))/P(i - 50) * 100$

18 financial indicators are also used in the model:

- Net turnover
- Net operating profit or loss
- Return on assets
- Equity-to-assets
- Share price performance

- Earnings to operating costs
- Equity per share
- Dividend per share
- Dividend payout
- Effective dividend yield
- Working Capital Ratio
- Quick Ratio
- Earnings per Share
- Price-Earnings Ratio
- Market Capitalization
- Trading Volume
- Debt-Equity Ratio
- Return on Equity

10 other technical indicators are used in the experiment. They are calculated as follows:

- Simple 10-day moving average:

$$\frac{C_t + C_{t-1} + \cdots + C_{t-10}}{10}$$

- Weighted 10-day moving average:

$$\frac{nC_t + (n-1)C_{t-1} + \cdots + C_{10}}{n + (n-1) + \cdots + 1}$$

- Momentum: $C_t - C_{t-n}$
- Stochastic K%: $\frac{C_t - LL_{t-n}}{HH_{t-n} - LL_{t-n}} \times 100$
- Stochastic D%: $\sum_{i=0}^{n-1} K_{t-i}\%/n$
- RSI (Relative strength index):

$$100 - \frac{100}{1 + \left(\sum_{i=0}^{n-1} Up_{t-i}/n\right) / \left(\sum_{i=0}^{n-1} DW_{t-i}/n\right)}$$

- MACD (Moving average convergence divergence):

$$MACD(n)_{t-1} + \frac{2}{n+1}\left(DIFF_t - MACD(n)\right)_{t-1}$$

- Larry William's R%: $\frac{H_n - C_t}{H_n - L_n} \times 100$
- A/D (Accumulation/Distribution): $\frac{H_t - C_{t-1}}{H_t - L_t}$

- CCI (Commodity Chanel Index): $\frac{M_t - SM_t}{0.015 D_t}$

C_t is the closing price, L_t the low price, H_t the high price at time t, DIFF: EMA $(12)_t - $ EMA$(26)_t$, EMA exponential moving average, EMA$(k)_t$: EMA$(k)_{t-1} + \alpha$ x $(C_t - $ EMA$(k)_{t-1})$, a smoothing factor: $2/1 + k$, k is time period of k day exponential moving average, LL_t and HH_t mean lowest low and highest high in the last t days, respectively, M_t : $H_t + L_t + C_t/3$; SM_t: $\left(\sum_{i=1}^{n} M_{t-i+1} \right)/n$, D_t : $\left(\sum_{i=1}^{n} |M_{t-i+1} - SM_t| \right)/n$; Up_t means the upward price change, Dw_t means the downward price change at time t.

Outliers affects the quality of the model. Outliers are replaced with a threshold fixed based on the standard variation. A second technique is used to accelerate the convergence speed of the SVM algorithm, it consists of the scaling to the range $[-1, 1]$ [23].

5.2 Experimental Design

The input used in this model consists of historical values of the stocks listed in the Casablanca S.E.

Firstly, KPCA reduces the dimension of the input by selecting the most significant principal component. The selected vectors are used in the SVM algorithm. The model performance is measured through the NMSE indicator. The model with the smallest NMSE is selected. The following figure explains the methodology used in this paper (Fig. 3).

5.3 Kernel Function and Parameters

The kernel function is a function that satisfy the mercer condition. The most used kernel functions are the polynomial and the gaussian. The gaussian function gives better results in the case of data centered around 0. The polynomial function takes more time in the learning process and is less performant than the gaussian.

The most important step in the KPCA implementation is the choice of the optimal number of principal components. This choice is based on the marginal contribution of the principal component. The number of principal components is chosen when the contribution of the principal component is less than 0, 5% and the global model explanation is higher than 80%.

The optimal parameters of SVM and KPCA are chosen based on grid search method. For each step, a combination of parameters is tested. The parameters (C and δ for SVM and C' and δ' for KPCA) that lead to the best performance are selected.

6 Results and Discussion

When the SVM algorithm is applied to a high dimensional database, the learning time becomes important. To decrease this duration, the KPCA algorithm is introduced to reduce the dimension. The number of principal components used as input to SVM lies

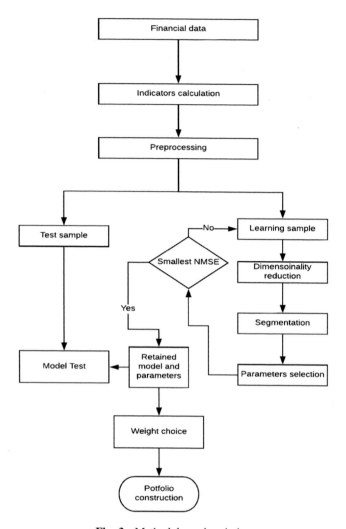

Fig. 3. Methodology description

to two factors, a global contribution higher than 80% and a marginal contribution higher then 0, 5%. The eigen vectors selected are used as input to the SVM model.

The choice of the parameters is also important. It increases the performance of the model. Consequently, parameters C and δ are meticulously chosen based on the grid search method.

At the first stage, the experiments for parameter setting were completed. The training performance of the SVM model for these parameter combinations was varied between 80.18 and 97.45%. On the other hand, the test performance of SVM model varied between 75.13 and 87.13%. It can be said that both the training and test performances of the SVM model are significant for parameter setting data set. However, it should be noted here that the best training performance and the best holdout performance were obtained at the same parameter combination. The couple (C, δ) = (1000, 0.1) leads to the best performance of the SVM model.

To analyze the obtained result, we construct an equal weighted portfolio with stocks selected by KPCA-SVM and do a comparison between the accumulated return gained by this model and MASI index of Casablanca Stock Exchange. The comparison is presented in Fig. 4. It manifests that KPCA-SVM has higher accumulated return over the MASI index, which means SVM classification method is accurate and highly efficient when dealing with complex and highly dimensional data.

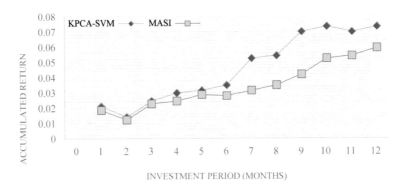

Fig. 4. KPCA-SVM versus MASI

7   Conclusion

Portfolio construction is important for the development of effective market trading strategies. It usually affects a financial trader's decision to buy or sell an instrument. Profitable portfolios may promise attractive benefits for investors. These tasks are highly complicated and very difficult.

The portfolio built from the model output is more profitable than MASI. Future researches should include the risk dimension in the study by analyzing the volatility of the returns.

References

1. Guo, M., Zhang, Y.-B.: A stock selection model based on analytic hierarchy process. In: Factor Analysis and TOPSIS. The International Conference on Computer and Communication Technologies in Agriculture Engineering, pp. 466–469 (2010)
2. Kuo, R.J., Chen, C.H., Hwang, Y.C.A.: Intelligent stock trading decision support system through integration of genetic algorithm based fuzzy neural network and artificial neural network. Fuzzy Sets Syst. **118**, 21–45 (2001)
3. Tsumato, S., Slowinski, S., Komorowsk, J., Grzymala-Busse, J.W.: In: The Fourth International Conference on Rough Sets and Current Trends in Computing. Lecture Notes in Artificial Intelligence (2004)

4. de Faria, E.L., Albuquerque, M.P., Gonzalez, J.L., Cavalcante, J.T.P., Albuquerque, M.P.: Predicting the Brazilian stock market through neural networks and adaptive exponential smoothing methods. Expert Syst. Appl. **36**, 12506–12509 (2009)
5. Zhang, Y., Wu, L.: Stock market prediction of S&P 500 via combination of improved BCO approach and BP neural network. Expert Syst. Appl. **36**, 8849–8854 (2009)
6. Vapnik, V.N.: Statistical Learning Theory. Publishing House of Electronics Industry (2004)
7. Yeh, C.-Y., Huang, C.-W., Lee, S.-J.: A multiple-kernel support vector regression approach for stock market price forecasting. Expert Syst. Appl. **38**, 2177–2186 (2011)
8. Huang, P.: Prediction of the Turnover Points in Stock Trend Based on Support Vector Machine. College of Software, Fudan University (2010)
9. Chen, A.S., Leung, M.T., Daouk, H.: Application of neural networks to an emerging financial market: forecasting and trading the Taiwan Stock Index. Comput. Oper. Res. **30**(6), 901–923 (2003)
10. Kim, K.: Financial time series forecasting using support vector machines. Neurocomputing **55**, 307–319 (2003)
11. Manish, K., Thenmozhi, M.: Forecasting stock index movement: a comparison of support vector machines and random forest. In: Proceedings of Ninth Indian Institute of Capital Markets Conference, Mumbai, India (2005)
12. Huang, W., Nakamori, Y., Wang, S.Y.: Forecasting stock market movement direction with support vector machine. Comput. Oper. Res. **32**, 2513–2522 (2005)
13. Manish, K., Thenmozhi, M.: Support vector machines approach to predict the S&P CNX NIFTY index returns. In: Proceedings of 10th Indian Institute of Capital Markets Conference, Mumbai, India (2006)
14. Hsu, S.H., Hsieh, J.J.P.A., Chih, T.C., Hsu, K.C.: A two-stage architecture for stock price forecasting by integrating self-organizing map and support vector regression. Expert Syst. Appl. **36**(4), 7947–7951 (2009)
15. Qiu, M.Y., Song, Y.: Predicting the direction of stock market index movement using an optimized artificial neural network model. PLoS ONE **11**(5) (2016)
16. Qiu, M.Y., Song, Y., Akagi, F.: Application of artificial neural network for the prediction of stock market returns: the case of the japanese stock market. Chaos Solitons Fract. **85**, 1–7 (2016)
17. Chen, Y.J., Hao, Y.: A feature weighted support vector machine and k-nearest neighbor algorithm for stock market indices prediction. Expert Syst. Appl. **80**, 340–355 (2017)
18. Zhang, X.D., Li, A., Pan, R.: Stock trend prediction based on a new status box method and adaboost probabilistic support vector machine. Appl. Soft Comput. **49**, 385–398 (2016)
19. Atsalakis, G.S., Valavanis, K.P.: Surveying stock market forecasting techniques—part II: soft computing methods. Expert Syst. Appl. **36**(3), 5932–5941 (2009)
20. Alcala, C.F., Qin, S.J.: Reconstruction-based contribution for process monitoring with kernel principal component analysis. Ind. Eng. Chem. Res. **49**, 7849–7857 (2010)
21. Lee, J.M., Yoo, C.K., Choi, S.W., Vanrolleghem, P.A., Lee, I.B.: Nonlinear process monitoring using kernel principal component analysis. Chem. Eng. Sci. **59**, 223–234 (2004)
22. Thomason, M.: The practitioner methods and tool. J. Comput. Intell. Financ. **7**(3), 36–45 (1999)
23. Juszczak, P., Tax, D.M.J., Duin, R.P.W.: Feature scaling in support vector data descriptions. In: Proceedings of the 8th Annual Conference on Advances in School Computing and Imaging (2002)

Sorting Decisions in Group Decision Making

Djamila Bouhalouan[1,2], Mohammed Frendi[1],
Abdelkader Ould-Mahraz[1,3], and Abdelkader Adla[1(✉)]

[1] Department of Computer Science, University of Oran 1 Ahmed
Ben Bella, Oran, Algeria
`Mi_departement@hotmail.fr`, `mohamedfrendi@yahoo.fr`,
{`mahrazaek`,`abdelkader.adla`}`@gmail.com`
[2] MI Department, University Center of Ain Temouchent,
Ain Temouchent, Algeria
[3] Departement of Computer Science, University of Ghardaia, Ghardaia, Algeria

Abstract. In the group decision making, alternatives amongst which a decision must be made can range from a few to a few thousand; the decision makers need to narrow the possibilities down to a reasonable number, and sort alternatives. Even when this is not the case, decision support approaches such as ontology-based frameworks potentially offer these capabilities and can assist the decision-makers in presenting the alternatives in a form that facilitates the decision making. In this research an ontology based approach is developed to screen and sort alternatives to the evaluation step. The resulting alternatives screening and sorting tool is based on ontologies whilst the evaluation tool is mainly based on Analytic Hierarchy Process. The ontologies have been built using the Web Ontology Language (OWL) which facilitates the sharing and integration of decision-making information between multiple decision makers.

Keywords: Group decision making · GDSS · Ontology · OWL

1 Introduction

Group Decision Making (GDM) is a multi-party decision problem where two or more independent concerned parties must make a joint decision. The alternatives amongst which a decision must be made can range from a few to a few thousand [1, 2]. The facilitator (or the decision makers) need(s) to narrow the possibilities down to a reasonable number, screen and sort alternatives, especially where the alternatives can be put into numerical terms. Even when this is not the case, decision support approaches such as ontology-based frameworks potentially offer these capabilities and can assist the decision-makers in presenting the alternatives in a form that facilitates the decision making.

In this research, an ontology based approach is developed to facilitate screening and organizing alternatives during the group decision making process. The resulting tool is based on two ontologies: application ontology and domain ontology.

The first ontology will allow structuring all documented possible decisions by specifying semantic inter-relations. The domain ontology defines the objects of the domain as well as their inter-relations. This second ontology will ensure another aspect

© Springer Nature Switzerland AG 2019
M. Ezziyyani (Ed.): AI2SD 2018, AISC 915, pp. 896–905, 2019.
https://doi.org/10.1007/978-3-030-11928-7_81

of the generalization link between decisions. As a result, these two ontologies are supplementary and each one ensures an aspect of the decision making.

We have built the ontologies using the Web Ontology Language (OWL) which facilitates the sharing and integration of decision-making information between multiple decision makers via the Web.

The remainder of this article is structured as follows: The Sect. 2 presents related works. In the Sect. 3, we develop our ontology-based approach to organize (screen and sort) alternatives decisions. In Sect. 4 an illustration with an example is given. Finally, in Sect. 5 we conclude and give future work.

2 Literature Review

Decision aid and decision making have greatly changed with the emergence of information and communication technology (ICT). Group Decision Making (GDM) is a multi-party decision problem where two or more independent concerned parties must make a joint decision [1].

Experience with group decision making has shown that an on-line "meeting" is generally used to represent a group decision process for the specific problem at hand and a recurring pattern of three stages occurs in the group decision process [2]. The three process phases are: Pre-meeting, during meeting, and post- meeting (see Fig. 1).

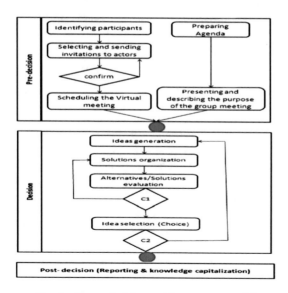

Fig. 1. Group decision making process model

In decision phase, a group can generate many alternatives in a short period of time. These alternatives may be similar or duplicated that need to be screened, organized, merged, sorted, classified and evaluated. The redundant alternatives can be retrieved for the facilitator to review, and then they can be merged or removed. Alternatives screening and organization in a distributed environment is mainly the facilitator's responsibility. It can be a very challenging task for the facilitator.

Supporting GDM consists of procedures to aggregate alternatives, since the final result typically balances the participants' points of view. To help decision makers and facilitator, some methods and tools have been developed (Table 1).

Table 1. Techniques and methods for group decision making

Phase	Step	Methods and techniques
Pre-decision	Identifying participants	Specialized databases
	Preparing agenda	Consensus + Mapping Tool
	Selecting and sending invitation to actors	Email
	Scheduling virtual meeting	TALA web service, Doodle, Framadate …
	Presenting and describing the purpose of the group meeting	Email
Decision	Ideas generation	Brainstorming, Problem mapping, Delphi method, Lateral thinking, Revolutionary Idea Generation, Brain writing, SCAMPER
	Alternatives organization	Categorizers or clustering methods/Algorithms, Ontology, screening and sorting methods.
	Alternatives/Solutions evaluation	Clarifying evaluation criteria, Multi-voting, Nominal Group Technique, Option Comparison Grid, AHP, ranking and sorting
	Idea selection (Choice)	Formal Consensus building, Stepladder technique, Paired comparisons and Option comparison grid
Post-decision		Reporting system + database

Screening consists of reducing a large set of alternatives to a smaller set that most likely contains the best choice. Screening techniques in GDM are studied to address a problem related to both choice and sorting. In practical applications of GDM, it is common for DMs facing complex choice problems to first identify those alternatives that do not appear to warrant further attention [3].

Alternatives screening techniques can be regarded as useful GDM methods, leading to a final choice. They apply when too many alternatives must be considered. The number of alternatives to be taken into account further is dramatically reduced if screening is carried out properly reducing the work load for the facilitator.

Sorting alternatives consists of arrange the alternatives into a few groups in preference order, so that the facilitator can manage them more effectively. A sorting problem is to sort the alternatives in A ($|A| = n$) into a ranked partition S ($|S| = m$), based on criteria set Q ($|Q| = q$). The goal of this research is to utilize the DM's alternatives to create a good sorting and to do so as efficiently as possible.

Sorting methods are used to assign alternatives to predefined groups (clusters, classes or categories). The groups are defined in an ordinal way based on decision-makers preferences. This means that classes are ordered from the most to the least preferred. This is the major difference with classification, where groups are nominal [4].

There are two kinds of sorting methods: (1) Direct judgment methods where a particular decision model is employed and the facilitator directly provides enough information to evaluate all preferential parameters in the model (e.g. ELECTRE TRI [5] and N-TOMIC [6] featuring some theoretical modifications to address sorting); (2) Case-based reasoning methods where the facilitator provides decisions for selected cases, which determine preferential parameters to grade a chosen procedure as consistently as possible (e.g. UTADIS, MHDIS [4] and the rough set method [7] which use the UTA [8] technique to sort alternatives.

3   The Ontology Approach

The alternatives proposed by the decision-makers may be:

- Redundant: the alternatives are syntactically identical;
- Synonyms: the alternatives are syntactically different, but semantically identical;
- Conflicting: two contradictory or conflicting alternatives mean that the application of one is incompatible with the application of the other;
- Generic: an alternative may be more general than another. In this case, the application of the most general includes the application of the most specific;

These alternatives must be screened and sorted before being evaluated and thus enabling the decision choice. The alternative screening and sorting tool contributes to retrieve and remove all the redundant, conflicting and synonymous decisions. The screening and sorting tool allows identifying semantic relationships between decisions then presents them to the decision-makers who will have the duty to decide among the suggested alternatives which will be removed and which have to be kept based on their expertise.

3.1   Ontologies Modelling

The purpose of our work is to integrate a screening and sorting tool (see Fig. 2) within a Group Decision Support System (GDSS) to support the facilitator during the alternatives organizing stage in the group decision making process. Our ontology based approach to support alternatives organizing uses two ontologies. The use of two distinct but smoothly coupled ontologies will enable to infer new useful knowledge for the alternatives organizing task.

The general approach cited in [9] is adopted to develop both ontologies (see Fig. 3). The three stages of the approach (conceptualization, ontologization and operationalization) are in general preceded of requirement analysis and knowledge domain delimitation. This process must however be entirely validated by a human expert. **Conceptualization.** The ontologies are represented in a conceptual model The ontology models allow represent domain concepts of classes and relations between the

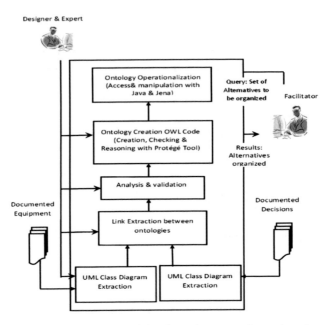

Fig. 2. Function architecture of the alternatives screening and sorting tool

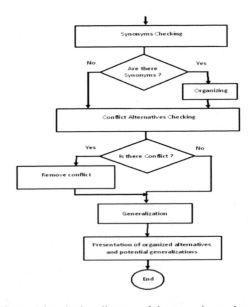

Fig. 3. General functioning diagram of the screening and sorting tool

classes. Every concept or instance may be identified by URI. These models will be of use as inputs of the ontoligization stage. In the application ontology each decision is indexed by one or several objects (components) implied by this decision.

Application ontology. It is a conceptual ontology where each object represents an alternative decision proposed by a decision-maker as a solution. The application ontology specifies all decisions and the relations between them.

We define four classes: (1) *Decision class:* represents decisions; (2) *DecisionEq class:* represents equivalent decisions; it is a sub-class of the decision class. Several equivalent decisions can be related by a synonymy link with a main decision. These equivalent decisions are all different expressing forms of the same decision. This group of decisions is represented by one decision in the main decisions class which contains no semantic redundancy; (3) *DecisionPr class:* represents all main decisions which are interrelated semantically; it is a sub-class of the decision class; (4) *Objetconcerned* representing objects (components) concerned by decisions.

We define three types of relations: (1) Conflict relations that link a main decision with all the main decisions which are conflicting. This relation is symmetrical; (2) Generalization relation that links a decision with its generic decisions. This relation is transitive; (3) Synonymy relations that identify synonymies between decisions. This relation is functional.

Domain ontology. This ontology specifies concepts of the domain. Relations between these concepts are of aggregation and inclusion. The domain ontology is considered to be an explicit specification of domain concepts as well as the relations existing between these concepts.

We define four classes: Composite class, Sub-system class, Auxiliary class, and element class. As for the semantic relations, we define: *"Is composed of" relation* which links the instances of element class, *Aggregation relations* representing the composite object formed of a group of sub-systems; each of which is formed in return of a group of auxiliary objects, and each of the latter contains a group of elements objects.

Ontologization. Ontologization consists of formalizing conceptual models developed at the previous stage, as far as possible. We use OWL (Ontology Web Language) [10] as formalizing language of our ontologies. OWL is a developing information technology of the Semantic Web and is based in Description Logic (DL) [11]. OWL represents ontology by building hierarchies of classes which describe the concepts in a domain and the properties which relate these classes to each other.

The creation of our ontologies is done using Protégé Ontology Editor [12] which is an ontology development tool developed by Stanford Medical Informatics. This allowed the classes and properties to be easily created in an OWL representation. We have also used it to check on our ontologies and the inconsistencies using to the reasoner FACT++. Partial views of application ontology and domain ontology are depicted in Figs. 4 and 5 respectively. The URI base is: http://www.ontoproject.org/ontologycomponents".

Operationalization. The sequence diagram (see Fig. 6) describes the functioning of the proposed screening and sorting module.

Ontology 1 is the application ontology while ontology 2 represents the domain ontology. To operationalize ontologies, we used NetBeans development environment and Java language. To exploit the ontologies, we used Jena framework [13, 14] which

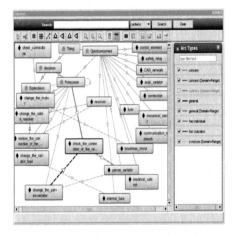

Fig. 4. The application ontology

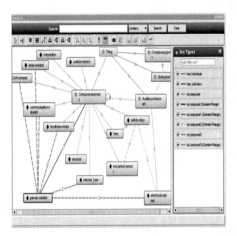

Fig. 5. The equipment domain ontology

provides a programming environment for RDF, RDFS [15] and OWL as well as a querying engine to execute SPARQL queries (Simple Protocol And RDF Query Language) [16] which is RDF querying language.

4   Example

We consider the breakdowns diagnosis application in a complex industrial system. In this kind of systems, decisions are known and listed in an appropriate documentation. The expert decision-makers propose all possible solutions to the problem.

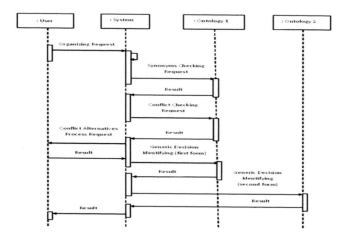

Fig. 6. Sequence diagram of the alternatives organizing step

Given the set of alternative generated by the group of decision makers, the screening and sorting tool will process these alternatives in two steps: the first one involves the application ontology. The outputs of this step are synonymous, conflict and generalized alternatives (see Fig. 7). When two alternatives are conflicting, the facilitator has to remove one. "restore_the_connection_of_the_resolver_plug" is conflicting with "change_the_cable_resolver", the facilitator has chosen to remove "change_the_cable_resolver". Thus, the latter don't appear in the following step (see Fig. 8).

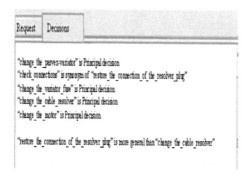

Fig. 7. Step 1: screening alternatives using application domain

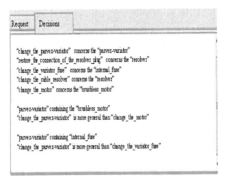

Fig. 8. Step 2: processing alternatives

5   Conclusion

In this paper an ontology-based approach is presented to support facilitator and tool supports the facilitator in the organizing stage of the process. We have developed two ontologies: an application ontology relating to alternatives screening task. It structures alternatives and their semantic relationships. As domain semantics are not entirely expressed by this ontology, the application ontology is connected to a domain ontology which supplements semantics by specifying the knowledge of the domain upon which alternatives are applied. The use of both ontologies jointly allows organizing the alternatives decisions. In future work, we plan to extend our approach by developing a third ontology: task ontology. The latter will express the context of the problem solving task.

References

1. Adla, A., Soubie, J.L., Zaraté, P.: A cooperative intelligent decision support system for boilers combustion management based on a distributed architecture. J. Decis. Syst. (JDS) **16** (2), 241–263 (2007)
2. Adla, A., Zarate, P., Soubie, J.L.: A Proposal of ToolKit for GDSS Facilitators, Group Decision and Negotiation (GDN), vol. 1, Springer (2011)
3. Hobbs, B.F., Meierm, P.: Energy Decision and the Environment: A Guide to the Use of Multicriteria Methods. Kluwer, Massachusetts (2000)
4. Zopounidis, C., Doumpos, M.: Multicriteria classification and sorting methods: a literature review. Eur. J. Oper. Res. **138**, 229–246 (2002)
5. Roy, B.: Multicriteria Methodology for Decision Aiding. Kluwer, Dordrecht (1996)
6. Massaglia, M., Ostanello, A.: N-TOMIC: A decision support for multicriteria segmentation problems. In: International Workshop on Multicriteria Decision Support, Lecture Notes in Economics and Mathematics Systems, vol. 356, pp. 167–174. Springer-Verlag, Berlin (1991)
7. Slowinski, R.: Rough set theory for multicriteria decision analysis. Eur. J. Oper. Res. **129**, 1–47 (2001)

8. Jacquet-Lagr`eze, E., Siskos, Y.: Assessing a set of additive utility functions for multicriteria decision-making, the UTA method. Eur. J. Oper. Res. **10** 151–164 (1982)
9. Mocko, G.M., Rosen, D.W., Mistree, F.: Decision retrieval and storage enabled through description logic. In: ASME IDTC/CIE, (2007)
10. Furst, F.: Contribution à l'ingénierie des ontologies: une méthode et un outil d'opérationalisation. Université de Nantes, Thèse de doctorat (2004)
11. http://www.w3.org/TR/owl-features/
12. Berners-Lee, T., Hendler, J., Lassila, O.: The Semantic Web, Scientific American Magazine (2001)
13. http://protege.stanford.edu/doc/users_guide/index.html
14. http://jena.sourceforge.net/
15. http://www.hpl.hp.com/semweb/jena.htm
16. http://www.w3.org/TR/rdf-schema/

Immune Based Genetic Algorithm to Solve a Combinatorial Optimization Problem: Application to Traveling Salesman Problem

Ahmed Lahjouji El Idrissi[1], Chakir Tajani[2($\boxtimes$)], Imad Krkri[2], and Hanane Fakhouri[2]

[1] Faculty of Science Meknes, Moulay Ismail University, Meknes, Morocco
idrissila@gmail.com
[2] Polydisciplinary Faculty of Larache, Abdelmalek Essaadi University, Tétouan, Morocco
Chakir_tajani@hotmail.fr

Abstract. We are interested in improving the performance of genetic algorithm (GA) to solve a combinatirial optimization problem. Several approaches have been developed based on the adaptation and improvement of different standard genetic operators. However, GA also has some significant drawbacks, for instance, the premature convergence of computations, expensive computation from evolutional procedures, and the poor capability of local search. Artificial immune system is a class of computational intelligence methods drawing inspiration from human immune system. As one type of popular artificial immune computing model, clonal selection algorithm (CSA) has been widely used for many optimization problems. In this paper, an immune based genetic algorithms are proposed to overcome these inconvenients for traveling salesman problem us a typical combinatirial optimization problem. Numerical results are presented for different standard instances from the TSPlib showing the performance of the proposed algorithms.

Keywords: Clonal selection algorithm · Artificial immune system · Optimization · Travelling salesman problem · Genetic algorithm

1 Introduction

The Traveling Salesman Problem (TSP) is one of the most famous problems in combinatorial optimization, which consists to solve the problem of visiting all cities by a salesman with the condition that each city can only be visited once. Hence, the problem is to minimize the distance of the complete tour that the salesman may take. Several real world application of the TSP can behind, such as Vehicle Routing, Scheduling, Image Processing and Pattern Recognition [1, 2].

The TSP problem is classified as NP-complete problem, which explain the number of research and the methods developed and exploited to resolve it. There are some methods to find the approximate solutions, but, these methods have exponential complexity, they take too much computing time or require too much memory. Then, metaheuristic methods should be exploited such as, artificial bee colony, genetic

© Springer Nature Switzerland AG 2019
M. Ezziyyani (Ed.): AI2SD 2018, AISC 915, pp. 906–915, 2019.
https://doi.org/10.1007/978-3-030-11928-7_82

algorithm, particle swarm optimization, ant colony optimization and Bat algorithm [2–4]. This technique does not guarantee the best solution; but, it is to come as close as possible to the optimum value in a reasonable amount of time which is at most polynomial time.

The genetic algorithm is a one of the family of evolutionary algorithms. The population of a genetic algorithm (GA) evolves by using genetic operators inspired by the evolutionary in biology. These algorithms were modeled on the natural evolution of species. We add to this evolution the concepts of observed properties of genetics (Selection, Crossover, Mutation), from which the name GA. They attracted the interest of many researchers starting with Holland [5] who developed the basic principles of GA, and Goldberg [6] that has used these principles to solve specific optimization problems.

In the general structure of a genetic algorithm, we find various steps: Encoding, selection method, crossover and mutation operators and their probabilities, insertion mechanism, and the stopping test. For each of these steps, there are several possibilities. The choice between these various possibilities allows creating several variants of GA, which can improve his performance. Several works are focused on the improvement of genetic operators, which has allowed the development of several adapted presentation, adapted crossover and mutation operators for TSP and the comparison of their performance, and even the hybridization between two operators to benefit of these specificities and make the GA more efficient and accurate [7, 8]. But, it is well known that GA get stuck in local optima very often, in addition to the expensive computation from evolutional procedures and the poor capability of local search.

Recently, artificial immune system (AIS) as a source of inspiration to the development of artificial computational systems, which were originally proposed by Jerne [9], have been widely studied and applied to a variety of optimization problems, usually of a combinatorial nature [10, 11]. Owing to numerous reports of successful applications of these innovative algorithms, AIS approaches have attracted more recent attentions than most other heuristic/metaheuristic methods in various field of optimization. Clonal selection algorithm (CLONALG), one of the most studied artificial immune systems based on the clonal selection theory, has received a great deal of interest in recent years [12] which can perform multimodal optimization while delivering good approximations of a global optimum.

In this paper, to overcome the disadvantages of GA and improve their performance in the resolution of the important TSP problem, we propose an Immune based genetic algorithm, which consist to combining the performance of the GA, and the Clonal selection algorithm. The importance of the application of the genetic algorithm based on immunity lies in these capabilities of recognition and memorization capabilities. As in immune approaches, variety is integrated by calculating the affinity between all antibody pairs, and self-adjustment of the immune response is accomplished by increasing or restricting antibody generations. Thus, in the studied optimization problem, the variety of feasible spaces can be better ensured so that optimal solutions are more likely to be reached.

The paper is organized as follows. The traveling salesman problem (TSP) is defined in Sect. 2. In Sect. 3, the genetic algorithm for TSP is described. The clonal selection algorithm is presented in Sect. 4. The proposed Immune based genetic algorithms are illustrated in Sect. 5. In Sect. 6, computational experiments were performed through many standard instances of TSPLIB [13] showing the performance of the proposed algorithms in comparison with the GA and CLONALG.

2   The Problem Description

Before describing the problem, it is important to mention that the reason behind choosing the above mentioned TSP is that, they are very common and are derived from real world applications. Hence, the TSP provide a very good platform for testing the impact of an elite pool on the performance and generality (consistency and efficiency) of our proposed genetic algorithm. The Traveling Salesman Problem (TSP) consist to finding the shortest closed route among n cities, having as input the complete distance matrix among all cities. Let d_{ij} be a non-negative integer that stands for the cost (distance) to travel from city i directly to city j. The TSP subject of this paper can formally be stated as follows:

Given a set of cities and the cost of travel (or distance) between each possible pairs, the TSP, is to find the best possible way of visiting all the cities and returning to the starting point that minimize the travel cost (or travel distance).

The objective is to find a tour of the minimum total length, where the length is the sum of the costs of each arc in the tour.

The search space for the TSP is a set of permutations of n cities and the optimal solution is a permutation which yields the minimum cost of the tour.

In other words, an TSP of size n is defined by:

We consider a set of points $v = \{v_1, v_2, \ldots, v_n\}$ which v_i is a city.

The mathematical formulation of the TSP is given by:

$$\text{Min}\{f(T), T = (T[1], T[1], \ldots, T[n], T[1]\} \tag{1}$$

where; f is the evaluation function calculates the adaptation of each solution of the problem given by the following formula:

$$f = \sum_{i=1}^{n-1}[d(T(i), T(i+1)), d(T(n), T(1))] \tag{2}$$

with d define a distance matrix and $d(i, j)$ the distance between the city v_i and v_j.

$T[i]$ is a permutation on the set $\{1, 2, \ldots, n\}$.

$T = (T[1], T[2], \ldots, T[n], T[1])$ is the scheduling form of a solution of the TSP.

d is as the Euclidean distance.

3   Genetic Algorithm for TSP

In a genetic algorithm, a population of individuals (possible solutions) is randomly selected. These individuals are subject to several operators inspired by the evolutionary in biology, called genetic operators (selection, crossover, mutation and insertion) to produce a new population containing in principle better individual. This population evolves more and more until a stopping criterion is satisfied and declaring obtaining optimal best solution. Thus, the performance of genetic algorithm depends on the choice of operators. Several works are focused on the improvement of genetic operators, which has allowed the development of several adapted crossover operators to TSP and the comparison of their performance, and even the hybridization between two operators to benefit of their specificity and make the GA more efficient. In this paper, we introduce some known operators presented below:

3.1   Representation Method

In this work, we consider the resolution of the TSP by GA where we will present each individual by the most adapted and natural method of data representation, the path representation method, which is the most natural representation of a tour (a tour is encoded by an array of integers representing the successor and predecessor of each city) (Figure 1).

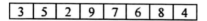

Fig. 1. Encoding using permutation representation

3.2   Crossover Operator (OX)

Crossover operator is a genetic operator that combines two chromosomes (parents) to produce a new chromosome (children) with crossover probability P_c. In this paper, we have chosen the order crossover operator "OX" which consist to: Given two parent chromosomes, two random crossover points are selected partitioning them into a left, middle and right portion. The ordered two-point crossover behaves in the following way: child1 inherits its left and right section from parent1, and its middle section is determined. The procedure illustrated in Fig. 2.

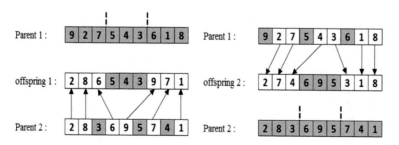

Fig. 2. Illustration of the OX crossover

3.3   Mutation Operator

The two individuals (children) resulting from each crossover operation will now be subjected to the mutation operator in the final step to forming the new generation. This operator randomly flips or alters one or more bit values at randomly selected locations in a chromosome. In this study, we chose as mutation operator the "Inversion muta-tion" where we select two positions within a chromosome at random and then invert the substring between these two positions. It is illustrated in Fig. 3.

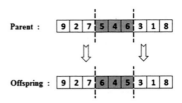

Fig. 3. Illustration of the inversion mutation

3.4   Insertion Method

We used the method of inserting elitism that consists in copy the best chromosome from the old to the new population. This is supplemented by the solutions resulting from operations of crossover and mutation, in ensuring that the population size remains fixed from one generation to another.

4   Clonal Selection Algorithm

Immune Algorithm is derived through the study of immune response. In short, it models how antibodies of the immune system learn adaptively the features of the intruding antigen and act upon. Clonal Selection Algorithm is a special class of Arti-ficial Immune Systems. In this work, CLONALG algorithm which was originally proposed by De Castro and Van Zuben [10] is used.

- **Step 1:** Generate a set of antibodies (generally created in a random manner) which are the current candidate solutions of a problem.
- **Step 2:** Calculate the affinity values of each candidate solution.
- **Step 3:** Sort the antibodies starting from the lowest affinity. Lowest affinity means that a better matching between antibody and antigen.
- **Step 4:** Clone the better matching antibodies more with some predefined ratio.
- **Step 5:** Mutate the antibodies with some predefined ratio. This ratio is obtained in a way that better matching clones mutated less and weakly matching clones mutated much more in order to reach the optimal solution.
- **Step 6:** Calculate the new affinity values of each antibody.
- **Step 7:** Repeat Steps 3 through 6 while the minimum error criterion is not met.

The algorithm starts by defining a purpose function $f(x)$ which needs to be optimized. Some possible candidate solutions are created, antibodies will be used in the purpose function to calculate their affinity and this will determine the ones which will be cloned for the next step. The cloned values are changed, mutated with a predefined ratio and the affinities are recalculated and sorted. After certain evaluations of affinity, affinity with the smallest value is the solution closest to our problem.

5 Proposed Immune-Based Genetic Algorithm

It has been demonstrated that hybridization is an effective way of combining the best properties of different algorithms to create novel hybrid methods. Then, in order to benefit from the advantages of both GA and CLONALG algorithms and to improve the GA performance, we propose three combinations of the two algorithms which consist in applying the immunity strategy either initially where the selected individuals undergoing mutation operator and subsequently apply the crossover operator of the genetic algorithm. For the second approach, the clonal selection algorithm is applied after crossing the selected individuals. In the third approach, the population is randomly divided into two parts. the GA operators and the second subpopulation will undergo the clonal selection algorithm. The three procedures are illustrated below (Fig. 4).

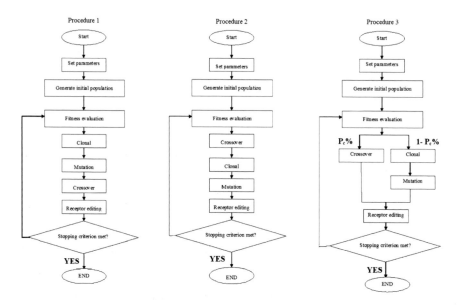

Fig. 4. Procedures of the immune based GA

6   Experimental Results and Discussion

In this paper, the GA, CLONALG and the three proposed immune based genetic algorithms for the resolution of the TSP problem are tested for small and large standard instances of the TSP from TSPLIB [13], especially: Bayes29, Berlin 52, EIL101... The effectiveness of the proposed approach in this paper, is demonstrated through comparisons with a *standard GA* and the clonal selection algorithm.

The parameters used in the proposed algorithms are adapted to each instances:

- Initial population: M = 50, 100, 150;
- Number of generations: 100, 500, 1000;
- Crossover: OX;
- Mutation: inversion mutation;
- Insertion: insertion elitism;
- Number of clones: 4, 10.

Figure 5. shows that the three proposed procedures give good results and especially the first procedure.

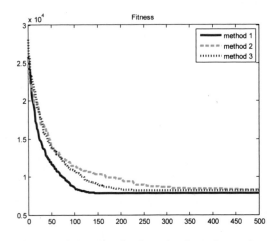

Fig. 5. Comparison result between the three developped procedures for berlin 52

Figure 6. and Table 1. illustrate the evolution of the cost function with respect to the number of iterations showing that the proposed approaches reduce the number of iterations needed in a very important way to obtain the optimal solution for the problem studied while surpassing the probable inconvenient in a standard GA or CLONALG, in particular the first procedure, which influences the execution time and resolution of the problem. For example, for Bayes29 instance the optimal solution obtained with the proposed procedure 1 is 9074.14 after 55 iterations which is better than the obtained results which are 9105.87 after 81 iteration with CLONALG and 9124.39 after 105 iteration with GA. The same conclusion for other instances, 7769.59 is obtained for

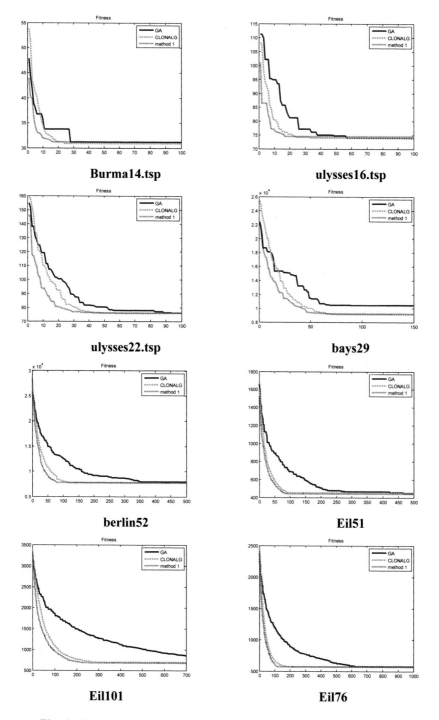

Fig. 6. Comparison result between CLONALG, GA and the first procedure

Table 1. Obtained results for different instances of TSP

Problem	M	Gen	Method 1		CLONALG		GA standard	
			Best	Iter	Best	Iter	Best	Iter
Burma14	30	100	30.79	37	30.79	70	30.79	81
Ulysses16	30	100	73.99	38	73.99	75	73.99	73
Ulysses22	30	100	75.30	35	75.30	51	75.30	105
Bayes29	50	100	9074.14	55	9105.87	81	9124.39	105
Berlin52	100	500	7769.59	88	7784.55	122	7930.78	127
Eil51	100	500	434.08	107	439.38	130	448.82	410
Eil101	200	1000	669.21	249	670.73	272	716.71	1194
EIL76	150	1000	570.04	151	577.70	161	578.47	723

berlin52 after 88 iterations with proposed procedure 1. However, we obtain 7784.55 as optimal solution after 122 with GA and 7930.78 after 127 with CLONALG.

7 Conclusion

In this work, hybridization between a genetic algorithm and Clonal Selection Algorithm is proposed in order to solve a specfic NP-complet combinatorial optimization problem which is the TSP problem. The numerical results performed for small and large standard instances show that, the three proposed procedures that are benefited from the advantages of the two approaches, give better results in comparison with a standard GA and CLONALG.

It is important to note that this algorithm can be applied to other transport optimization problem since the TSP problem is a reference problem, has several applications in different domains, and has several variants.

References

1. Savla, K., Frazzoli, E., Bullo, F.: Traveling salesperson problems for the dubins vehicle. Autom. Contr. IEEE Trans. **53**(6), 1378–1391 (2008)
2. Marinakis, Y., Marinaki, M., Dounias, G.: A hybrid particle swarm optimization algorithm for the vehicle routing problem. Eng. Appl. Artif. Intell. **23**(4), 463–472 (2010)
3. Karaboga, D., Gorkemli, B.: A combinatorial artificial bee colony algorithm for traveling salesman problem. In: 2011 International Symposium on Innovations in Intelligent Systems and Applications (INISTA), pp. 50–53 (2011)
4. Osaba, E., Yang, X.S., Diaz, F., Garcia, P., Carballedo, R.: An improved discrete bat algorithm for symmetric and asymmetric traveling salesman problems. Eng. Appl. Artif. Intell. **48**, 59–71 (2016)
5. Holland, J.H.: Adaptation in Natural and Artificial Systems, The University of Michigan Press, Ann Arbor, (1975). Goldberg, D.: Genetic Algorithm in Search, Optimization, and Machine Learning, Addison Wesley (1989)

6. Goldberg, D.E.: Genetic Algorithms in Search, Optimization and Machine Learning. Addisson-Wesley, Reading, MA (1989)
7. Abdoun, O., Tajani, C., Abouchabaka, J., El Khatir, H.: Improved genetic algorithm to solve asymmetric traveling salesman problem. Int. J. Open Problems Compt. Math. 9(4), 42–55 (2016)
8. Tajani, C., Abdoun, O., Lahjouji, A.I.: Genetic algorithm adopting immigration operator to solve the asymmetric traveling salesman problem. Int. J. Pure Appl. Math. 115(4), 801–812 (2017)
9. Jerne, N.K.: The immune system. Sci. Am. 229(1), 52–60 (1973)
10. De Castro, L.N., Von Zuben, F.J.: The clonal selection algorithm with engineering applications. In: Workshop Proceedings of the GECCO 2000, 36–37 (2000)
11. De Castro, L.N., Timmis, J.: Artificial Immune Systems: A New Computational Intelligence Approach. Springer, New York (2002)
12. Gong, M., Jiao, L., Zhang, L.: Baldwinian learning in clonal selection algorithm for optimization. Inf. Sci. 180(8), 1218–1236 (2010)
13. Reinelt, G.: The TSPLIB symmetric traveling salesman problem instances. (1995) Available in: http://elib.zib.de/pub/mp-testdata/tsp/tsplib/tsp/index.htm

A Comparative Study of Vehicle Detection Methods

S. Baghdadi$^{(\boxtimes)}$ and N. Aboutabit

IPOSI Laboratory, National School of Applied Sciences, Hassan 1stUniversity,
Settat, Morocco
sara92.baghdadi@gmail.com

Abstract. Our project aims to tackle one of the most famous violation on the road; when a vehicle crosses to the wrong side of the road to overtake another vehicle traveling in the same direction. So, we aim to develop a computer vision system to detect robustly the prohibited overtaking observed from a static camera. Our approach is based on two main stages: Line Detection and Vehicle Detection. For each stage, several techniques can be used. In the presented work, we will focus on vehicle detection stage. Here, features are extracted from image and then classified using machine learning algorithms such as SVM (Support Vector Machines), kNN (K-nearest neighbor) and Decision Tree. We used two different kinds of features HOG (Histogram of Oriented Gradient) and SURF (Speeded up Robust Features) we constructed different combinations for vehicle detection. Finally, various parameters are calculated to evaluate the performance of each algorithm used in order to carry out a comparative study. The experiments reveal that the results vary according to each combination.

Keywords: Vehicle detection · Overtaking prohibited · HOG · SIFT · SURF · SVM · KNN · Decision tree

1 Introduction

1.1 A Subsection Sample

Up to 90% of vehicle accidents are caused by human faults [1]. In most cases, they are due to a vehicle trying to overtake another on a single track or on a turn. That is, when the overtaking is prohibited. This is usually indicated by a solid white or yellow line painted on the roadway marking the left limit of traffic (centerline). Every vehicle must not exceed this line to not pass in the opposite direction of the traffic. Thus, prohibited overtaking is especially a hard problem that still remains a challenging task.

Actually, the technology may reduce the huge number of human fatalities by using many techniques based on artificial visual information to increase security and comfort of transport [1]. In doing so, we aim to develop a computer vision system that aims to detect the prohibited overtaking observed from a stationary camera. Detection of vehicles in traffic scenes is of fundamental importance for surveillance system [2]. One of the most challenging research problems in computer vision is vehicle detection.

© Springer Nature Switzerland AG 2019
M. Ezziyyani (Ed.): AI2SD 2018, AISC 915, pp. 916–927, 2019.
https://doi.org/10.1007/978-3-030-11928-7_83

Due to the different views, lighting and complex background, vehicle detection becomes a problem even more difficult [3]. There are many possible views of a vehicle: the side-view, the forward and rear views.

The vehicle side-views have obvious and consistent characteristics in their structure such as wheels, oblique windows and bumpers, which provide crucial cues for detection [4]. We find a very active area of research that was focused on side-view vehicle detection. However, there isn't too many forward and rear-view vehicle detection works.

In our project, we focus on overtaking vehicle setting from forward and rear views. There are two approaches to resolve the vehicle detection problem. The first one called Machine Learning and the second one called Deep Learning. Machine learning starts with features being manually extracted from images. The features are then used to train a classifier that categorizes the objects in the image. With a deep learning, features are automatically extracted from images.

In vehicle detection, two main phases can be identified feature extraction step and classification step. The first step in vehicle detection is to simplify the image by extracting the important information contained in the image taken by camera. The step is called feature extraction using techniques and algorithms such as: HOG, SIFT, SURF, Local binary patterns (LBP), Haar-like. Once features have been extracted, they may be used to build machine learning models for vehicle detection such as SVM, kNN and Decision Trees.

The present article aims to compare Different combinations between feature extraction methods and machine learning models HOG + SVM, HOG + kNN, HOG + Decision Tree, SURF + SVM, SURF + KNN, and SURF + Decision Tree.

The paper is organized as follows: Sect. 2 presents a survey of the main related works. Section 3 describes the vehicle detection methods. Section 4 describes the results and discussion.

2 Related Work

This section presents some related works to vehicle detection, highlighting the methods used in the feature extraction step and classification step.

In [3, 5, 6], the authors used different descriptors to train the SVM classifier. Sun et al. [5] used optimized Gabor filter, here, the author concluded that the experimental results illustrate that the set of Gabor filters, specifically optimized for the problem of vehicle detection, yield better performance than using traditional filter banks. Lin et al. [6] used many feature extraction methods, such as the local energy shape histogram, the LBP model and the HOG. [3] presented an approach for identifying a vehicle shape in high quality image using Active Shape Model (ASM). The landmarks of ASM are detected by a two stages pipeline of Support Vector Machines (SVM), where the result of the first is presented to the another one. The first SVM classifier has a high Recall rate and the second one has high Precision.

References [7–13] used many descriptors like SIFT, GLOH, SURF, HOG, LBP and GIST. Meng et al. [7] combined HOG with LBP features to realize vehicle detection. Lowe [8] proposed the scale invariant feature transform (SIFT), which uses a rectangular location grid. The SIFT features are invariant concerning illumination, rotation and scaling [9, 10] proposed gradient location and orientation histogram (GLOH) descriptor similar to SIFT and replaces the rectangular location grid used by SIFT with a log-polar one. SURF features can be compared and computed much faster than SIFT. HOG is similar to both SIFT and GLOH, because it uses both rectangular and log-polar location grids. The main difference between HOG and SIFT is that HOG is computed on a dense grid of uniformly spaced cells, with overlapping local contrast normalization [11]. In [12], the features of the vehicle are extracted by the proposed GIST image processing algorithm and recognized by Support Vectors Machine classifier. In [13], due to the distinct features of two types of vehicles the author used different approaches to detect vehicles in different directions. The author used optical flow to detect vehicles in the opposite direction because the coming traffics shows salient motions and Haar-like feature detection for vehicles in the same direction, because the traffics represent relatively stable shape (car rear) and little motion.

In [14], the author proposed a way to detect vehicles at different perspective front, back, side, and oblique. For front/back vehicle, he used the symmetrical feature of the vehicle. For side vehicles, he used a side-view car detection algorithm based on template detection. [15] proposed a new feature type called "connected control-points", for adaBoost training of visual object classifiers to detect cars and pedestrians. In [16], the authors proposed a hybrid method of vehicle detection based on Haar-like feature with Adaboost. The next section is devoted to the description of the methods used in vehicle detection.

3   Methods

3.1   Descriptors

Histogram of Oriented Gradient HOG Features. Introduced in the year 2005 by Dalal and Trigg, the histogram of oriented gradients (HOG) is a feature descriptor utilized to detect objects [6, 16]. As we see in the Fig. 1, the image is segmented into small regions called cells, which are interconnected. HOG directions are compiled for each pixel within these cells by using gradient extraction operator. A histogram is formed in different orientations based on the accumulated value of the gradient, the HOG features of each cell are extracted to the series, and a one-dimensional feature vector of the vehicle image is obtained.

Speeded Up Robust Features (SURF). SURF is a Hessian matrix based unique scale and rotation-invariant interest point descriptor and detector [16, 17]. It is used mainly for object recognition. SURF was built on another feature extraction algorithm, Scale invariant feature transform (SIFT), which was one of first algorithms used in the late 90's. SURF is faster in getting the results than SIFT and also very robust in nature. The feature descriptor used in SURF is based on the sum of the Haar wavelet response around the point of interest, which makes it proficient to be computed with the aid of internal image.

SURF descriptors have been used to locate and recognize objects, people or faces, to track objects and to extract points of interest.

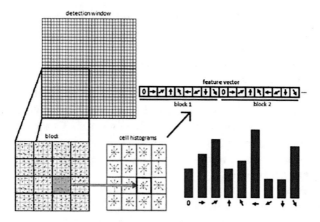

Fig. 1. HOG Descriptor

3.2 Classifiers

Support Vector Machines (SVM). SVM was initially proposed by Cortes and Vapnik [6]. The principle of SVM classification is to find a hyper plane, which makes the classification of multidimensional space is maximized. Suppose that each sample in the training data is composed of an eigenvector and a class label, that is $D_i = (x_i, y_i)$, where x_i represents the eigenvector of sample i, y_i represents the class label of sample i. Multi-class classification can be regarded as a combination of a number of binary classification. In the linear binary classification, the category labels are only two values, respectively, 1 and −1. Assuming that the new data points are classified according to the equation, the margin between samples to a hyperplane is defined as,

$$M_i = y_i(wx_i + b) \tag{1}$$

w represents a spatial conversion of one function, b represents the offset parameter. After normalizing w and b, the margin can be expressed as

$$M_i = |wx_i + b| / ||w|| \tag{2}$$

The geometrical margin is shown in Fig. 2.

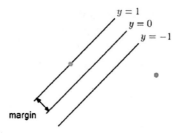

Fig. 2. Geometrical margin of SVM classfier

In Fig. 2, y = 0 is the Classification-plane, both y = 1 and are y = −1 parallel to y = 0, and they are through the sample point which is nearest to y = 0. The interval between y = 1 or y = −1 and y = 0 is the geometrical margin. In order to minimize errors, it is necessary to maximize the geometrical margin.

K-nearest neighbor (kNN). K-nearest neighbor (kNN) was proposed by Cover and Hart. It is the extension of the minimum distance method and the nearest neighbor method. It calculates the distance between testing sample x and all the training samples and makes the distances in descending order. Then it selects k training samples which are nearest to the testing sample x and counts the category of the k training samples selected. The testing sample belongs to the category which has the largest number of votes in the same category [6].

Decision-Tree. The classification structure defined by a decision tree is estimated from training data using a statistical procedure [18]. The 'tree' is made of a root node, internal nodes and leaves. Nodes are where trees branch or split the dataset; terminal nodes are called leaves which contain most homogeneous classes. If in a training set T, there is k number of classes (C) and a total of |T| cases, the expected information from such a system is,

$$\text{info}(T) = -\sum_{j-1}^{K} \frac{\text{freq}(C_j, T)}{|T|} \log_2 \left(\frac{\text{freq}(C_j, T)}{|T|} \right)$$

where, $\frac{\text{freq}(C_j, T)}{|T|}$ is the probability of occurrence of class Cj in training set T.

3.3 Evaluation Critaria

Results were evaluated through statistical analysis, for this, first we calculate True Positive, False Positive, False Negative and True Negative. From this, Runtime rate, True Detection rate, Extra Detection rate, and Missed Detection rate are calculated as follows:

$$\text{True Detection} = (TP + TN)/(TP + TN + FP + FN)$$

$$\text{Extra Detection} = FN$$

$$\text{Missed Detection} = FP$$

We calculated two other parameters Rloss and Kloss. Rloss examine the resubstitution loss; it is the fraction of misclassifications from the predictions of the classifier. Kloss examine the cross-validation loss, which is the average loss of each cross-validation model when predicting on data that is not used for training.

4   Experimental Results

4.1   Materials

We have conducted an experiment using a dataset having 875 images. The dataset includes two classes of images, the first class contains the positive images (Fig. 3), and the other class contains the negative images. From the dataset two sets are created a training set and a test set. 80% of these positives were included in the training set. The remaining 20% were included in the test set.

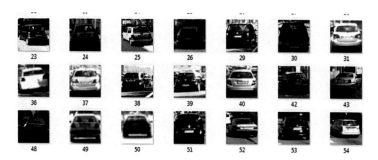

Fig. 3. Samples from Vehicle class

We executed our algorithms on a machine with a processor of 4,39 GHz Intel Cerelon CPU and a Memory of 2 GB.

4.2   Results and Discussion

This paper aims at comparing the combinations of the classifiers SVM, kNN and Decision Tree and the descriptors HOG and SURF to find which of these combinations provides significant and faster results. To accomplish this, we implemented the algorithms in Matlab. The parameters are set as follows: the kernel function of SVM is the linear kernel, the parameter of kNN k is set to 4 and 1 (by default) and the distance metric is either Euclidean (default) or cosine.

To evaluate the performance of these algorithms, we tested all of them by the same image list to keep the same evaluation conditions. This evaluation was based on runtime and detection rate.

The average runtime per image for each combination is shown in Table 1.

As shown in the Table 1, the combination HOG + Decision Tree is the faster one. The HOG is faster than the SURF because the SURF is too slow; it is based on a bag of features which contains different phases such as the extraction of features, the coding of features, the pooling of features, and the spatial information preservation. Thus, the decision tree is extremely simple. Because the complexity of this method depends on the depth and the depth of this tree is 1 (A depth-1 decision tree is called a decision stump). This classifier is simpler than a linear classifier.

Table 1. Average runtime of each combination

Vehicle detection methods									
HOG+ SVM	HOG + KNN			HOG+ Decision Tree	SURF + SVM	SURF + KNN			SURF + Decision Tree
	$k = 1$ $D = 'euclicean'$	$k = 4$ $D = 'euclicean'$	$k = 1$ $D = 'cosine'$			$k = 1$ $D = 'euclicean'$	$k = 4$ $D = 'euclicean'$	$k = 1$ $D = 'cosine'$	
0.1046	0.205	0. 228	0.375	0.0496	0. 3139	0.2410	0. 3102	0.3168	0.3164

Runtime/Image (s)

As we see, the SVM classifier is a fair bit faster than kNN classifier when they are combined with the HOG descriptor. However, these classifiers achieve the same runtime when they are combined with the SURF descriptor. As the parameter k increases, the classifier is averaging over more neighbors, and then more time required classifying data. The same observation if we modify the kNN classifier to use cosine distance instead of the default.

And finally, we checked whether the results are correct or not. The Table 2 shows the percentage of true detection, the number of extradetection followed by the number of missed vehicles. To simplify the comparison between the models, we computed the receiver operating characteristic (ROC) graph of each algorithm. The ROC curve is a popular and powerful tool for evaluating classifier performance. It is created by plotting the true positive rate against the false positive rate at various threshold settings. The ROC curves obtained are shown in the Fig. 4.

As Table 2 shown, the descriptor HOG performs much better than SURF. Because HOG is a dense grid; it is used as low-level features. HOG works very well in combination with SVM and kNN classifier. SURF performs less well with kNN and Decision Tree, but when it is combined with SVM classifier, it provides better results. We can observe that the Decision Tree classifier works well in combination with HOG.

For the classifier kNN, if we increase slightly the parameter k, the classifier performs similarly. The kNN classifier with the cosine distance performs slightly better than the one using the Euclidean distance function. Basing on the ROC curves (the Fig. 4) and the Table 2, the order of these combinations according to the accuracy in descending is as follows: HOG + kNN, HOG + SVM, HOG + Decision Tree, SURF + SVM, SURF + Decision Tree, SURF + kNN.

For the model SURF + Decision Tree, Rloss = 0.10. It means that this model predicts incorrectly for 10% of the training data. As we see, the classifier kNN with cosine distance has lower resubstitution error than the first one.

During the execution of our algorithms, we observed that with the increase of training samples, the accuracy of the model rises and the error rate seems to decrease. For kNN classifier, if we increase k, the error on training data starts to increase. And we also observed that the kNN works well with the new data because it just use the training data as a look up table and search to classify the new data.

We can improve the SURF performances by adding more features. Thus, we concatenated SURF features with HOG features into a single feature vector and train a single classifier and finally we calculated the parameters of evaluation the detection rate.

Figure 5 summarizes the fusion technique that we used. The SURF and HOG descriptors are applied separately. Then, the obtained features are concatenated and provided as an input of the classification step (SVM, KNN and Decision-Tree are used).

The results are displayed in the Table 3. We observed that this hybrid descriptor is better than the SURF descriptor (the accuracy and Runtime).

In most cases, the fusion technique provides better results than using a single technique

Table 2. Evaluation parameters of each combination

	Vehicle detection methods									
	HOG+ SVM	HOG + KNN			HOG+ Decision Tree	SURF + SVM	SURF + KNN			SURF + Decision Tree
		$k=1$ $D=$ 'euclicean'	$k=4$ $D=$ 'euclicean'	$k=1$ $D=$ 'cosine'			$k=1$ $D=$ 'euclicean'	$k=4$ $D=$ 'euclicean'	$k=1$ $D=$ 'cosine'	
True detection	96%	97.71	96.57%	98.29%	85.71%	82.86%	62.29%	54.68%	66.86%	67.43%
Number of extradetection (%)	0	7	10.2	5.4	24.1	12.9	57	61	55	52
Number of missed vehicles (%)	5.4	0	0	0	9.9	18.1	18.2	16.9	25	15.1
Rloss Kloss	Rloss = 0 Kloss = 0.01	Rloss = 0.0194 Kloss = 0.030	Rloss = 0.0194 Kloss = 0.034	Rloss = 0.018 Kloss = 0.014	Rloss = 0.015 Kloss = 0.118	Rloss = 0.149 Kloss = 0.173	Rloss = 0.115 Kloss = 0.233	Rloss = 0.216 Kloss = 0.278	Rloss = 0.0266 Kloss = 0.16	Rloss = 0.108 Kloss = 0.234

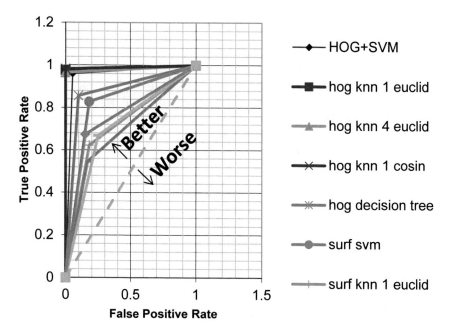

Fig. 4. The graph shows the ROC curves of the models

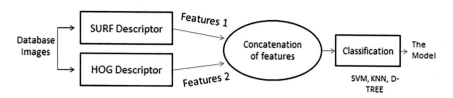

Fig. 5. The fusion technique scheme

Table 3. Evaluation parameters of fusion technique

	SURF/HOG +SVM	SURF/HOG + KNN	SURF/HOG+ Decision Tree
True detection (%)	84.86	63.93	84.71
Number of extradetection (%)	0	54	0.9
Number of missed vehicles (%)	17.8	0	17.9
Runtime (s)	0.213	0.198	0.201

5 Conclusion

This paper presented a comparative study of vehicle detection methods. We compared six combinations HOG + SVM, HOG + kNN, HOG + D-Tree, SURF + SVM, SURF + kNN, SURF + D-Tree. From the comparison results, we can conclude that the method based on HOG and SVM provides the best results with an accuracy and runtime per frame of about 96% and 0.1083 s respectively. HOG with kNN is slightly better than the first one but it is the slower one. The combination HOG with Decision Tree is the faster one with an accuracy and runtime per frame of about 85.71% and 0.0496 s respectively. We have shown that we can improve the SURF descriptor by concatenating his features with the HOG's features. This fusion technique provides interesting results. We will extend our comparative study by adding others descriptors and classifiers and exploring hybrid methods by merging more than one feature and classifier.

References

1. Aly, M.: Real time Detection of Lane Markers in Urban Streets Computational Vision, p. 1 (2014)
2. Liu, L., Xing, J., Ai, H.: Multi-view Vehicle Detection and Tracking in Crossroads, p. 1
3. Gessica, M., Meneses, R., Nogueira, L.: Vehicle Shape Recognition Using SVM and ASM, p. 1
4. Vinoharan, V., Ramanan, A., Kodituwakku, S.R.: A Wheel-based Side-view Car Detection using Snake Algorithm, p. 1. (1963)
5. Sun, Z., Bebis, G., Miller, R.: Evolutionary gabor filter optimization with application to vehicle detection. In: Proceedings of the 3rd IEEE International Conference on Data Mining, Florida, pp. 307–314 (2003)
6. Lin, S., Zhao, C., Qi, X.: Comparative analysis of several feature extraction methods in vehicle brand recognition. In: 10th International Conference on Sensing Technology (ICST), Nanjing, China (2016)
7. Meng, J., Liu, J., Li, Q. Zhao, P.: Vehicle detection method based on improved HOG-LBP. In: 3rd International Conference on Vehicle, Mechanical and Electrical Engineering (ICVMEE) (2016)
8. Lowe, D.: Distinctive image features from scale-invariant keypoints. Int. J. Comput. Vis. **60** (2) (2004)
9. Mikolajczyk, K., Schmid, C.: A performance evaluation of local descriptors. In: Proceedings of 2003 IEEE Computer Society Conference Computer Vision and Pattern Recognition (2003)
10. Ke, Y., Sukthankar, R.: PCA-SIFT: a more distinctive representation for local image descriptors. In: Proceedings of the 2004 IEEE Computer Society Conference on Computer Vision and Pattern Recognition (CVPR 2004), pp. II-506–II-513 (2004)
11. Rani, R., Kumar, R., Singh, A.P.: A comparative study of object recognition techniques. In: 7th International Conference on Intelligent Systems Modelling and Simulation (ISMS) (2016)
12. El Jaafari, I., El Ansari, M., Koutti, L., Ellahyani, A., Charfi, S.: A novel approach for on-road vehicle detection and tracking. Int. J. Adv. Comput. Sci. Appl. (IJACSA) **7**, 594–601 (2016)

13. Choi, J.: Real time on road vehicle detection with optical flows and haar-like feature detectors. Technical Report, CS Department, University of Illinois at Urbana-Champaign (2006)
14. Cai, B., Tan, F., Lu, Y., Zhang, D.: Knowledge template based multi-perspective car recognition algorithm. Int. J. Inf. Eng. Electron. Bus. **2**, 38–45 (2010)
15. Moutarde, F., Stanciulescu, B., Breheret, A.: Real-time visual detection of vehicles and pedestrians with new efficient adaBoost features. Workshop of International Conference on Intelligent Robots Systems (2008)
16. Wang, H., Zhang, H.: Hybrid method of vehicle detection based on computer vision for intelligent transportation system. Int. J. Multimed. Ubiquitous Eng. (IJMUE) **9**(6), 105–118 (2014)
17. Raj, N.S., Niar, V.: Comparison study of algorithms used for feature extraction in facial recognition. Int. J. Comput. Sci. Inf. Technol. **8**(2), 163–166 (2017)
18. Prasad S., Ramkumar, B.: Passive copy-move forgery detection using SIFT, HOG and SURF features. In: IEEE International Conference on Recent Trends in Electronics, Information & Communication Technology (RTEICT), Bangalore, pp. 706–710 (2016)

Connected Car & IoT: A Review

Asmaa Berdigh[1(✉)], Kenza Oufaska[2], and Khalid El Yassini[1]

[1] Informatics and Applications Laboratory, Department of Mathematics
and Computer Sciences, Faculty of Sciences,
Moulay Ismail University, Meknes, Morocco
{asmaberdigh, khalid.elyassini}@gmail.com
[2] TICLab, Faculty of Computer Science and Logistics,
International University of Rabat, Rabat, Morocco
kenza.oufaska@uir.ac.ma

Abstract. The introduction of large numbers of sensors and ECU to provide driver assistance applications and the associated high-bandwidth, weight and cost requirements have accelerated the demand for faster and more flexible network communication within the vehicle. This paper identifies a promising IoT application within intra-vehicular network and presents a comprehensive overview of current research on IoV applications, by describing different communication scenarios (V2V, V2I, V2R). This paper highlighted also the most recurrent transport issues and the IoT outcome solutions, there characteristics and challenges.

Keywords: Connected car · IoV · Intra-vehicle connectivity · V2V · V2I · V2R · Wireless technologies · CO_2 emission

1 Introduction

The number of ECU (Electronic Control Unit) and sensors in a modern vehicle has increased significantly due to the various safety and convenience applications. Since, the wired architecture is not flexible nor scalable because of the internal vehicle structure. Therefore, there is an increasing appeal to design a system where the wired connections between ECUs or ECU and sensors are replaced within wireless links. To this end, we investigated the possibility to use the IoT concept inside the Intra-vehicular network. And instead of using the knowns automotive wire technologies such FlexRay, Local Interconnect Network (LIN) and Controller Area Network (CAN) substitute them with wireless technologies, such as Radio Frequency IDentification (RFID), Bluetooth and Zigbee.

The idea of this paper will be structed by starting first and foremost by defining the keywords needed, namely the IoV the In-vehicular network and a connected car, then evaluating the current IoV applications in the inter-vehicle network by illustration the most investigated applications in the literature such as V2V, V2I and V2R. and lastly present the purpose of this research, which moving from a wire to wireless network in the intra-vehicle network communication and identify the candidate wireless communication alternatives.

© Springer Nature Switzerland AG 2019
M. Ezziyyani (Ed.): AI2SD 2018, AISC 915, pp. 928–940, 2019.
https://doi.org/10.1007/978-3-030-11928-7_84

1.1 Internet of the Vehicle

The Internet of vehicles (IoV) is an Internet of things (IoT) application in the transport system, and which has prompted a lot of research. The IoV can be used to collect, transmit, identify, integrate and make use of information from cars.

Nowadays, the vehicles sales have increased dramatically around the world and will continue to increase [1], as shown in the Fig. 1. Moreover, 90% will be connected, by 2020 [2].

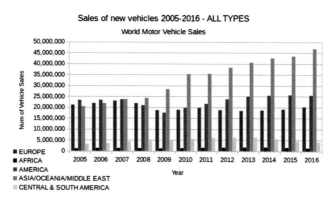

Fig. 1. Sales of new vehicles 2005–2016—All Types

This char is based on the statistics file "total-sales-2016.xlsx" available [3].

This section provides an overview of to the connected car notion and the in-vehicle networking.

1.2 In-vehicle Network

The recent vehicle consists of 50–100 embedded computers [3], called electronic control units (ECUs), connected to sensors and actuators inside an in-vehicle network. ECUs receive the environment information from sensors and send commands to actuators, to perform their tasks [4].

The in-vehicular network is built through different bus system technologies constitute sub-networking interconnected by special gateway ECUs: FlexRay, Local Interconnect Network (LIN) and Controller Area Network (CAN) [5].

A comparison between the listed above bus, per the main criteria could be found in the bellow Table 1. This table done based on automotive Trier2 inputs [6].

1.2.1 Media Oriented System Transport (MOST)

MOST is a high-speed network classified into Class D networks devoted to multimedia data [7], developed in 1998 by MOST cooperation which. This protocol can provide point-to-point data transfer with data rate up to 24.8 Mb/s. MOST defines separately data channels and control channels used to set up the data channels for each link. Once the connection is established, data can flow continuously stream.

Table 1. Classic in-vehicle networking bus

Specification	CAN	LIN	FlexRay
Data rate	1 Mbps	20 Kbps	10 Mbps
Physical layer	Dual wire	Single wire	Dual wire, optical fiber
Architecture	Multi-master, typically 10–30 nodes	Single master, typically 2–10 slaves	Multi-master, up to 64 nodes
Message transmission type	Asynchronous	Synchronous	Synchronous and Asynchronous
Message identification	Identifier	Identifier	Time slot
Usage	Soft real time	Subnets	Hard real time
Latency	Load dependent	Constant	Constant

1.2.2   IEEE 802.3 Ethernet

is a commonly utilized CSMA/CD communication bus protocol due to its low cost, fast speed and high flexibility [8]. Not surprisingly, Ethernet is the technology of choice for much of the Internet and the most popular technology for local area network (LAN) in computer networking. The motivation to implement Ethernet in in-vehicle network is the ever-increasing bandwidth demanded by automotive applications, especially video-based Advance Drive Assistance System (ADAS).

The vehicle network should meet different requirements. For instance, the infotainment systems require higher bandwidth, where other systems require fault-tolerant networks. Therefore, a variety of network topologies are combined [9] (Fig. 2):

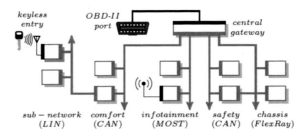

Fig. 2. Schematic overview of various in-car networks

1.3   Connected Car

The connected car can be considered as a multi-layered platform or an embedded system equipped with a wireless network gateway connecting the in–vehicle network to an external network via Over-the Air (OTA) technologies, and data collection/processing systems.

The connected vehicle allows the exchange of several information between the vehicle and its surroundings using WIFI, Bluetooth, GPS. The connection of the vehicle to the Internet is ensured either by as transmitter/receiver unit integrated with the vehicle itself, or via third-party systems such as smart phones.

The Fig. 3, illustrates routing of information between a connected vehicle and data center or OTA center and point out the steps to control the software updates and assure security of each level [10, 11].

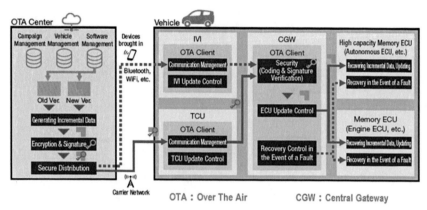

OTA : Over The Air   CGW : Central Gateway

ECU : Electronic Control Unit IVI : In-Vehicle Infotainment

TCU : Telematics Control Unit

Fig. 3. Connected car architecture & information flow

A critical challenge for connected cars is the need to prevent damage from cyber-attacks. As in all distributed applications or sever-client models, the key to security is an efficient encryption keys management strategy, which ensures the mutual verification of authenticity and protects the communication channels between the center and the vehicle, as well as between the ECUs of the vehicle.

The Introduction section, gives a state of the art concerning the IoT in transportation as well as definition of serval key concept were defined starting from Internet of Vehicle, In-vehicle Network and the car connected.

In second section, will briefly define the most popular architecture Inter-Network vehicle communication.

While the third section extend the intra-vehicle connectivity the most technologies used. The last section, present the discussion of the IoV solutions already adopted and challenges to be overcome.

2   Inter-Vehicle Communications

As shown in Fig. 4, the connected cars have multiple communication possibilities to connect to other vehicles (Vehicle-to-Vehicle) or exchange information with the external environments (Vehicle-to-road infrastructure), networks and services (Vehicle To Internet). These interactions, provide a promising opportunity to address the increasing transportation issues, such as heavy traffic, congestion, and vehicle safety.

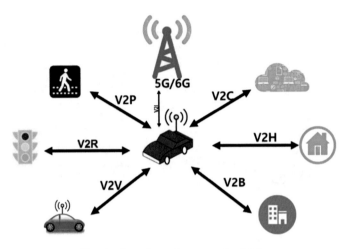

Fig. 4. Overview of connected vehicles

In this section, we listed succinctly the various types of communications for a connected car detailed in the literature [12, 13].

2.1   Vehicle-to-Vehicle (V2V)

V2V help improve road safety and improve the efficiency of traffic. In V2V scenario, vehicles exchange wirelessly relevant information to make the driving experience more enjoyable, for example drivers can take steps to reduce the severity or avoid the collision if a sudden brake warning is received earlier. That what affirms The National Highway Traffic Safety Administration (NHTSA) [14]: "V2V technology has the potential to address approximately 80 percent of multi-vehicle crashes" (Fig. 5).

2.2   Vehicle to Internet (V2I)

The connected vehicle shall be able to connect to internet in order to access to different multimedia services. the most common way is using cellular network infrastructures like Subscriber Identity Module (SIM) to allow the vehicle to get connected to the 3G/4G network.

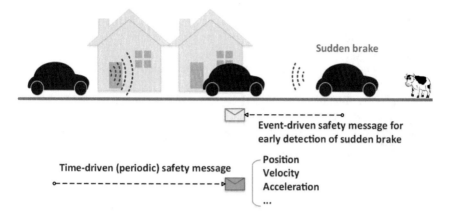

Fig. 5. Application of V2V to avoid collision

The Data centers can query the location using 3G/4G & LTE network, of vehicles at any time, analysis of historical data, video playback, oil and weight loss; this application is illustrated in the in the Fig. 6.

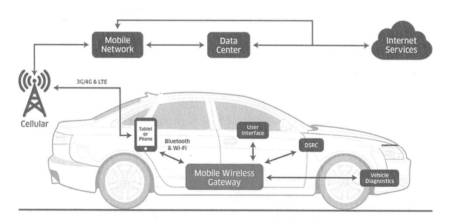

Fig. 6. 3G vehicle monitoring solution

2.3 Vehicle-to-Road Infrastructure (V2R)

V2R connectivity is crucial nowadays for efficient management of intelligent transportation system. The reception of real time road information help in mitigate or avoid the effects of the accidents. An application example could be a parking lot with infrared devices, WIFI network, and parking belts to detect miss parked cars, illustrated in the literature [15].

Scenario description:

- When a car enters the parking lot and heads to the reserved parking slot, the entrance booth will validate the reservation.
- If the parking spot is validated, a direction-related guidance will be uploaded to the car for finding the reserved spot.
- The road infrastructure engaged: parking belt, lights and infrared device, collaborate to prevent and detect the mismarking. As shown in Fig. 7, when the front wheel presses the belt-a, the Bluetooth communication enhanced.

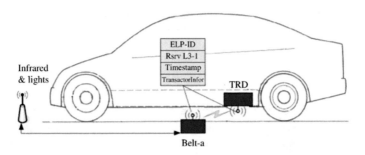

Fig. 7. Vacancy of parking slot detections by sensors

- The belt-a and tamper-resistant device (TRD) illustrated in Fig. 4 will validate, as necessary, the reservation confirmation
- For temporary purpose to validate the parked car the infrared device is used instead of the slot

The previous section place the IoT concept in automotive context it presented the definition and infrastructure of a connected car and different scenarios of IoT application engaging the inter-vehicular network.

The idea of the Sect. 3, is to evaluate the possibility of applying the IoT concept inside the Vehicle by transforming the wire intra-vehicular networks to Wireless Inter-vehicular networks, with the objective to lighten the vehicle weight, reduce the cost of development, harness placements as well as the cost of maintenance and make use of the information technologies advances. So, rethinking the automotive industry to provide a complete intelligent connected vehicle. And therefore, propelling automotive industry toward a new era.

The section start by summarizing the most potential wireless communication standards used to perform automotive functions inside a vehicle such as: "IEEE 802.15.1—Bluetooth", "IEEE 802.15.3—Ultra Wideband (UWB), high data rate", and "IEEE 802.15.4—ZigBee, low data rate", "Radio-frequency identification (RFID) "," IEEE 802.11—WIFI".

Continuing with the opportunities and proposals for solutions, features and challenges, end up with an advantage example of this approach, reduce the reduction of CO_2 emissions through the weight lighten.

3   Intra-Vehicle Connectivity

A forecasted increasing number of sensors deployed in cars, up to 200 per vehicle by 2020 [16] is required to report time-driven or event-driven messages to the electrical control units (ECU). Consequently, a growing interest is given to the intra-vehicle communication network design [17].

We present below the main candidate wireless technologies to build intra-vehicle wireless sensor networks, that have been investigated extensively in the literature.

3.1   Wireless Technologies

Bluetooth. is a short-range wireless technology based on the IEEE 802.15.1 standard allows a data rate communication up to 3 Mb/s between portable devices [18]. The Bluetooth devices are common in current vehicles, such as the rearview mirror and Bluetooth headset. However, a Bluetooth network can support just eight active devices, [19] and the transmission requires a high-power level, major disadvantage for battery-driven sensors [12].

ZigBee. is a short-range wireless technology based on the IEEE 802.15.4 physical radio standard. The ZigBee devices operate in ISM bands at 2.4 GHz and have transmission rates of 250 Kb/s at the 2.4 GHz band with 16 channels, 40 Kb/s at the 915 MHz band with 10 channels and 20 Kb/s at the 868 MHz band with 1 channel. Transmission range varies depending on the chosen transmission power [20], from 10 to 1600 m.

Radio-Frequency Identification. The feasibility of using the radio-frequency identification (RFID) technology. The rationale of the considered passive RFID solution is that each sensor is equipped with an RFID tag and a reader connected to the ECU, which periodically retrieves the sensed data by sending an energizing pulse to each tag [17].

Ultra Wideband(UWB). operates on unlicensed frequency band between 3.1 and 10.6 GHz, can support a STA with mobility of 10 kph. It supports low power operation, low power dissipation, robustness for multi-path fading and higher throughput of up to 480 Mbps. Like Bluetooth, it has a transmission range of 10 m. In Vehicular Ad hoc Networks (VANET), it can be used for collision avoidance [21].

Wi-Fi. WLAN is based on the IEEE 802.11standard family. The most common current versions are 802.11b and 802.11 g standards operating in 2.4 GHz bandwidth and capable of up to 54 Mbps or 11 Mbps data speeds, respectively. Recently also some devices supporting forthcoming standard have been published, expected to be able to provide up to hundreds of Mbps data speeds [19] (Table 2).

Table 2. The key comparison criteria of the listed wireless technologies

Standard	Bluetooth	UWB	ZigBee	Wi-Fi
IEEE spec.	802.15.1	802.15.3a[a]	802.15.4	802.11b and 802.11g
Frequency band	2.4 GHz	3.1–10.6 GHz	868/915 MHz; 2.4 GHz	2.4 GHz; 5 GHz
Max signal rate	1 Mb/s	110 Mb/s	250 Kb/s	54 Mb/s
Nominal range	10 m	10 m	10–100 m	100 m
Nominal TX power	0–10 dBm	−41.3 dBm/MHz (−25)	(−25)–0 dBm	15–20 dBm
Modulation type	GFSK[b]	BPSK, QPSK[c]	BPSK (+ SK), O-QPSK[d]	BPSK, QPSK COFDM, CCK, M-QAM[e]
Max number of cell nodes	8	8	>65,000	2007
Data protection	16-bit CRC	32-bit CRC	16-bit CRC	32-bit CRC
Application	Multimedia	Multimedia	Monitoring & control	Multimedia

[a]draft status
[b]GFSK (Gaussian frequency SK)
[c]BPSK/QPSK (binary/quadrature phase SK)
[d]O-QPSK (offset-QPSK)
[e]OFDM (orthogonal frequency division multiplexing), COFDM (coded OFDM)
MB-OFDM (multiband OFDM), M-QAM (M-ary quadrature amplitude modulation), CCK (complementary code keying)

3.2   Solution and Opportunities

The evolution of automotive technology, Advanced Driver Assistance Systems (ADAS) integrates dedicated functions into more complete systems, require additional components, more sensors and more cameras and more wires and therefore more weight is needed to build larger smarter systems.

Cables and other accessories nowadays can add significant weight (up to 50 kg) to the vehicle mass [12]. Recent advances in wireless sensor communication and networking technologies have paved the way for an intriguing alternative of using cable connection, leading to a significant reduction of the cost and complexity, where ECU and sensors build an intra-vehicle wireless sensor network.

As result, more functions could be added to enhance the safety and the intelligence of the vehicle without introducing additional weight, Fig. 8.

There are advantages to the hybrid wireless concept [21], such as:

- The weight reduction due to the wires replacement
- A simpler electrical wiring
- The easiest maintenance of the electrical submodules.
- A systemic approach to this idea replaced an initial component-level approach.
- Availability and reliability of the off-the-shelf components (ECU, Sensor, actuator…) including wireless communication ability.

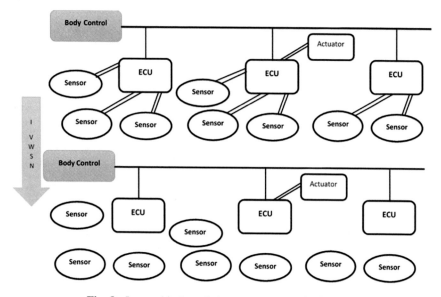

Fig. 8. Intra-vehicular wireless sensor networks(IVWSN)

3.3 Characteristics and Challenges

- The intra-vehicle wireless sensor networks have specific characteristics:
- Sensors are stationary so that the network topology does not change over time.
- Sensors are typically connected to ECU through one hop, which yields a simple star-topology.
- There is no energy constraint for sensors having wired connection to the vehicle power system.

3.4 CO$_2$ Reduction as Fundamental Driver for Weight Reduction in Automotive

Nowadays, the regulations are forcing OEMs to reduce significantly the car's CO$_2$ emissions. The average emissions, in Europe as an example, of all models sold by an OEM in one year must drop down from about 140 g CO$_2$ per kilometer to 95 g in 2020 and to 75 g in 2025 and beyond (with some exceptions/adaptations regarding the vehicle class).

The precise formula for the value curve is [23]:

$$Permitted\ specific\ emissions\ of\ CO_2 = 130 + a \times (M - M0) \tag{1}$$

where: M = mass in kg, M0 = 1289 kg, a = 0.0457 g CO$_2$/kg

However, this slope does not reflect the physical correlation between weight and CO$_2$ emissions, which is at about 0.08 g CO$_2$ reduction per kilogram saved. Therefore, reducing weight does help reach CO$_2$ target as shown in the Fig. 9.

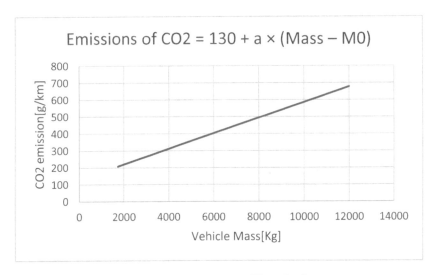

Fig. 9. Weight impact on CO_2 reduction

4 Discussion

The open-up of automotive sector to adopt IoT approach is a promoted area of solutions to the increasing transportation problems such as energy consumption, urban
congestion and environmental pollution. The table illustrate the application of IoT cited
in some papers for inter-Network and Intra-Network communication solutions provided versus the challenges to overcome (Table 3).

One of the major challenges for developing intelligent and green transportation
system, to accelerate the development of connected vehicles is data security, because of
the consequence severity of data security indecent. For example, once the traffic

Table 3. Resume of the IoV applications intra/Inter Network communication

	Papier	Transport problem	IoT application Solution	IoT application Challenge
Inter-network communication	[21]	Reduce accident and avoid Traffic congestion	V2V application	Data security and Delay constraints.
	[12]	Increase a traffic Safety	V2I application	bandwidth constraint and Data Security
	[15]	Smarter car and more intelligent systems in the vehicle	V2R application	The Roadside infrastructure involves additional installation costs.
Intra-network communication	[21] / [22]	Weight, maintenance cost reduction and fuel consumption	Intra-Vehicular Wireless Sensor Networks	Interferences, malicious attack, Real-time requirements.

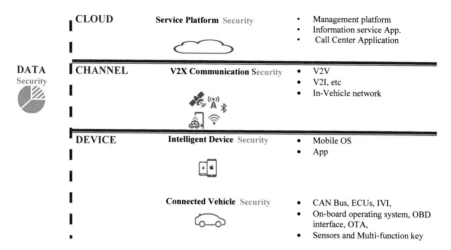

Fig. 10. Security through IoV architecture

management data, or data related to automobile operating, such as brake data, speed, fuel consumption, tire pressure, etc.is falsified or tampered, it will threat the safety of vehicle, passengers and the road management.

To assure IoV security we need to fulfill security requirements through the IoV Architecture [24] (Fig. 10).

5   Conclusion & Perspectives

This paper present of the state-of- the-art of Internet of vehicle. we have discussed the potential challenges of building an intra-vehicle wireless sensor networks and identified the space for future improvement reduce the future car weight, thereby to increase the margin to meet the regulations of CO_2 emission continuously tightened by the governments, In addition, our future work will extend the reliable IoT modeling and simulating a vehicle system (ECU and Sensors eventually actuators) applying the IoT architecture to migrate it from wire communication to a wireless communication system to demonstrate that cable removal is possible while ensuring the same safe functionality.

References

1. Alam, K.M.: Toward Social Internet of Vehicles: Concept, Architecture, and Applications. Fellow, IEEE, vol. 3, pp. 343. 27 April 2015
2. Fool.com: Internet of Things in 2016: 6 Stats Everyone Should Know. Online. Available: https://www.fool.com/investing/general/2016/01/18/internet-of-things-in-2016-6-stats-everyone-should.aspx
3. International Organization of Motor Vehicle Manufacturers.: Sales Statistic 3 2017 © OICA. Online. Available: http://www.oica.net/cookie-policy/

4. Kleberger, P., Javaheri, A., Olovsson, T., Jonsson, E.: A Framework for Assessing the Security of the Connected Car Infrastructure. 236, Chalmers University of Technology ISBN: 978-1-61208-166-3, 8 Nov 2011

5. Coppola, R., Morisio, M.: Connected car: technologies, issues, future trends Connected, car: Technologies, issues, future trends. ACM Comput. Surv. **49**(3), 36 (2016) (Article 46)

6. Freescale: In-Vehicle Networking. March 2013 Online. Available: https://www.nxp.com/docs/en/brochure/BRINVEHICLENET.pdf

7. Hergenhan, A., Heiser, G.: Operating Systems Technology for Converged ECUs. In: Proceedings of the 7th escar Embedded Security in Cars Conference, Nov 2008

8. IEEE standard for Ethernet IEEE Std 802.3-2012 (Revision to IEEE Std 802.3-2008), Dec 2012

9. Bosch.: OSI Layers in Automotive Networks. March 2013. Online. Available: http://www.ieee802.org/1/files/public/docs2013/new-tsn-diarra-osi-layers-in-automotive-networks-0313-v01.pdf

10. Kleberger, P., Olovsson, T., Jonsson, E.: Security aspects of the in-vehicle network in the connected car. In: Intelligent Vehicles Symposium (IV), IEEE, p. 528–533. IEEE, (2011)

11. Sagstetter, F., Lukasiewycz, M., Sebastian, S., Wolf, M., Bouard, A., Harris, W.R., Jha, S., Peyrin, T., Poschmann, A., Chakraborty, S.: Security challenges in automotive hardware/software architecture design. In: Proceedings of the Conference on Design, Automation and Test in Eu-rope, pp. 458–463. EDA. Consortium, (2013)

12. Qu, F., Wang, F.-Y., Yang, L.: Intelligent transportation spaces: Vehicles, traffic, communications, and beyond. IEEE Commun. Mag. **48**(11), 136–142 (2010)

13. Faezipour, M., Nourani, M., Saeed, A., Addepalli, S.: Progress and challenges in intelligent vehicle area networks. Commun. ACM **55**(2), 90–100 (2012)

14. National Highway Traffic Safety Administration NHTSA: Online. (2017) Available: https://www.nhtsa.gov/technology-innovation/vehicle-vehicle-communications

15. He, W., Yan, G., Da Xu, L.,: Developing Vehicular Data Cloud Services in the IoT Environment. IEEE Trans. Ind. Inf. **10**(2) (2014)

16. Pinelis, M.: Automotive Sensors and Electronics: Trends and developments in 2013 in Automot. Sensors Electron. Expo, Detroit, MI, USA (2013)

17. Lu, N., Cheng, N., Zhang, N., Shen, X., Mark, J.W.: Connected vehicles: solutions and challenges. IEEE Internet Things J. **1**(4) (2014)

18. Wang, D., O'Keefe, K., Petovello, M.G.: Decentralized Cooperative Positioning for Vehicle-to-Vehicle (V2V) Application Using GPS Integrated with UWB Range. In: Proceedings of the ION 2013 Pacific PNT Meeting, Honolulu, Hawaii pp. 793–803 April 2013

19. Gandhi, A., Jadhav, B.T.: Role of wireless technology for vehicular network. (IJCSIT) Int. J. Comput. Sci. Inf. Technol. **3**(4), 4823–4828 (2012)

20. Blasius, J.T.: Short-range wireless communications for vehicular Ad hoc networking. In: Proceedings of the National Conference on Undergraduate Research (NCUR) 2014 University of Kentucky, Lexington, KY, 3–5 April 2014

21. Bickel, G.S.: Inter/Intra-vehicle Wireless Communication. http://www.cse.wustl.edu/~jain/cse574-06/ftp/vehicular_wireless.pdf

22. Huo, Y., Tu, W., Sheng, Z., Leung, C.M.: A Survey of In-vehicle Communications: Requirements, Solutions and Opportunities in IoT, IEEE 2015

23. Lightweight, Heavy Impact Advanced Industries Designed by Visual Media Europe Copyright © McKinsey & Company, pp. 11–12. Feb 2012

24. Tian, H.: Introduction of IOV Security. Security Research Institute, CAICT, 2 Nov 2017

An Enhanced Localization Approach for Three-Dimensional Wireless Sensor Networks

A. Hadir[1]($^{(\boxtimes)}$), K. Zine-Dine[1], M. Bakhouya[2], and J. El Kafi[1]

[1] LAROSERI Lab, Chouaib Doukkali University, El Jadida, Morocco
{hadir.a,zinedine,elkafi.j}@ucd.ac.ma
[2] TIC Lab, Faculty of Computing and Logistics, International University of Rabat, Sala El Jadida, Morocco
mohamed.bakhouya@uir.ac.ma

Abstract. In most of Wireless Sensor Network (WSN) applications, it is important to associate each event's information with its location's information. If sensors are accurately located, the identified event (e.g., fire, accident) could be of most important in order to figure out and understand the context or situation. However, sensors localization is still an important issue in order to develop context-driven applications. This paper introduces a new scheme for sensor nodes localization in three-dimensional WSNs, denoted 3DeDV-Hop. We have implemented both algorithms the 3DeDV-Hop and 3DDV-Hop in OMNET++, and studied their performance in three dimensional wireless sensor networks. Simulation results show that the 3DeDV-Hop outperforms the basic 3DDV-Hop localization algorithm in terms of localization accuracy and the number of localized nodes.

Keywords: WSNs · Sensors localization · 3DV-Hop · Performance evaluation

1 Introduction

Recent advances in microelectronics have enabled the design and manufacturing of inexpensive, small and smart sensor components having multiple functions (e.g., sensing, actuating). Every sensor incorporates several modules, such as a processor, a memory, and a power module [1]. In addition to their small size, sensors have limited power and low computational capabilities, which require adaptable software and tools (e.g., OS). Furthermore, these sensor components have the ability to communicate with each other via wireless network protocols [2]. In fact, in many applications, a collection of tiny sensor nodes could be deployed in dedicated area, and are able to communicate with each other via wireless network protocols. They have the capabilities to collect, compute and send the physical data accordingly i.e. temperature, pressure, light, humidity, etc [3] Besides, if an event occurs in the area of interest, sensors gather and broadcast related data to a dedicated platform, where data can be analyzed, processed and used [4].

© Springer Nature Switzerland AG 2019
M. Ezziyyani (Ed.): AI2SD 2018, AISC 915, pp. 941–954, 2019.
https://doi.org/10.1007/978-3-030-11928-7_85

WSNs have attracted a lot of attention in the past few years and are now widely used in many applications [3], such as in smart buildings, healthcare, commerce, logistics, smart transportations, military, disaster management, underwater applications and in environment monitoring [5–11]. In most of these applications of WSNs, it is important to associate each event's information with its location's information. For instance, in fire detection applications both events and positions where fire is detected are needed. Thus, the localization of sensors is one of most critical tasks in WSN applications. In fact, if sensor nodes are accurately located, the identified event (e.g., fire, accident) could be of most important in order to figure out and understand the actual context or situation. In addition the nodes' localization is useful in order to operate nodes communication, such as data routing using, for example geographic routing techniques [12].

Equipping sensors with Global Positioning System (GPS) modules is one of the simplest solutions that can be used for sensors localization. But unfortunately, using GPS modules is not always a good solution in many fields. For example, sensor nodes in underwater applications are not always stable and they can float around even if they are physically anchored. In addition, GPS signals are severely attenuated underwater, and also very expensive and power consuming, especially in applications that need hundreds or thousands of sensor nodes. Recent solutions put more emphasize on collaborative localization techniques. These solutions assume that only a small number of sensor nodes know their exact location (e.g., via GPS) and are commonly called anchors. The positions of these nodes are used as references to help unknown sensor nodes estimating their locations by using exchanged packets.

Many localization solutions for wireless sensor networks have been introduced to estimate sensors' locations. These solutions can be classified into two main classes: range-free and range-based localization. Range-based localization techniques use exact measurements based techniques and generally require costly equipment to find distance or angle information between neighboring nodes in order to determine with high accuracy location information. Some of range-based localization algorithms are received signal strength indicator (RSSI) [13], time of arrival (TOA) [14], time difference of arrival (TDOA) [15], and angle of arrival (AOA) [16]. Range-free localization techniques apply distance approximation algorithms to determine sensors' location that does not require any expensive hardware. Range-free localization algorithms mainly use nodes that are aware of their location (anchors) to find the location of unknown nodes. There are many range-free localization algorithms, examples are centroid algorithm [17], DV-Hop [18], amorphous [19], Multidimensional Scaling (MDS) [20] and Approximate Point-In-Triangulation (APIT) [21]. Although range-based algorithms give accurate results, still range-free localization algorithms are main candidates due to their low cost and feasibility for large-scale wireless sensor networks.

In this work, we focus on the range-free DV-Hop algorithm that is more popular among all other range-free localization algorithms for two-dimensional due to its simplicity, low cost and robustness. But, DV-Hop algorithm also has some limitations, such as low localization accuracy, high power consumption and high communication overhead. Previous works have tried to improve localization error in DV-Hop algorithm for two-dimensional, but very little work has been done to enhance DV-Hop for three-dimensional WSNs (3DWSNs). In this paper, we present an enhanced scheme of the basic 3DDV-Hop, denoted 3DDeDV-Hop. Mainly, we implemented both 3DDV-Hop and 3DeDV-Hop in OMNeT++, instead of using MATLAB, to study their performance in terms of localization accuracy. Obtained results show that 3DeDV-Hop provides better localization accuracy. Especially, the main contribution of this work is: (i) enhance DV-Hop in three-dimensional WSNs using the average hop size weighted mean technique as a new formula for computing the basic average hop size and the hyperbolic location technique instead of the trilateration, (ii) implement both 3DDV-Hop and 3DeDV-Hop techniques in OMNeT++ and study their performance in static 3D WSNs.

The rest of this paper is organized as follows. Section 2 presents the state of the art review of existing work from literature. Section 3 introduces the 3DeDV-Hop, an extended scheme of the basic DV-Hop for 3DWSNs. Section 4 presents the simulation environment, parameters and metrics used to assess on the performance of 3DDV-Hop and 3DeDV-Hop together with obtained results. Section 5 provides some conclusions and perspectives.

2 Related Work

In the last decade, many solutions schemes for localization in WSNs have been presented to improve range-free techniques, such as DV-Hop, APIT, and MDS. However, the localization in three-dimensional WSNs is still a critical issue that needs to be addressed. This section is dedicated mainly to localization techniques that have been proposed for 3DWSNs [22–25]. For instance, DV-Hop has attracted more attention due to its simplicity, stability, feasibility and less hardware requirement. For instance, Xu et al. [25] introduced an improved 3D localization technique based on the degree of co-planarity. The RSSI method was applied to measure the distance and the concept of co-planarity was used in order to minimize localization error generated by co-planar anchors. Authors also used the Quasi-Newton technique to calculate the final location of sensor nodes. The simulation results showed that the introduced algorithm can improve the localization accuracy and localization coverage. Chen et al. in [26] proposed an enhanced 3DDV-Hop localization algorithm. In the first stage of this algorithm, the location of unknown sensors is calculated using the basic DV-hop localization technique. In the second stage, the Particle Swarm Optimization (PSO) was used to improve the localization accuracy. Obtained results showed that this algorithm has a significant localization accuracy compared to the 3DDV-Hop.

Yang et al. [27] presented a new sequence localization correction algorithm based on Voronoi diagram in three dimensional WSNs. The main idea of the proposed algorithm is based on divides area with 3D Voronoi and the correction of the calculated distance by fixing location sequences of target sensor nodes. In fact, the authors select an optimal number of virtual anchors in order to improve the accuracy and to reduce the effects of real number of anchor nodes. Wang et al. [28] proposed a range-free localization algorithm (denoted as a PMDV-Hop) based on DV-Hop. The basic average hop size of the anchor is modified by using the root-mean-square error and dynamically correct by the weighted RMSE based on group hops. However, the authors used a PSO technique to get a more accurate estimated location of sensor nodes. Simulation results showed that PMDV-Hop outperforms the basic DV-hop localization algorithm. However, despite the importance of the proposed DV-hop extension for 3DWSNs there is a room for enhancement to get more localization accuracy. Therefore, the work presented in this paper introduces an enhanced 3DDV-Hop algorithm based on average hop size weighed mean and 2D-hyperbolic techniques. In summary, DV-Hop [18], as stated above, is one of widely used range-free localization algorithm in 2DWSNs. 3DV-Hop algorithms have been proposed as an extension of DV-Hop but for 3DWSNs. Many of these algorithms are based on DV-Hop because is very simple and can localize unknown nodes, which have neighboring anchor nodes. However, the accuracy of the proposed algorithms needs to be enhanced. In our work, we have introduced a technique aiming at further increasing the accuracy of 3DV-Hop.

3   3DeDV-Hop: An Enhanced Extension of DV-Hop

The localization problem in 3DWSNs can be presented as follows. We assume a 3DWSNs composed of $Net = \{SN1, SN2 \dots SNm+n\}$ with m anchor nodes and n unknown nodes (i.e., sensor nodes) and denote the location of each sensor node as $A_i = \begin{pmatrix} x_i \\ y_i \\ z_i \end{pmatrix} M_i = \begin{pmatrix} x_{Mi} \\ y_{Mi} \\ z_{Mi} \end{pmatrix}$ for $i=1\dots m+n$. It is considered that the m anchor nodes, $\{A1, A2 \dots Am\}$ know their position but the positions of the n unknown nodes have to be estimated. The only available information is the distance and the number of hop counts between anchor nodes. Let us define the geographic distance between two sensor nodes M_i and M_j as $d_{ij} = \sqrt{(x_i - x_j)^2 + (y_i - y_j)^2 + (z_i - z_j)^2}$ and denote the estimate information between the ith node and the jth node as $hop_{ij} = \{0, 1, 2, 3 \dots\}$, which represents the value of hop counts between the two nodes. Alike DV–Hop, in the proposed enhanced scheme for 3DWSNs, the average hop size is based on the average hop size weighted mean. The average hop size weighted mean is a measure of central tendency, a special case of weighted mean, where weighting coefficient for each average hop size is computed as the inverse sum of distances between this average hop size and the other average hop sizes [29]. An important property of the distance-weighted mean is that computing weighting coefficients does not require mean or other parameters of the original distribution. It is worth noting that, the average hop size weighted mean is less sensitive to outliers than the arithmetic mean and many other measures of central tendency.

Basically, the proposed schemas, denoted 3DeDV-Hop, is divided into the following three improved stages: (i) anchor nodes flood their positions, (ii) the calculation of the average hop size is modified, and (iii) the 2D hyperbolic technique is used, instead of the trilateration, to estimate the nodes' locations. More precisely, the first stage of 3DeDV-Hop is similar to the basic 3DDV-Hop. Every anchor node broadcasts a message containing the position of per anchor and initializes the hop count between anchor nodes by 0. In the second stage, we use the weighted mean technique [29] to calculate the average hop size following a new formula. To calculate the average hop size in 3DeDV-Hop, we used the mean square error technique [30]. Thus, the formula used to obtain $AvgHopSize_i$, is computed by the following formula:

$$e_1 = \frac{1}{m-1} \sum_{j \neq i} \left(d_{ij} - AvgHopSize_i \times hop_{ij}\right)^2 \tag{1}$$

where m is the number of anchor nodes and $AvgHopSize_i$ can be calculated as follows by considering that $\partial e1 / AvgHopSize_i = 0$, d_{ij} represents the distance from A_i to A_j and hop_{ij} represents the minimum hop counts number between A_i and A_j:

$$AvgHopSize_i = \frac{\sum_{j \neq i} hop_{ij} \times d_{ij}}{\sum_{j \neq i} hop_{ij}^2} \tag{2}$$

So, the average hop size is calculated using the following formula

$$AvgHopSize_{new} = \frac{\sum_{i=1}^{m} w_i \times AvgHopSize_i}{\sum_{i=1}^{m} w_i} \tag{3}$$

where

$$w_i = \frac{1}{\sum_{j \neq i}^{m} \left| AvgHopSize_i - AvgHopSize_j \right|} \tag{4}$$

In the third stage, instead of using the trilateration or the multilateration location method to estimate nodes location, we have used the 2D hyperbolic location method [31]. It is assumed that (x_i, y_i, z_i) are the coordinates of anchor node A_i and (x_M, y_M, z_M) are the coordinates of unknown node M. The estimated distance d_{iM} is calculated as follows:

$$d_{iM}^2 = (x_i - x_M)^2 + (y_i - y_M)^2 + (z_i - z_M)^2 \tag{5}$$

If $R_i = x_i^2 + y_i^2 + z_i^2$ and $K_i = x_M^2 + y_M^2 + z_M^2$ can be rewritten as follows:

$$d_{iM}^2 - R_i = -2 \times x_i \times x_M - 2 \times y_i \times y_M - 2 \times z_i \times z_M + K_i \tag{6}$$

The matrix form of eq. 6 is:

$$L \times A = b \tag{7}$$

where

$$A = [x_M, y_M, z_M, K_M]^T \quad L = \begin{bmatrix} -2x_1 & -2y_1 & -2z_1 & 1 \\ -2x_2 & -2y_2 & -2z_2 & 1 \\ ... & ... & ... & ... \\ -2x_n & y & -2z_n & 1 \end{bmatrix}$$

$$b = \begin{bmatrix} d_{1M}^2 - R_1 \\ d_{2M}^2 - R_2 \\ \cdots \\ d_{nM}^2 - R_n \end{bmatrix}$$

According to eq. 7, using the least mean square estimation method, A can be obtained by the following formula:

$$A = \left(L^T L\right)^{-1} L^T b \tag{8}$$

Thus, M unknown sensor node coordinates are calculated as follows:

$$\begin{cases} x_M = A(1) \\ y_M = A(2) \\ z_M = A(3) \end{cases} \tag{9}$$

The process of 3DeDV-Hop algorithm is summarized as follows:

S_1.	For Each anchor, A_i diffuses from the network a packet containing the position of A_i and also a hop-count initialized to 0.	
	$S_{1.1.}$	Update anchors packet to compare with the new packet received {d_{ij}, hop-counts, x_j, y_j, z_i} from new anchor.
	$S_{1.2}$	If the anchor A_i receives a new packet from anchor A_j with a new hop-count A_i save the minimum hop count.
S_2.	If ISANCHORS then	
	$S_{2.1.}$	Anchor A_i can calculate it average hop size $AvgHopSize_i$.
	$S_{2.2.}$	The anchor nodes can calculate the optimized average hop size $AvgHopSize\_new$.
S_3.	$Node\_i$ receives the packet from anchor	
	$S_{3.1.}$	$Node\_i$ estimates the distance $d_i = AvgHopSize\_new \times hop\text{-}counts_i$
	$S_{3.2.}$	$Node\_i$ estimates the position using 2D-Hyperbolic method.

4 Simulation Results

In this section, we mainly focus on the performance evaluation of DV-Hop and its proposed enhancing version for 3DWSNS. We have decided to develop these algorithms in OMNET++ [32] in order to evaluate their performances in terms of localization accuracy and number of localized nodes. In our simulations, sensor nodes are randomly deployed in a 500 m × 500 m × 500 m monitored space and all sensor nodes are located within static WSN, i.e., sensors are not mobile. The localization error is used for evaluating the localization accuracy as follows:

$$Localization\ error = \frac{\sum_i^N d(estimated_i, real_i)}{n}$$

where $estimate_i$ is the estimated position of sensor i by the respective localization algorithm, $real_i$ is the actual position of sensor i, $d(estimated_i, actual_i)$ is the Euclidean distance between sensor i's actual position and its estimated position, n represents the number of nodes. The localization coverage is defined as the ratio of the localized unknown nodes to the total number of nodes in the networks as follows:

$$Localization\ coverage = \frac{Localizednodes}{n}$$

However, In order to study the performance of 3DDV-Hop and 3DeDV-Hop localization techniques we have considered several scenarios using the following parameters. The network topology was generated according to the number and communication range of sensor nodes. All sensor nodes have the same communication range and are randomly distributed in an area of 500 m × 500 m × 500 m. We have studied the effect of these parameters (e.g. communication range, number of anchor nodes, and number of unknown sensor nodes) on the performance of these two algorithms in terms of the localization error and the percentage of localized nodes.

4.1 Influence of Anchor Nodes

In this subsection, we study the impact of the number of anchor nodes on the localization error and percentage of localized nodes. We have evaluated, mainly, the impact of the number of anchor nodes on the localization accuracy of 3DDV-Hop and 3DeDV-Hop algorithms. We have fixed the number of anchor nodes to 100, 110, 120, 130 and 140, the total number of sensor nodes is fixed to 400, 600 and 800 and the communication radius R is equal to 100 m. We show the results of 400, 600 and 800 sensor nodes by varying the number of anchor nodes. Figure 1a–c show the performance of localization algorithms according to the total number of anchor nodes in the network. However, when the number of anchor nodes increases beyond a certain threshold only a slight enhancement can be noticed. But, 3DeDV-Hop outperforms the basic 3DDV-Hop localization algorithm. We can also see that 3DeDV-Hop outperforms the basic 3DDV-Hop algorithm, but both algorithms scale in the same way as the number of anchor nodes increases.

Figure 2a–c present the localization coverage, which is defined as the percentage of localized nodes according to the number of anchor nodes. We can see that both algorithms perform well and scale as the number of anchor nodes increases, i.e., the number of localized nodes reaches almost 100% become more preponderant over unknown nodes, but 3DDV-Hop converges is better. In fact, Figure 2b, c shows that the 3DeDV-Hop outperforms 3DDV-Hop in terms of the localization coverage when the number of total sensor nodes equals 600 and 800.

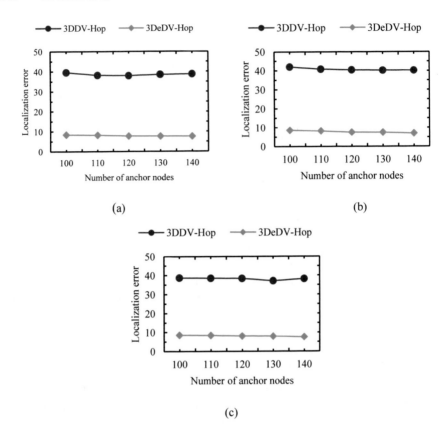

Fig. 1. Localization error versus number of anchor nodes: **a** 400 sensor nodes, **b** 600 senor nodes, and **c** 800 sensor nodes.

4.2   Influence of the Communication Range

In this subsection, we study the effect of the communication range of all sensor nodes on the localization error and percentage of localized nodes. We have mainly evaluated the effect of the communication range of sensor nodes on the localization accuracy of 3DDV-Hop and 3DeDV-Hop algorithms. We fixed the total number of sensor nodes to 400, 600 and 800, the total number of anchor nodes is fixed to 100, and the communication radius R is equal to 100, 110, 120, 130 and 140m. We show the results of 400, 600 and 800 sensor nodes by varying the communication radius. Figure 3a–c show the performance of localization algorithms according to the communication range of sensor nodes within the network. However, when the communication radius of sensor nodes increases the localization error of both 3DDV-Hop and 3DeDV-Hop decreases slowly. But, 3DeDV-Hop outperforms the basic 3DDV-Hop localization algorithm.

We can also see that 3DeDV-Hop outperforms the basic 3DDV-Hop algorithm, but both algorithms scale well as the number of anchor nodes increases. Figure 4a–c present the localization coverage of both algorithms according to the communication

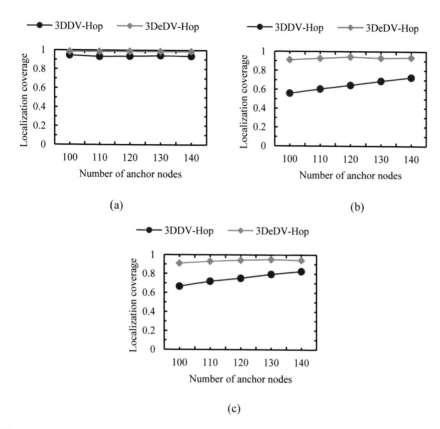

Fig. 2. Localization coverage versus number of anchor nodes: **a** 400 sensor nodes, **b** 600 senor nodes, and **c** 800 sensor nodes.

range. We can see that both algorithms perform well and scale as the communication range of sensor nodes increases, but 3DDV-Hop converges well. In fact, as depicted in Figure 4b, c it is observed that the 3DeDV-Hop outperforms 3DDV-Hop in terms of the localization coverage when the number of total sensor nodes is equal 600 and 800.

4.3   Influence of Total Number of Sensor Nodes

In this subsection, we have evaluated both algorithms according to the total number of unknown nodes. The total number of sensor nodes is fixed to 400, 500, 600, 700, and 800, the number of anchor nodes is fixed to 100 anchor nodes, and the communication range is set to 100 m. As depicted in Figure 5, the localization error given by 3DeDV-Hop is reduced by almost 30% compared to the basic 3DDV-Hop algorithm. As the number of nodes increases, the localization error slightly decreases in both 3DDV-Hop and 3DeDV-Hop.

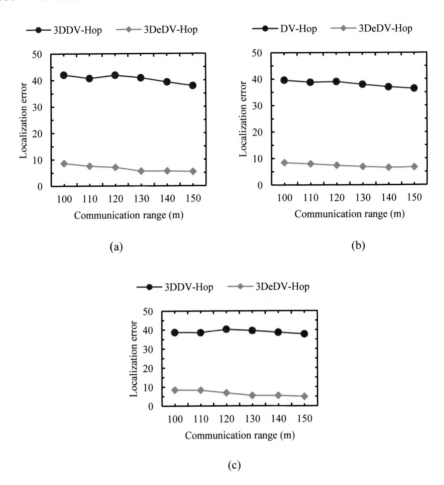

Fig. 3. Localization error versus communication range of sensors: **a** 400 sensor nodes, **b** 600 senor nodes, and **c** 800 sensor nodes.

We have also evaluated the localization error per node for both algorithms and results presented in Figure 6 show that the localization error for each unknown node of 3DeDV-Hop is lower compared to 3DDV-Hop.

5   Conclusions and Future work

Several localization approaches for WSNs have been presented in the past few years to accurately estimate sensor nodes location in two-dimensional. In this paper, an enhanced version of DV-Hop, named 3DeDV-Hop, is introduced to improve the localization error of node for three-dimensional wireless sensor networks. 3DeDV-Hop uses the average hop–size weighted mean to estimate average hop–size for networks and 2D hyperbolic techniques. The algorithms have been implemented in OMNeT++

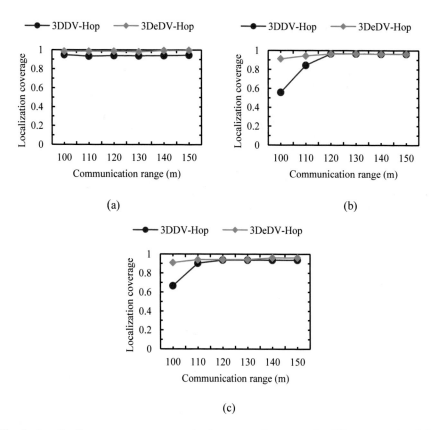

(a)   (b)

(c)

Fig. 4. Localization error versus communication range of sensors **a** for 400 sensor nodes, **b** for 600 senor nodes, and **c** for 800.

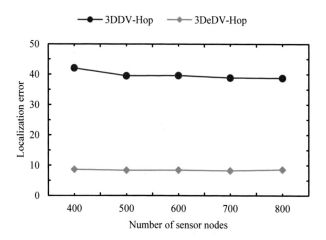

Fig. 5. Localization error versus number of sensor nodes.

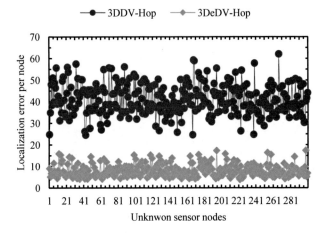

Fig. 6. Localization error versus unknown nodes.

simulator. The aim was to assess both algorithms in terms of localization accuracy and localization coverage for static WSNs. Simulations have been conducted and results are presented and showed that 3DeDV-Hop outperforms 3DDV-Hop. More simulations will be done to compare 3DDV-Hop with those from literature [33–37], mainly for Mobile Wireless Sensor Networks (MWSNs).

References

1. Akyildiz, I.F., Su, W., Sankarasubramaniam, Y., Cayirci, E.: A survey on sensor networks. IEEE Commun. Mag. **40**(8), 102–114 (2002)
2. Boukerche, A., Oliveira, H.A., Nakamura, E.F., Loureiro, A.A.: Localization in time and space for wireless sensor networks: A Mobile Beacon approach. In: 2008 International Symposium on a World of Wireless, Mobile and Multimedia Networks, WoWMoM 2008, pp. 1–8 (2008)
3. Yalgashev, O., Bakhouya, M., Nait-Sidi-Moh, A., Gaber, J.: Wireless sensor networks: basics and fundamentals. Book Cyber-Physical System Design with Sensor Networking Technologies ISBN, pp. 978–1 (2016)
4. Malek, Y.N., et al.: On the use of IoT and big data technologies for real-time monitoring and data processing. Procedia Comput. Sci. **113**, 429–434 (2017)
5. Kaiwen, C., Kumar, A., Xavier, N., Panda, S.K.: An intelligent home appliance control-based on WSN for smart buildings. In: 2016 IEEE International Conference on Sustainable Energy Technologies (ICSET), pp. 282–287 (2016)
6. Bhuiyan, M.Z.A., Wang, G., Cao, J., Wu, J.: Deploying wireless sensor networks with fault-tolerance for structural health monitoring. IEEE Trans. Comput. **64**(2), 382–395 (2015)
7. Antolín, D., Medrano, N., Calvo, B., Pérez, F.: A wearable wireless sensor network for indoor smart environment monitoring in safety applications. Sensors **17**(2), 365 (2017)
8. Viani, F., Robol, F., Polo, A., Rocca, P., Oliveri, G., Massa, A.: Wireless architectures for heterogeneous sensing in smart home applications: concepts and real implementation. Proc. IEEE **101**(11), 2381–2396 (2013)

9. Abrardo, A., Martalò, M., Ferrari, G.: Information fusion for efficient target detection in large-scale surveillance wireless sensor networks. Inf. Fusion **38**, 55–64 (2017)
10. Malekian, R., Moloisane, N.R., Nair, L., Maharaj, B.T., Chude-Okonkwo, U.A.K.: Design and implementation of a wireless OBD II fleet management system. IEEE Sens. J. **17**(4), 1154–1164 (2017)
11. Al-Turjman, F.: Cognitive routing protocol for disaster-inspired Internet of Things. Future Gener. Comput. Syst. Mar 2017
12. Hadir, A., Zine-Dine, K., Bakhouya, M., El Kafi, J., El Ouadghiri, D.: Towards an integrated geographic routing approach using estimated sensors position in WSNs. In: 2018 International Conference on High Performance Computing Simulation (HPCS), 2018
13. Fang, Z., Zhao, Z., Geng, D., Xuan, Y., Du, L., Cui, X.: RSSI variability characterization and calibration method in wireless sensor network. In: 2010 IEEE International Conference on Information and Automation (ICIA), pp. 1532–1537 (2010)
14. Niculescu, D., Nath, B.:"Ad hoc positioning system (APS) using AOA," in INFOCOM 2003. Twenty-Second Annual Joint Conference of the IEEE Computer and Communications. IEEE Societies, vol. 3, pp. 1734–1743. (2003)
15. Gustafsson. F., Gunnarsson, F.: Positioning using time-difference of arrival measurements. In: ICASSP (6), pp. 553–556 (2003)
16. Doğançay, K., Hmam, H.: Optimal angular sensor separation for AOA localization. Signal Process. **88**(5), 1248–1260 (2008)
17. Bulusu, N., Heidemann, J., Estrin, D.: GPS-less low-cost outdoor localization for very small devices. IEEE Pers. Commun. **7**(5), 28–34 (2000)
18. Niculescu, D., Nath, B.: DV based positioning in ad hoc networks. Telecommun. Syst. **22**(1–4), 267–280 (2003)
19. Nagpal, R.: Organizing a global coordinate system from local information on an amorphous computer (1999)
20. Shang, Y., Ruml, W.: "Improved MDS-based localization," in INFOCOM 2004. Twenty-third AnnualJoint Conference of the IEEE Computer and Communications Societies, vol. 4, pp. 2640–2651 (2004)
21. Yong, Z., Shixiong, X., Shifei, D., Lei, Z., Xin, A.: An improved APIT node self-localization algorithm in WSN based on triangle-center scan. J. Comput. Res. Dev. **46**(4), 566–574 (2009)
22. Zhang, L., Peng, F., Cao, P., Ji, W.: An improved three-dimensional DV-Hop localization algorithm optimized by adaptive cuckoo search algorithm. Int. J. Online Eng. IJOE **13**(02), 102–118 (2017)
23. Chaurasiya, V.K., Jain, N., Nandi, G.C.: A novel distance estimation approach for 3D localization in wireless sensor network using multi dimensional scaling. Inf. Fusion **15**, 5–18 (2014)
24. Sharma, G., Kumar, A.: Fuzzy logic based 3D localization in wireless sensor networks using invasive weed and bacterial foraging optimization. Telecommun. Syst. **67**(2), 149–162 (2018)
25. Xu, Y., Zhuang, Y., Gu, J.: An improved 3D localization algorithm for the wireless sensor network. Int. J. Distrib. Sens. Netw. **11**(6), 315714 (2015)
26. Chen, X., Zhang, B.: 3D DV–hop localisation scheme based on particle swarm optimisation in wireless sensor networks. Int. J. Sens. Netw. **16**(2), 100–105 (2014)
27. Yang, X., Yan, F., Liu, J.: 3D localization algorithm based on Voronoi diagram and rank sequence in wireless sensor network. Sci. Program (2017)
28. Wu, W., Wen, X., Xu, H., Yuan, L., Meng, Q.: Accurate Range-free Localization Based on Quantum Particle Swarm Optimization in Heterogeneous Wireless Sensor Networks. KSII Trans. Internet Inf. Syst. **12**(3) (2018)

29. Dodonov, Y.S., Dodonova, Y.A.: Robust measures of central tendency: weighting as a possible alternative to trimming in response-time data analysis. Psikhologicheskie Issledovaniya, 5(19) (2011)
30. Zhang, X.: Modern Signal Processing [M], pp. 40–42. (2002)
31. Chan, Y.T., Ho, K.C.: A simple and efficient estimator for hyperbolic location. IEEE Trans. Signal Process. 42(8), 1905–1915 (1994)
32. OMNeT++ Discrete Event Simulator—Home. [Online]. Available: https://www.omnetpp. org/
33. Cui, H., Wang, Y.: Four-mobile-beacon assisted localization in three-dimensional wireless sensor networks. Comput. Electr. Eng. 38(3), 652–661 (2012)
34. Jia, Z., Wu, C., Li, Z., Zhang, Y., Guan, B.: The Indoor localization and tracking estimation method of mobile targets in three-dimensional wireless sensor networks. Sensors 15(11), 29661–29684 (2015)
35. Hadir, A., Zine-Dine, K., Bakhouya, M., El Kafi, J., El Ouadghiri, D.: Performance evaluation of DV-Hop localization algorithm for geographical routing in wireless sensor networks. Procedia Comput. Sci. 113, 261–266 (2017)
36. Zhou, J., Chen, Y., Leong, B., Sundaramoorthy, P.S.: Practical 3D geographic routing for wireless sensor networks. In: Proceedings of the 8th ACM Conference on Embedded Networked Sensor Systems, pp. 337–350. New York, NY, USA, (2010)
37. Huang, H., Yin, H., Luo, Y., Zhang, X., Min, G., Fan, Q.: Three-dimensional geographic routing in wireless mobile ad hoc and sensor networks. IEEE Netw. 30(2), 82–90 (2016)

Neural Networks Architecture for Amazigh POS Tagging

Samir Amri[✉] and Lahbib Zenkouar

ERSC Laboratory, EMI School, Med V University, Rabat, Morocco
amri.samir@gmail.com, zenkouar@emi.ac.ma

Abstract. Morphosyntactic processing of natural languages is mainly restricted by the lack of labelled data sets. Deep Learning methods proved their efficiency in domains such as imaging or acoustic process. Part-of-speech tagging is an important preprocessing step in many natural language processing applications. Despite much work already carried out in this field, there is still room for improvement, especially in Amazigh language. We propose here architectures based on neural networks and word embeddings, and that has achieved promising results in English. Furthermore, instead of extracting from the sentence a rich set of hand-crafted features which are the fed to a standard classification algorithm, we drew our inspiration from recent papers about the automatic extraction of word embeddings from large unlabelled data sets. On such embeddings, we expect to benefit from linearity and compositionality properties to improve our Amazigh POS Tagging system performances.

Keywords: Deep learning · CNN · Amazigh · POS tagging

1 Introduction

In recent years there were a large number of works trying to push the accuracy of the PoS-tagging task forward using new techniques, mainly from the deep learning domain. All these studies are mainly devoted to show how to find the best combination of new neural network structures and character/word embeddings for reaching the highest classification performances, and typically present solutions that do not make any use of specific language resources.

Furthermore, Part-of-speech tagging could be viewed as a classification problem, which merits the exploration of methods that are successful in solving similar types of problems. The method of choice in this work is the use of artificial neural networks using a purely contextual representation of words (Word2Vec) as a possible solution for part-of-speech tagging [1]. Artificial neural networks also allow the concept of deep learning, meaning they can create highly abstract representations of the data with the addition of more hidden layers. These networks should be able to excel in part-of-speech tagging without the drawbacks listed above. For example, no handcrafted features would be required; those features will be automatically discovered by the network. The network itself will not be language dependent, although the model will have to be trained on the new language, but no part of the code will have to be changed for it to be successful. One drawback of this method is that training the model would

© Springer Nature Switzerland AG 2019
M. Ezziyyani (Ed.): AI2SD 2018, AISC 915, pp. 955–965, 2019.
https://doi.org/10.1007/978-3-030-11928-7_86

require a huge amount of text, where each word is marked with their corresponding part-of-speech tag by experts. These data sets are very expensive to produce, which poses a problem for languages that are used only by a small amount of people, such as Amazigh language.

The methods exploiting the theory of deep neural network or deep learning have proved their robustness on complex tasks of the fields of the imagery and the acoustic treatment [2]. In this study, still work-in-progress, we set-up a PoS-tagger for Amazigh able to gather the highest classification performances by using Amazigh language resource and Deep Neural Network/Convolutional Neural Network (DNN/CNN).

To the best of our knowledge, this work is the first of its type to comprehensively cover the deep learning methods in Amazigh PoS Tagging research today.

The structure of the paper is as follows: Sect. 2 presents NLP and POS Tagging in Amazigh language. Section 3 describes a linguistic background. Section 4 is devoted to our approach for Amazigh POS Tagging using neural networks and word embedding. The conclusions are given in Sect. 5.

2   NLP and Amazigh POS Tagging

Part-of-speech (POS) tagging is the process of assigning to each word in a sentence.

Natural language processing (NLP) is a subfield within the broader field of language technology. NLP is mainly interested in the interaction between computers and natural language [3]. This relates NLP to several other disciplines within the field of cognitive science, such as artificial intelligence, linguistics and computer science.

Within the context of NLP the task of part-of -speech (POS) tagging focuses on the automation of POS tagging. This is done with various techniques, such as handcrafted features, Bayesian statistics and various machine-learning approaches [4]. Since natural language is extremely flexible and dynamic words usually have different meanings in different contexts, the context is included by tagging words where the naturally occur, in sentences. The tagging process itself is performed by the system being provided with a sentence and the assignment to tag each word in a sentence with the correct POS tag (e.g. noun, verb...). To be able to assess whether the assigned tag is correct or not, it is required to have pre-tagged data that is tagged by human experts. To a human this might not seem as a difficult task to perform, but the vast amount of ambiguous words that exists in natural languages makes this a difficult task for a computer.

For this work, we focus on Amazigh POS tagging, Amazigh is a difficult morphological language; it uses different dialects in its standardization (Tassousiyt, Tarifiyt and Tamazight the three used in Morocco).

Amazigh, like most of the languages which have only recently started being investigated for NLP, still suffers from the scarcity of language processing tools and resources. In this sense, Amazigh language presents interesting challenges for NLP researchers.

Furthermore, Amazigh word segmentation and part-of-speech tagging tasks can be formulated as assigning labels to characters of an input sentence. The performance of the traditional tagging approaches is heavily dependent on the choice of features, for example, Hidden Markov Models (HMMs), often with a set of feature templates [5].

For that reason, much of the effort in designing such systems goes into the feature engineering, which is important but labor-intensive, mainly based on human ingenuity and linguistic intuition.

The previous works of POS tagging can be divided into three categories; rule based tagging [6], statistical tagging and hybrid tagging [7, 8]. A set of hand written rules are applied along with it the contextual information is used to assign POS tags to words in the rule based POS. The disadvantage of this system is that it doesn't work when the text is not known.

In the literature, many machine learning methods have been successfully applied for POS tagging, namely: the Hidden Markov Models (HMMs) [9], the transformation-based error driven system [10], the decision trees [11], the maximum entropy model [12], SVMs [13], CRFs [14]. Results produced by statistical taggers obtain about 95–97% of correctly tagged words.

3   Linguistic Background

3.1   Amazigh Language

Amazighe language belongs to the Hamito-Semitic/"Afro-Asiatic" languages, with rich morphology [15]. In linguistic terms, the language is characterized by the proliferation of dialects due to historical, geographical and sociolinguistic factors. It is spoken in Morocco, Algeria, Tunisia, Libya, and Siwa (an Egyptian Oasis); it is also spoken by many other communities in parts of Niger and Mali.

Amazighe is used by tens of millions of people in North Africa mainly for oral communication and has been introduced in mass media and in the educational system in collaboration with several ministries in Morocco. In Morocco Amazigh language uses different dialects in its standardization (Tachelhit, Tarifit and Tamazight).

Amazigh NLP presents many challenges for researchers. Its major features are:

- It has its own script: the Tifinagh, which is written from left to right.
- It does not contain uppercase.
- Like other natural language, Amazigh presents for NLP ambiguities in grammar classes, named entities, meaning, etc. For example, grammatically; the word (illi) depending on the context can mean a noun in this sentence (tfulki illi: my daughter is beautiful) or a verb in this sentence (ur illi walou: there is nothing).
- As most languages whose research in NLP is new, Amazigh is not endowed with linguistic resources and NLP tools.
- Amazigh, like most of the languages which have only recently started being investigated for NLP, still suffers from the scarcity of language processing tools and resources.

3.2   Amazigh Script

Like any language that passes through oral to written mode, Amazigh language has been in need of a graphic system. In Morocco, the choice ultimately fell on Tifi-naghefor technical, historical and symbolic reasons. Since the Royal declaration on

2003, Tifinaghe has become the official graphic system for writing Amazigh. Thus, IRCAM has developed an alphabet system called Tifinaghe-IRCAM. This alphabet is based on a graphic system towards phonological tendency. This system does not retain all the phonetic realizations produced, but only those that are functional. It is written from left to right and contains 33 graphemes which correspond to:

- 27 consonants including: the labials (ⵝ, ⴱ, ⵛ),dentals (ⵜ, ⵏ, ⴹ, ⴻ, ⵉ, ⵓ, ⵇ, ⵀ), the alveolars (ⵣ,ⵥ, ⵚ, ⵤ), the palatals (ⵛ, ⵊ), the velar (ⴽ, ⵅ), the labiovelars (ⴽ ˮ, ⵅ ˮ), the uvulars (ⵇ, ⵅ, ⵯ), the pharyngeals (ⵄ, ⵃ) and the laryngeal (ⵁ);
- 2 semi-consonants: ⵢ and ⵡ;
- 4 vowels: three full vowels ⵄ, ⵅ, ⵙ and neutral vowel (or schwa) ⵉ.

3.3 Amazigh Morphological Properties

Language morphology is knowledge of the ways in which the language's words can have different surface representations. Hence, the Amazigh morphology is considered rich and complex in terms of its inflections involving infixation, prefixation and suffixation. The Amazigh morphology covers five main lexical categories, which are noun, verb, adverb, pronoun, and preposition [16].

- Noun is a lexical unit, formed from a root and a pattern. It could occur in a simple form ('izm' the lion), compound form ('ighsdis'the rib), or derived one ('amkraz' the labourer). This unit varies in gender (masculine, feminine), number (singular, plural) and case (free case, construct case).
- Verb has two forms: basic and derived forms. The basic form is composed of a root and a radical, while the derived one is based on the combination of a basic form and prefixes. Whether basic or derived, the verb is conjugated in four aspects: aorist, imperfective, perfect, and negative perfect.
- Particle is a function word that is not assignable to noun neither to verb. It contains pronouns, conjunctions, prepositions, aspectual, orientation and negative particles, adverbs, and subordinates. Generally, particles are uninflected words. However in Amazigh, some of these particles are flectional, such as the possessive and demonstrative pronouns (Table 1).

3.4 POS Tagging Challenges

There are two challenges that we need to tackle to be able to predict part-of-speech tags. Some words can have different labels depending on their role in the sentence. For instance, "illi" in Amazigh is used as a verb (exist) (base form VB and present form VBP) and a as noun (NN) (daughter). The second problem is unseen words for which we don't know in advance their tags. For instance number are given the CD tag. But there is an infinity of numbers which are not in the training data.

Our classifier will have to learn to deal with both problems. In HMM taggers, this is generally handled by estimating the probability for a word to have a given tag (to help with the ambiguity problem) and the probability for a tag to be followed by another tag

Table 1. Amazigh tagset

N	TAG	Designation
1	NN	Common noun
2	NNK	Kinship noun
3	NNP	Proper noun
4	VB	Verb, base form
5	VBP	Verb, participle
6	ADJ	Adjective
7	ADV	Adverb
8	C	Conjunction
9	DT	Determiner
10	FOC	Focalizer
11	IN	Interjection
12	NEG	Particle, negative
13	VOC	Vocative
14	PRED	Particle, predicate
15	PROR	Particle, orientation
16	PRPR	Particle, preverbal
17	PROT	Particle, other
18	PDEM	Demonstrative pronoun
19	PP	Personal pronoun
20	PPOS	Possessive pronoun
21	INT	Interrogative
22	REL	Relative
23	S	Preposition
24	FW	Foreign word
25	NUM	Numeral
26	DATE	Date
27	ROT	Residual,other
28	PUNC	Punctuation

(to help with generalization on unseen words). We can do similarly by defining a feature for the current word and the associated tag, and a feature for the current tag given the previous tag.

4 Our Approaches

Deep learning is a new area of machine learning research since 2006 [17]. Deep learning is a set of machine learning algorithms which attempt to learn multiple-layered models of inputs, commonly neural networks. The deep neural networks are composed of multiple levels of non-linear operations (Fig. 1). Searching the parameter space of deep architectures is a nontrivial task, but recently deep learning algorithms have been proposed to resolve this problem with notable success, beating the state-of-the-art in certain areas [18].

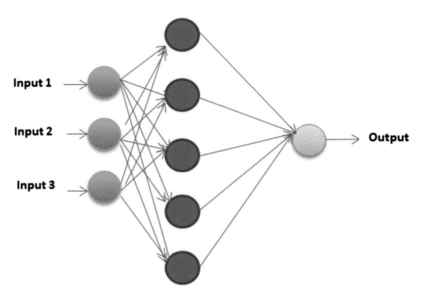

Fig. 1. The generic architecture of neural deep learning

During the past several years, the deep learning techniques have already been impacting a wide range of machine learning and artificial intelligence. It is thought that moving machine learning closer to one of its original goals: Artificial Intelligence. It has been successfully applied to several fields such as images, sounds, text and motion. The rapid increase in scientific activity on deep learning has been motivated by the empirical successes both in academia and in industry.

In this section we describe the approaches that we have adopted for Amazigh POS tagging, we propose two kinds of approaches: one by using CNN and another one by using DNN. The aim of this work is to evaluate how well deep learning algorithms, such as CNN and DNN, work for POS tagging taking in input a raw Amazigh texts. The data have been collected from different sources and different topics. We have extracted 80% for the definition of the training set and the 20% for the testing set. The TD has been used to train both the deep neural network (DNN) and convolutional neural network (CNN).

4.1   Word Embeddings

Word embeddings essentially follow the distributional hypothesis, according to which words with similar meanings tend to occur in similar context. Thus, these vectors try to capture the features of the context of a word. The main advantage of distributional vectors is that they capture similarity between words. Measuring similarity between vectors is possible, using measures such as cosine similarity. Word embeddings are often used as the first data processing layer in a deep learning model. Typically, word-embeddings are pre-trained by optimizing an auxiliary objective in a large unlabeled corpus, such as predicting a word based on its context [19], where the learnt word vectors can capture general morpho-syntactical information. Thus, these embeddings have proven to be efficient in capturing context similarity, analogies and due to its smaller dimensionality, are fast and efficient in computing core NLP tasks. Over the years, the models that create such embeddings have been shallow neural networks and there has not been need for deep networks to create good embeddings. However, deep learning based NLP models invariably represent their words, phrases and even sentences using these embeddings.

4.2 Deep Neural Network

Robust methods to extract morphological information from words must take into consideration all characters of the word and select which features are more important for the task at hand. For instance, in the POS tagging task, informative features may appear in the beginning (like the prefix "am" in "amkraz"), in the middle (like the hyphen in "ighs-diss" and the "h" in "10h30"), or at the end (like suffix "awn" in "izmawn"). In order to tackle this problem we propose a DNN approach. Our approach produces local features around each character of the word and then combines them using a max operation to create a fixed-sized character-level embedding of the word.

Moreover, the first step is to define a suitable training dataset (TD) from the training set for the DNN. In our scenario the TD is composed of a set of vector of features fi extracted from a temporal windows wi, with i = 1...N. The selected features are described. For each features we have assigned the correct grammatical class: {Verb (VB), Noun (NN), Adjective (ADJ), ...}.

Figure 2 shows a piece of the training dataset that we have created. Each line is a vector of features fi. The second step is the building of the DNN. Basically, a generic neural network is formed in three layers, called the input layer, hidden layer, and output layer. Each layer consists of one or more nodes, represented in this diagram by the small circle. The nodes of the input layer receive a single value on their input and duplicate the value to their output. The hidden layers are in charge to get the data and analyzed them and provide results to the next layer.

The output layers show the results of the learning process (e.g. a prediction/classification). In our paper, the numbers of the nodes of the output layers are 28 (the Amazigh tagset). The size of the input layer is equal to the size of the features vectors. The number of the units of each hidden layer and the number of the hidden layers are two hyper parameters that we have considered for the tuning of the DNN. In order to find the best hyper-parameters setting, we plan in the next step to perform a set of experiments changing the values of the hyper-parameters, and to test the number of hidden layer in a range from 2 to 4 layers.

For each layer in a range from 5 to 20 units. The configuration that given the best performance in terms of accuracy was with 2 hidden layers with 10 units for each layer. Other configurations with a higher numbers of both layers and units have produced the same results of the selected one.

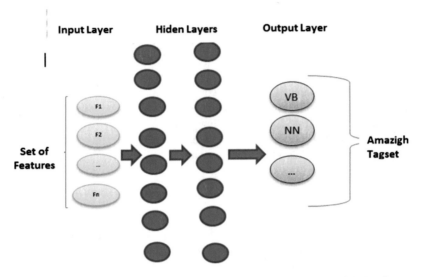

Fig. 2. Deep Neural network architecture proposed for Amazigh POS Tagging

4.3 Convolutional Neural Network

In this section, we describe the second proposed approach based on CNN structure, which is formed on tree basic type of layers: convolutional layers (CL), polling (P) and fully-connected (FC) layers [20]. The convolutional layers are in charge to perform the features extraction stage. Each input of the unit in this layer is connected to a local receptive file of the previous one. The pooling layers perform the features reducing from the results of the previous CL. The fully-connected layer finally takes all output/neurons in the previous layer and connects it to every single neuron it has as in a classic neural network, an overall view of the generic structure of a CNN is shown in Fig. 3. In this approach we have chosen as pooling function the max-pool, in other words, for each temporal window, the network considers only the point with max values from the output of the CL. The hyper-parameters take in account for this strategy are:

Learning rate
Number of Convolutional Layers
Number of the units of Convolutional Layers
Number of the Fully-connected Layers
Dropout

The Learning rate is a training parameter that controls the size of the steps of the changes during the learning process.

Generic Structure of a Convolutional Neural Network training algorithm (e.g. Stochastic Gradient Descent) [15]. The Dropout is a regularization technique for reducing over-fitting in neural networks by preventing complex coadaptations on training data. In order to find the best configuration for the hyper-parameters of the

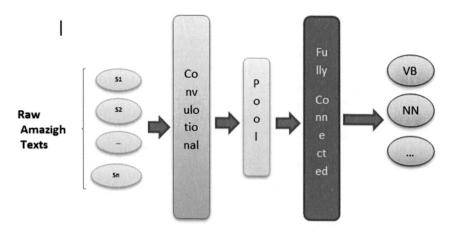

Fig. 3. The proposed architecture of CNN approach

CNN, we plan to perform a set of experiments by combining them and changing their values. The range of the values is:

Learning rate = {0.01, 0.001, 0.0001}
Number of Convolutional Layers = {1, 2, 3}
Number of the units of Convolutional Layers = {1, 2, 3}
Number of the Fully-connected Layers = {1, 2, 3}
Dropout {YES, NO} The deeper configuration of our network reach a number of levels composed of 3 level of CL, 3 levels of FC and 1 level of dropout, for an amount of 7 levels.

4.4 The Comparison Between CNN and DNN Approaches

DNNs are typically designed as Feedforward Networks. However, research has applied Recurrent Neural Networks very successfully, for other applications like language modeling. On the other hand, the Convolutional Deep Neural Networks (CNNs) are used in computer vision and automatic speech recognition where their success is well-documented and accepted.

Therefore, it is important to highlight a different between DNN and CNN about how they have been trained. In CNN approach we have not proposed the TD defined for the DNN, instead, we have proposed the raw data of the training set for the training of the CNN. The reason of that is because we want to use one of the most important properties of the CNN, the capability of finding local connections between data [21]. We have applied the same procedure for the setting the number of output of the FC layers with a number of inputs of the first layer set to 1028 neurons. After the training of the networks, we have chosen the test set for the evaluation of the performance of the two algorithms. For the DNN we have proposed to create a set of vector features from a temporal window extracted from the test set, for the CNN they have used directly the data of the test set.

5   Conclusion and Perspectives

In this paper, we have studied two famous approaches for the application of Deep Learning for the Amazigh POS Tagging: Deep Neural Network and Convolution Neural Network. We have collected an Amazigh corpus of 60,000 tokens and we have created a data set for both training and testing process.

The preliminary results of this study look like shown that CNN performs a better evaluation for the classification of grammatical classes in Amazigh text.

As future, we have several issues to face such as:—increasing the size of our corpus —evaluating training dataset by changing type of features—evaluating the application of the recurrent neural network—incorporating some common techniques, such as cascading, voting, and ensemble—introducing specific linguistic features that are helpful for the tasks.

References

1. Goldberg, Y., Levy, O.: Word2vec explained: Deriving Mikilov et al.'s negative-sampling word embedding metod. arXiv preprint arXiv:1402.3722 (2014)
2. Collobert, R., Weston, J., Bottou, L., Karlen, M., Kavukcuoglu, K., Kuksa, P.: Natural language processing (almost) from scratch. J. Mach. Learn. Res. 12, 2493–2537 (2011)
3. Manning, C.D.: Part-of-speech tagging from 97% to 100%: Is it time for some linguistics? In: Proceedings of the 12th International Conference on Computational Linguistics and Intelligent Text Processing, CICLing'11, pp. 171–189 (2011)
4. Bengio, Y.: Practical recommendations for gradient based training of deep architectures. In: Montavon, G., Orr, G.B., Müller, KR. (eds.) Neural Networks: Tricks of the Trade, volume 7700 of Lecture Notes in Computer Science, pp. 437–478. Springer Berlin Heidelberg, (2012) ISBN 978-3- 642-35288-1
5. Collobert, R., Weston, J., Bottou, L., Karlen, M., Kavukcuoglu, K., Kuksa, P.: Natural language processing (almost) from scratch. J. Mach. Learn. Res. 12, 2493–2537 (2011)
6. Martin, J.H, Jurafsky, D.: Speech and Language Processing, International Edition (2010)
7. Van Guilder, L.: Automated Part of Speech Tagging: A Brief Overview. Handout for LING361, Georgetown University, (1995)
8. Nakagawa, T., Uchimoto, K.: A hybrid approach to word segmentation and pos tagging. In: The 45th Annual Meeting of the ACL on Interactive Poster and Demonstration Sessions, pp 217–220
9. Charniak, E.: Statistical Language Learning. MIT Press, Cambridge (1993)
10. Brill, E.: Transformation-Based Error-Driven Learning and Natural Language Processing: A Case Study in Part-of-Speech Tagging (1995)
11. Schmid, H.: Improvements in Part-of-speech tagging with an application to German. In: Proceedings of the ACL SIGDAT-Workshop, pp. 13–26. Academic Publishers, Dordrecht (1999)
12. Ratnaparkhi, A.: A Maximum entropy model for part-of-speech tagging. In: Proceedings of EMNLP, Philadelphia, USA (1996)
13. Kudo, T., Matsumoto, Y.: Use of Support Vector Learning for Chunk Identification (2000)
14. Lafferty, J., McCallum, A., Pereira, F.: Conditional random fields: probabilistic models for segmenting and labeling sequence data. In: Proceedings of ICML 2001, pp. 282–289 (2001)

15. Dahl, G.E., Yu, D., et al.: Context-dependent pre-trained deep neural networks for large vocabulary speech recognition. IEEE Trans. Audio Speech Lang. Process. 20(1):30–42 (2012)

16. Boukhris, F., Boumalk, A., Elmoujahid, E., Souifi, H.: La nouvelle grammaire de l'amazighe. Rabat, Maroc: IRCAM, (2008)

17. Yoshua, B.: Representation learning: a review and new perspectives. IEEE Trans. Pattern Anal. Mach. Intell. 35(8):1798–1828 (2013)

18. Bengio, Y.: Learning Deep Architectures for AI. Found. Trends Mach. Learn. 2(1), 1–127 (2009)

19. Mikolov, T., Chen, K., Corrado, G., Dean, J.: Efficient Estimation of Word Representations in Vector Space. arXiv preprint arXiv:1301.3781 (2013)

20. Collobert, R., Weston, J., et al.: Natural language processing (almost) from scratch. J. Mach. Learn. Res. 12 2493–2537 (2011)

21. Mikolov, T., Deoras, A., et al.: Empirical evaluation and combination of advanced language modeling techniques. INTERSPEECH (2011)

22. Chafiq, M.: [Forty four lessons in Amazigh]. éd. Arabo-africaines (1991)

23. Chaker, S.: Textes en linguistique berbère -introduction au domaine berbère, éditions du CNRS, pp 232–242 (1984)

A Comparative Study of RF MEMS Switch Test Methods

H. Baghdadi[1]([⊠]), M. Lamhamdi[1], K. Rhofir[1], and S. Baghdadi[2]

[1] ISERT Laboratory, National School of Applied Sciences, Hassan 1st
University, Settat, Morocco
h.baghdadi@uhp.ac.ma
[2] IPOSI Laboratory, National School of Applied Sciences, Hassan 1st
University, Settat, Morocco

Abstract. Micro-ElectroMechanical Systems, often abbreviated as MEMS are miniaturized elements, multiplied components and microelectronics that can capture and act on the environment in order to perform a number of missions. They have a small size, limited energy capacity and low memory capacity. MEMS applications exceed the scaling limits of current computational paradigms, posing serious challenges and new opportunities for information technology. The heart of the MEMS switches is a moving electrode that, by contacting a fixed electrode, creates modifications in an RF circuit. The movable electrode is often formed of a suspended beam exerting movement. Another form of the moving electrode is a thin disk suspended above the electrode system disposed on the substrate. The movement of the moving electrode is generated by an actuating force that is often electrostatic, but it can be thermal, piezoelectric, or magnetic. The purpose of the test is to discriminate between the good devices that respect its specifications and the faulty ones that are not functional. In general, the failures occur due to deviations in the parameters of the manufacturing process or the presence of manufacturing defects. This problem cannot be solved by a single method, but requires several complementary techniques. This paper will present a comparison between the test techniques of RF MEMS Switches. Thus, the proposed method is based on machine learning to create predictive models for testing devices. This reliable test strategy helps to overcome the necessity of sophisticated test equipment, as well as the access difficulties to measure embedded points.

Keywords: RF MEMS · Switch · Test · Reliability

1 Introduction

The semiconductor industry has now reached the integration of hundreds of millions of transistors into a single chip. In the field of telecommunications, these chips integrate digital blocks, analog and mixed blocks, and RF[1] blocks.

Numerous researches are underway in the field of design for testing and MEMS production testing. In general, a device fails when it does not correspond to its

---

[1] Radio Frequency.

© Springer Nature Switzerland AG 2019
M. Ezziyani (Ed.): AI2SD 2018, AISC 915, pp. 966–975, 2019.
https://doi.org/10.1007/978-3-030-11928-7_87

specifications. A defect is a bad construction at one of the parts of the circuit. Modeling the faulty behavior of a circuit is called a fault. In analog circuits and devices (mixed, RF, MEMS) we distinguish two major classes of faults:

- Parametric fault: the variation of a physical or geometrical parameter of the device under test, which causes the violation of at least one of the specifications of this device.
- Catastrophic fault: abrupt or wide variation of a parameter (for example, the breakage of a suspended part after or during manufacture).

In order to establish a list of faults, it is necessary to study the defects that engender them. Thus, the manufacturing technology must be taken into consideration. From a list of all possible faults, we can start looking for the test technique that can detect these faults. During fault simulation, faults are injected into the device and test techniques are checked and evaluated. Therefore, an ideal test technique must pass all faultless circuits and specifications (good devices) and must reject any faulty and out-of-specification devices (bad devices).

The testing of analog and mixed components is particularly difficult for many reasons:

- Stimulus generation/response analysis in the analog domain
- Lack of models of faults
- Failure modes are numerous and difficult to model
- Considering the tolerances and the noise of the circuit

This paper explores firstly an overview of the main topic of microelectromechanical systems (MEMS) in Sect. 2 and a look at the different methods used to test the MEMS devices in Sect. 3. Section 4 describes the alternative strategy, outlines the machine learning techniques and ends with a description of the proposed method for testing RF MEMS Switches. Finally, Sect. 5 draws conclusions and any future work that will be pursued following this research.

2 Mems

The origin and the heart of the explosion of the electronics industry is, of course, microelectronics which categorically depend on computation. In fact, MEMS change our daily lives. Yet, there are various computational tools and techniques that lie behind.

The key to success for the MEMS is the possibility of bringing electronics and mechanics closer. These microsystems are made using the fabrication techniques and materials of microelectronics (MEMS technologies). Indeed, the MEMS are characterized by a reduction of the scale which modifies the ratio of the forces existing in the macro-monde, a collective fabrication (thus, it possible to fabricate ten thousand or a million MEMS components as easily and quickly as one and to reduce unit costs), and a very large use of the resonant structures. These three characteristics: miniaturization, multiplicity and microelectronics were the reasons laying behind the success of the MEMS.

MEMS systems have thousands of integrated sensors, actuators, and computers to sense the physical world and act upon it, as illustrated by the example in Fig. 1. So, we must compute and communicate distributed devices in order to work together effectively on global goals, while keeping interaction and adaptation to the environment in real time. This coupling to the physical world (such as fluid flow, pressure, light, inertia) is one of the things that makes MEMS systems different because the differential equations built by the physical world emerge in our computer programs. In essence, the challenge presented by MEMS on information technology is not only to coordinate sets of tiny computers, but rather to add a bit of computational behavior to materials and the environment.

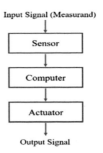

Fig. 1. The distributed MEMS approach consists integrated sense–act–compute modules

– Measurand is the quantity being measurand by sensor.
– Sensor is a device that converts a non-electrical quantity into an electrical signal.
– Actuator is a device that converts an electrical signal into a non-electrical quantity.
– Computer is a device that performs a set of logical or mathematical operations.

In fact, from a computer point of view, coupling computing with the physical world might not seem new or terribly difficult at first glance. Still significant computational challenges come out.

A radio frequency microelectromechanical system (RF MEMS) is a microelectromechanical systems with electronic components comprising moving sub-millimeter-sized parts that provide radio frequency functionality (see Fig. 2). More details of these components are given in [1, 2].

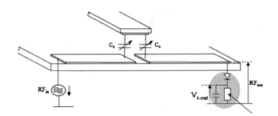

Fig. 2. RF MEMS with capacitive contact [3]

3   MEMS Test Methods

In general, depending on the manufacturing steps, a device must pass different types of tests described in Table 1.

Table 1. Test Types

Test types	Description
Validation test	The test is performed after device design to verify the design and define the required specifications. The step builds a list of faults for the simulation of faulty behaviors
Characterization test	If in general the first samples or prototypes do not satisfy the specifications, the design must be redone
Wafer test	The test is performed at the Wafer level in order to avoid the encapsulation of defective chips and thus reducing the production costs
Test after packaging	The chips are encapsulated in order to avoid environmental influences and clashes
Test after integrating the devices	Testing the system before being marketed
Test during the operation	During the operation, it is possible to perform tests in the chip like the integrated Self-Test (BIST)

Built-In Self-Test

The main test types of a microsystem are the functional test and the structural test during production. The other tests are mainly the reliability test and the packaging test. Structural testing is the process of analyzing and controlling the devices for errors due to manufacturing processes or errors due to the characteristics of the materials used.

3.1   Functional Test

The purpose of the functional test is to check all the specifications described in the user requirements of the device. During the test, we applied test vectors to the inputs and examined the responses on the outputs in order to obtain the device performances. If any performance is out of specification, the device is faulty (see Fig. 3). For analog and mixed circuits, the functional test is the most favored because it is difficult to have adequate fault models and fault simulation tools. For digital circuits, it appears that it is almost impossible to check the functionality of a chip. For example, a circuit having n inputs can have 2^n combinations of the test vectors. For this reason, structural tests are used in electronic circuits to reduce the amount of test vectors.

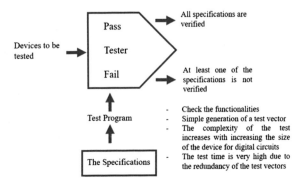

Fig. 3. Functional test principle

3.2   Structural Test

The purpose of the structural test is to detect if the devices have defects. These defects may be originated during manufacture or during the operation. To detect these faults, the structural test generates the test vectors using a predefined list of faults (see Fig. 4). This requires a detailed knowledge of faults and fault mechanisms in order to build fault models that allow us to simulate bad circuit behavior. So, this simulation will be used to generate the set of necessary test vectors. The structural test is widely used for testing digital circuits. In general, structural tests are more difficult to generate than functional tests, but they make it possible to use an optimal set of test vectors. This effectively reduces the time and cost of the test.

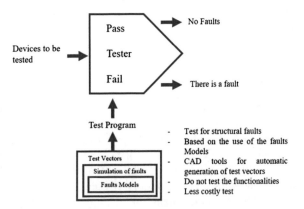

Fig. 4. Structural test principle

3.3   Alternative Test

The purpose of the alternative test is to measure indirectly the performance of the system or analog, mixed and RF circuits. In this case, one will try to predict the performances values from a reduced set of test measurements realized at low cost. The alternative test constructs a non-linear correlation between a set of measurements and the performances defined in the user requirements. This technique requires the use of statistical regression methods (in particular, nonlinear multiple regression for the case of RF circuits). In general, we aim to use a single analog test vector that optimize the performances prediction. Thus, the alternative test can effectively replace the standard specifications test procedure by checking the performances of the circuit implicitly (see Fig. 5).

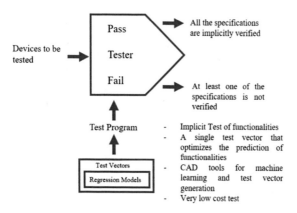

Fig. 5. Alternative test principle

4   Alternative Test

The traditional test of analog circuits is to check their functional specifications, which requires a complete evaluation of these specifications. This constraining operation makes the test very costly in terms of test time as well as consumption and resources. These traditional methods are particularly are not suitable to complex RF systems having functional specifications defined at very high frequencies.

Recently, many researches have proposed the replacement of the traditional specification test with other tests. The challenge of the alternative test is to avoid the complexity of direct measurements of the specified performances by building a non-linear interdependence relationship between low cost measurements and system performances. The use of the alternative test accelerates the test procedure by replacing the long and costly measurements of the specified performance with a direct non-linear relationship between the (less expensive) measurements space and the performances space.

4.1   Machine Learning Techniques

When we have a complex problem involving a lots variables and data without a formula or equation. To handle situations like these, we use machine learning techniques because the nature of the data keeps changing and thus the program needs to adapt. In fact, machine learning uses two types of techniques: supervised and unsupervised learning (see Fig. 6).

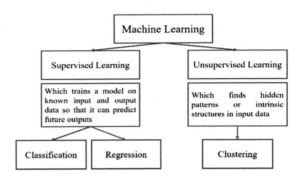

Fig. 6. Machine learning techniques include both unsupervised and supervised learning

We will focus on the supervised learning because we have known outputs that can predict future outputs.

4.2   Supervised Learning

We want to build a model that generate reasonable predictions for the response to new data. A supervised learning algorithm takes a known set of input data and known responses to the data (output) and trains a model. Indeed, classification method predicts discrete response and classifies input data into categories. Although, Regression techniques predict continuous responses. Indeed, to develop predictive models, supervised learning uses classification and regression techniques (see Fig. 7).

4.3   Alternative Test for RF MEMS Switch

The production test of RF integrated circuits requires very sophisticated and expensive ATE[2]. In addition, measuring RF performance also consumes a lot of test time. In [3], the proposed RF MEMS Switch is performed using low frequency measurements, eliminating the need to use a very expensive RF ATE (see Fig. 8).

Estimation of S-Parameters. One of the very first presentations of the alternative test is made by Variyam and Chatterjee in [4]. From an initial series of linearly independent measurements, the proposed method generates a new series of data to decide if the analog circuit under test checks all its specifications or not. The proposed method requires the construction of a non-linear function to project the space of accessible measurements into the specified performance space. A regression algorithm of the MARS[3] type is used for this purpose.

---

[2] Automatic Test Equipment.
[3] Multivariate Adaptive Regression Splines.

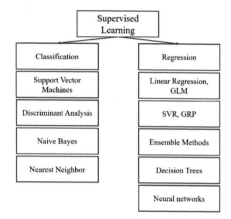

Fig. 7. Supervised learning techniques

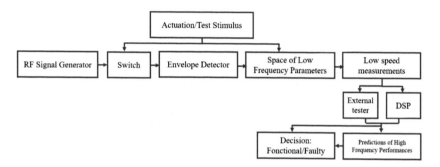

Fig. 8. Schematic diagram of the proposed method

In order to improve the accuracy of the circuit performances prediction, Voorakaranam and al. present in [5] an algorithm for generating the test stimulus and selecting the appropriate measurements to promote the (non-linear) correlation between functional performances and accessible measurements. This method generates a single test stimulus constructed to minimize the prediction error. To simplify the optimization procedure, the test generation is first performed using a simple linear model. The non-linear model is needed only during the final step of the algorithm, in order to refine the accuracy of the final prediction. In [3], the proposed method combines Monte Carlo simulation with a nonlinear regression algorithm to generate functions (see Fig. 9).

- Step 1: Generation of a set of 1000 switches by Monte Carlo simulation (Gaussian distribution on each physical parameter).
- Step 2: Calculation of low frequency characteristics and high frequency performance for each of the 1000 switches.
- Step 3: Identification and elimination of switches that do not work (with trivially detectable catastrophic faults).

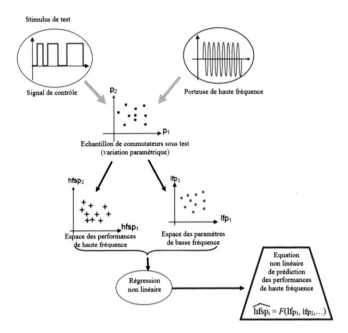

Fig. 9. Estimation of S-Parameters [3]

- Step 4: Divide the rest of the functional switches into two subsets: the first subset for learning and the second set for validation.
- Step 5: Generation of the regressive models from the learning subset.
- Step 6: Determination and choice of the best regression model in the sense of LSM.[4]
- Step 7: Applying the best regression model over the entire validation, and calculating the residual variance.

5 Conclusion and Perspectives

We have briefly described the testing of analog devices. Then, we focused on the MEMS test in general, and the RF MEMS switch test in particular. A bibliographic review of the testing techniques of these devices has been carried out. The proposed method is based on machine learning to create predictive models for testing devices: access and load the data, preprocess the data, derive features using the preprocessed data, train models using the features derived in previous step, iterate to find the best model, and integrate the best-trained model into a production system.

Simulation Matlab/Simulink requires too long computing times, especially for the Monte Carlo statistical simulation. Thus, the simulation with other algorithms such as

---

[4] Least Square method.

Neural Networks seems to be reliable. Although, the envelope detector is an important element for monitoring the switch, allowing observation of the degradation of this before catastrophic behavior is triggered. However, the use of this detector alone at the output of the switch is insufficient to allow accurate prediction of performance. Thus, it is desirable to study other measurements that can be performed also at low frequency, at the input and at the output of the switch, allowing an improvement in the performance prediction.

Acknowledgements. The authors wish to acknowledge all the members of the scientific committee.

References

1. Tembo, S., El-Baz, D.: Distributed resolution of a trajectory optimization problem on a MEMS-based reconfigurable modular surface. In: 2014 IEEE International Parallel & Distributed Processing Symposium Workshops (IPDPSW), pp. 1591–1598 (2014)
2. Lucyszyn, S.: Review of radio frequency microelectromechanical systems technology. IEEE Proc. Sci. Meas. Technol. **151**(2), 93–103 (2004)
3. Nguyen, H.N.: Technique alternative de test pour les interrupteurs MEMS RF. Thèse du Laboratoire TIMA, Novembre 2009
4. Variyam P.N., Cherubal S., Chatterjee A.: Prediction of analog performance parameters using fast transienttesting. IEEE Trans. CAD Integr. Circ. Syst. **21**(3), 349–361 (2002)
5. Voorakaranam R., et al.: Production deployment of a fast-transient testing methodology for analog circuits: case study and results. In: International Test Conference (ITC'03), vol.1, pp. 1174–1181 (2003)

A Deep Learning Model for Intrusion Detection

Taha Ait Tchakoucht[(✉)] and Mostafa Ezziyyani

Faculty of Sciences and Techniques, Abdelmalek Essaâdi University, Tangier,
Morocco
{taha.ait,ezziyyani}@gmail.com

Abstract. Intrusion detection systems have the ability to analyze data and monitor traffic to detect malicious behaviors. Many research studies have been conducted to increase the performance of such systems in order to enforce security policy of information systems. In this paper we investigate the efficiency of deep neural networks in intrusion detection. We evaluate the performance of the proposed technique with respect to KDD'99 and NSL-KDD both in binary classification and multiclass classification. Furthermore, we compare the model to some of the recent state-of-the-art models. Experiments show that deep learning can efficiently detect intrusions, and compare very well with the existing techniques.

Keywords: Neural networks · Deep learning · Intrusion detection

1 Introduction

Confidentiality, integrity and availability (CIA) are the three fundamentals of information security. An intrusion is a malicious activity that affects the CIA by having access to an unauthorized computer resource, by altering or destructing data, or by interrupting a service. An intrusion detection system (IDS) corresponds then, to a set of tools, made to identify and prevent activities that threatens the CIA. In general, there are two major families of intrusion detection; Anomaly detection and Misuse detection. The misuse detection approach attempts to recognize attacks that follow intrusion patterns that have been recognized and reported by experts. Misuse detection systems are vulnerable to intruders who use new patterns of behavior or who mask their illegal behavior to deceive the detection system. Anomaly detection methods were developed to counter this problem. Anomaly detection is based on the behavior of the user and/or application; it is called user profile or behavior of an application. It was proposed by Anderson in 1980 and taken over by Denning in 1987. Anderson proposed to describe the user profile by a set of relevant measures modeling its behavior to detect subsequent deviation from the usual behavior already learned. Anomaly detection systems then seek to answer the question: "Is the current behavior of the user and/or application coherent with its past behavior?" (For more details on the various tools of the behavioral approach. An hybrid intrusion detection which combines both techniques in the same time can be added as a third approach of the IDS Often, these two approaches are based on Data-mining techniques. Data-mining Techniques is a set of techniques

© Springer Nature Switzerland AG 2019
M. Ezziyyani (Ed.): AI2SD 2018, AISC 915, pp. 976–983, 2019.
https://doi.org/10.1007/978-3-030-11928-7_88

for the extraction of motifs from large data sets, combining statistical and machine learning methods with database management. Those techniques involve learning association rules, cluster analysis, classification and regression. Applications include clients data mining to determine the segments that most likely respond to an offer, the mining of human resources data to identify the characteristics of employees who are more successful, or analysis of the market basket for modeling the purchasing behavior of clients.

Another criterion for differentiating IDSs is whether it is a Network-based IDS (NIDS) or Host-based IDS (HIDS). The objective of HIDS is to focus on a single machine while he NIDSs look at the packets that pass through the whole network to determine if an attack occurs. In Anomaly-based approach, they consist of establishing a network profile that separates between normal and abnormal activity. NIDSs are easy to install.

In this paper, we model a deep learning intrusion detection system based on artificial neural networks using Adam gradient descent as a training technique. The main contributions are:

(1) Using deep learning for intrusion detection.
(2) Adopting a deep learning architecture to model an anomaly-based intrusion detection system; we present the general scheme, we choose the best hyperparameters and assess the model on the datasets both in binary classification and multilabel classification.
(3) Evaluating the model w.r.t the performance metrics and comparing it with some of the existing techniques from the literature. The proposed model achieves a high performance and compares very well with the recent studies on the field

The remainder of this paper is organized as follows: Sect. 2 represents some studies related to the subject. Section 3 enumerates data preparation steps, and defines the performance metrics. In Sect. 4, experimental results and performance comparison are discussed. Finally, Sect. 5 describes conclusion and opens to some perspectives.

2   State of the Art

Many research studies have been proposed to advance the field of intrusion detection. They use machine learning techniques such as Support Vector Machine (SVM), Artificial Neural Networks (ANN), Decision Trees, Random Forest, Bayesian Networks, Ensemble techniques, etc.....

Most of the proposed techniques are assessed with KDDCup99 [6] and NSL-KDD [16] datasets.

2.1   NSL-KDD

Manekar and Waghmare [15] used SVM to design an intrusion detection system. Their model consist of leveraging Particle Swarm Optimization (PSO) to train the classifier and reducing the dimension of the problem. SVM is then used to classify different types of events. To speed up convergence and increase accuracy, Pervez and Md. Farid [17] used 36 features out of 41 from NSL-KDD as the feature set, and SVM as the detection approach. Extreme Learning Machine (ELM) is employed as a training technique for a single-hidden layer neural network (SLFN) [13]. Authors have also used Principal Components Analysis (PCA) to reduce the problem's dimension and set the best architecture. Ingre and Yadav [5] used BFGS quasi-Newton gradient descent to train an ANN intrusion classifier, and assessed their model both in binary and multiclass classification. In [11] Li et al. used Convolutional Neural Networks (CNN) to build an intrusion detection system, which consist of encoding data into an image from which features are extracted and fed to the CNN classifier.

2.2   KDD'99

Malik et al. [14] chose the best set of features using binary PSO, then applied Random Forest (RF) as a classifier to detect intrusions. Restricted Boltzmann Machine (RBM) was used by Alrawashdeh and Purdy [2] to create a Deep Belief Network (DBN). The method included logistic regression architecture and multiclass softmax classifier.

2.3   NSL-KDD and KDD'99

Recurrent Neural Networks (RNN) was recently widely explored in the field of intrusion detection. Yin et al. [20] proposed an IDS based on Neural Networks architecture. Authors used back-propagation through time (BPTT) as a technique for training an RNN classifier. Shone et al. [19] used stacked nonsymmetric deep autoencoder (S-NDAE) and DBN as deep learning model for intrusion detection. Ait Tchakoucht and Ezziyyani [1] designed an intrusion classifier for fast probe and DoS attacks detection. The technique consists of applying various features selection approaches using different wrappers and filters. The outcome is a reduced set of features for each type of attack.

3   Proposed Model

Machine learning applications have known a quantum leap after the introduction of deep learning by Professor Hinton in 2006 [9]. This paradigm has yielded great performance results in multiple research areas including but not limited to Computer Vision, Speech Recognition, Face Recognition, Translation, etc. The latter fact motivated this research study as promising results in the literature have been achieved.

In this study, we used multiple layers of fully connected neural networks to build an intrusion detection classifier. Input Data from both NSL-KDD and KDD'99 are preprocessed then fed to the network to perform a feed-forward propagation. A cross-entropy cost function is then computed and Adam Stochastic Gradient Descent [8] is used as an efficient backpropagation training method. The latter is optimized

and corresponding updated weights are used to test the model. The general architecture of the model is described in Fig. 1.

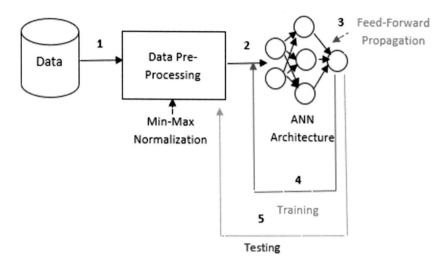

Fig. 1. The general architecture of the proposed model

3.1 Datasets Benchmarks

KDD'99 is a widely used intrusion detection data benchmark as it is the most cited dataset in the field. The data contains almost 4 GB of data, encompassing network traffic provided by DARPA [12] in tcpdump format, and converted by Lee et al. [10] into 5 million training instances and 2 million test instances. Data observations are represented as arrays of 41 features, each corresponding to normal activity or a specific attack. The data include 'kddcup.data_10_percent_corrected' and 'corrected' files as training and test sets respectively. There are 49,4021 instances in training set, with 97,278 normal instances, and 22 types of attacks for an overall of 396,744. Additional 14 types of attacks are present in the test set. All attacks are regrouped in four categories, namely, Probe, Dos R2L and U2R. In this study we used 49,402 training records ("10% KDD" file) and extracted 31,104 testing records from "Corrected KDD".

NSL-KDD is a dataset that is processed from the original KDD'99. It is created to solve some of the main problems in the KDD'99. The authors removed duplicate records from both train and test sets so that the most frequent records do not affect classification. Moreover, it is affordable to assess models on the complete dataset, since the number of records is reasonable as shown in Table 1. The benchmark is composed of *KDDTrain+* as the train set, and *KDDTest+* and *KDDTest-21* as the test sets. The latter is a subset of the former and is more difficult to classify. Additional attack patterns are included in the test sets to evaluate the ability to detect novel attacks. Each record is labeled as normal or intrusion based on 41 features.

For both KDD'99 and NSL-KDD, features are classified into 3 categories: Basic features (N°. 1–9) which contain all the attributes that can be extracted from a TCP/IP Connection. Content features category (N°. 10–22) allow to capture intrusion patterns that are embedded in the data (R2L and U2R). Traffic features category (N°. 23–41)

Table 1. Features of KDD'99 and NSL-KDD

N°—Feature	N°—Feature	N°—Feature
1—Duration	15—Su_attempted	29—Same_srv_rate
2—Protocol_type	16—Num_root	30—Diff_srv_rate
3—Service	17—Num_file_creations	31—Srv_diff_host_rate
4—Flag	18—Num_shells	32—Dst_host_count
5—Src_bytes	19—Num_access_files	33—Dst_host_srv_count
6—Dst_bytes	20—Num_outbound_cmds	34—Dst_host_same_srv_rate
7—Land	21—Is_hot_login	35—Dst_host_diff_srv_rate
8—Wrong_fragment	22—Is_guest_login	36—Dst_host_same_src_port_rate
9—Urgent	23—Count	37—Dst_host_srv_diff_host_rate
10—Hot	24—Srv_count	38—Dst_host_serror_rate
11—Num_failed_logins	25—Serror_rate	39—Dst_host_srv_serror_rate
12—Logged_in	26—Srv_serror_rate	40—Dst_host_rerror_rate
13—Num_compromised	27—Rerror_rate	41—Dst_host_srv_rerror_rate
14—Root_shell	28—Srv_rerror_rate	

incorporate features that are calculated with respect to a window interval. All features are numerical, except N°. 2, 3, 4, which are categorical. Table 1 show the features of both KDD'99 and NSL-KDD (for detailed description of feature subset, see [6]).

3.2 Pre-processing

Numericalization. Input data fed to Neural Networks must be numerical, therefore, categorical data such as *protocol_type*, *Service* and *Flag* are encoded into dummy values (binary). *protocol_type* counts 3 values, Service vary in an interval of 70 values, and Flag regroups 11 values. A set of 122 features are processed from the original 41 features.

Normalization. Features range in distinct intervals. *duration* varies in [0, 58,329], while *protocole_type* ranges in [13, 15]. This causes a very slow convergence. We then used the same normalization method as in [20]. The logarithmic scaling is first applied, so that for example we obtain a range of [0, 4.77] for *duration*. Then, the features are scaled to obtain values between 0 and 1, according to the following equation:

$$x_i = \frac{x_i - min}{max - min} \tag{1}$$

where x_i is the feature value at time i, *max* is the maximum value of feature x over all dataset's instances, and *min* is the minimum value of feature x over all dataset's instances.

4 Experiments and Discussion

We run the experiments on a PC i7 intel(R) 2.00, 2.6 GHz processor and 12 GB of RAM. We implemented the system using python programming language, taking benefit of some of its machine learning packages (Keras) [7]. The proposed model is evaluated both in binary classification and multilabel classification. The best results were obtained after 200 epochs. Parameters settings are described in Tables 2 and 3.

Table 2. Parameters settings for binary classification

Parameter	Value for KDD99	Value for NSL-KDD
Number of hidden layers	2	3
Number of hidden nodes	250	200
Activation function (hidden layers)	Sigmoid	Tanh
Activation function (output layer)	Softmax	Softmax
Optimizer	Adam	Adam
Cost function	Cross-entropy	Cross-entropy
Batch size	49,402	125,973

Table 3. Parameters settings for multiclass classification

Parameter	Value for KDD99	Value for NSL-KDD
Number of hidden layers	3	3
Number of hidden nodes	200	200
Activation function (hidden layers)	Relu	Relu
Activation function (output layer)	Softmax	Softmax
Optimizer	Adam	Adam
Cost function	Cross-entropy	Cross-entropy
Batch size	49,402	125,973

4.1 Binary Classification

To study the performance of the model in binary classification, we run the experiments using 122 input nodes for KDD'99 and NSL-KDD. We compare the system with the literature as indicated in Tables 4 and Table 5.

Table 4. Performance comparison in binary classification (KDD99, in %)

Model	Detection rate
2012—reduced-size RNN [18]	94.1
2015—CFA [3]	91.5
2017—RNN [20]	97.09
Proposed model	100

Table 5. Performance comparison in binary classification (NSL-KDD in %)

Model	Detection rate
2014—SVM-PSO [15]	82
2014—SVM [17]	82.37
2015—ANN [5]	81.2
Proposed model	92

4.2   Multiclass Classification

In the second part of the experiments, we used 122 input nodes and 5 output class labels to refers to normal behaviors and the four types of intrusions, Tables 6 and 7 compare the results with some of the state-of-the-art techniques evaluated in 5-class classification

Table 6. Detection rate in multiclass classification (KDD99, in %)

Model	Normal	DoS	Probe	R2L	U2R
2013—SVM [4]	98.73	96.38	58.34	16.35	21.43
2018—DBN [19]	99.49	99.65	14.19	89.25	7.14
2018—NDAE [19]	99.49	99.79	98.74	9.31	0
Proposed model	89	96	80	100	92

Table 7. Detection rate in multiclass classification (NSL-KDD, in %)

Model	Normal	DoS	Probe	R2L	U2R
2015—ANN [5]	–	77.7	76.6	34.4	10.5
2018—DBN [19]	95.64	87.96	72.97	0	0
2018—NDAE [19]	97.73	94.58	94.67	3.82	2.7
Proposed model	68	91	85	97	87

5   Conclusion and Perspectives

In this work we designed an intrusion detection system based on deep artificial Neural Networks trained with Adam Stochastic Gradient Descent. Multiple layers of neural network with a softmax activation function in the output layer provides an accurate intrusion detection. Performance evaluation show competitive results that outperforms some of the aforementioned state-of-the art models and compare with others some. In a future work we will address the problem of high speed networks, in which large amounts data are processed which raises the problem of scalability. Hence, the intrusion detection system should analyze data and perform classification in a very brief time. Moreover, false positive rate is to be reduced in order to increase the F-Score metric.

References

1. Ait Tchakoucht, T., Ezziyyani, M.: Building a fast intrusion detection system for high-speed-networks: probe and DoS attacks detection. Proc. Comput. Sci. **127**, 521–530 (2018)
2. Alrawashdeh, K., Purdy, C.: Toward an online anomaly intrusion detection system based on deep learning. In: Proceedings of 15th IEEE International Conference on Machicine Learning and Applications, pp. 195–200, Anaheim, CA, USA (2016)
3. Eesa, A.D., Orman, Z., Brifcani, A.M.A.: A novel feature selection approach based on the cuttlefish optimization algorithm for intrusion detection systems. Expert Syst. Appl. **42**(5), 2670–2679 (2014)
4. Hasan, Md.A.M., Nasser, M., Pal, B., Ahmad, S.: Intrusion detection using-combination of various kernels based support vector machine. Int. J. Sci. Eng. Res. **4**(9) (2013)
5. Ingre, B., Yadav, A.: Performance analysis of NSL-KDD dataset using ANN. In: International Conference on Signal Processing and Communication Engineering Systems, pp. 92–96 (2015)
6. KDD Cup 1999.: http://kdd.ics.uci.edu/databases/kddcup99/kddcup99.html. Last accessed Feb 2018
7. Keras.: The python deep learning library. https://keras.io/. Last accessed 3 Aug 2018
8. Kingma, D.P., Ba, J.L.: ADAM: a method for stochastic optimization. In: Proceedings of the 3rd International Conference on Learning Representations (ICLR 2015), Ithaca, NY, USA (2015)
9. LeCun, Y., Bengio, Y., Hinton, G.: Deep learning. Nature **521**(7553), 436–444 (2015)
10. Lee, W., Stolfo, W.: A framework for constructing features and models for intrusion detection systems. ACM Trans. Inf. Syst. Sec. **3**(4), 227–261 (2000)
11. Li, Z., Qin, Z., Huang, K., Yang, X., Ye, S.: Intrusion detection using convolutional neural networks for representation learning. In: Liu, D., Xie, S., Li, Y., Zhao, D., El-Alfy, E.S. (eds.) Lecture Notes in Computer Science 2017, vol. 10638, pp. 858–866 (2017)
12. Lippmann, R. P., D.Fried, Graf, I., Haines, J., Kendall, K., Mcclung, et al.: Evaluating intrusion detection systems: the 1998 DARPA off-line intrusion detection evaluation. In: Proceedings of the DARPA Information Survivability Conference and Exposition (DISCEX'00), pp. 12–26. IEEE Computer Society Press, Hilton Head (2000)
13. Liu, Q., Yin, J., Leung, V.C.M., Zhai, J.-H., Cai, Z., Lin, J.: Applying a new localized generalization error model to design neural networks trained with extreme learning machine. Neural Comput. Appl. **27**(1), 59–66 (2014)
14. Malik, A.J., Shahzad, W., Khan, F.A.: Network intrusion detection using hybrid binary PSO and random forests algorithm. Security Comm. Networks **8**(16), 2646–2660 (2012)
15. Manekar, V., Waghmare, K.: Intrusion detection system using support vector machine (SVM) and particle swarm optimization (PSO). Int. J. Adv. Comput. Res. **4**(16), 808–812 (2014)
16. NSL-KDD.: http://www.unb.ca/research/iscx/dataset/iscx-NSL-KDD-dataset.html. Last accessed Feb 2018
17. Pervez, M.S., Md. Farid, D.: Feature selection and intrusion classification in NSL-KDD Cup 99 dataset employing SVMs. In: Proceedings of 8th International Conference on Software, Knowledge, Information Management and Applications, Dhaka, Bangladesh, pp. 1–6 (2014)
18. Sheikhan, M., Jadidi, T., Farokhi, A.: Intrusion detection using reduced-size RNN based on feature grouping. Neural Comput. Appl. **21**(6), 1185–1190 (2012)
19. Shone, K., Ngoc, T.N., Phai, V.D., Shi, Q.: A deep learning approach to network intrusion detection. IEEE Trans. Emerg. Topics Comput. Intell. **2**(1), 41–50 (2018)
20. Yin, C., Zhu, Y., Fei, J., He, X.: A deep learning approach for intrusion detection using recurrent neural networks. IEEE Access **5**, 21954–21961 (2017)

Dynamic Adaptation and Automatic Execution of Services According to Ubiquitous Computing

Marwa Zaryouli[✉] and Mostafa Ezziyyani

LMA Laboratory, Faculty of Sciences and Techniques of Tangier, Abdelmalek Essaâdi University, Tétouan, Morocco
{zaryouli.marwa, ezziyyani}@gmail.com

Abstract. Many current devices have network connections that allow access to their functionality through a computer network, so ubiquitous applications aim to structure these features to put them to the users' services. Therefore, the behavior of ubiquitous applications depends on the state and availability of entities (software and devices) that make up the environment in which they evolve, the latter characterized by a dynamic availability of functionalities and a heterogeneity of hardware and software devices, and depends on user preferences and locations. In addition, these applications must adapt according to the context of the user. In this future article, we present an infrastructure dedicated to ubiquitous computing services. These services are in the form of assembly of distributed software components and dynamically discovered according to the location of the terminal and these characteristics. We have implemented this infrastructure, with an example of services to benchmark the performance of services in this environment.

Keywords: Ubiquitous computing · Context of the user · Distributed software components

1 Introduction

Ubiquitous computing is a new vision, in which several devices (sensors, processors, and actuators) included in different physical objects participate in a global information network. Indeed, mobility and dynamical configuration are the most important features of these systems, requiring permanent adaptation of applications. This raises several issues such as the heterogeneity of equipment with limited resources, application distribution, device mobility, security, dynamic discovery of services, and automatic deployment of the software on the user terminal.

In this paper, we will present ubiquitous contextual services consisting of assemblies of components distributed and dynamically discovered according to the location of the user's terminal and these characteristics, then automatically deployed on the terminal of the user.

Then we will propose a global approach based on software components for the design, the dynamic discovery, the automatic deployment and the execution of these services for the mobile users.

M. Ezziyyani (Ed.): AI2SD 2018, AISC 915, pp. 984–990, 2019.
https://doi.org/10.1007/978-3-030-11928-7_89

This article is organized as follows: Sect. 2 describes the problems to be solved in the context of ubiquitous computing using an example in the aeronautical field. Section 3 discusses related work. Section 4 describes the methodology chosen in our work. Section 5 details the component infrastructure for discovery, automatic deployment of contextual services, and Sect. 6 concludes our contribution.

2 Context

This section discusses issues related to ubiquitous applications through an illustrative example.

2.1 Contextual Service

With the help of a simple example in the field of aeronautics. A traveler with a WIFI digital assistant arrives at the airport to catch the plane, his PDA automatically detects the location and launches a service providing information about the terminal, flight schedules, terminal locations and the way to follow etc. This service can be designed with different user interfaces (Fig. 1).

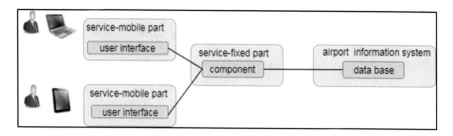

Fig. 1. User case of service

2.2 Problems to Solve

- The variety of equipment: the user can have a laptop, a PDA or a Smartphone. Indeed, all these devices operate with separate operating systems.
- Limited resources: the first problem encountered is the energy consumption of mobile equipment. Indeed smartphones and PDAs have a little memory and limited power.
- Distributed applications: the problem arises here because the communication between the two parties (fixed and mobile) is via a wireless network, so it is certainly necessary to use a communication middleware.
- Service discovery: First, you have to allow a user to discover all the available services according to the location, in order to deploy them according to the type of device that the user owns. Therefore, for this the system must have information on the characteristics of the terminal to present the user with suitable services that can run on his terminal.

– Deploying services: the infrastructure must be ready to deploy the code of any service on the user's terminal as needed by the user.

3 Related Work

There is a lot of research on infrastructure for ubiquitous computing. By limiting itself to CORBA-based infrastructure. The project AMPROS [1] studies and develops middleware for the mobile environment. This work is based on the OpenCCM [2] platform. A set of tools is developed to allow the adaptation of the applications to the execution.

The Appear Provisioning Server product [3] from Appear Networks is an infrastructure for discovery and deployment of services [4]. The product makes it possible to deploy applications or documents on mobile terminals when the users are in specific places. Applications are developed independently of the broadcast platform.

The broker OMG/ISO trader [5] and the trader RM-ODP [6] manage the publication and discover of services. Our SR component can be implemented using these technologies. JINI [7], developed by Sun Microsystems, offers different ways to discover services. The Multicast Request Protocol allows a user terminal to send multicast requests to find a server. The response is returned to the user terminal as a TCP message.

The work of [8] on the Satin model aims to provide component assemblies with safety properties.

All these works are complementary to our proposal.

4 Methodologies

In order to meet the above challenges, we have chosen to adapt the methodology to a component approach. Indeed, a service is composed of a set of distributed and interconnected software component assemblies. Here we have two types of assembly (fixed and mobile).

The fixed assembly represents the main part of a service: it is deployed on the fixed machines of the ubiquitous environment when the service is started up and is present as long as the service is available.

The mobile assembly represents the part of the service dedicated to a user: it is automatically deployed at the user's request and is automatically destroyed when the user leaves the contextual coverage area.

Each component has a set of configurable attributes and ports identifying the features offered or required by the component.

Indeed, we chose the CORBA [9] component model, which is dedicated to the design, development, packaging, assembly, deployment and execution of heterogeneous hardware components. Here we will use the four port types of the CORBA component model (facets, receptacles, sinks, and event sources).

- A facet and a receptacle expose an interface, a set of methods, respectively implanted or required by the component.
- A well and a source identify that a component can respectively consume or produce a certain type of event.
- The connection of a receptacle to a facet and a well on a source allows the implementation of respectively synchronous and asynchronous interactions between components (Fig. 2).

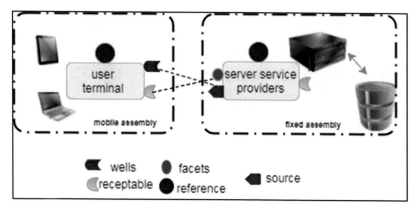

Fig. 2. Assembly of service components

5 Our Infrastructure

5.1 Dynamic Discovery of Services

Service discovery is a fundamental part of ubiquitous computing. The idea is to inform a user entering the specific area of the existence of services. To reveal this challenge, we will introduce a component called Service Registry, hosted on the fixed part of the ubiquitous environment (the server of the airport). This component has the role of managing the list of services (add, delete, modify...) and it transfers a unique identifier in order to distinguish the service providers. Another role of the Service Registry component is to calculate the mobile assembly of the service adapted to the terminal of the user according to the hardware and software capacity of the terminal, and then send the list of available services.

At the user's terminal, a component called Service Activator is started and listens to the credentials that Service Registry sends. With these credentials, the Service Activator component can query the Service Registry to know what services are available.

The Services Activator component also passes the hardware and software characteristics of the device to the selected Services Register. Finally, this component receives and displays the adapted services on the user's timeline.

This architecture allows the fixed server to host the Service Registry. Then once the terminal discovers the Service Register, the Service Activator issues a request and obtains the list of services adapted to the equipment. For this, a negotiation protocol has been defined between the service provider's server and the mobile terminal. After discovering the Service Register, the terminal characteristics are sent to the Service Register. This calculates the appropriate assemblies and sends a list to the terminal that contains only the appropriate contextual services (Fig. 3).

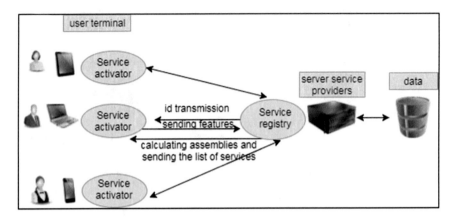

Fig. 3. Service discovery and negotiation protocol

5.2   Automatic Deployment and Execution

Once a user chooses a discovered service, the infrastructure will deploy the code on its terminal. This consists in downloading the components binaries from a repository to the terminal, instantiating the components, configuring them and finally interconnecting them with the components of the fixed part of the service (the airport information system). We will then introduce a new component named Deployed. The latter is deployed on the user terminal, as for the service activator (Fig. 4).

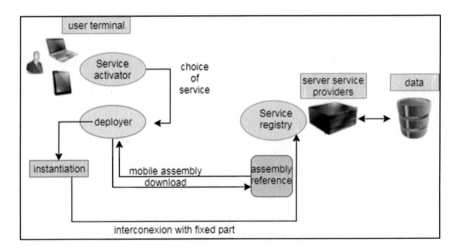

Fig. 4. Choice of service and deployment on the terminal

Indeed, Deplorer's role in the infrastructure is not limited to the deployment of mobile assemblies. It also manages the application lifecycle in a ubiquitous context when a user enters or leaves the network coverage area.

On the other hand, if a user would like to immediately take advantage of the service on a future visit without going through all of the previous steps, the infrastructure must cache the entire mobile assembly in order to reinstate it later. For service version management, a unique identifier must be assigned for each version and service.

6 Conclusion

The main objective of this article is to solve the problem of dynamic discovery and service execution for ubiquitous applications; we presented a design model based on distributed software components, with an infrastructure for execution ubiquitous contextual services. Among other things, this solution deals with issues related to discovery and automatic deployment on user terminals. The architecture is based on the CORBA component model. This work opens several perspectives. First, we want to experiment architecture by implementing it on a platform. Another objective is to focus on the negotiation protocol, specifically the calculation of the assemblies adapted to the terminals according to their characteristics, based on the existing works among other things.

Indeed the work on the improvement of the loading time of the archives will be carried out then this will take into account the possible weakness of flow of the wireless network and the size of the archives of the components. We also have the idea of moving towards a dynamic generation of containers at runtime. As regards the deployment of the services, it is assumed that the client part is already installed on the user's terminal. Currently, this installation is done by hand on each terminal.

Finally, we want to study other examples of ubiquities services in order to propose a model approach that will be independent of the execution platforms.

References

1. Ayed, D., Taconet, C., Bernard, G.: Deployment and reconfiguration of component-based applications in AMPROS. In: Proactive Computing Workshop (PROW 2004). Finland, 2004
2. Briclet, F., Contreras, C., Merle, P.: OpenCCM: une infrastructure à composants pour le déploiement d'applications à base de composants CORBA. In: Actes Conférence DECOR'04. France (2004)
3. Appear Networks: The appear provisioning server. http://www.appearnetworks.com
4. https://www.researchgate.net/scientific-contributions/8076645_Robert_E_McGrath
5. Object Management Group: Trading Object Service Specification, Version 1.0. OMG TC Document formal/2000-06-27, USA (2000)
6. Leydekkers, P.: Multimedia services in open distributed telecommunications environments. Ph.D. thesis. CTIT (1997)
7. Edwards, W.K.: Core Jini Introduction. Prentice Hall PTR (1999)

8. Occello, A., Dery-Pinna, A.M.: Sûreté de fonctionnement d'applications nomades construites par assemblage de composants, UbiMob'05. Grenoble, France (2005)
9. Object Management Group: CORBA Components Specification, Version 3.0, OMG TC Document formal/2002-06-65, USA (2002)

Security and Risks for Cloud Environments

Ahmed Ziani[1(✉)] and Abdellatif Medouri[2]

[1] Information Systems and Telecommunications Laboratory FST,
Abdelmalek Essaadi University, Tetuan, Morocco
zianiahmed@gmail.com
[2] Modeling and Information Theory Group, PFT,
Abdelmalek Essaadi University, Tetuan, Morocco
amedouri@uae.ma

Abstract. Cloud computing has been considered a revolutionary approach towards the computing and a promising solution to increasing demand for using resources provisioned over the Internet which becomes more risky than ever. The cloud computing is a powerful technology in IT environment to provide cost effective, easy to manage, elastic, and powerful resources over the Internet. The Cloud computing offers several advantages and conveniences for today's organizations. Personnel can work together in documents in real time from their phone or tablet from any location, and communicate instantly with teammates via video, voice, instant message, or email. Even though there are innumerable advantages to approaching the cloud computing, security standards are emerging —and constantly evolving—that directly address many of the challenges we already see today. This paper explores the key issues surrounding cloud security for providers, and passes on valuable guidance about not only information security, but more broadly risk. Also, it will help providers to make informed security decisions about their diverse cloud set-ups and better understand how to reap all the benefits of cloud without compromising their organizations' security.

Keywords: Cloud computing · Cloud security · Security challenges · Risks issues

1 Introduction

Cloud computing Cloud computing is a powerful technology to carry out massive-scale and complex computing, it can be seen as an emerging trend to deploy and maintain software, and it is the delivery of computing services both hardware (storage, servers and networking) and software (databases, applications and analytics) over the Internet. Cloud computing is based on a group of many new and old concepts of various areas like distributed computing, grid computing and virtualization. It has grown so much in the last few years. Simply we can say, cloud computing is the computing that is based on internet. Earlier, users download the application or software on a physical system, but with cloud computing, users can access the same kind of application or software through the net. Cloud Computing can be a key computing platform for sharing resources including infrastructure, software, applications and business processes [1, 2].

© Springer Nature Switzerland AG 2019
M. Ezziyyani (Ed.): AI2SD 2018, AISC 915, pp. 991–1002, 2019.
https://doi.org/10.1007/978-3-030-11928-7_90

According to a recent report from IT research and advisory firm Gartner, Cloud Computing has a significant impact on the economy, although it is a new technology. The report predicts global cloud services revenues will surpass $ 68.3 billion in 2010 and reach $ 148.8 billion in 2014. Cloud computing is expected to reach $ 162 billion by 2020 [4, 5].

Cloud Computing can be defined as one or more unified computing resources based on service-level agreements and has been presented as a distributed and parallel system consisting of a pool of interconnected and virtualized computers that are dynamically provisioned [5].

Cloud computing structures typically use a Web client to serve as a user interface to perform certain functions such as accessing applications and exploring data stored on off-site servers.

However, cloud computing raises such an amount of questions concerning security guarantees that potential users are waiting for clear answers before moving into the cloud. Cloud is the combination of work of server and connections. It is easy to access information stored in the cloud. Cloud computing collects all the computing resources and software required to work on them. It provides an efficient technique to provide an accurate information and proper service to users and enterprises. Cloud computing is also described as "On-demand computing" because the user can access as per their requirement and demand.

So it is essential to secure data from any illegitimate user access or any other attack such as denial of service, modification and forgery of document etc. Cloud Computing enables ubiquitous, convenient, on-demand network access to a shared pool of configurable computing resources (e.g., networks, servers, storage, applications, and services) that can be rapidly provisioned and released with minimal management effort or service provider interaction [2]. There are numerous benedictions to adopt cloud computing but still there are few loop holes that make adoption difficult to adopt. Cloud computing providers must ensure their users.

This paper is organized as follows. Section 2 gives an overview Cloud computing. The security issues in the cloud computing detailed in Sect. 3. Section 4 shows the Security Challenges for Cloud Environments. The Security characteristics of different types of cloud are detailed in Sect. 5. The conclusion and future work are presented in Sect. 6.

2   Cloud Computing

Cloud Computing is a powerful technology in IT environment to perform massive-scale and complex computing by eliminating the need to maintain expensive computing hardware, dedicated space, and software, and that refers to the recent advancement to the recent advancement of distributed computing by providing 'computing as a service' for end users in a 'pay-as-you-go' mode; like a mechanism had been a long-held dream of distributed computing and has now become a reality [1] [8].

The National Institute of Standards and Technology (NIST) defines cloud computing as '… a model for enabling convenient, on-demand network access to a shared pool of configurable computing resources (e.g. networks, servers, storage, applications and services) that can be rapidly provisioned and released with minimal management effort or service provider interaction [8].

2.1 Cloud Computing Models

Cloud Computing is a powerful technology in IT environment to perform massive-scale and complex computing by eliminating the need to maintain expensive computing hardware, dedicated space, and software, and that refers to the recent advancement of distributed computing by providing 'computing as a service' for end users in a 'pay-as-you-go' mode; like a mechanism had been a long-held dream of distributed computing and has now become a reality [1, 8].

The National Institute of Standards and Technology (NIST) defines cloud computing as '… a model for enabling convenient, on-demand network access to a shared pool of configurable computing resources (e.g. networks, servers, storage, applications and services) that can be rapidly provisioned and released with minimal management effort or service provider interaction [8].

Cloud Computing Models

Cloud computing may be deployed with four models: private, public, community and hybrid. These deployment models shows who owns, manages and is responsible for the services.

Private cloud.

Private clouds refer to cloud computing on private networks. They are built for the exclusive use of one client, offering full control over data, security, and quality of service. Private clouds may be built and managed by a cloud provider or by a company's own IT department.

Public cloud.

Public clouds are owned by service providers, and they built over the Internet. Public clouds are accessed by subscription and can be accessed by any user who has paid for the service. Several companies have built public clouds, namely Google App Engine, Amazon AWS, Microsoft Azure and IBM Blue Cloud.

Community cloud.

The community clouds combine aspects of the private and public clouds: resources are shared, but only with organizations/users that have the same requirements (e.g., mission, security requirements, policy, and compliance considerations). Also, they can be managed by the organizations or a third party.

Hybrid cloud.

Hybrid Clouds are usually a combination of private clouds and public clouds that interoperates. Generally, in this model, users farm out no business—critical information and processing to the public cloud, while keeping business–critical services and data in their command. A hybrid cloud also can be used to handle planned workload spikes and to perform periodic tasks that can be deployed easily on a public cloud (Fig. 1).

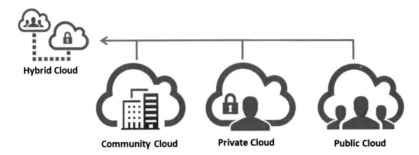

Fig. 1. Cloud computing deployment models

2.2 Cloud Service Models

Cloud Computing is a powerful technology in IT environment to perform massive-scale and complex computing by eliminating the need to maintain expensive computing hardware, dedicated space, and software, and that refers to the recent advancement to the recent advancement of distributed computing by providing 'computing as a service' for end users in a 'pay-as-you-go' mode; like a mechanism had been a long-held dream of distributed computing and has now become a reality [1, 8].

The National Institute of Standards and Technology (NIST) defines cloud computing as '… a model for enabling convenient, on-demand network access to a shared pool of configurable computing resources (e.g. networks, servers, storage, applications and services) that can be rapidly provisioned and released with minimal management effort or service provider interaction [8].

Cloud Service Models

Cloud computing is provided through at least four types of services: Infrastructure as a Service (IaaS), Platform as a Service (PaaS), Software as a Service (SaaS), and Data as a Service (DaaS) [1, 4, 6].

Infrastructure as a Service (IaaS)

Iaas provides many competences to the clients such as provision processing, storage, networks, and other fundamental computing resources where the client is capable to deploy and run arbitrary software, which can include operating systems and applications. The user does not manage or control the underlying cloud physical infrastructure but has control over operating systems, storage, deployed applications, and possibly limited control of select networking components.

Software as a Service (SaaS)

Saas allows the user, via several capabilities, to use the provider's applications running on a cloud infrastructure. The applications are accessible from various devices through a client interface such as a web browser. The user does not manage or control the underlying cloud infrastructure including network, servers, operating systems, storage, or even individual application capabilities, with the possible exception of provider-defined user-specific application configuration settings.

Platform as a Service (PaaS)

The capability provided to the user is to organize onto the cloud infrastructure user-created or acquired applications created using programming languages and tools supported by the provider. The user has control over the deployed applications and possibly application hosting environment configurations, but does not manage or control the underlying cloud infrastructure including network, servers, operating systems, or storage.

Data as a Service (DaaS).

Daas is an information distribution and provision web based model in which data files are accessed by users during some defined API layer over a network, typically the Internet. The delivery of virtualized storage on demand becomes a separate Cloud service—data storage service. Notice that DaaS could be seen as a special type IaaS. DaaS services are frequently considered as a dedicated subset of Software as a service offering.

3   Cloud Security

Cloud security can seem dauntingly complex, involving many different aspects that touch all parts of an organization. Provider's teams need to plot effective management strategies as well as understand the implications for operations and technology [7, 8]:

- Management
- Operation
- Technology

It provides an at-a-glance reference to the issues organization's need to address if they are to put in place effective cloud security strategies backed up with appropriate processes and technologies. On the following, there is a drill-down into each of these. The following is a brief explanation of each of the elements highlighted on the Fig. 2 [8, 9].

3.1   Management

- Updated security policy: Amendments to the organization are overarching security policy.
- Cloud security strategy: Organization's strategy for security with respect to cloud. This should complement or be part of the organization's existing overarching security strategy.
- Cloud security governance: The process for ensuring cloud security strategy and policy updates are adhered to.
- Cloud security processes: The security processes associated specifically with cloud and/or the amendments required to existing security processes in order to incorporate cloud.
- Security roles and responsibilities: Who is responsible for what with respect to ensuring the different elements of cloud security are implemented effectively.

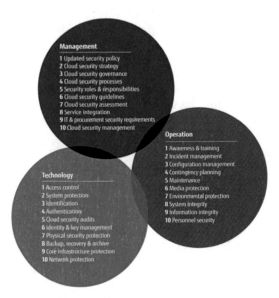

Fig. 2. Aspects of cloud security

- Cloud security guidelines: Advice and guidance provided to both business and IT teams regarding all aspects of security that affect them.
- Cloud security assessment: The ability to objectively measure the effectiveness of a given cloud service provider's security.
- Service integration: The integration of several cloud services at a management level.
- IT and procurement security requirements: Specific cloud security requirements that would need to be included in any procurement and/or IT project's overall requirements.
- Cloud security management: The overall day-to-day management of cloud security.

3.2   Operation

- Awareness and training: Educating employees about the security impact of cloud on their individual functions and roles.
- Incident management: Managing cloud-related problems and incidents.
- Configuration management: Ensuring the configuration of an organization's service is appropriate and secure.
- Contingency planning: A pre-planned approach to business continuity, disaster recovery and the ongoing management (up and down) of cloud usage.
- Maintenance: The processes ensuring that anything in a cloud environment (or consumed from a cloud environment) is properly maintained and up to date.
- Media protection: Ensuring any data stored in a cloud environment is managed appropriately.

- Environmental protection: Ensuring an organization's cloud service provider (and using that provider rather than internal IT) improves that organization's environmental credentials.
- System integrity: Ensuring all cloud systems remain secure.
- Information integrity: Ensuring all information stored in a cloud environment is secure.
- Personnel security: Ensuring all personnel (both internal staff and employees of the cloud provider) are trustworthy and do not have the ability to compromise the service.

3.3   Technology

- Access control: Technology and software (including its configuration) that ensures the right person has access to the right data (and only the right data) for them.
- System protection: Technology to protect individual cloud systems from security risks such as distributed denial-of-service (DDoS) attacks.
- Identification: Technology to identify employees and other authorised personnel accessing a cloud service.
- Authentication: Technology to verify that an individual accessing a cloud system is who they claim to be.
- Cloud security audits: The tools and processes by which organizations ensure security (and associated systems and processes) are adequately maintained.
- Identity and key management: The management of security keys (e.g. encryption keys, SSL keys) and identities of the organization's personnel.
- Physical security protection: Ensuring a provider has appropriate security controls for access to its buildings.
- Backup, recovery and archive: The tools and procedures for ensuring that data stored in a cloud system is available in the event of a catastrophic failure on the part of the provider.
- Core infrastructure protection: Protection of servers and other core infrastructure.
- Network protection: Protection of the internal network and the boundary of the network (where it connects to a cloud environment).

4   Security Challenges for Cloud Environments

The Cloud computing providers promoting cloud computing security best practices and standards, has identified seven areas of security risk. Five of these apply directly to focus on protecting data and platform [11–13]:

- Abuse and nefarious use of cloud services
- Multitenancy and shared technology issues
- Data loss
- Account hijacking
- Unknown risk.

4.1   Abuse and Nefarious Use of Cloud Services

Many infrastructure-as-a-service (IaaS) providers make it easy to take advantage of their services. With a valid credit card, users can register and start using cloud services right away. Cybercriminals actively target cloud services providers, partially because of this relatively weak registration system that helps obscure identities, and because many providers have limited fraud-detection capabilities. Stringent initial registration and validation processes, credit card fraud monitoring, and subsequent authentication are ways to remediate this type of threat [12, 13].

4.2   Multitenancy and Shared Technology Issues

Clouds deliver scalable services that provide computing power for multiple tenants, whether those tenants are business groups from the same company or independent organizations. That means shared infrastructure—CPU caches, graphics processing units (GPUs), disk partitions, memory, and other components—that was never designed for strong compartmentalization. Even with a virtualization hypervisor to mediate access between guest operating systems and physical resources, there is concern that attackers can gain unauthorized access and control of your underlying platform with software-only isolation mechanisms. Potential compromise of the hypervisor layer can in turn lead to a potential compromise of all the shared physical resources of the server that it controls, including memory and data as well as other virtual machines (VMs) on that server.

Experience at Intel found that virtualization brings with it an aggregation of risks to the enterprise when consolidating application components and services of varying risk profiles onto a single physical server platform. This is a key limiter faced by most IT organizations in achieving their virtualization goals—and subsequently in moving workloads to the cloud [15, 16].

4.3   Data Loss

Protecting data can be a headache because of the number of ways it can be compromised. Some data—customer, employee, or financial data, for example—should be protected from unauthorized users. But data can also be maliciously deleted, altered, or unlinked from its larger context. Loss of data can damage your company's brand and reputation, affect customer and employee trust, and have regulatory compliance or competitive consequences [17].

4.4   Account or Service Hijacking

Attacks using methods such as phishing and fraud continue to be an ongoing threat. With stolen credentials, hackers can access critical areas of your cloud and potentially eavesdrop on transactions, manipulate or falsify data, and redirect your clients to illegitimate sites. IT organizations can fight back with strong identity and access management, including two-factor authentication where possible, strong password requirements, and proactive monitoring for unauthorized activity [16, 17].

4.5   Unknown Risk

Releasing control of your data to a cloud service provider has important security ramifications. Without clearly understanding the service provider's security practices, your company may be open to hidden vulnerabilities and risks. Also, the complexity of cloud environments may make it tempting for IT managers to cobble together security measures. Unfortunately, that same complexity and the relatively new concept of cloud computing and related technologies make it difficult to consider the full ramifications of any change, and you may be leaving your cloud open to new or still undiscovered vulnerabilities [17, 18].

5   Security Characteristics of Different Types of Cloud

It is important to know that the type of cloud an organization chooses is one of the biggest factors affecting risk. As defined early, cloud are types as private, public, community or hybrid clouds to refer to a combination of approaches. Each types of cloud have different security characteristics. Figure 3 shows a simple comparison; The

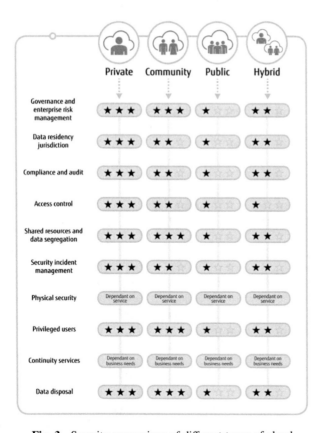

Fig. 3. Security comparison of different types of cloud

number of stars indicates how suitable each type of cloud is for each area. Organizations with defined controls for externally sourced services or access to IT risk-assessment capabilities should still apply these to aspects of cloud services where appropriate.

But while many of the security risks of cloud overlap with those of outsourcing and offshoring, there are also differences that organizations need to understand and manage [17–19].

5.1   Processing Sensitive or Business-Critical Data

Outside the enterprise introduces a level of risk because any outsourced service bypasses an organization's in-house security controls. With cloud, however, it is possible to establish compatible controls if the provider offers a dedicated service. An organization should ascertain a provider's position by asking for information about the control and supervision of privileged administrators [19, 20].

5.2   Organizations Using Cloud Services

Remain responsible for the security and integrity of their own data, even when it is held by a service provider. Traditional service providers are subject to external audits and security certifications. Cloud providers may not be prepared to undergo the same level of scrutiny [19–21].

5.3   When an Organization Uses a Cloud Service

it may not know exactly where its data resides or have any ability to influence changes to the location of data.

5.4   Most Providers Store Data in a Shared Environment

Although this may be segregated from other customers' data while it's in that environment, it may be combined in backup and archive copies. This could especially be the case in multi-tenanted environments [19–21].

5.5   Providers Teams Responsibilities

They will be able to support electronic discovery or internal investigations of inappropriate or illegal activity. Cloud services are especially difficult to investigate because logs and data for multiple customers may be either co-located or spread across an ill-defined and changing set of hosts [19–21].

5.6   Organizations Need to Evaluate the Long-Term Viability of Any Cloud Provider

They should consider the consequences to service should the provider fail or be acquired, since there will be far fewer readily identifiable assets that can easily be transferred in-house or to another provider. In short, no one security method will solve all these data protection problems so it is important to consider multiple layers of defence. Ideally, organizations should compartmentalize their cloud infrastructure and applications to apply the right controls in the right places and help contain the impact of security incidents [19–21].

6 Conclusion

Organizations new to cloud consider security is their number one concern. So, the protection of user data is a primary design consideration for all providers' infrastructures.

While security is just as important for them, it is no longer a source of worry or apprehension. It has simply become another consideration in their risk management strategies, processes and future decisions about moving other services into a cloud environment.

In this paper, we have tried to pass on the insights to ease transitions to cloud. Extensive analysis has led to the following conclusions: The type of cloud (public, trusted, private or hybrid) has the biggest single impact on the level of risk and its manageability. To assure confidentiality, organizations need to define approaches for identifying the data to be protected and ascertaining how to access that data.

To do that, organizations should consider an access-control approach that incorporates and integrates in-house, outsourced and cloud systems. And they should build relationships with trusted cloud service providers who will continue to invest in security, innovation to evolve Organizations platform to allow users to benefit from services in a secure and transparent manner.

References

1. Murugesan, S., Bojanova, I.: Encyclopedia of Cloud Computing. Wiley, Hoboken (2016)
2. Pourabbas, E.: Geographical Information Systems: Trends and Technologies. CRC press (2014)
3. Zhu, X.: GIS for Environmental Applications: A Practical Approach. Routledge, London (2016)
4. Rafaels, R.: Cloud Computing: From Beginning to End. CreateSpace Independent Publishing Platform (2015)
5. Zheng, D.: Future Intelligent Information Systems, vol. 1. Springer, Heidelberg (2011)
6. Furht, B., Escalante, A.: Handbook of Cloud Computing. Springer Science & Business Media, Heidelberg (2010)
7. Mell, P., Grance, T.: The NIST Definition of Cloud Computing. NIST, USA (2011)
8. Vance, T.C., Merati, N., Yang, C., Yuan, M.: Cloud Computing in Ocean and Atmospheric Sciences. Elsevier
9. Yang, C., Huang, Q.: Spatial Cloud Computing: A Practical Approach. CRC Press (2013)

10. Ziani, A., Medouri, A.: Use of cloud computing technologies for geographic information systems. In: Ezziyyani, M., Bahaj, M., Khoukhi, F. (eds.) Advanced Information Technology, Services and Systems. AIT2S 2017. Lecture Notes in Networks and Systems, vol. 25, pp. 315–323. Springer, Cham. https://doi.org/10.1007/978-3-319-69137-4_28. 978-3-319-69136-7

11. Ivan, I., Singleton, A., Horák, J., Inspektor, T.: The Rise of Big Spatial Data. Springer, Heidelberg (2016)

12. Bhat, M.A., Shah, R.M., Ahmad, B., Bhat, I.R.: Cloud computing: a solution to information support systems (ISS). Int. J. Comput. Appl. **11**(5), 0975–8887 (2010)

13. Sehgal, N.K., Bhatt, P.C.P.: Cloud Computing: Concepts and Practices. Springer International Publishing, Heidelberg (2018)   ﹗

14. Peng, S., Wang, S., Balas, V.E., Zhao, M.: Security with Intelligent Computing and Big-data Services. Springer International Publishing, Heidelberg (2018)

15. Turuk, A.K., Sahoo, B., Kanti, A.S.: Resource Management and Efficiency in Cloud Computing Environments. IGI Global (2016)

16. Gupta, P.K., Tyagi, V., Singh, S.K.: Predictive Computing and Information Security. Springer, Singapore (2017)

17. Kumar, V., Chaisiri, S., Ko, R.: Data Security in Cloud Computing. Institution of Engineering and Technology (2017)

18. Peng, S., Wang, S., Balas, V.E., Zhao, M.: Security with Intelligent Computing and Big-data Services. Springer International Publishing, Heidelberg (2018)

19. Krutz, R., Vines, R.: Cloud Security: A Comprehensive Guide to Secure Cloud Computing, p. 384. Wiley, Hoboken (2010)

20. Mishra, B.S.P., Das, H., Dehuri, S., Jagadev, A.K.: Cloud Computing for Optimization: Foundations, Applications, and Challenges. Springer, Heidelberg (2018)

21. Le, D., Kumar, R., Nguyen, G., Chatterjee, J.M.: Cloud Computing and Virtualization. Wiley, Hoboken (2018)

Author Index

© Springer Nature Switzerland AG 2019
M. Ezziyyani (Ed.): AI2SD 2018, AISC 915, pp. 1003–1005, 2019.
https://doi.org/10.1007/978-3-030-11928-7

Printed in the United States
By Bookmasters